T0175041

Insomnia

MEDICAL PSYCHIATRY

Series Editors Emeritus

William A. Frosch, M.D.
Weill Medical College of Council University, New York, New York, U.S.A.

Advisory Board

Jonathan E. Alpert, M.D., Ph.D.
Massachusetts General Hospital and Harvard University School of Medicine Boston, Massachusetts, U.S.A.

Bennett Leventhal, M.D.
University of Chicago School of Medicine Chicago, Illinois, U.S.A.

Siegfried Kasper, M.D.
Medical University of Vienna Vienna, Austria

Mark H. Rapaport, M.D.
Cedars-Sinai Medical Center Los Angeles, California, U.S.A.

Recent Titles in Series

Bipolar Disorders: Basic Mechanisms and Therapeutic Implications, Second Edition, *edited by Jair C. Soares and Allan H. Young*

Neurogenetics of Psychiatric Disorders, *edited by Akira Sawa and Melvin G. McInnis*

Attention Deficit Hyperactivity Disorder: Concepts, Controversies, New Directions, *edited by Keith McBurnett, Linda Pfiffner, Russell Schachar, Glen Raymond Elliot, and Joel Nigg*

Insulin Resistance Syndrome and Neuropsychiatric Disorders, *edited by Natalie L. Rasgon*

Antiepileptic Drugs to Treat Psychiatric Disorders, *edited by Susan L. McElroy, Paul E. Keck, Jr., and Robert M. Post*

Asperger's Disorder, *edited by Jeffrey L. Rausch, Marie E. Johnson, and Manuel F. Casanova*

Depression and Mood Disorders in Later Life, Second Edition, *edited by James E. Ellison, Helen Kyomen, and Sumer K. Verma*

Depression: Treatment Strategies and Management, Second Edition, *edited by Thomas L. Schwartz and Timothy Peterson*

Schizophrenia, Second Edition, *edited by Siegfried Kasper and George N. Papadimitriou*

Insomnia: Diagnosis and Treatment, *edited by Michael J. Sateia and Daniel J. Buysse*

Insomnia
Diagnosis and Treatment

Edited by

Michael J. Sateia
Dartmouth Medical School
Lebanon, New Hampshire, U.S.A.

Daniel J. Buysse
University of Pittsburgh School of Medicine
Pittsburgh, Pennsylvania, U.S.A.

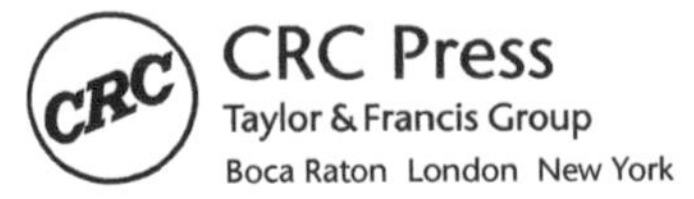

CRC Press is an imprint of the
Taylor & Francis Group, an **informa** business

CRC Press
Taylor & Francis Group
6000 Broken Sound Parkway NW, Suite 300
Boca Raton, FL 33487-2742

First issued in paperback 2019

© 2010 by Taylor & Francis Group, LLC
CRC Press is an imprint of Taylor & Francis Group, an Informa business

No claim to original U.S. Government works

ISBN-13: 978-0-367-38416-6

This book contains information obtained from authentic and highly regarded sources. While all reasonable efforts have been made to publish reliable data and information, neither the author[s] nor the publisher can accept any legal responsibility or liability for any errors or omissions that may be made. The publishers wish to make clear that any views or opinions expressed in this book by individual editors, authors or contributors are personal to them and do not necessarily reflect the views/opinions of the publishers. The information or guidance contained in this book is intended for use by medical, scientific or health-care professionals and is provided strictly as a supplement to the medical or other professional's own judgement, their knowledge of the patient's medical history, relevant manufacturer's instructions and the appropriate best practice guidelines. Because of the rapid advances in medical science, any information or advice on dosages, procedures or diagnoses should be independently verified. The reader is strongly urged to consult the relevant national drug formulary and the drug companies' and device or material manufacturers' printed instructions, and their websites, before administering or utilizing any of the drugs, devices or materials mentioned in this book. This book does not indicate whether a particular treatment is appropriate or suitable for a particular individual. Ultimately it is the sole responsibility of the medical professional to make his or her own professional judgements, so as to advise and treat patients appropriately. The authors and publishers have also attempted to trace the copyright holders of all material reproduced in this publication and apologize to copyright holders if permission to publish in this form has not been obtained. If any copyright material has not been acknowledged please write and let us know so we may rectify in any future reprint.

Except as permitted under U.S. Copyright Law, no part of this book may be reprinted, reproduced, transmitted, or utilized in any form by any electronic, mechanical, or other means, now known or hereafter invented, including photocopying, microfilming, and recording, or in any information storage or retrieval system, without written permission from the publishers.

For permission to photocopy or use material electronically from this work, please access www.copyright.com (http://www.copyright.com/) or contact the Copyright Clearance Center, Inc. (CCC), 222 Rosewood Drive, Danvers, MA 01923, 978-750-8400. CCC is a not-for-profit organization that provides licenses and registration for a variety of users. For organizations that have been granted a photocopy license by the CCC, a separate system of payment has been arranged.

Trademark Notice: Product or corporate names may be trademarks or registered trademarks, and are used only for identification and explanation without intent to infringe.

A CIP record for this book is available from the British Library.

Library of Congress Cataloging-in-Publication Data available on application

Visit the Taylor & Francis Web site at
http://www.taylorandfrancis.com

and the CRC Press Web site at
http://www.crcpress.com

This book is dedicated to our families – Holly, Heather, and Caitlin; and Sandy, Caitlin, Allison, and Evan – whose love and support allow us to write about insomnia rather than experience it.

Preface

As the field of sleep medicine has matured in recent decades, it has become increasingly apparent that disruption or failure of normal sleep function, not unlike failure of other essential physiologic functions, has sweeping adverse consequences. Chronic insomnia is arguably the most common form of sleep disruption, although its significance as a serious health problem has been, and continues to be, largely overlooked. Much of this neglect seems to arise from the tacit assumption that this condition is, in effect, more a benign existential problem than a disorder deserving serious medical attention. Yet, investigations of chronic insomnia over the past 20 years underscore the importance of addressing this issue as a component of the patient's overall health care. Not only is it clear that chronic insomnia is associated with impairments in quality of life and function, comparable to those seen in disorders such as major depression and congestive heart failure, but emerging data also indicate that insomnia may be a significant risk factor for development of major psychiatric and possibly medical disorders. The availability of effective therapies that can produce clinically meaningful and durable improvement or resolution of symptoms lends further weight to the importance of identifying insomnia.

Although a small and dedicated group of sleep researchers and clinicians have made significant strides in addressing this problem, an enormous knowledge and awareness gap exists among most health care providers with respect to insomnia. Although we have made substantial efforts to address this through educational means, clearly the work has only begun. A necessary foundation of sound educational efforts is a detailed, accessible body of knowledge that addresses the pathophysiology, evaluation, and treatment of the disorder. Although many excellent books have been published on insomnia, somewhat surprisingly, there have been only limited efforts to produce a comprehensive reference text in this area. Our hope is that this volume will help to meet this need.

Insomnia is relevant to virtually all aspects of medicine. For this reason, researchers and clinicians from all fields must have access to detailed information. The subject matter of this book will certainly be of considerable interest and importance to all sleep medicine clinicians. However, its relevance and utility should extend well beyond this audience. As data increasingly underscore the important and complex interaction between insomnia and mental illness, it is incumbent upon psychiatrists, psychologists, and other mental health workers to not only identify but also actively intervene when chronic insomnia complicates psychiatric disease. Although the evidence that compels effective management of insomnia in comorbid medical and neurological disease is not yet as well developed as that for mental illness, there is, nonetheless, ample basis for internists, family practice physicians, neurologists, and other specialists to appreciate the significant role that insomnia may play in the pathogenesis and maintenance of physical illnesses.

The past 20 years have seen enormous progress in our understanding of the nature and characteristics of chronic insomnia and in our ability to accurately assess and effectively treat the problem. These advances have profoundly affected our view of chronic insomnia—most importantly, transitioning its position from that of "secondary" symptom of other disorders to a condition comorbid with other disorders. This paradigm shift is important because most chronic insomnia is, in fact, comorbid with other medical or psychiatric disease. This perspective suggests that chronic insomnia exhibits its own unique and somewhat independent pathophysiology, which is not only influenced by comorbid disorders but also, in turn, has major influence on those disorders.

This book is intended to provide the reader with a comprehensive and detailed overview of the current research and state-of-the-art practice parameters related to insomnia in three parts. The first section, *Fundamentals*, addresses the characteristics and consequences of chronic insomnia and, in effect, speaks about the nature of the disorder and the question of why it deserves medical attention. The *Evaluation* section provides the clinician with a detailed description of causes and comorbidities and offers clinicians specific guidelines and tools for evaluating the disorder in its varied and often complex presentations. Finally, the section on *Management* represents what we believe to be the most detailed and comprehensive description of treatment modalities for chronic insomnia that is currently available. Each of the chapters in this book is authored by recognized experts in the field whose research and writing have collectively defined this area of sleep medicine.

In the modern era, medicine has moved progressively toward a multideterminant model of causation of disease and multimodal treatment. It has become increasingly apparent that sleep is one of the critical determinants of health and well-being. It is no longer possible for researchers to effectively study disease or clinicians to effectively treat it without considering the potential role of sleep and circadian factors. We believe that this comprehensive volume will serve to stimulate interest and further inquiry in this area by scientists and clinicians from many fields, and will provide practitioners with a guide for the management of this common malady.

We welcome your thoughts, comments, and suggestions on the text to help us prepare for the Second Edition.

Michael J. Sateia
Daniel J. Buysse

Contents

Contributors

Sonia Ancoli-Israel Department of Psychiatry, University of California, San Diego, La Jolla, California, U.S.A.

Donna Arand Dayton Department of Veterans Affairs Medical Center, Wright State University, Wallace Kettering Neuroscience Institute, and Kettering Medical Center, Dayton, Ohio, U.S.A.

J. Todd Arnedt Department of Psychiatry and Neurology, University of Michigan, Ann Arbor, Michigen, U.S.A.

Alan N. Bateson Institute for Membrane and Systems Biology, Faculty of Biological Sciences, University of Leeds, Leeds, U.K.

Ruth M. Benca Department of Psychiatry, University of Wisconsin-Madison, Madison, Wisconsin, U.S.A.

Michael Bonnet Dayton Department of Veterans Affairs Medical Center, Wright State University, Wallace Kettering Neuroscience Institute, and Kettering Medical Center, Dayton, Ohio, U.S.A.

Richard R. Bootzin Departments of Psychology and Psychiatry, University of Arizona, Tucson, Arizona, U.S.A.

Kirk J. Brower Department of Psychiatry, University of Michigan, Ann Arbor, Michigan, U.S.A.

Daniel J. Buysse Neuroscience Clinical and Translational Research Center, University of Pittsburgh School of Medicine, Pittsburgh, Pennsylvania, U.S.A.

Colleen E. Carney Department of Psychology, Ryerson University, Toronto, Ontario, Canada

Nancy A. Collop Division of Pulmonary and Critical Care, Johns Hopkins University School of Medicine, Baltimore, Maryland, U.S.A.

Scott E. Cologne American Sleep Medicine, St. Louis, Missouri, U.S.A.

Deirdre A. Conroy Department of Psychiatry, University of Michigan, Ann Arbor, Michigan, U.S.A.

Kimberly Cote Department of Psychology, Brock University, St. Catharines, Ontario, Canada

Natalie D. Dautovich Department of Psychology, The University of Florida, Gainesville, Florida, U.S.A.

Haley R. Dillon Department of Psychology, The University of Alabama, Tuscaloosa, Alabama, U.S.A.

Karl Doghramji Jefferson Sleep Disorders Center and the Department of Psychiatry and Human Behavior, Thomas Jefferson University, Philadelphia, Pennsylvania, U.S.A.

Joseph M. Dzierzewski Department of Clinical and Health Psychology, University of Florida, Gainesville, Florida, U.S.A.

Jack D. Edinger Psychology Service, VA Medical Center, Department of Psychiatry and Behavioral Sciences, Duke University Medical Center, Durham, North Carolina, U.S.A.

Jason Ellis Northumbria Centre for Sleep Research, School of Psychology and Sports Science, Northumbria University, Newcastle upon Tyne, U.K.

Colin A. Espie University of Glasgow Sleep Centre, Sackler Institute of Psychobiological Research, Southern General Hospital, Glasgow, Scotland, U.K.

Leah Friedman Department of Psychiatry and Behavioral Sciences, Stanford University, Stanford, California, U.S.A.

Kelleen N. Flaherty Department of Biomedical Writing, University of the Sciences in Philadelphia, Philadelphia, Pennsylvania, U.S.A.

Peter L. Franzen Sleep Medicine Institute and Department of Psychiatry, University of Pittsburgh School of Medicine, Pittsburgh, Pennsylvania, U.S.A.

Philip Gehrman Department of Psychiatry, University of Pennsylvania, Philadelphia, Pennsylvania, U.S.A.

Anne Germain Department of Psychiatry, University of Pittsburgh School of Medicine, Pittsburgh, Pennsylvania, U.S.A.

Daniel Glaze Baylor College of Medicine, Texas Children's Hospital Children's Sleep Center, Houston, Texas, U.S.A.

Paul B. Glovinsky Cognitive Neurosciences Doctoral Program, Department of Psychology, The City College of New York, City University of New York, New York, and Department of Medicine, Section of Psychology, St. Peter's Hospital, St. Peter's Sleep Center, Albany, New York, U.S.A.

Glen P. Greenough Dartmouth-Hitchcock Medical Center, Lebanon, New Hampshire, U.S.A.

Emily A. Grieser Department of Psychology, University of North Texas, Denton, Texas, U.S.A.

Allison G. Harvey Department of Psychology, University of California, Berkeley, California, U.S.A.

Bobbi Hopkins Baylor College of Medicine, Texas Children's Hospital Children's Sleep Center, Houston, Texas, U.S.A.

Brooke G. Judd Dartmouth-Hitchcock Medical Center, Lebanon, New Hampshire, U.S.A.

Andrew D. Krystal Insomnia and Sleep Research Laboratory, Department of Psychiatry and Behavioral Sciences, Duke University School of Medicine, Durham, North Carolina, U.S.A.

Damien Leger Sleep and Vigilance Center, Hotel Dieu de Paris, Assistance Publique Hopitaux de Paris and University Paris Descartes, Faculty of Medicine, Paris, France

Kenneth L. Lichstein Department of Psychology, The University of Alabama, Tuscaloosa, Alabama, U.S.A.

Rachel Manber Psychiatry & Behavioral Sciences, Stanford, California, U.S.A.

W. Vaughn McCall Department of Psychiatry and Behavioral Medicine, Wake Forest University School of Medicine, Winston-Salem, North Carolina, U.S.A.

Christina S. McCrae Department of Clinical and Health Psychology, University of Florida, Gainesville, Florida, U.S.A.

Douglas E. Moul Department of Psychiatry, Louisiana State University at Shreveport School of Medicine, Shreveport, Louisiana, U.S.A.

Martin S. Mumenthaler Department of Psychiatry and Behavioral Sciences, Stanford University, Stanford, California, U.S.A.

David N. Neubauer Department of Psychiatry, Johns Hopkins Bayview Medical Center, Johns Hopkins University School of Medicine, Baltimore, Maryland, U.S.A.

Eric A. Nofzinger Sleep Neuroimaging Research Program, University of Pittsburgh School of Medicine, Pittsburgh, Pennsylvania, U.S.A.

Jason C. Ong Department of Behavioral Sciences, Rush University Medical Center, Chicago, Illinois, U.S.A.

Slobodanka Pejovic Sleep Research and Treatment Center, Department of Psychiatry, Penn State University College of Medicine, Hershey, Pennsylvania, U.S.A.

Michael Perlis Department of Psychiatry, University of Pennsylvania, Philadelphia, Pennsylvania, U.S.A.

Wilfred R. Pigeon Sleep and Neurophysiology Research Lab, University of Rochester Medical Center, Rochester, New York, U.S.A.

Kathryn J. Reid Department of Neurology, Feinberg School of Medicine, Northwestern University, Chicago, Illinois, U.S.A.

Dieter Riemann Center for Sleep Research and Sleep Medicine, Department of Psychiatry, Freiburg University, Freiburg, Germany

Timothy Roehrs Sleep Disorders and Research Center, Henry Ford Hospital, and Department of Psychiatry and Behavioral Neuroscience, School of Medicine, Wayne State University, Detroit, Michigan, U.S.A.

Thomas Roth Sleep Disorders and Research Center, Henry Ford Hospital, and Department of Psychiatry and Behavioral Neuroscience, School of Medicine, Wayne State University, Detroit, Michigan, U.S.A.

Meredith E. Rumble Department of Psychiatry, University of Wisconsin-Madison, Madison, Wisconsin, U.S.A.

Bruce Rybarczyk Department of Psychology, Virginia Commonwealth University, Richmond, Virginia, U.S.A.

Robert L. Sack Oregon Health and Science University, Portland, Oregon, U.S.A.

Michael J. Sateia Department of Psychiatry, Dartmouth Medical School, Lebanon, New Hampshire, U.S.A.

Michael H. Silber Center for Sleep Medicine and Department of Neurology, Mayo Clinic College of Medicine, Rochester, Minnesota, U.S.A.

Shauna L. Shapiro Department of Counseling Psychology, Santa Clara University, Santa Clara, California, U.S.A.

Leisha J. Smith Department of Psychology, University of Arizona, Tucson, Arizona, U.S.A.

Michael T. Smith Department of Psychiatry and Behavioral Sciences, Behavioral Sleep Medicine Program, Johns Hopkins University School of Medicine, Baltimore, Maryland, U.S.A.

Arthur J. Spielman Cognitive Neurosciences Doctoral Program, Department of Psychology, The City College of New York, City University of New York, New York; Center for Sleep Medicine, Department of Neurology, New York Presbyterian Hospital, Weill Cornell Medical College, New York; and Center for Sleep Disorders Medicine and Research, Department of Pulmonary Medicine, New York Methodist Hospital, Brooklyn, New York, U.S.A.

Lisa S. Talbot Department of Psychology, University of California, Berkeley, California, U.S.A.

JoLyn I. Tatum Department of Psychology, University of North Texas, Denton, Texas, U.S.A.

Daniel J. Taylor Department of Psychology, University of North Texas, Denton, Texas, U.S.A.

Mario Terzano Department of Neurology, University of Parma, Parma, Italy

Alexandros N. Vgontzas Sleep Research and Treatment Center, Department of Psychiatry, Penn State University College of Medicine, Hershey, Pennsylvania, U.S.A.

Emerson M. Wickwire Center for Sleep Disorders, Pulmonary Disease and Critical Care Associates, Columbia, Maryland, U.S.A.

Chien-Ming Yang Department of Psychology, The Research Center for Mind, Brain & Learning, National Cheng-Chi University, Taipei, Taiwan

Gary K. Zammit Clinilabs, Inc., Sleep Disorders Institute, Columbia University College of Physicians and Surgeons, New York, New York, U.S.A.

Phyllis C. Zee Department of Neurology, Feinberg School of Medicine, Northwestern University, Chicago, Illinois, U.S.A.

Jamie M. Zeitzer Department of Psychiatry and Behavioral Sciences, Stanford University, Stanford, and Psychiatry Service, VA Palo Alto Health Care System, Palo Alto, California, U.S.A.

1 Introduction: History, Definition, and Epidemiology

Michael J. Sateia
Department of Psychiatry, Dartmouth Medical School, Lebanon, New Hampshire, U.S.A.

The worst thing in the world is to try to sleep and not to.

F. Scott Fitzgerald

HISTORY

Fitzgerald succinctly captured the feelings of many chronic insomnia sufferers who labor nightly to achieve the solace and restoration of a good night's sleep. History is replete with examples of the tragedies and anguish wrought as a result of insomnia. In one of the earliest known pieces of literature, the Epic of Gilgamesh, the epic hero and ruler of the first known civilization is beset by sleeplessness (1). In the biblical tale of Job, God inflicts insomnia on Job, causing him to lament: "When I lie down, I say, 'when shall I arise, and the night be gone?' and I am full of tossings to and fro unto the dawning of the day."

The earliest recorded discussion of insomnia as a medical symptom can be traced to Hippocrates (2), who recognized perturbations of sleep as a sign of disease. However, it is likely that insomnia was being treated with opium and herbal preparations well prior to the rise of Greek civilization (3). During much of the past two millennia, insomnia has been viewed as a secondary phenomenon, attributable to a variety of causes. Disturbances of sleep have, for millennia, been associated with an unquiet mind, in the form of guilt, vexation or rumination. Examples of this are commonly cited in literature, such as in the works of Shakespeare, when Romeo's advisor, Friar Lawrence, notes: "Care keeps his watch in every old man's eye, and where care lodges, sleep can never lie." Environmental factors such as noise, light, temperature, or characteristics of the bed have been blamed. Benjamin Franklin, a noted insomniac, would remove himself from bed and allow it to air so that the sheets might cool (4). Charles Dickens, another insomnia sufferer, would sleep only in the exact middle of north-facing beds (5). Dickens often wandered the streets of London during the night, providing a source of inspiration for many of his characters and scenes. Insomnia became the subject of increasing medical attention in Victorian England, when the queen herself was reportedly prescribed cannabis for sleep. An article from the British Medical Journal of 1894 (6) lamented: "The hurry and excitement of modern life is held to be responsible for much of the insomnia of which we hear; and most of the articles and letters are full of good advice to live more quietly and of platitudes concerning the harmfulness of rush and worry. The pity of it is that so many people are unable to follow this good advice and are obliged to lead a life of anxiety and high tension."

As Horne (5) points out in a 2008 essay, it is remarkable that, despite the widely held notion that sleep disturbance was the product of psychological factors, "cures" for the affliction were overwhelmingly pharmacological in nature. Opiates, alcohol, and herbals, such as valerian, were likely used to treat insomnia in Sumerian and Greek civilizations, and continued to occupy a central role in this respect (e.g., laudanum, a combination of opioid and alcohol) until the late 19th century when they gradually became supplanted by newer compounds such as bromides, chloral hydrate, and later, barbiturates.

The conceptualization of insomnia in the first half of the 20th century was largely dominated by the psychoanalytic view of insomnia as a psychoneurotic symptom, treatable, in theory, through analysis. This view perpetuated the long-standing perception of insomnia as a symptom secondary to psychological distress or other primary conditions. Nevertheless, the most widely used therapies during this period were barbiturate and like compounds such as glutethimide or ethchlorvynol. Development of benzodiazepine drugs in the 1960s subsequently gave rise to the current pharmacological approach to insomnia.

The view of insomnia as a secondary symptom has largely persisted, even to the present day. However, as our understanding of the biological and psychobehavioral characteristics of the condition has grown, greater emphasis has been placed on insomnia as a disorder in its own right, with a pathophysiology that may be, in many respects, independent of the identified "primary" condition. This view was elaborated in the NIH Consensus Statement (7) on chronic insomnia, which recommended that the term "comorbid" replace "secondary" in describing associated conditions. This important operational distinction is discussed later in this volume.

DEFINING INSOMNIA

For much of the modern era of sleep medicine, the field has suffered from a lack of a comprehensive, widely accepted and utilized definition of insomnia. This absence has resulted in a considerable degree of heterogeneity in definitions and, hence, difficulties in comparing clinical or research samples of "insomnia." There are a number of components that may be considered in a general definition of insomnia. These include: (1) symptom profile—most definitions have historically included problems getting to sleep and staying asleep, the latter including early awakening. There continues to be debate as to whether nonrestorative sleep complaints should be included in this definition; (2) chronicity—most modern-day definitions have distinguished between acute and chronic insomnia, although the exact durations that separate these have varied significantly from as short as two weeks to as long as six months. Historically, some have suggested that the term insomnia be reserved only for chronic disturbances; (3) subjective versus objective findings—although it has long been recognized that insomnia is in many respects, a highly subjective experience, researchers and some clinical approaches have attempted to define insomnia by means of objective parameters such as sleep latency, number of awakenings, wake time after sleep onset or total sleep time. At present, quantitative, objective criteria are employed primarily in research settings, while clinical diagnostic criteria rely solely on subjective complaints; (4) frequency—there has been wide variability with respect to application of frequency criteria. Presently, neither the Diagnostic and Statistical Manual of Mental Disorders, fourth edition (DSM-IV) (8) nor the International Classification of Sleep Disorders, second edition (ICSD-2) (9) include a frequency criterion; (5) presence of daytime consequences–while it has long been understood that complaints of daytime symptoms and dysfunction are one of the major complications of insomnia, inclusion of these consequences has not been a standard component of many research criteria until recent years. Both DSM-IV and ICSD-2 include a requirement of daytime dysfunction.

The modern-day definitions of insomnia can be traced to the 1979 publication of the Diagnostic Classification of Sleep and Arousal Disorders (10). It is of note that this volume does not, in fact, offer a general definition of insomnia but only describes features specific to each particular diagnosis. The insomnia diagnoses are clumped within a single category of disorders of initiating and maintaining sleep (DIMS). There are no specific diagnostic criteria other than presence of a DIMS and descriptors of key characteristics that are focused largely on presumed etiologies. The first edition of the International Classification of Sleep Disorders (11) did not offer a general definition of insomnia, other than to describe degrees of severity in terms of "a . . . complaint of an insufficient amount of sleep or not feeling rested." ICSD-1 does include a requirement of "a complaint of decreased functioning during wakefulness" with some (though, curiously, not all) insomnia related diagnoses.

The Diagnostic and Statistical Manual of Mental Disorders, Fourth Edition (DSM-IV) specifically includes difficulty initiating or maintaining sleep, as well as nonrestorative sleep in its insomnia criteria. It also includes minimum one-month duration and a requirement that the disturbance results in "clinically significant distress or impairment in social, occupational, or other important areas of function." The 2005 revision of the ICSD (second edition) was the first to include explicit general criteria for insomnia (Table 1). The criteria include the unique addition of a requirement of adequate opportunity and circumstances to sleep, drawing a bright line between insomnia and insufficient sleep syndromes. All insomnia disorders must be of at least one-month duration, excepting adjustment insomnia, which must be of less than

Table 1 Standardized Criteria for Defining Insomnia

A. A complaint of difficulty initiating sleep, difficulty maintaining sleep, or waking up too early, or sleep that is chronically nonrestorative or poor in quality. In children the sleep difficulty is often reported by the caretaker and may consist of observed bedtime resistance or inability to sleep independently.
B. The above sleep difficulty occurs despite adequate opportunity and circumstances for sleep.
C. At least one of the following forms of daytime impairment related to the nighttime sleep difficulty is reported by the patient:
   i Fatigue/malaise;
   ii Attention, concentration, or memory impairment;
   iii Social/vocational dysfunction or poor school performance;
   iv Mood disturbance/irritability;
   v Daytime sleepiness;
   vi Motivation/energy/initiative reduction;
   vii Proneness for errors/accidents at work or while driving;
   viii Tension, headaches, and/or GI symptoms in response to sleep loss; and
   ix Concerns or worries about sleep.

Source: From Ref. 9.

three months duration. These criteria also identify specific daytime consequences, which must occur as a result of the sleep disturbance. A companion of sorts to the ICSD-2 criteria is the Research Diagnostic Criteria (RDC) (12) for insomnia. The general criteria of the RDC are essentially identical to those of the ICSD-2. The extensive review of criteria undertaken as part of the development of the RDC examined the frequency with which various diagnostic criteria were utilized for subject selection in the 165 insomnia papers selected. These data are reproduced in Figure 1. Research studies have typically included objective PSG criteria as criteria for inclusion in insomnia studies. This begs the question of whether objective criteria should be applied to clinical populations as well. In research environments, such criteria allow for establishment of more uniform and highly specific populations, essential to the research. In the clinical setting, however, effective application of such objective criteria is fraught with significant problems. These complications are best encapsulated by the oft-cited observation that not every (objectively) poor sleeper has insomnia and not every insomniac has (objectively) poor sleep. Indeed, there are many individuals who suffer great distress as a result of perceived sleep disturbance who would not meet typical objective (e.g., PSG) criteria for "insomnia" (e.g., patients with paradoxical insomnia), while many others who would meet such criteria have no insomnia complaints. Thus, degree of distress, perhaps to a greater extent than any objective changes, seems to dictate the presence or severity of this condition.

Investigations of insomnia have, for some time, identified this discrepancy between objective findings and subjective perception of sleep in patients with insomnia as characteristic of the condition (13,14). Persons with insomnia most often overestimate the degree of sleep disturbance in comparison to objective (polysomnographic or actigraphic) criteria. Thus, sleep latency, frequency of awakening and amount of wake after sleep onset are overestimated, while total sleep time is underestimated. This discrepancy is observed at its greatest magnitude in paradoxical insomnia, a condition in which sleep is objectively normal or near normal (by standard PSG scoring criteria), while subjective perception suggests very little or no sleep. While there is no well-established explanation for this discrepancy, emerging data on alteration of biological and cognitive activity in the sleep of chronic insomnia patients (discussed in later sections) may help explain why PSG-defined sleep may be misperceived as wake in this population.

Nonrestorative Sleep

Nonrestorative sleep (NRS) represents a little-investigated complaint that has been categorized in both ICSD-2 and DSM-IV with more standard insomnia symptoms of initiation and maintenance problems. ICSD-2 references sleep that is "chronically nonrestorative and poor in quality" (9). Thus, the affected individual is required to invoke a causal relationship between

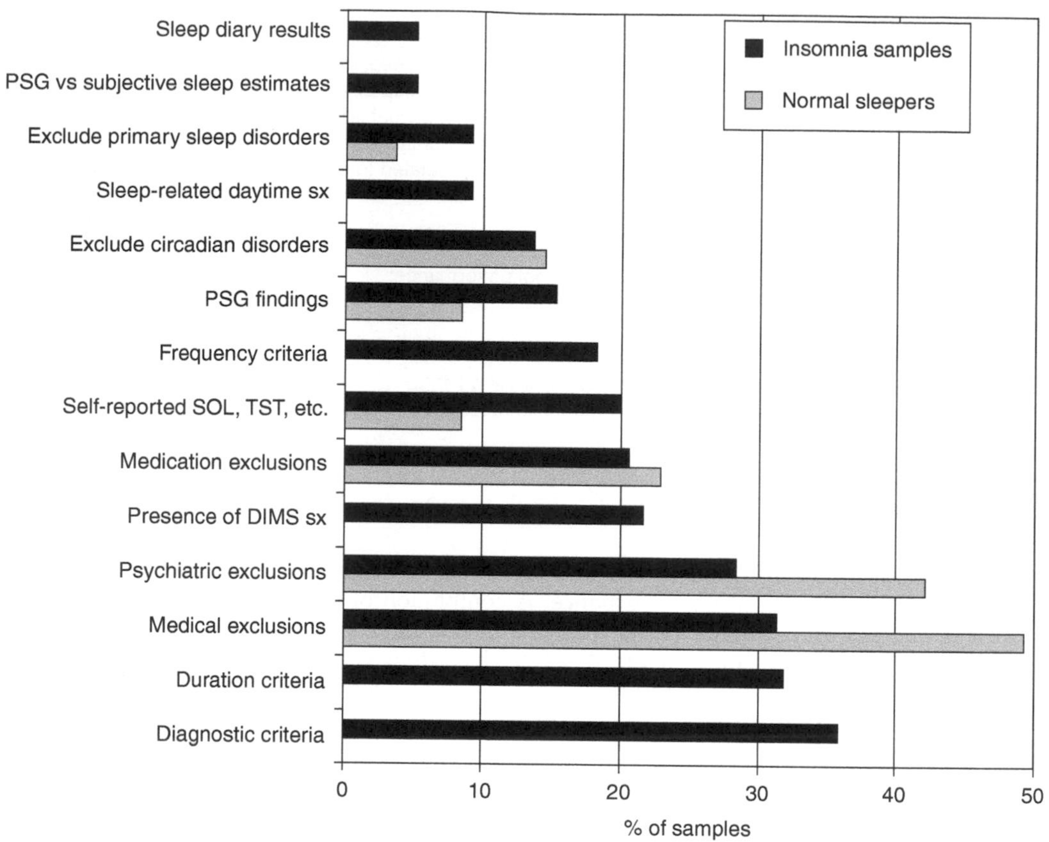

Figure 1 Criteria used for Sample Selection. *Source*: From Ref. 12.

the poorly defined nocturnal disturbance and daytime symptoms. When complaints of non-restorative sleep are associated with other insomnia complaints (trouble falling or staying asleep), this etiologic leap may seem relatively straightforward. In the absence of these more typical insomnia complaints, patients may experience "light" sleep (a vaguely defined sense of partial/intermittent wakefulness) or no specific nocturnal complaints at all. In these cases, the etiologic association would seem significantly more tenuous. Much of the available data on NRS is epidemiologic in nature (15,16). The subject has also been recently reviewed (17). Although the definitions applied in such studies typically include the criterion that the complaint occurs "despite normal sleep duration," this may not adequately account for individuals with longer sleep requirements who are, in effect, sleep-deprived. Absent objective assessment of sleep, the possibility of other, unidentified sleep disorders must also be considered. In this regard, it is noteworthy that one survey of NRS (16) found that this group has a threefold higher rate of excessive daytime sleepiness complaints, a finding more often associated with sleep disorders other than insomnia. Many of the questions utilized to define NRS focus on morning symptoms ("not feeling rested on awakening," "ease in getting started" or "waking up exhausted or fatigued"), perhaps reflecting more of an issue of high sleep inertia in some, as opposed to truly nonrestorative sleep.

The estimated prevalence of nonrestorative sleep is in the range of approximately 10% (16). However, when the prevalence of NRS, in the absence of any other insomnia symptoms, is examined, the prevalence drops to approximately 1% to 2%. Thus, it seems likely that there is a subgroup of individuals who may manifest psychophysiologic disturbance and daytime consequences similar to those of the more well-defined insomnia population, absent the usual insomnia complaints. However, this remains poorly characterized and appears likely to represent a relatively small percentage of the total population of "insomnia" patients.

CONCLUSION

It seems clear that work remains in achieving a comprehensive and broadly applied definition of insomnia. While insomnia definitions have varied considerably in the clinical and clinical research arenas, even greater variability in definition can be found in the epidemiological research on insomnia. This is discussed below. Although psychological and behavioral aspects of insomnia will likely remain important components in defining the disorder, current research in the biology of insomnia holds the promise that more physiologically based definitions may hold greater sway as we move forward.

EPIDEMIOLOGY

The earliest identified epidemiologic study of insomnia in the modern era of sleep research was published by Bixler and colleagues in 1979 (18). This study surveyed around 1000 residents of the Los Angeles area and found a prevalence of "insomnia" of 42.5%. The survey relied solely on respondents endorsing "insomnia" as a symptom. Since that time, epidemiologic surveys have become progressively more sophisticated, including criteria that assess symptom profile, frequency, severity, consequences and other characteristics (e.g., "dissatisfaction with sleep") that are considered germane in the current understanding of the disorder. With this increasing refinement of definition, prevalence data have diminished from the remarkably high percentage originally described by Bixler.

Detailed discussions of the epidemiology of insomnia have been published elsewhere (19,20). The influence of varying criteria on prevalence of insomnia has also been reviewed at length (21,22). Ohayon categorizes the approaches into four major categories: (1) insomnia as a symptom, with or without frequency and/or severity criteria; (2) insomnia with daytime consequences; (3) dissatisfaction with quality of sleep; (4) application of formal insomnia diagnostic criteria such as DSM-IV or ICSD (Fig. 2). Broadly speaking, use of a symptom criterion alone expectedly produces the highest prevalence—roughly in the 30% to 40% range. Addition of severity and/or frequency criteria reduces this to a range of approximately 15% to 25%. Requirement of daytime consequences produces prevalence rates in the 10% to 15% range. Similar, if perhaps, slightly lower estimates are observed when "dissatisfaction with quality or quantity of sleep" is applied. Formal diagnostic criteria yield the lowest estimates—in the 5% to 6% range.

As discussed above in the *Definition* section, identifying those characteristics that accurately define this condition can be elusive. Currently, the clear trend in epidemiologic research is toward requirement of daytime consequences and application of formal diagnostic criteria. A survey (22) of nearly 25,000 Europeans found that 16.8% of those sampled reported one or more symptoms of insomnia (difficulty with sleep initiation or maintenance, or nonrestorative sleep). Addition of a one-month duration criterion reduces this to 15.8%, while further requirement of associated daytime consequences yields 11.1% meeting all three criteria. Quite similar results were reported for a Canadian population (15), beginning with an initial criterion of dissatisfaction with sleep (17.8%). Addition of an insomnia symptom requirement (sleep initiation and/or maintenance disturbance) yielded a prevalence of 11.2%. Addition of duration and daytime consequences criteria further reduces this to 4% to 5%. The complete criteria in both of the studies cited above approximate DSM-IV/ICSD criteria for chronic insomnia. While some variability exists, most recent studies have reported similar prevalence when comparable criteria are employed.

Risk Factors

Numerous factors are associated with higher rates of chronic insomnia. In almost all surveys, insomnia is reported to be more frequent in women than in men (23–31). Explanations for this are not clear, although hypotheses range from reporting bias to endocrine differences to higher prevalence of certain mental disorders (e.g., depression) in women. Likewise, older age has been found to be highly associated with chronic insomnia (24,25,32). This is certainly not surprising in light of the multiple factors that also covary with age, including medical illness, pain, medication use, and increased prevalence of other sleep disorders. In fact, some data suggest that it is largely these covariates, rather than age itself, that are responsible for the increased prevalence observed in later life (33).

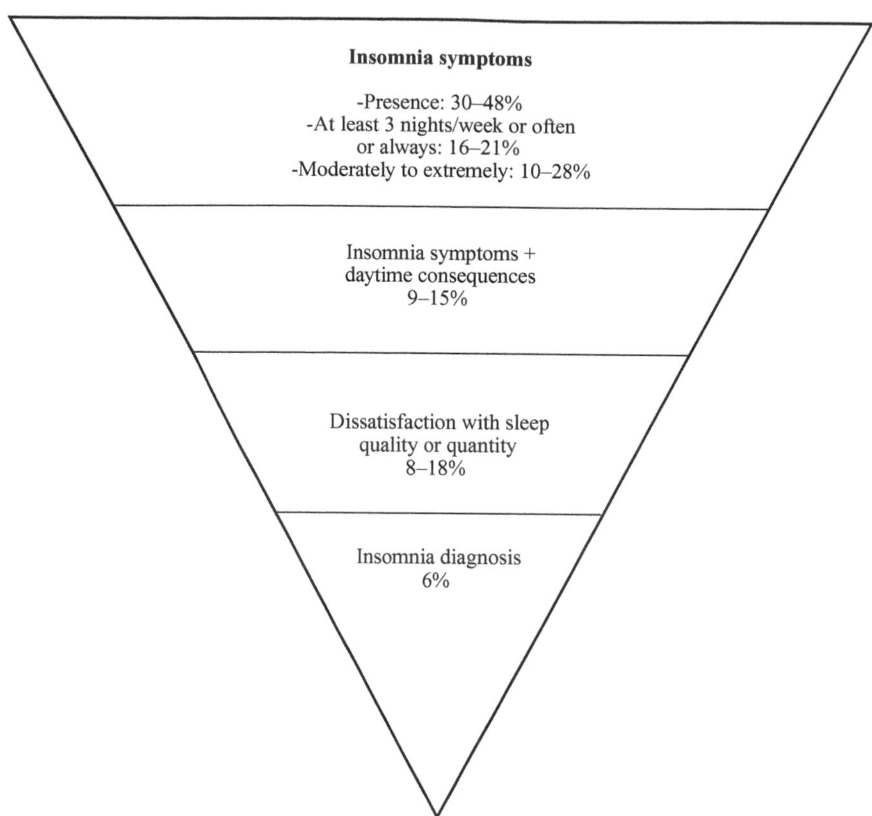

Figure 2 Average prevalence of insomnia symptoms and diagnoses. *Source*: From Ref. 21.

Unemployment and socioeconomic deprivation have been strongly associated with chronic insomnia (34). Various markers such as educational level and income have been employed as socioeconomic markers (35). However, confounders such as higher rates of other medical and psychiatric comorbidities, limited access to health care, medications, ethnicity, and occupational status that covary with SE status must be considered in interpreting this association.

Mental disorders are the most commonly associated comorbid conditions in chronic insomnia. Early epidemiologic studies generally reported significant associations between insomnia and depression and anxiety (18,25). Data from the 1989 National Institute of Mental Health (NIMH) Epidemiologic Catchment Area study (36) found a prevalence of insomnia (≥ 2 weeks of sleep initiation, maintenance or early awakening plus report to health professional or treatment or daytime consequences) of 10.2%. Forty percent of those had a comorbid psychiatric disorder, predominantly major depression and anxiety disorders. A large-scale (N = 5622) survey (31) of the French population found an overall prevalence of insomnia (initiation, maintenance or nonrestorative sleep complaint of > 1 month plus daytime consequences) of 18.6%. More than 40% of these individuals exhibited comorbid psychopathology (DSM-IV Insomnia related to mental disorder = 16.6%; DSM-IV depression or anxiety disorder = 27.9%). Pooled data from several European studies indicate that 48% of respondents meeting criteria for insomnia also met criteria for a DSM-IV psychiatric disorder diagnosis (21).

The primary interpretation of this strong association between insomnia and mental disorders was, for many years, that psychopathology is a key element in the genesis and maintenance of chronic insomnia. While that interpretation remains valid, numerous epidemiologic studies (36–38) exploring the chronological relationship between insomnia and psychiatric illness have raised the important alternative hypothesis that chronic insomnia may be a key element in the genesis and maintenance of psychiatric disorders. This issue is addressed in greater detail in Chapter 4.

Numerous medical comorbidities have likewise been associated with insomnia. In most cases, the characteristics of the relationship have not been well-investigated. Chronic pain is a common condition frequently associated with insomnia (16). A multinational study of almost 19,000 persons found that 40% of those with insomnia complaints reported at least one chronic pain problem. In this population, chronic pain was associated with greater difficulty getting back to sleep and shorter duration of sleep, as well as more prominent daytime consequences. Other medical conditions frequently associated with insomnia include lung disease, cardiovascular diseases and various neurological disorders, especially degenerative diseases and stroke (39–42). As with mental disorders, the causal relationship between these conditions is undoubtedly complex and is yet to be fully elucidated. Some recent studies (43,44) have explored potential predisposition to cardiovascular disease as a result of chronic insomnia, but results are preliminary and a causal link between chronic insomnia and incident hypertension is yet to be clearly established.

DURATION AND COURSE

Chronic insomnia is variously defined as sleep disturbance that lasts longer than one to six months. However, duration of chronic insomnia is typically measured in years or even decades. The longitudinal course of insomnia has not been studied extensively. Early epidemiologic studies (24,45,46) based on retrospective reports indicated that the vast majority of patients had at least one-year duration, while approximately 40% reported durations of five years or more. Subsequent longitudinal studies suggest that from 30% to 80% of chronic insomnia patients show no significant remission over time.

More recent investigations confirm that most affected individuals suffer with this condition for very long periods. Three-year follow-up of a sample of nearly 400 individuals selected for insomnia at baseline revealed that the problem was present for a minimum of one year in almost 75% of the sample (47). Nearly half had the maximum three-year duration. Greater likelihood of persistence was associated with increasing severity and age as well as female gender. A recent analysis of data from the long-term Zurich study (48) examined the course of insomnia among young adults. Interview intervals ranged from two to six years over the study course. Of subjects with insomnia duration of one month or longer, 30% had the same diagnosis at a previous interview, while 99% had some insomnia diagnosis (shorter duration or intermittent insomnia) previously. Thirty-five percent of one-month insomnia subjects had the diagnosis at a subsequent interview and 82% had some type of insomnia diagnosis.

In assessing these data, one should bear in mind the fact that only a small percentage of these patients are actually diagnosed and appropriately treated. Therefore, one can reasonably assume that much of the chronicity reflects relatively low rates of spontaneous remission, rather than refractoriness to treatment.

CONCLUSION

Chronic insomnia is a highly prevalent and unremitting condition characterized by complaints of difficulty initiating or maintaining sleep or sleep that is not restorative. General agreement exists that the definition must also include the presence of daytime symptoms attributable to the insomnia. Women, older adults, and persons with psychiatric or medical comorbidities are at increased risk for chronic insomnia. As discussed elsewhere, chronic insomnia may, in turn, represent a risk for development of these comorbidities. The duration of chronic insomnia is generally long, with many individuals experiencing fluctuating levels of sleep disturbance over decades. Failure of patients to report the problem, and health care providers to identify and treat it, contributes to persistence of the condition.

REFERENCES

1. Summers-Bremner E. Insomnia: A Cultural History. London: Reaktion Books, 2008.
2. Hippocrates. *Aphorisms*. eBooks@Adelaide. 2009. http://ebooks.adelaide.edu.au/h/hippocrates/aphorisms/index.html

3. Schiff P Jr. Opium and its alkaloids. Am J Pharm Educ 2002; 66:186–194.
4. *The History of Insomnia*. http://www.bbc.co.uk/dna/h2g2/A294031. Accessed 5, 2008.
5. Horne J. Insomnia—Victorian Style. Psychologist 2008; 21(10):910–911.
6. Anonymous. Sleeplessness. Br Med J 1894; 2(1761):719.
7. NIH State of the Science Conference statement on Manifestations and Management of Chronic Insomnia in Adults. J Clin Sleep Med 2005; 1(4):412–421.
8. American Psychiatric Association. Diagnostic and Statistical Manual of Mental Disorders (DSM-IV). Washington DC: American Psychiatric Association, 1994.
9. American Academy of Sleep Medicine. International classification of sleep disorders, 2nd ed. Diagnostic and coding manual. Westchester, IL: American Academy of Sleep Medicine, 2005.
10. Association of Sleep Disorders Centers and the Association for the Psychophysiological Study of Sleep. Diagnostic classification of sleep and arousal disorders. 1979 first edition. Sleep 1979; 2(1):1–154.
11. American Sleep Disorders Association, International Classification of Sleep Disorders. ed. Diagnostic Classification Steering Committee. 1990, Rochester MN.
12. Edinger JD, Bonnet MH, Bootzin RR, et al. Derivation of research diagnostic criteria for insomnia: Report of an American Academy of Sleep Medicine Work Group. Sleep 2004; 27(8):1567–1596.
13. Carskadon M, Dement W, Mitler M, et al. Self report versus sleep laboratory findings in 122 drug-free subjects with the complaint of chronic insomnia. Am J Psychiatry 1976; 133:1382–1388.
14. Frankel BL, Coursey RD, Buchbinder R, et al. Recorded and reported sleep in chronic primary insomnia. Arch Gen Psychiatry 1976; 33(5):615–623.
15. Ohayon MM, Caulet M, Guilleminault C. How a general population perceives its sleep and how this relates to the complaint of insomnia. Sleep 1997; 20(9):715–723.
16. Ohayon MM. Relationship between chronic painful physical condition and insomnia. J Psychiatr Res 2005; 39(2):151–159.
17. Stone KC, Taylor DJ, McCrae CS, et al. Nonrestorative sleep. Sleep Med Rev 2008; 12(4):275–288.
18. Bixler E, Kales A, Soldatos C, et al. Prevalence of sleep disorders in the Los Angeles metropolitan area. Am J Psychiatry 1979; 136:1257–1262.
19. Lichstein KL, Riedel BW, Taylor DJ. Epidemiology of sleep: Age, gender, and ethnicity. Mahwah, New Jersey: Lawrence Erlbaum Associates, 2004.
20. Partinen M, Hublin C. Epidemiology of sleep disorders. In Kryger MH, Roth T, Dement WC, eds. Principles and Practice of Sleep Medicine. Elsevier Saunders: Philadelphia, 2005:626–647.
21. Ohayon MM. Epidemiology of insomnia: What we know and what we still need to learn. Sleep Med Rev 2002; 6(2):97–111.
22. Ohayon MM, Roth T. What are the contributing factors for insomnia in the general population? J Psychosom Res 2001; 51(6):745–755.
23. Hajak G. Epidemiology of severe insomnia and its consequences in Germany. Eur Arch Psychiatry Clin Neurosci 2001; 251(2):49–56.
24. Hohagen F, Rink K, Käppler C, et al. Prevalence and treatment of insomnia in general practice: A longitudinal study. Eur Arch Psychiatry Clin Neurosci 1993; 242:329–336.
25. Mellinger G, Balter M, Uhlenhuth E. Insomnia and its treatment: Prevalence and correlates. Arch Gen Psychiatry 1985; 42:25–232.
26. Weyerer S, Dilling H. Prevalence and treatment of insomnia in the community: Results from the Upper Bavarian Field Study. Sleep 1991; 14:392–398.
27. Chevalier H, Los F, Boichut D, et al. Evaluation of severe insomnia in the general population: Results of a European multinational survey. J Psychopharmacol 1999; 13(4 Suppl 1):S21–S24.
28. Hatoum HT, Kania CM, Kong SX, et al. Prevalence of insomnia: A survey of the enrollees at five managed care organizations. Am J Manag Care 1998; 4(1):79–86.
29. Leger D, Guilleminault C, Dreyfus JP, et al. Prevalence of insomnia in a survey of 12,778 adults in France. J Sleep Res 2000; 9(1):35–42.
30. Ohayon MM, Caulet M, Priest RG, et al. DSM-IV and ICSD-90 insomnia symptoms and sleep dissatisfaction. Br J Psychiatry 1997; 171:382–388.
31. Ohayon MM. Prevalence of DSM-IV diagnostic criteria of insomnia: Distinguishing insomnia related to mental disorders from sleep disorders. J Psychiatr Res 1997; 31(3):333–346.
32. Ohayon M. Epidemiological study on insomnia in the general population. Sleep 1996; 19(3 Suppl):S7–S15.
33. Ohayon MM, Zulley J, Guilleminault C, et al. How age and daytime activities are related to insomnia in the general population: Consequences for older people. J Am Geriatr Soc 2001; 49(4):360–366.
34. Regenstein Q, Dambrosia J, Hallett M, et al. Daytime alertness in patients with primary insomnia. Am J Psychiatry 1993; 150:1529–1534.
35. Gellis LA, Lichstein KL, Scarinci IC, et al. Socioeconomic status and insomnia. J Abnorm Psychol 2005; 114(1):111–118.

36. Ford D, Kamerow D. Epidemiologic study of sleep disturbances and psychiatric disorders. JAMA 1989; 262:1479–1484.
37. Breslau N, Roth T, Rosenthal L, et al. Sleep disturbance and psychiatric disorders: A longitudinal epidemiological study of young adults. Biol Psychiatry 1996; 39(6):411–418.
38. Weissman MM, Greenwald S, Nino-Murcia G, et al. The morbidity of insomnia uncomplicated by psychiatric disorders. Gen Hosp Psychiatry 1997; 19(4):245–250.
39. Gislason T, Reymisdötter H, Kritbjarnarson H, et al. Sleep habits and sleep disturbances among the elderly—An epidemiological survey. J Intern Med 1993; 234:31–39.
40. Klink M, Quan S. Prevalence of reported sleep disturbances in general adult population and their relationship to obstructive airway disease. Chest 1987; 91:540–546.
41. Klink M, Quan S, Kaltenborn W, et al. Risk factors associated with complaints of insomnia in a general adult population. Arch Intern Med 1992; 152:1634–1637.
42. Elwood P, Hack M, Pickering J, et al. Sleep disturbance, stroke, and heart disease events: Evidence from the Caerphilly cohort. J Epidemiol Community Health 2006; 60(1):69–73.
43. Phillips B, Buzkova P, Enright P. Insomnia did not predict incident hypertension in older adults in the cardiovascular health study. Sleep 2009; 32(1):65–72.
44. Lanfranchi PA, Pennestri MH, Fradette L, et al. Nighttime blood pressure in normotensive subjects with chronic insomnia: Implications for cardiovascular risk. Sleep 2009; 32(6):760–766.
45. Foley DJ, Monjan A, Simonsick EM, et al. Incidence and remission of insomnia among elderly adults: An epidemiologic study of 6,800 persons over three years. Sleep 1999; 22(Suppl 2):S366–S372.
46. Morgan K, Clarke D. Longitudinal trends in late life insomnia: Implications for prescribing. Age Ageing 1997; 26(3):179–184.
47. Morin CM, Belanger L, LeBlanc M, et al. The natural history of insomnia: A population-based 3-year longitudinal study. Arch Intern Med 2009; 169(5):447–453.
48. Buysse DJ, Angst J, Gamma A, et al. Prevalence, course, and comorbidity of insomnia and depression in young adults. Sleep 2008; 31(4):473–480.

2 Subjective and Objective Daytime Consequences of Insomnia

Michael Bonnet and Donna Arand

Dayton Department of Veterans Affairs Medical Center, Wright State University, Wallace Kettering Neuroscience Institute, and Kettering Medical Center, Dayton, Ohio, U.S.A.

The International Classification of Sleep Disorders Second Edition (ICSD-2) (1) requires both poor sleep and daytime functional compromise for the diagnosis of insomnia. Patients report numerous consequences of their insomnia, and the ICSD-2 lists the following as diagnostically sufficient examples:

Fatigue or malaise
Poor attention or concentration
Social or vocational dysfunction
Mood disturbance
Daytime sleepiness
Reduced motivation or energy
Increased errors or accidents
Tension, headache or gastrointestinal symptoms
Continuing worry about sleep

Insomnia produces numerous medical, psychological, and economic deficits in addition to changes in subjective state and performance, but only the latter two factors, specifically related to the diagnostic criteria required for a diagnosis of insomnia, will be considered in this chapter. A section reviewing subjective deficits will be followed by a section examining objective deficits.

SUBJECTIVE MOOD AND PERFORMANCE DECREMENTS ASSOCIATED WITH INSOMNIA

Medications for sleep have historically been developed to produce efficacy based on decreasing sleep latency or increasing sleep time at night. Mood and performance testing have been conducted primarily to rule out hangover sedation rather than to demonstrate improvement of the daytime symptoms reported by patients. In recent years, however, researchers have realized that successful treatment for insomnia should both improve sleep parameters and reverse the daytime consequences reported by patients (2). Numerous measures have been developed to document subjective deficits in patients with insomnia. Categories that have been measured include mood, anxiety or depression, quality of life, and work-related performance. Sections reviewing significant subjective deficits will be followed by available data showing treatment response.

Mood

Dysphoria is commonly reported by patients with insomnia. A number of studies have assessed various mood components in these patients.

Sleepiness/Fatigue

The most commonly reported mood dimensions have been subjective fatigue and sleepiness. In a review of studies prior to 2000 (3), it was reported that 7 of 12 studies using the Stanford Sleepiness Scale in insomnia patients found significantly greater sleepiness in patients as compared to controls. However, as the evaluation of insomnia has evolved, investigators began to differentiate frank sleepiness (by asking patients if they would actually fall asleep in a given circumstance using a questionnaire such as the Epworth Sleepiness Scale—ESS) from fatigue (feeling tired or without energy but not likely to fall asleep). In recent years, the Stanford

Sleepiness Scale has been used less frequently in insomnia patients, and a number of more fatigue-related mood scales and measures have appeared (4). For example, in a study that compared sleepiness measured by the ESS and fatigue measured by the Tiredness Symptoms Scale (TSS), insomnia patients had sleepiness levels on the ESS that were nonsignificantly lower than controls and significantly lower than sleep apnea patients whereas their TSS scores were nonsignificantly higher than sleep apnea patients and significantly higher than controls (5). These findings of lower sleepiness despite increased fatigue are consistent with objective sleepiness data from the Multiple Sleep Latency Test. A recent review found that none of 12 studies comparing objective daytime sleepiness in insomnia patients with controls found significantly greater objective sleepiness in the insomnia patients (6). These findings suggest that sleepiness and fatigue can be diagnostically differentiated if patients are given sufficient descriptive latitude and that insomnia patients view their problem as more of a fatigue problem rather than excessive sleepiness.

Fatigue has been measured from general mood scales such as the Profile of Mood States (POMS), which has a specific fatigue scale, in addition to more recently developed specific scales such as the Fatigue Severity Scale (FSS). Significant increases in fatigue have been reported in insomnia patients in four (3,7–9) of seven studies (10–12).

Other Mood Changes

Insomnia patients frequently have more negative mood on a number of dimensions. Other scales from the POMS that have been significantly different in insomnia patients compared with controls include elevated Confusion, Tension/Anxiety, and Depression and reduced Vigor (3,10–12).

Recent studies have begun to report changes in mood associated with insomnia treatment. For example, studies of eszopiclone 2 and 3 mg have found that there was a significant increase in daytime alertness, physical well-being, and ability to function but no improvement in morning sleepiness at the end of treatment compared with parallel placebo groups in primary and comorbid insomnia (13,14). Krystal et al. (15), in a six-month study of eszopiclone 3 mg, reported significantly improved daytime subjective alertness and physical well-being in their treatment group that continued until the end of medication administration compared with a parallel placebo group. Another study (16) has shown that zolpidem extended release 12.5 mg prn for six months was effective in reducing morning sleepiness (and ESS scores) and improving concentration, with changes that were statistically significant for each of the six months of the study (except for the sixth month for the ESS).

Anxiety and Depression

Most research studies have examined patients with primary insomnia, thereby excluding patients with specific clinical mood disorders such as anxiety or depression. However, even with exclusions for such clinical pathology, studies that have utilized traditional measures of personality such as the Minnesota Multiphasic Personality Inventory (MMPI), Hamilton Depression Rating Scale, Beck Depression Inventory, and the depression scale from the POMS have consistently shown that patients with primary insomnia have significantly elevated scores on the depression subscale compared to controls. Nine of 12 studies reviewed reported significantly higher scores in insomnia patients compared with controls (17–25) [negative studies (26–28)]. One of the studies found equivalent elevations in the MMPI in insomnia patients regardless of whether their insomnia was psychologically based (psychophysiological insomnia) or medically based (including insomnia with sleep apnea, periodic limb movements, or restless legs) (24). However, these MMPI scale elevations typically do not place the insomnia patients into the realm of clinical pathology, as such patients have typically been excluded.

Anxiety is also frequently elevated in patients with insomnia. Six of 12 studies have reported significantly elevated anxiety in insomnia patients based on the MMPI (17,21,23–25,29) [negative (18–20,26–28)] and two have reported elevations based on the Spielberger State-Trait Anxiety Inventory (30,31). Studies have not reported decreases in anxiety or depression after insomnia treatment. However, in clinically depressed patients, treatment of both depression and insomnia has been shown to produce a more rapid improvement in depression (32).

Quality of Life

There are several means of assessing quality of life (QOL) in patients. Some studies have used one or two specific questions whereas others have used QOL scales such as the Quality of Life in Insomnia Scale (4). One QOL scale that has been widely used in diverse patient populations is the Medical Outcomes Study Short Form (SF-36) (33). The SF-36 assesses physical functioning, limitations due to physical health problems, bodily pain, general health perception, vitality, social functioning, limitations due to emotional health problems, and mental health. Patients with insomnia reported decreased QOL compared with normal controls on all dimensions of the SF-36 ($P < 0.0001$) (34,35) and SF-12 (36). One study (37) compared SF-36 results in a group of mild and severe insomnia patients with groups of patients diagnosed with depression or congestive heart failure (CHF). Severe insomnia patients had numerically greater loss of function than patients with CHF on all of the SF-36 scales except physical functioning. Insomnia patients also reported more physical problems (the first four scales of the SF-36) than patients with depression (37). Such findings suggest that the subjective dysphoria and loss of function associated with insomnia is similar to that seen in other significant chronic illness.

Research studies have also begun to examine changes in QOL with insomnia treatment. One study found significantly improved ability to function during the day and physical well-being throughout six months in patients receiving eszopiclone 3 mg compared with placebo in a double-blind design (15). A study of eszopiclone 1 and 2 mg in elderly insomnia patients found improved QOL on some subscales at the 2 mg but not the 1 mg dose over two weeks of medication administration (13). Another study (38) tracked the 3-item subscale of the Insomnia Severity Index that deals with QOL and functioning in patients receiving indiplon 10 mg, indiplon 20 mg, or placebo in a double-blind study and found that patients receiving either dose of medication were significantly improved compared to the placebo group during each of the three months of the study. The percentage of patients reporting minimal to no daytime impairment was significantly higher in the active treatment group (73%) versus the placebo group (60%). At the end of the study approximately 2/3 of the patients in the medication treatment conditions scored within the normal range on the complete Insomnia Severity Index compared with 38% in the placebo group, also a significant difference (38). Finally, in a study that evaluated eszopiclone 3 mg or matching placebo under double-blind conditions for six months (39), the complete SF-36 was administered at baseline and after one, three, and six months. At baseline, patients had significantly lower values on the SF-36 Vitality, Social Functioning, and Mental Health scales compared with healthy U.S. population norms. After six months of treatment, patients taking eszopiclone had significantly improved on these three scales in comparison with the insomnia patients receiving placebo and were at or above the U.S. population norms. QOL has also been assessed in a behavioral treatment paradigm (40). In this study, patients with chronic insomnia who had been treated with pharmacotherapy for 10 years on average were given cognitive-behavioral therapy or no additional therapy (patients were allowed to either continue or be withdrawn from their current sleeping medications). At intake, patients were found to have significantly worse QOL compared with population norms, and this was significant for all scales on the SF-36 for younger subjects (age 30–49). However, the oldest subjects (age 70–100) were much closer to population norms and were significantly worse than those norms only on physical functioning, mental health, vitality, and bodily pain. By the end of the six-month trial, patients across all ages in the cognitive-behavioral therapy group had significantly better scores than the control population on physical functioning, mental health, and limitations due to emotional health problems. Unfortunately, these improvements occurred primarily because QOL deteriorated in control patients rather than truly improving in the patients with behavioral therapy.

The studies of QOL are consistent in showing that decrements in insomnia patients can be reversed with return to normal levels after treatment for as long as six months (the duration of study trials). There has also been improvement in parallel placebo groups, but improvement in medication treatment groups has been significantly greater than that seen in the placebo groups. Improved QOL has implications for decreased health care utilization and improved work performance. One study has actually used QOL improvement as a basis for a determination of cost effectiveness for long-term treatment of primary insomnia (41).

Work Performance

Another means of assessing QOL is to assess job performance or career success in patients compared to controls. One study found that self-reported poor sleepers in the Navy received significantly fewer promotions and were less likely to be recommended for reenlistment (42). Questionnaire studies have shown that subjectively identified patients with insomnia felt more fatigued and irritated with their children and had more health care consequences on a number of dimensions (43). Insomnia patients also reported consequences at work including significantly more errors, significantly more accidents, more absenteeism, and poor efficiency (43,44). However, a recent study that attempted to replicate the finding of increased absenteeism in insomnia patients found, in a logistic regression model, that absenteeism based on company sick leave records was determined only by sex, profession, and depression (45). To some extent these results may reflect a limitation of questionnaire studies of sleep problems (in which patients with sleep apnea, other sleep pathology, or untreated depression may also be included in insomnia groups). Moreover, subjective responses to queries about accidents and sick leave further confound results.

Fortunately, careful studies have begun to more clearly identify patients with primary insomnia. One recent study used the Work Limitations Questionnaire (46) to assess time demands, physical demands, mental demands, output demands, and work productivity loss in primary insomnia patients given eszopiclone 3 mg or placebo in a double-blind design for six months. Patients receiving medication were significantly improved compared with placebo on all scales for the one to six month average score. Scores at the end of the study were in the range of normal scores on all of the scales except time demands, but there was large variability. In another study using the same questionnaire (47), patients given zolpidem extended release 12.5 mg versus placebo in a double-blind study for 12 weeks showed significant improvement on the time demands and output demands scales at the end of the study. The magnitude of improvement on these scales was similar in both studies.

OBJECTIVE MEASURES OF PERFORMANCE

Subjective measures clearly support the common perception of poor performance in insomnia patients. However, it is also important to understand the extent to which these subjective reports of poor performance are linked to objectively measured psychomotor performance. At least 21 studies have compared performance in patients with insomnia to matched controls on more than 30 different performance tasks (7–12,17–19,26,28,48–57). One review has compared the results of these insomnia studies with those reported from sleep deprivation studies (one presumption is that both insomnia patients and sleep deprived individuals have some accumulated sleep loss) because many of the tests used to compare insomnia patients with normal sleepers have been used and found sensitive in sleep deprivation studies (6). For convenience, that review divided the many performance measures into several broad categories: memory, balance, math, vigilance, hand/eye coordination, and reasoning tasks. These same categories were retained for the current review.

Memory

Numerous memory tasks have been used to document differences between insomnia patients and controls. Common short-term memory tasks that have been used include the Digit Symbol Substitution Task (NS in seven of seven studies), digit span (NS in three of five studies), the MAST (NS in six of seven reports from two studies), and simple short-term memory (NS in six of nine studies). The nine studies reporting number of words recalled in an immediate memory task were reviewed, and data from the four of those that included means plus standard deviations in comparable patient and control groups were combined to calculate an effect size (58). From those studies (7–9,53), mean words recalled from normals and insomnia patients were 10.8 and 8.4 words respectively (combined standard deviation of 2.69 with 105 and 185 Ss) giving a combined t-value of $t_{288} = 7.51$ ($P < 0.01$) and effect size (ES) of 0.91. However, ESs for other types of memory measures were lower (in the range of 0.28). In studies with long-term recall, insomnia subjects performed significantly worse than controls in only one of four studies. More recently, primary insomnia was associated with impairment of procedural memory in comparison to controls (52). The number of studies showing significant results for various memory variables is low, but the combination of studies with largely nonsignificant results to increase the sample size produced a significant effect that also had a large ES. Therefore, examination of memory effects in larger studies is indicated.

Balance

Two studies that have examined balance in insomnia patients and controls have both reported statistically significant decreases in balance in insomnia patients (10,12) compared with controls, and ES from the one study with data sufficient to calculate the statistic was 3.1 (12). One implication of these results is a recent finding that insomnia, in elderly nursing home residents, is associated with a greater risk of falls, and this risk is not based on the use of sleeping medication (59). These data also imply that further examination of balance could be important.

Math

Computational ability has been infrequently examined in insomnia patients. None of the three studies that have examined ability to perform additions have found significant decrements in insomnia patients compared with controls.

Vigilance

True vigilance tasks and simple and choice reaction time tasks were included with vigilance tasks. Two significant vigilance results were found from six studies; two significant 4-choice reaction time results were found from four studies, and one significant simple reaction time result was found from eight studies. Of studies reporting mean and standard deviation for simple reaction time (10,11), reaction times from normals and insomnia patients were 290 and 364 msec, respectively (combined standard deviation of 256 msec with 56 Ss in both groups), giving a small ES of 0.288. One study that reported nonsignificant differences for simple reaction time in large groups (60) did report significantly slower response latencies for insomnia patients compared with controls for responses to more complex decisions.

Hand/Eye Coordination

Hand/eye coordination tasks included tremor, card sorting, Purdue pegboard, tapping, line tracing, trail making, and visual resolution. Of 13 total studies in this area, only one statistically significant result, for the single study of line tracing (17), was found.

Reasoning

Four studies reported logical reasoning or proofreading in insomnia patients versus controls but no statistically different results were reported.

Sleepiness/Alertness

Objective sleepiness/alertness is commonly measured with the Multiple Sleep Latency Test (MSLT) or Maintenance of Wakefulness Test (MWT). A number of studies have examined the ability of insomnia patients to fall asleep using the MSLT. These studies are of particular interest because, if patients suffer mainly from reduced sleep at night, their daytime nap latencies should be significantly reduced (61). However, if patients primarily suffer from physiological hyperarousal, their daytime nap latencies should be increased. Twelve studies were found where daytime nap latency was compared between insomnia patients and study controls (7,9,17–19,26,49–51,62–64). Sleep latency was not significantly reduced in insomnia patients as compared to controls in any study. Sleep latency was significantly increased in insomnia patients as compared to controls in 6 of the 12 studies. Of the 12 studies, 7 used a relatively standard protocol and reported both means and standard deviations for the groups. When the data for these seven studies were combined, the average sleep latency for insomnia patients ($N = 192$) was 13.5 (±4.9) minutes and for controls ($N = 167$) was 12.1 (±5.3) minutes. This difference was statistically significant ($t_{357} = 2.586$, $P = 0.01$). The ES, based on these group data, was 0.27. The t-value and ES value are both somewhat lower than in studies for which subjects were required to meet both a subjective and objective sleep criterion to be included (6). In general, these data are consistent with subjective data that show insomnia patients report increases in subjective sleepiness and more specifically, fatigue, without objective sleepiness.

SUMMARY

Extensive psychomotor performance and sleepiness data recorded from insomnia patients over the past 25 years have shown that these patients have marginal decreases in performance. Of functions assessed, decrements in balance accompanied by increased falls in elderly insomnia patients are the most persuasive. Several individual studies and the pooled analysis of short-term memory data do suggest the likelihood of some memory deficits in patients. Unfortunately, objective performance indicators have only been reported in treatment studies in the negative sense (absence of decrements shortly after awakening rather than improved performance during the day). The large number of nonsignificant results along with the finding that insomnia patients are significantly less sleepy than controls on the MSLT suggests that insomnia is not the same as sleep deprivation. Since many of the tests used to compare insomnia patients with controls have been selected secondary to their sensitivity to sleep deprivation, it is possible that the psychomotor tests employed have not been the optimal measures for assessment of impairment and that different or more specific tests might provide additional information. In addition, the results from memory tests suggest that future studies of performance in insomnia patients can benefit from larger sample sizes to more easily demonstrate deficits.

It is also the case that the picture of performance in patients with the insomnia is much different when one examines objective performance measures than when one examines subjective measures such as mood or QOL. It will be important to reconcile the differences between data sets that should reasonably be expected to correlate with one another. One means of doing this is to compare objective and subjective results from within the same study. For example, one study (8) both asked patients to subjectively rate their performance ability and employed several objective performance measures. As expected, insomnia patients subjectively rated their performance compared with their real capacity as significantly worse than did control subjects with a large effect size (ES = 1.20). However, of eight objective performance measures including memory tests, motor tests, reaction time, and executive function, insomnia patients performed significantly worse than normals on only one of the four memory tests (digit span), and the median ES for the performance tests was low (around 0.4). In the same study, insomnia patients had reported a significantly longer subjective sleep latency compared to the controls (ES = 1.32) while their objective PSG sleep latency was actually nonsignificantly shorter than the controls (ES = −0.05). Similarly, the insomnia patients reported subjectively that their total sleep time was significantly shorter than the controls (ES = 2.15) while their actual total sleep time was not significantly different from the controls (ES = 0.4). These objective and subjective sleep data are very consistent with the objective and subjective performance data reported above and suggest that the same mechanism that results in patients subjectively reporting much worse sleep than is corroborated objectively may also operate similarly when subjective performance is compared with objective psychomotor performance measures.

CONCLUSIONS AND RECOMMENDATIONS FOR FURTHER RESEARCH

Patients with insomnia are differentiated from normal sleepers with a short sleep requirement based on their complaint of daytime dysphoria and poor performance. Subjective report measures have consistently shown that insomnia patients have reduced QOL in all dimensions and believe that their work and social performance is greatly limited. Recently, treatment studies have begun to focus on QOL and have shown that pharmacological treatment and, possibly, behavioral treatment can produce improvement in QOL with a return to baseline levels. The inability to show consistent decrements in objective daytime alertness and performance has limited more effective evaluation and treatment of insomnia for many years. Objective performance deficits, like objective sleep deficits, have been difficult to identify in these patients. A common limitation of these studies is smaller sample size (60). The ability to observe an overall significant decrement in short-term memory performance by pooling over a number of largely nonsignificant previous studies suggests that evaluation of memory and balance, at least, in multicenter studies could provide evidence of significantly improved psychomotor performance secondary to treatment. Furthermore, the extent to which the subjective and objective deficits reported by the patients are associated with partial sleep deprivation/sleepiness versus hyperarousal requires additional investigation. In a study that correlated MSLT results with sleep, demographic, and performance/mood variables (65), it was found that insomnia patients with longer MSLT values (higher daytime alertness) also had longer subjective sleep latency at night and higher anxiety scores on the POMS. Such findings link dysphoria and poor subjective sleep with hyperarousal rather than sleepiness and suggest that performance deficits in insomnia patients will be more apparent on psychomotor performance tasks that are sensitive to central activation rather than sleepiness. Because many of the tests used in insomnia research have evolved from sleep deprivation research, they may simply be inappropriate or irrelevant for use in insomnia patients. The development of more appropriate and sensitive tests for insomnia-related impairment may allow us to better define the relationship between objective and subjective consequences of the condition.

ACKNOWLEDGMENT

This study was supported by the Dayton Department of Veterans Affairs Medical Center, Wright State University School of Medicine, and the Sleep-Wake Disorders Research Institute.

REFERENCES

1. American Academy of Sleep Medicine. International Classification of Sleep Disorders: Diagnostic and Coding Manual. 2nd ed. Westchester, IL: American Academy of Sleep Medicine, 2005.
2. Krystal AD. Treating the health, quality of life, and functional impairments in insomnia. J Clin Sleep Med 2007; 3(1):63–72.
3. Riedel B, Lichstein K. Insomnia and daytime functioning. Sleep Med Rev 2000; 4:277–298.
4. Buysse DJ, Ancoli-Israel S, Edinger JD, et al. Recommendations for a standard research assessment of insomnia. Sleep 2006; 29(9):1155–1173.
5. Schneider C, Fulda S, Schulz H. Daytime variation in performance and tiredness/sleepiness ratings in patients with insomnia, narcolepsy, sleep apnea and normal controls. J Sleep Res 2004; 13(4):373–383.
6. Bonnet MH, Arand DL. Consequences of insomnia. Sleep Med Clin 2006; 1:351–358.
7. Rosa R, Bonnet M. Reported chronic insomnia is independent of poor sleep as measured by electroencephalography. Psychosom Med 2000; 62:474–482.
8. Vignola A, Lamoureux C, Bastien CH, et al. Effects of chronic insomnia and use of benzodiazepines on daytime performance in older adults. J Gerontol B Psychol Sci Soc Sci 2000; 55(1):P54–P62.
9. Pedrosi B, Roehrs T, Rosenthal L, et al. Daytime function and benzodiazepine effects in insomniacs compared to normals. Sleep Res 1995; 24:48.
10. Hauri PJ. Cognitive deficits in insomnia patients. Acta Neurol Belg 1997; 97(2):113–117.
11. Crenshaw MC, Edinger JD. Slow-wave sleep and waking cognitive performance among older adults with and without insomnia complaints. Physiol Behav 1999; 66(3):485–492.
12. Mendelson WB, Garnett D, Linnoila M. Do insomniacs have impaired daytime functioning? Biol Psychiatry 1984; 19(8):1261–1264.
13. Scharf M, Erman M, Rosenberg R, et al. A 2-week efficacy and safety study of eszopiclone in elderly patients with primary insomnia. Sleep 2005; 28(6):720–727.
14. Soares CN, Joffe H, Rubens R, et al. Eszopiclone in patients with insomnia during perimenopause and early postmenopause: a randomized controlled trial. Obstet Gynecol 2006; 108(6):1402–1410.
15. Krystal AD, Walsh JK, Laska E, et al. Sustained efficacy of eszopiclone over 6 months of nightly treatment: results of a randomized, double-blind, placebo-controlled study in adults with chronic insomnia. Sleep 2003; 26(7):793–799.
16. Krystal AD, Erman M, Zammit GK, et al. Long-term efficacy and safety of zolpidem extended-release 12.5 mg, administered 3 to 7 nights per week for 24 weeks, in patients with chronic primary insomnia: a 6-month, randomized, double-blind, placebo-controlled, parallel-group, multicenter study. Sleep 2008; 31(1):79–90.
17. Schneider-Helmert D. Twenty-four-hour sleep-wake function and personality patterns in chronic insomniacs and healthy controls. Sleep 1987; 10(5):452–462.
18. Mendelson WB, Garnett D, Gillin CG, et al. The experience of insomnia and daytime and nighttime functioning. Psychiatry Res 1984; 12:235–250.
19. Bonnet MH, Arand DL. 24-Hour metabolic rate in insomniacs and matched normal sleepers. Sleep 1995; 18:581–588.
20. Beutler L. Psychological variables in the diagnosis of insomnia. In: Williams RL, Karacan I, eds. Sleep Disorders: Diagnosis and Treatment. New York: John Wiley & Sons, 1978:61–100.
21. Coursey RD, Buchsbaum M, Frankel BL. Personality measures and evoked responses in chronic insomniacs. J Abnorm Psychol 1975; 84:239–249.
22. Szelenberger W, Niemcewicz S. Severity of insomnia correlates with cognitive impairment. Acta Neurobiol Exp (Wars) 2000; 60:373.

23. Kales A, Caldwell AB, Soldatos CR, et al. Biopsychobehavioral correlates of insomnia. II. Pattern specificity and consistency with the Minnesota Multiphasic Personality Inventory. Psychosom Med 1983; 45(4):341–355.
24. Kalogjera-Sackellares D, Cartwright RD. Comparison of MMPI profiles in medically and psychologically based insomnias. Psychiatry Res 1997; 70:49–56.
25. Bliwise NG, Bliwise DL, Dement WC. Age and psychopathology in insomnia. Clin Gerontol 1985/1986; 4:3–9.
26. Seidel WF, Ball S, Cohen S, et al. Daytime alertness in relation to mood, performance, and nocturnal sleep in chronic insomniacs and noncomplaining sleepers. Sleep 1984; 7(3):230–238.
27. Hauri P, Fisher J. Persistent psychophysiologic (learned) insomnia. Sleep 1986; 9(1):38–53.
28. Bonnet MH. Recovery of performance during sleep following sleep deprivation in older normal and insomniac adult males. Percept Mot Skills 1985; 60(1):323–334.
29. Freedman RR, Sattler HL. Physiological and psychological factors in sleep-onset insomnia. J Abnorm Psychol 1982; 91:380–389.
30. Chambers M, Keller B. Alert insomniacs: are they really sleep deprived? Clin Psychol Rev 1993; 13:649–666.
31. Morin CM, Gramling SE. Sleep patterns and aging: comparison of older adults with and without insomnia complaints. Psychol Aging 1989; 4(3):290–294.
32. Fava M, McCall WV, Krystal A, et al. Eszopiclone co-administered with fluoxetine in patients with insomnia coexisting with major depressive disorder. Biol Psychiatry 2006; 59:1052–1060.
33. McHorney CA, Ware JE Jr., Lu JF, et al. The MOS 36-item Short-Form Health Survey (SF-36): III. Tests of data quality, scaling assumptions, and reliability across diverse patient groups. Med Care 1994; 32:40–66.
34. Zammit GK, Weiner J, Damato N, et al. Quality of life in people with insomnia. Sleep 1999; 22 (suppl):S379–S385.
35. Leger D, Scheuermaier K, Philip P, et al. SF-36: evaluation of quality of life in severe and mild insomniacs compared with good sleepers. Psychosom Med 2001; 63(1):49–55.
36. LeBlanc M, Beaulieu-Bonneau S, Merette C, et al. Psychological and health-related quality of life factors associated with insomnia in a population-based sample. J Psychosom Res 2007; 63(2):157–166.
37. Katz D, McHorney C. The relationship between insomnia and health-related quality of life in patients with chronic illness. J Fam Pract 2002; 51:229–235.
38. Scharf MB, Black J, Hull S, et al. Long-term nightly treatment with indiplon in adults with primary insomnia: results of a double-blind, placebo-controlled, 3-month study. Sleep 2007; 30(6): 743–752.
39. Walsh JK, Krystal AD, Amato DA, et al. Nightly treatment of primary insomnia with eszopiclone for six months: effect on sleep, quality of life, and work limitations. Sleep 2007; 30:959–968.
40. Dixon S, Morgan K, Mathers N, et al. Impact of cognitive behavioral therapy on health-related quality of life among adult hypnotic users with chronic insomnia. Behav Sleep Med 2006; 4:71–84.
41. Botteman MF, Ozminkowski RJ, Wang S, et al. Cost effectiveness of long-term treatment with eszopiclone for primary insomnia in adults: a decision analytical model. CNS Drugs 2007; 21(4):319–334.
42. Johnson LJ, Spinweber CL. Good and poor sleepers differ in Navy performance. Mil Med 1983; 148:727–731.
43. Leger D, Guilleminault C, Bader G, et al. Medical and socio-professional impact of insomnia. Sleep 2002; 25:625–629.
44. Leger D, Massuel MA, Metlaine A. Professional correlates of insomnia. Sleep 2006; 29(2):171–178.
45. Philip P, Leger D, Taillard J, et al. Insomniac complaints interfere with quality of life but not with absenteeism: respective role of depressive and organic comorbidity. Sleep Med 2006; 7(7):585–591.
46. Lerner D, Amick BC, Rogers WH, et al. The Work Limitations Questionnaire. Med Care 2001; 39:72–85.
47. Erman M. Ambien cr work performance. In: US Psychiatric and Mental Health Congress; 2008; Orlando.
48. Church MW, Johnson LC. Mood and performance of poor sleepers during repeated use of flurazepam. Psychopharmacology 1979; 61:309–316.
49. Edinger JD, Fins AI, Sullivan RJ, et al. Do our methods lead to insomniacs' madness? Daytime testing after laboratory and home-based polysomnographic studies. Sleep 1997; 20(12):1127–1134.
50. Sugerman JL, Stern JA, Walsh JK. Daytime alertness in subjective and objective insomnia: some preliminary findings. Biol Psychiatry 1985; 20(7):741–750.
51. Stepanski E, Zorick F, Roehrs T, et al. Daytime alertness in patients with chronic insomnia compared with asymptomatic control subjects. Sleep 1988; 11(1):54–60.
52. Nissen C, Kloepfer C, Nofzinger EA, et al. Impaired sleep-related memory consolidation in primary insomnia—a pilot study. Sleep 2006; 29(8):1068–1073.

53. Orff HJ, Drummond SP, Nowakowski S, et al. Discrepancy between subjective symptomatology and objective neuropsychological performance in insomnia. Sleep 2007; 30(9):1205–1211.
54. Raymann RJ, Van Someren EJ. Time-on-task impairment of psychomotor vigilance is affected by mild skin warming and changes with aging and insomnia. Sleep 2007; 30(1):96–103.
55. Varkevisser MG, Kerkhof GA. Chronic insomnia and performance in a 24-h constant routine study. J Sleep Res 2005; 14:49–59.
56. MacMahon K, Broomfield N, Espie C. Attention bias for sleep-related stimuli in primary insomnia and delayed sleep phase syndrome using the dot-probe task. Sleep 2006; 29:1420–1427.
57. Semler C, Harvey A. Daytime functioning in primary insomnia: does attentional focus contribute to real or perceived impairment? Behav Sleep Med 2006; 4:85–103.
58. Cohen J. Statistical power analysis for the behavioral sciences. 2nd ed. Hillsdale: Lawrence Erlbaum Associates, 1988.
59. Avidan AY, Fries BE, James ML, et al. Insomnia and hypnotic use, recorded in the minimum data set, as predictors of falls and hip fractures in Michigan nursing homes. J Am Geriatr Soc 2005; 53(6):955–962.
60. Edinger JD, Means MK, Carney CE, et al. Psychomotor performance deficits and their relation to prior nights' sleep among individuals with primary insomnia. Sleep 2008; 31:599–607.
61. Bonnet MH, Arand DL. The consequences of a week of insomnia. Sleep 1996; 19:453–461.
62. Lichstein KL, Wilson NM, Noe SL, et al. Daytime sleepiness in insomnia: behavioral, biological and subjective indices. Sleep 1994; 17(8):693–702.
63. Stepanski E, Lamphere J, Badia P, et al. Sleep fragmentation and daytime sleepiness. Sleep 1984; 7(1):18–26.
64. Haynes SN, Fitzgerald SG, Shute GE, et al. The utility and validity of daytime naps in the assessment of sleep-onset insomnia. J Behav Med 1985; 8(3):237–247.
65. Bonnet MH, Rosa RR. Predictors of objective sleepiness in insomniacs and normal sleepers. Sleep 2001; 24(suppl):A79–A80.

3 Socioeconomic Impact of Insomnia

Damien Leger

Sleep and Vigilance Center, Hotel Dieu de Paris, Assistance Publique Hopitaux de Paris and University Paris Descartes, Faculty of Medicine, Paris, France

INTRODUCTION

Insomnia is now widely recognized as one of the major complaints associated with numerous psychological and physical diseases in the general population and in primary care patients around the world (1–4). Despite insomnia's high prevalence, it is still frequently unrecognized as a serious health threat by health professionals. One challenge is the fact that insomnia is frequently considered as a symptom, rather than as a true disease, and it is not clear to practitioners whether it is a symptom or a disease. Another challenge is that it is often difficult for patients and for health professionals to understand when insomnia is severe enough to require a treatment. In addition, there is still insufficient knowledge about the management of insomnia. In the last decade, several consensus meetings about insomnia and its recognition, diagnosis, and treatment have published recommendations (5–10). All these consensus groups have underlined the effect of insomnia on public health and the need to better encompass the consequences of insomnia on work, economics, and health-related quality of life (QOL).

The aim of this chapter was to carefully describe the possible links between insomnia and public health concerns and to point out what are the certitudes and the missing data on the consequences of insomnia on work, economics, and health-related QOL.

EPIDEMIOLOGY OF INSOMNIA AND CONSEQUENCES ON ECONOMICS

Insomnia is very prevalent in the general population, and this prevalence contributes to the global economic impact of insomnia. In the last decade, several national and international studies have underscored the universal presence of insomnia.

At the national level, to assess the prevalence of insomnia, Ohayon and Smirne (11) conducted in 2002 a study with a representative sample of the U.K. population composed of 3970 individuals aged 15 years or older. In this study, insomnia symptoms were reported by 27.6% of the sample. Sleep dissatisfaction was found in 10.1% of the sample and insomnia disorder was diagnosed in 7% of the sample. The use of sleep-enhancing medication was reported by 5.7% of the sample. Leger et al. (12) in an epidemiological questionnaire survey of a representative sample of the French population that included 12,778 individuals found a prevalence of insomnia in 19% of the individuals surveyed, with 9% presenting severe insomnia [at least two symptoms of insomnia according to the DSM-IV (*Diagnostic and Statistical Manual of Mental Disorders*, 4th edition) definition]. Kim et al. (13), in a study with a representative sample of the general population of Japan that included 3000 individuals, found a prevalence of insomnia in 21.4% of the individuals. In the United States, the most recent study was conducted in 2004 by the National Sleep Foundation on a representative sample of 1506 subjects older than 18 years. Twenty-one percent of the sample complained of insomnia, according to the ICSD (International Classification of Sleep Disorders) definition, but only 9% had insomnia and daytime consequences (14). A compilation of the recent studies was conducted in 2002 by Ohayon (1), who reported the prevalence of insomnia in one-third of the general population. However, from 16% to 21% of the general population have insomnia only at least three times a week, from 13% to 17% of the general population qualify their trouble as important or major, and from 9% to 13% of the general population have insomnia and its daytime consequences.

International comparisons have also been made using the same protocol. They demonstrated the universality of the insomnia complaint: Ohayon (15), in a survey of 25,580 individuals from seven European countries, observed that the prevalence of nonrestorative sleep seems to follow a north-south line, with the United Kingdom having the highest prevalence and Spain the lowest. He identified factors such as sleeping habits, climate, and cultural impact on responses to questionnaires to explain these differences (14). Soldatos et al. (2), in a survey that included 35,327 questionnaires and subjects from 10 countries, found that 31.6% of subjects had "insomnia" while another 17.5% could be considered as having "subthreshold insomnia." More recently, Leger et al. (3) in a survey comparing sleep disorders among representative samples of 3962 North Americans, 5005 Europeans, and 1165 Japanese found that insomnia was significantly higher in the United States (39%) than in Europe (28%) and Japan (21%).

SOCIODEMOGRAPHICS FACTORS CONTRIBUTING TO INSOMNIA

Almost all studies show an increasing prevalence of insomnia with age and a sex ratio in favor of women (1–7). In a 12,778 sample, Leger et al. (12) found that severe insomnia was almost twice as high for women as for men (12% vs. 6.3%; $p < 0.0001$). Older subjects have usually more severe complaints than do younger subjects. In a representative sample ($n = 5622$) of the general population of France aged 15 or older, Ohayon and Lemoine (16) found that the prevalence of insomnia was more frequent (twice) in subjects 65 years of age or older compared with subjects younger than 45 years. Moreover, in this last study, 47.1% of subjects older than 65 years reported three symptoms of insomnia compared with 32.2% of subjects younger than 44 years ($p < 0.001$). However, younger subjects (under 45 years) and females had significantly more daytime consequences of insomnia than did older subjects and males.

There are few studies which support the link between perceived job stress and the prevalence of insomnia. Nakata et al. (17) surveyed 1161 male white-collar employees of a Japanese electric equipment company by a mailed questionnaire. This study found an overall prevalence rate of 23.6% for insomnia. Workers with high intragroup conflict [odds ratio (OR): 1.6] and high job dissatisfaction (OR: 1.5) had a significantly increased risk of insomnia after adjusting for multiple confounding factors. Low employment opportunities, physical environment, and low coworker support were also found to be weakly associated with a risk of insomnia among workers.

The prevalence of insomnia is also generally higher in persons of low socioeconomic status (17). In the French population, the prevalence of insomnia has been found to be the highest in the white-collar group (20, 8%) (12). A trend toward lower rates of insomnia in upper level executives, in liberal professions, and in the farmers group was also found. In a cross-sectional study including 4868 daytime white-collar workers, Doi et al. (18) similarly showed that poor sleep was significantly more prevalent in white-collar workers (30–45%) than in the Japanese general working population. Recently, Gellis et al. (19) investigated the likelihood of insomnia and insomnia-related health consequences among a sample of at least 50 men and 50 women in each age decade from 20 to 80+ years old and of different socioeconomic status. Results indicated that individuals of lower individual and household education were significantly more likely to experience insomnia, even after researchers accounted for ethnicity, gender, and age. In addition, individuals with fewer years of education, particularly those who had dropped out of high school, experienced greater subjective impairment because of their insomnia.

SEEKING HELP FOR INSOMNIA AND ACCESS TO TREATMENTS

Insomniacs, even severe insomniacs, often do not seek treatment. Years ago, a Gallup study found that only 5% of insomniacs had ever visited a physician to discuss specifically their sleeping problem and that only 21% had ever taken a prescription medication for sleep (20). In France, 53% of severe insomniacs versus 27% of subjects with occasional sleep problems reported that they had ever visited a doctor specifically for insomnia ($p < 10^{-4}$) (21). Many individuals with sleep dissatisfaction just watch television, read, use nonprescription medication, or drink alcohol to promote sleep (1). In a survey in the Detroit area of a representative sample of 2181 adults aged between 18 and 45, Johnson et al. (22) found that 13.3% of the sample had used alcohol as a sleep aid in the past year and 10.1% of the sample an over-the-counter prescription. Fifteen percent of those who used alcohol as a sleep aid did it for at least one month; however, the duration of use was short for the majority of users (<1 week). Only 5.3% of the sample used a prescription medication. However, it was found that 10.8% of French adults regularly used prescription medication to promote sleep (20). Recently, a consecutive sample ($n = 700$) of U.S. adults attending a nonurgent primary care appointment was screened for sleep problems. A follow-up mailed survey then assessed insomnia symptoms, daytime impairment, beliefs about sleep, medication use, sleepiness and fatigue, and medical help-seeking (23). Aikens and Rouse conversely found that a high percentage (52%) of patients with probable insomnia reported discussing this with a physician. Multivariate logistic regression analyses indicated that discussing one's probable insomnia with a physician was independently associated with having a greater number of medical conditions [OR: 2.19 (95% CI: 1.13–4.22)], being more highly educated [OR: 1.67 (95% CI: 1.11–2.51)], sleeping less per night [OR: 0.71 (95% CI: 0.52–0.96)], and greater perceived daytime impairment due to insomnia [OR: 2.07 (95% CI: 1.06–4.03)]. Pires et al. (24) compared two studies carried out in Brazil in 1987 and 1995. They showed that only 12.5% of the Brazilian insomniacs had sought medical help for their sleep problems or had informed their physician of sleep problems during evaluation of other problems in 1987; this was even less (10.8%) in 1995. In a study carried out in the United States at five managed care organizations, Hatoum et al. (25) found that only 0.9% of American patients were seeing physicians due to sleep problems. Of these, only 11.6% were taking prescription medications specifically for sleep problems and 21.4% were taking over-the-counter medications for sleep. Moreover, the diagnosis of insomnia is not always followed by treatment. In Germany, a Nationwide Insomnia Screening and Awareness Study (NISAS-2000) found that close to 50% of all patients with insomnia did not receive a prescription for a specific insomnia therapy (26).

COMORBIDTY WITH DEPRESSION AND ANXIETY: RESPECTIVE IMPACT ON ECONOMICS

Insomnia is associated with various medical and psychiatric conditions. It is easier to understand how insomnia might result from a medical problem than to understand how insomnia is a cause or a consequence of psychiatric diseases. Comorbidities with depression and anxiety are estimated to occur in 35% to 60% of chronic insomniacs (1,7,11,21,27,28). Several longitudinal studies have shown that insomnia may represent a substantial and statistical risk for the development of depressive disorders (1,27). However, there is actually increasing evidence that the coexistence of these two diseases reflects a common pathology rather than two separate diseases. However, in order to clarify public health consequences due to insomnia, independent of psychiatric disorders, it seems important to clearly identify insomniacs with psychiatric diseases in the design of the studies. Depression and anxiety have indeed a well-documented impact on economics and QOL (29–31).

INSOMNIA AT THE WORKPLACE

As previously stated, insomnia is very prevalent in adults and is therefore also frequently found in professionals. There are very few studies that are specifically devoted to insomnia at the workplace. However, it is commonly reported that insomnia affects daytime functioning and working ability in professionals (32). Riedel and Lichstein (33) have, for example, recommended using objective measures of work performance (absenteeism, promotion, etc.) to clarify the impact of insomnia on daytime functioning. Insomnia is not a visible handicap in the workplace, and it is difficult for insomniacs to explain to their colleagues and managers that they have had a poor night and that they need to rest. Insomniacs have to face a regular work load, and they often complain of difficulties in their professional life (35,36). However, there are few data assessing the true impact of insomnia on daily work. It is essential that the impact of insomnia on absenteeism and other work measures be evaluated in a real-world setting.

Absenteeism

In economic and epidemiological studies, overall measures of the respondent's health appeared to be the most important covariate of absenteeism (36,37). In a large, cross- sectional, national probability sample of 1308 workers in the United States, Leigh (37) demonstrated that complaining of insomnia was the most predictable factor of absenteeism from among 36 variables. In a study comparing 80 insomniacs at work to 135 good sleepers, it was found that insomniacs had double the control rate of absenteeism (21). Lavie (38) also found a higher rate of absenteeism in insomniacs, which is significantly linked to a higher rate of work accidents in insomniacs. He hypothesized that coworkers of the absentee insomniacs are more exposed to accidents because of their work overload.

However, these preliminary studies were based on general population samples: insomnia was not always clearly defined and the groups of insomniacs were heterogeneous. Moreover, the absenteeism data were mainly based on the patients' declaration and not on objective data.

In a recent study (39), we specifically surveyed the absenteeism of a group of insomniacs at work compared to a matched group of good sleepers. Insomniacs showed almost twice as much absenteeism as good sleepers. The difference between insomniacs and good sleepers was particularly high for managers (OR = 2.29) and women (OR = 2.31). We believe that this study is of particular interest because (*i*) we processed objective (rather than subjective) data on absenteeism, (*ii*) insomnia was defined according to international classifications, (*iii*) subjects with depression and anxiety were excluded, (*iv*) subjects were all full-time workers and representative of the active population in the area, and (*v*) subjects with chronic disease (which may interfere with sleep) and pregnant women were excluded from the study. Hence, in the group studied here, it seems more probable that significant differences between insomniacs and good sleepers reflect the impact of insomnia itself, rather than the effects of comorbidities. In another study also assessing long-term absenteeism (including absence more than six months) and comparing insomniac subjects ($n = 986$) with control subjects ($n = 584$), subjects with insomnia complaints (with or without mood or behavioral/physiologic sleep complaints) reported poorer QOL and had a higher absenteeism rate than did controls (9.6 ± 31 vs. 5.8 ± 19 days; $p < 0.01$). Logistic regression analysis of insomniacs with depressive complaints indicated that absenteeism was more significantly associated with depression than insomnia itself (40).

Other Occupational Characteristics

The earliest study of this issue was conducted by Johnson et al. (41), who demonstrated that, in a population of U.S. Navy workers, insomniacs performed more slowly and had poorer career advancement than good sleepers. The difficulty of comparing the respective work loads of insomniacs and good sleepers is a major concern in the discussion of these results. Insomniacs' impairment at the workplace has been assessed by very few authors. Lavie, in a large and detailed study of the lifestyle, health, sleep, and work habits of 1502 employees, concluded that sleep habits directly affect the workplace. They showed that workers with daytime fatigue had significantly more complaints of somnolence during work breaks (14.2% vs. 3.5%; $p < 0.001$), higher frequency of napping at work (16.8% vs. 1.4%; $p < 0.0001$), and significantly less job satisfaction (38) than other workers. However, this study was not directly focused on insomnia but on sleep disorders. In a study comparing 240 severe insomniacs (SI) with 391 good sleepers (GS), Leger et al. explored the consequences of insomnia on work (21). Fifteen percent of SI versus 6% of GS ($p < 0.001$) reported having made errors at work over the past month, which could have resulted in serious consequences. For 6% of SI versus 2% of GS, errors had occurred more than once during the past month ($p = 0.0032$). Twelve percent of insomniacs versus 6% of GS reported being late to work during the past month ($p =$ NS). Moreover, 18% of SI versus 8% of GS ($p = 0.0004$) felt that they had exhibited poor efficiency at work. Thirteen percent of SI versus 9% of GS reported difficulties completing complicated tasks at work ($p =$ NS). In a recent work, Daley et al. questioned 930 adults from the province of Quebec about sleep and professional consequences. Reduced productivity was assessed by using the visual analogue scale (VAS). Thirty-five percent of insomniacs versus 9.8% of the GS group reported reduced productivity (42). These preliminary findings must be confirmed by more thorough and well-designed studies which investigate insomniacs and GS working in the same field.

Accidents

The impact of sleep disorders on automobile accidents is a crucial issue from a public health point of view. Public authorities and the media are well-informed on the risk of sleepiness at the wheel during the night and on the effects of sleep debt and sleep pathologies (sleep apnea, hypersomnia) on accidents. However, there are very few data on the risk of accidents due to insomnia by itself.

Insomnia may impact the risk of accident in different ways: sleep deprivation, lack of attention, and side effects of hypnotics. Motor vehicle accidents (MVA) and work accidents (WA) have been the primary areas of investigation.

In the French study comparing 240 SI with 391 GS (21), WA were found to occur eight times more commonly over the past 12 months in SI (8%) than in GS (1%) ($p = 0.0150$), with an average number of 0.07 (±0.25) accidents per SI versus 0.01 ± 0.11 per GS ($p = 0.0550$). There was, however, no statistical difference for MVA over the past 12 months between the groups (9% vs. 10%). The authors explained the discrepancy between WA and MVA by the fact that SI may have avoided driving or driven shorter distance: 65.8% of SI versus 72.5% of GS drove a car ($p = 0.012$). Lavie also showed a higher rate of WA in insomniacs (in their lifetime) than in GS (52.1% vs. 35.6%; $p < 0.01$) (38). The rate of MVA due to fatigue (5% vs. 2%; $p =$ NS) was found to be slightly, but not significantly, increased in insomniacs.

Similarly, Daley et al., in a group of 930 adults in Quebec, did not find a different rate of MVA in the last six months between insomniacs and GS. However, 23.5% of drivers reporting an accident felt that insomnia played an important role in this event (42). Moreover, 39.5% of participants described a link between their sleep difficulties and other types of accidents ($p < 0.001$).

In Japan, in a study collecting data on occupational injuries in 1298 workers of small-scale manufacturing firms, Nakata et al. (43) found that insomnia symptoms were significantly associated with occupational injuries in both genders [OR = 1.64 (95%CI: 1.23–2.18)].

Regarding the effects of treatments on driving ability, it is usually generally held that long-term half-life hypnotics (medium to long-term benzodiazepines and antihistamines) may induce a risk of accidents, while driving, in the morning and a risk of falls in the night in older adults. In Europe, the vast majority of hypnotics are labeled with a sign indicating the possible risk of accidents due to the treatment. There are, however, very few published studies on the effects of common hypnotics on driving ability. Partinen et al. (44) recently performed a double-blind, randomized, placebo-controlled, three-treatment three-period crossover study investigating the effects of zolpidem (10 mg) and temazepam 20 mg versus placebo in 18 insomniacs in a real-life condition on driving performance. After polysomnography at baseline and each treatment night, patients underwent, a STISIM driving simulator test at 7:30 a.m., 5.5 hours after drug intake. There were no differences between treatments for the primary outcome measure (mean time to collision; baseline: 0.120 s, P: 0.124, T: 0.118, Z: 0.124; $p \geq 0.12$ for all pairwise comparisons). No differences were recorded for speed deviation and reaction time to tasks for the verum treatments; however, lane position deviation was greater after administration of zolpidem in comparison with both placebo and temazepam ($p = 0.025$ and 0.05, respectively). They underlined the necessity to strongly advocate against the late intake of hypnotics if patients intend to drive a car early the next morning. Using a mathematical model, Menzin et al. calculated the potential effects of sleep medications on MVA and costs, and applied the model to the French setting. They used the model of standard deviation of a vehicle's lateral position (SDLP) and hypothesized that compared with zaleplon, the use of zopiclone over 14 days would be expected to result in 503 excess accidents per 100,000 drivers (45).

COMORBIDITIES AND HEALTH CARE USE

Several studies have looked at the links between insomnia and general health status. Although insomnia appears to be associated with poorer health status, it is difficult to know whether insomnia is the result or cause of the poorer health status. Comorbid insomnia, which includes not only psychological but also physical diseases, accounts for at least 50% of chronic insomnia. It is likely that the high prevalence of comorbidity contributes to increased utilization of medical services, including visits to doctors and other health professionals, intake of medications, and the number and duration of hospitalizations.

Wereyer and Dilling (46) found a significantly higher average annual consultation rate among mild and moderate SI than among those without sleep disorders (10.61 and 12.87 consultations per year, respectively, vs. 5.25 per year for GS). They also reported a hospitalization rate of 21.9% (SI) versus 12.2% (GS). Lavie (38) also found a higher rate of hospitalizations for insomniacs, as did Kales et al. (47), who found an annual hospitalization rate of 15.7%. In the study by Leger et al. (21), 18% of SI and 9% of GS had been hospitalized during the past 12 months ($p = 0.0017$), with an average of 0.17 (±0.40) hospitalizations for SI versus 0.11 (±0.45) hospitalizations for GS ($p =$ NS). The average duration of stay in hospital was 1.19 (± 3.45) days for SI versus 0.76 (±3.83) days for GS ($p =$ NS). Fifty-nine percent of SI and 49% of GS had undergone a medical evaluation in the past six months ($p = 0.0138$), with an average of 2 (±3.0) evaluations for SI versus 1.2 (±2.2) evaluations for GS ($p = 0.0198$). SI had had more blood studies (48% vs. 34%; $p = 0.0005$) and radiological procedures (17% vs. 10%; $p = 0.0142$) than GS. SI also had more outpatient visits and used more medications (particularly cardiovascular, central nervous system, genitourinary, and gastrointestinal) than GS. However, there was no difference in the use of analgesic medications, despite the fact that 46% of insomniacs versus 29% of GS ($p < 0.001$) said that they were particularly sensitive to pain. This is an important point, as pain may be an obvious cause of sleep disturbance. Katz and McHorney (48) have reported that poor mental and physical health were far more prevalent among insomniacs than among controls. Recently, Katz and McHorney (49) calculated the odds ratio between chronic diseases and complaints of insomnia. Severe insomnia was strongly linked to current depression (OR = 8.2), as well as to congestive heart failure (OR = 2.5), obstructive airway disease (OR = +1.6), and prostrate problems (OR = 1.6). Darko et al. (58) showed in a prospective study that fatigue and sleep disturbance were frequent symptoms of advanced HIV infection and emphasized the significance of these complaints in assessment of patients' clinical status.

Finally, the fact that insomnia can be a risk factor for psychiatric diseases and alcoholism (3–7,33) was also firmly demonstrated by Katz and McHorney (49). These findings have two implications. First, insomnia seems to be associated with poorer health status; indeed, insomniacs should be routinely evaluated for psychiatric and somatic disorders. Second, although we cannot conclude whether insomnia is the cause of or the result of worsened health status, insomniacs are clearly at increased risk for certain diseases and a higher use of medical services. Many of the findings reported to be consequences of insomnia are actually correlates. Until a cause–effect relationship is established, correlate or comorbidity may be a more accurate term to describe the relationship between insomnia and poor medical status. Finally, taking care of insomnia may significantly reduce the severity of comorbidities as Dirksen and Epstein (50) demonstrated: Women receiving cognitive-behavioral therapy for insomnia had significant improvements in fatigue, trait anxiety, depression, and QOL.

COSTS OF INSOMNIA

At this time, there are very little published studies to address the economic consequences of insomnia. The National Commission of Sleep Disorders Research (NCSDR) in the United States estimated the direct cost of insomnia in 1990 to be $15.4 billion, extrapolating from available data (51). However, in the judgment of the Commission, "the absence of hard epidemiological data makes it impossible to calculate the precise cost of sleep disorders, but some data do exist to show that the costs are substantial." In 1988 Leger (52) examined, the cost of accidents related to sleep disorders in the United States for the NCSDR and estimated its cost between $43.15 billion and $56.02 billion. Stoller (53) made an estimate of the total cost of insomnia in the United States in 1988, based on a literature review on the economic costs and effects associated with insomnia. Her cost estimate ranged from $92.5 billion to $107.5 billion (53). All consensus reports agree on the lack of socioeconomic data to better understand the burden of insomnia on society. One difficulty is the paucity of information about insomnia-related use of health care services. Another is the degree of overlap between insomnia and many somatic and psychiatric diseases. The following sections summarize the work that has been accomplished in the field and define what could be undertaken to better understand the economic consequences of insomnia.

The economic impact of insomnia can be divided into direct costs, indirect costs, and related costs. Direct costs of insomnia are charges for medical care or self–treatment that are borne by patients, government, organized health care providers, or insurance companies. Indirect costs refer to patient– and employer–borne costs that result from insomnia–related morbidity and mortality. Related costs are other costs that can be rationally associated with the illness, such as the cost of property damage resulting from accidents associated with insomnia.

Direct Costs of Insomnia

Direct costs of insomnia include those incurred for outpatient visits, sleep recordings, and medications directly devoted to insomnia. There is very little knowledge about this kind of cost. In 1999, Walsh and Engelhardt (54) estimated (using 1995 dollars) direct costs of insomnia to be $13.93 billion, which consisted of health care services ($11.96 billion), including nursing home care ($10.9 billion), and medications/substances used for treatment ($1.97 billion). Leger et al. (55) also made an estimate of the direct costs of insomnia in France in 1995 (based on 1995 dollars values). They gave a $2.067 billion value divided mainly into $1.75 billion for outpatient visits and $310,59 million for substances used for insomnia. It was of particular interest to observe the very limited costs of sleep centers in this estimate, $1.75 million. In both estimates, the cost of prescriptions was very little compared with other costs. However, the direct costs related to sleep disorders evaluation by practitioners seem to be a small part of the total cost of insomnia. Recently, an update of the direct and indirect costs of untreated insomnia in adults was made in the United States (56). With the help of a self-insurer, employer-sponsored plan, the authors compared direct costs of insomnia (including inpatient, outpatient, pharmacy, and emergency department costs for all diseases) for six months before the diagnosis of insomnia or the first prescription of hypnotics was made. They compared 138,820 younger adults and 75,558 older adults with insomnia to control groups. After logistic regression they found $924 greater direct costs per six months for insomniacs versus controls and $1143 greater estimated direct costs in older adult insomniacs.

INDIRECT COSTS OF INSOMNIA

The indirect costs of insomnia are the costs associated with the potential consequences of insomnia on society, such as health problems, professional consequences (loss of productivity and absenteeism), and accidents. The only estimate of the cost of accidents related to sleep disorders ($46–$52 billion in 1988) was more focused on sleepiness at the wheel than on insomnia (52). We previously reported that Johnson et al. demonstrated that insomniacs from a sample of U.S. Navy men were slower at work and had poorer career advancement than did good sleepers (41). On the basis of this last study, Stoller (53) estimated the loss of productivity due to insomnia in the United States to be $41.1 billion in 1988 (53). The cost of absenteeism was evaluated among nonmanagerial personnel and was estimated to be approximately $143 per day, or more than $57 billion per year. We recently conducted a study on the indirect costs of absenteeism due to insomnia in a sample of 369 employees of the Ile de France area with insomnia and 369 good sleeper professionals (57) The costs of absenteeism at work associated with insomnia were estimated by comparing the two matched groups in terms of the number and duration of work absences. We considered that work absences incurred costs relating to salary replacement and loss of productivity: these were given a monetary value on the basis of the added value per hour worked. The percentage of employees with at least one work absence was 50% and 34% for insomniacs and GS, respectively. The work absenteeism [expressed in days, per employee, per year ± confidence intervals (CI)] differed significantly between insomniacs and GS: 5.8 (±1.1) and 2.4 (±0.5), respectively ($p < 0.001$). The extra cost (±CI) to the national health insurance system of insomnia-associated absenteeism was estimated at €77 (±€39) per employee per year. The extra cost (±CI) to employers was estimated at €233 (±€101) for salary replacement and €1062 (±€386) for loss of productivity. Finally, employees themselves bore a cost (+CI) of €100 (€54). Ozminkowski et al. (56) also assessed the indirect costs of insomnia in their impressive survey of 138,820 younger adults. Indirect costs included costs related to absenteeism from work and the use of short-term disability programs. They found an average additional cost of absenteeism over a 6-month period of $405 in patients eventually diagnosed with or treated for insomnia (on a six-month period). The total short-term disability expenditures were, however, $86 lower in insomniacs than in the control group.

Discussion About the Costs of Insomnia

Despite these several evaluations on the topic, the total costs of insomnia remain largely unknown, and it is actually difficult to have a general view on the impact of insomnia on economics. The studies on direct costs have been carried out only in two countries (54–57), and it is difficult to apply these results to other parts of the world. The studies on indirect costs are based on hypotheses that have limited empirical support and must be confirmed by larger studies in more representative samples. The same degree of insomnia may not necessarily have the same impact in different countries and there is a need for cross-cultural studies to better understand the daily economic impact of diseases in insomniacs around the world. Future studies might try to adopt economical values such as the national gross product for a better and more comprehensive implication of the results at each country level.

QUALITY OF LIFE

There were very few studies specifically designed to assess the impact of insomnia on QOL. Most of these were devoted to the impact of sleep disorders on the QOL of patients suffering from cancer. Some of the QOL studies have also been performed to explore the relationship of poor sleep with diabetes, depression, Parkinson disease, chronic renal diseases with hemodialysis, and HIV or chronic psychiatric diseases. QOL is also sometimes used to evaluate pharmacological and nonpharmacological treatments of insomnia.

The Impact of Insomnia on QOL

The World Health Consensus report on sleep and health strongly recommends more studies on the QOL of insomniacs (6). Surprisingly, until recently, there were relatively few works specifically devoted to the subject (58–62). Four of them used the SF-36 [Short Form (36) Health Survey] (58,59,61,62), a very widely used scale in QOL (63).

Zammitt et al. (62) used several instruments to evaluate the impact of insomnia on QOL in a sample of 261 insomniacs compared to a control group of 101 GS. Insomniacs were recruited by advertisements and had to fulfill the DSM criteria for insomnia. Individuals with criteria of irregular sleep patterns, sleep apnea, restless leg syndrome, periodic limb movement disorders, history of psychiatric illness, alcohol or substance abuse, epilepsy, and HIV-positive infection were excluded from the study. They used the SF-36 and the QOL inventory, a 31-item questionnaire specifically designed for the study which includes items related to sleep, cognitive function, daytime performance, social and family relationships, and health. The authors showed a significant difference between the two groups ($p < 0.0001$; MANOVA) on all eight SF-36 subscales. Insomniacs reported more health concerns that limit physical activity, greater interference of physical or emotional problems with normal social activities, more bodily pain, poorer general health, less vitality, more emotional difficulties, and more mental health problems than did the GS group. Using the QOL inventory, they also found a significant impact on the QOL of insomniacs. The authors suggested that the SF-36 can be used to assess differences between subjects with insomnia and healthy controls and that the SF-36 may have clinical utility as a measure of impairment associated with insomnia.

Leger et al. (64) also used the SF-36 to evaluate the QOL of three matched groups of 240 SI, 422 mild insomniacs, and 391 GS selected from the general population. They eliminated those meeting DSM-IV criteria for anxiety and depression from the original group. They found that SI had lower scores in eight dimensions of the SF-36 than did mild insomniacs and GS. Mild insomniacs also had lower scores in the same eight dimensions than GS. No dimension was more altered than the other. However, the mental health status and the emotional state were worse in severe and mild insomniacs than in GS. This result demonstrates a clear interrelationship between insomnia and emotional state, despite the fact that we had eliminated the subjects with DSM-IV criteria of anxiety. The authors concluded that SF-36 was sensitive to the severity of insomnia and seemed to be a reliable instrument to assess the impact of insomnia on QOL.

In a telephone interview study conducted as part of a five-year follow-up examination of the Epidemiology of Hearing Loss Study, Schubert et al. (65) found the same kind of relationship between the severity of insomnia and the decreased QOL in a group of 2800 older adults (aged from 53 to 97 years). Participants were asked about symptoms of poor sleep. A response of "often" or "almost always" was coded as positive for an insomnia trait. The SF-36 was administrated to assess QOL of these subjects. Twenty-six percent of the population reported one insomnia trait, 13% reported two, and 10% reported three. The eight domains of the SF-36 were found to be significantly decreased as the number of insomnia traits increased. The authors concluded that insomnia is common among older adults and is associated with a decreased QOL.

Idzikowski (58) discussed the concept of QOL applied to sleep and introduced the fact that short sleep is not necessarily deleterious but that abnormally shortened or fragmented sleep can reduce an individual's QOL. Smith and Shneerson (61) used the SF-36 in a sample of

223 subjects explored for snoring or daytime somnolence. They showed that the SF-36 score is sensitive to sleep disruption.

Finally, Katz and McHorney (49) demonstrated that insomnia acts by itself on the QOL of patients suffering from chronic illness. Insomnia was found to be severe in 16% and mild in 34% of these patients. Differences between patients with mild insomnia versus no insomnia showed small-to-medium decrements across SF-36 subscales ranging from 4.1 to 9.3 points (on a scale of 100) and for severe insomnia from 12.0 to 23.9 points. Insomnia appeared in this study as an independent factor of a worsened QOL to almost the same extent as chronic conditions such as congestive heart failure and clinical depression.

Sleep in Comorbid Insomnia and QOL

In patients suffering from cancer, the quality of sleep has been recognized as a powerful factor acting on the QOL (66). In a sample of 263 cancer patients undergoing chemotherapy, the authors found that insomnia was negatively correlated to the QOL, probably by the way of depression. Insomnia explained only 4% of the variance of QOL and depression 47%. Stark et al. (67) also reported in 178 cancer subjects that insomnia was significantly and independently associated with a deficit of QOL. They recommended that subjects with cancer be interviewed about sleep to better discriminate subjects with anxiety. Lindley et al. (68) considered insomnia as a good reflection of QOL in women following adjuvant therapy for early stage breast cancer. Treating insomnia by cognitive-behavioral therapy in 72 women with breast cancer also statistically significantly increased QOL, with a trend suggestive of lower depression at posttreatment (50).

In other chronic illness, several studies have shown that insomnia influences the QOL of patients with Parkinson disease (69), hemodialysis patients (70), or patients with anxiety and depression (71). In HIV infection, Nokes and Kendrew (72) also found that there was a correlation between sleep quality (assessed by the Pittsburgh Sleep Quality Index) and positive general well-being.

QOL in the Treatment of Insomnia

Goldenberg et al. (73) and Leger et al. (60) have shown that the QOL of insomniacs, as assessed by questionnaires on professional, relational, sentimental, domestic, leisure, and safety aspects, does not differ significantly from that of good sleepers. Walsh et al. (74) also reported an improvement in the physical functioning, vitality, and social functioning dimensions of the SF-36 of patients treated with eszopiclone versus placebo for the month one to six average ($p < 0.005$). Baca et al. (75) also showed that zolpidem improved patients' QOL assessed by a questionnaire including four factors: social support, general satisfaction, physical and psychological well-being, and the absence of work overload/free time. However, to our knowledge, there is no extensive survey comparing the effects of several hypnotics with well-validated QOL instruments. Regarding nonpharmacological therapies, Quesnel et al. (76) showed the efficacy of cognitive-behavioral therapy in insomnia in 10 women treated for nonmetastatic breast cancer. They found an improvement in sleep assessed by polysomnography and in the global and cognitive subscales of the QLQ-C30. In a study comparing data from different studies using cognitive-behavioral therapy on QOL, Dixon et al. (77) stated that after cognitive-behavioral therapy intervention, statistically significant differences in SF-36 scores in favor of the intervention were present for physical functioning, emotional role limitation, and mental health over six months.

Insomnia affects the daily lives of patients. However, it is often difficult to evaluate the impact of insomnia and the effect of treatments on patients' everyday lives. QOL seems to be a good way to better understand the complaints of insomniacs regarding their day-to-day functioning. Several studies have shown the sensitivity of the SF-36 in evaluating the impact of insomnia by itself or in relationship with other associated chronic diseases. We also recommend the development of more accurate QOL tools specifically designed for insomnia.

HD-16: A Specifically Designed QOL Scale for Insomniacs

In many other chronic diseases, it has been shown that a disease-focused QOL instrument was useful to accurately evaluate its impact on the daily lives of patients and to show the efficacy of some treatments. In the field of insomnia, there is a need for specific instruments to better encompass the QOL of patients. This is why HD-16, a QOL scale specifically designed for insomniacs, has been proposed (78). On the basis of interviews with SI patients, a 43-item questionnaire on QOL has been built and tested on three groups composed of 240 SI, 422 mild insomniacs, and 391 GS. Ten steps led to the construction of a specific QOL scale. Five dimensions have been validated as both relevant and independent from each other: physical role, psychological role, social relationships with the others, cognitive (concentration, attention, memorization), and energy. Sixteen items out the 43 initially tested were retained and were found to be significantly different within the groups in each dimension. On the basis of these 16 items selected, we called the scale Hotel Dieu-16 (HD-16). The score's specificity (correlation score: 0.36) and reliability (Cronbach coefficient alpha: 0.78) were verified.

CONCLUSION

Insomnia affects the daily lives of millions of people around the world. The economic impact of insomnia on society seems enormous. There is also increasing evidence linking insomnia to several severe public health concerns: obesity, diabetes, depression, and cardiovascular diseases. Besides the patients themselves, their family and work relatives are also affected by the consequences of poor sleep. Public authorities are becoming increasingly focused on sleep education and the protection of sleepers' environment against noise. However, much work has to be done to convince them that having good nights of sleep may deeply benefit individuals as well as society.

REFERENCES

1. Ohayon MM. Epidemiology of insomnia: what we know and what we still need to learn. Sleep Med Rev 2002; 6:97–111.
2. Soldatos CR, Allaert FA, Ohta T, et al. How do individuals sleep around the world? Results from a single-day survey in ten countries. Sleep Med 2005; 6:5–13.
3. Leger D, Poursain B, Neubauer D, et al. An international survey of sleeping problems in the general population. Curr Med Res Opin 2008; 24:307–317.
4. Alattar M, Harrington JJ, Mitchell CM, et al. Sleep problems in primary care: a North Carolina Family Practice Research Network (NC-FP-RN) study. J Am Board Fam Med 2007; 20:365–374.
5. Roth T, Hajak G, Ustun TB. Consensus for the pharmacological management of insomnia in the new millennium. Int J Clin Pract 2001; 55:42–52.
6. World Health Organization. Insomnia: an international consensus conference report. Versailles, October 13–15, 1996. WHO Publications MSA/MDN/98.2, 1998:55.
7. Buysse DJ. Diagnosis and assessment of sleep and circadian rhythm disorders. J Psychiatr Pract 2005; 11:102–115.
8. Kupfer DJ, Reynolds CF. Management of insomnia. N Eng J Med 1997; 336:341–346.
9. Schenck CH, Mahowald MW, Sack RL. Assessment and management of insomnia. JAMA 2003; 19: 2475.
10. Edinger JD, Bonnet MH, Bootzin RR, et al. Derivation of research diagnostic criteria for insomnia: report of an American Academy of Sleep Medicine Work Group. Sleep 2004; 27:1567–1596.
11. Ohayon MM, Smirne S. Prevalence and consequences of insomnia disorders in the general population of Italy. Sleep Med 2002; 3:115–120.
12. Leger D, Guilleminault C, Dreyfus JP, et al. Prevalence of insomnia in a survey of 12,778 adults in France. J Sleep Res 2000; 9:35–42.
13. Kim K, Uchiyama M, Okawa M, et al. An epidemiological study of insomnia among the Japanese general population. Sleep 2000; 23:41–47.
14. National Sleep Foundation (NSF). Sleep in America 2004. Gallup Organization. www.sleepfoundation.org
15. Ohayon MM. Prevalence and correlates of nonrestorative sleep complaints. Arch Intern Med 2005; 165:35–41.
16. Ohayon MM, Lemoine P. Daytime consequences of insomnia complaints in the French general population. Encephale 2004; 30:222–227.
17. Nakata A, Haratani T, Takahashi M, et al. Job stress, social support, and prevalence of insomnia in a population of Japanese daytime workers. Soc Sci Med 2004; 59:1719–1730.
18. Doi Y, Minowa M, Tango T. Impact and correlates of poor sleep quality in Japanese white-collar employees. Sleep 2003; 26:467–471.

19. Gellis LA, Lichstein KL, Scarinci IC, et al. Socioeconomic status and insomnia. J Abnorm Psychol 2005; 114:111–118.
20. National Sleep Foundation (NSF). Sleep in America. Princeton, NJ: Gallup Organization, 1991.
21. Leger D, Guilleminault C, Bader G, et al. Medical and socio-professional impact of insomnia. Sleep 2002; 25:625–629.
22. Johnson EO, Roehrs T, Roth T, et al. Epidemiology of alcohol and medication as aid sleep in early adulthood. Sleep 1998; 21:178–186.
23. Aikens JE, Rouse ME. Help-seeking for insomnia among adult patients in primary care. J Am Board Fam Pract 2005; 18:257–261.
24. Pires ML, Benedito-Silva AA, Mello MT, et al. Sleep habits and complaints of adults in the city of São Paulo, Brazil, in 1987 and 1995. Braz J Med Biol Res 2007; 40:1505–1515.
25. Hatoum HT, Kania CM, Kong SX, et al. Prevalence of insomnia: a survey of the enrollees at five managed care organizations. Am J Manag Care 1998; 4:79–86.
26. Wittchen HU, Krause P, Hofler M, et al. NISAS-2000: the "Nationwide Insomnia Screening and Awareness Study". Prevalence and interventions in primary care. Fortschr Med Orig 2001; 119:9–19.
27. Buysse DJ, Angst J, Gamma A, et al. Prevalence, course, and comorbidity of insomnia and depression in young adults. Sleep 2008; 31:473–480.
28. Roth T, Jaeger S, Jin R, et al. Sleep problems, comorbid mental disorders, and role functioning in the national comorbidity survey replication. Biol Psychiatry 2006; 60:1364–1371.
29. Gjesdal S, Ringdal PR, Haug K, et al. Long-term sickness absence and disability pension with psychiatric diagnoses: a population-based cohort study. Nord J Psychiatry 2008; 14:1–8.
30. Kessler RC, Heeringa S, Lakoma MD, et al. Individual and societal effects of mental disorders on earnings in the United States: results from the national comorbidity survey replication. Am J Psychiatry 2008; 165:703–711.
31. Wang PS, Aguilar-Gaxiola S, Alonso J, et al. Use of mental health services for anxiety, mood, and substance disorders in 17 countries in the WHO world mental health surveys. Lancet 2007; 370:841–850.
32. Stepanski E, Zorick F, Roehrs T, et al. Daytime alertness in patients with chronic insomnia compared with asymptomatic control subjects. Sleep 1988; 11:54–60.
33. Riedel BW, Lichstein KL. Insomnia and daytime functioning. Sleep Med Rev 2000; 4:277–298.
34. Schneider-Helmert D. Twenty four hour sleep/wake function and personality patterns in chronic insomniacs and healthy controls. Sleep 1987; 11:54–60.
35. Manocchia M, Keller S, Ware JE. Sleep problems, health-related quality of life, work functioning and health care utilization among the chronically ill. Qual Life Res 2001; 10:331–345.
36. Lerner D, Henke RM. What does research tell us about depression, job performance, and work productivity? J Occup Environ Med 2008; 50:401–410.
37. Leigh P. Employee and job attributes and predictors of absenteeism in a national sample of workers: the importance of health and dangerous working conditions. Soc Sci Med 1991; 33:127–131.
38. Lavie P. Sleep habits and sleep disturbances in industrial workers in Israel: main findings and some characteristics of workers complaining of daytime sleepiness. Sleep 1981; 4:147–158.
39. Leger D, Massuel MA, Comet D; the SISYPHE group. Consequences of insomnia on professional activity in the Paris Region. Sleep 2004; 27:A270.
40. Philip P, Leger D, Taillard J, et al. Insomniac complaints interfere with quality of life but not with absenteeism: respective role of depressive and organic comorbidity. Sleep Med 2006; 7: 585–591.
41. Johnson LC, Spinweber CL, Gomez SA, et al. Daytime sleepiness, performance, mood, nocturnal sleep: the effect of benzodiazepine and caffeine on their relationship. Sleep 1990; 13:121–135.
42. Daley ME, LeBlanc M, Morin CM. The impact of insomnia on absenteeism, productivity and accidents rate. Sleep 2005; 28:A247.
43. Nakata A, Ikeda T, Takahashi M, et al. The prevalence and correlates of occupational injuries in small-scale manufacturing enterprises. J Occup Health 2006; 48:366–376.
44. Partinen M, Hirvonen K, Hublin C, et al. Effects of after-midnight intake of zolpidem and temazepam on driving ability in women with non-organic insomnia. Sleep Med 2003; 4:553–561.
45. Menzin J, Lang KM, Levy P, et al. A general model of the effects of sleep medications on the risk and cost of motor vehicle accidents and its application to France. Pharmacoeconomics 2001; 19:69–78.
46. Wereyer S, Dilling H. Prevalence and treatment of insomnia in the community: results from the Upper Bavarian field study. Sleep 1991; 14:392–398.
47. Kales JD, Kales A, Bixler EO, et al. Biopsychobehavioral correlates of insomnia. Clinical characteristics and behavior correlates. Am J Psychiatry 1984; 141:1371–1376.
48. Katz DA, McHorney CA. Clinical correlates of insomnia in patients with chronic illness. Arch Intern Med 1998; 159:1099–1107.

49. Katz DA, McHorney CA. The relationship between insomnia and health-related quality of life in patients with chronic illness. J Fam Pract 2002; 51:229–235.
50. Dirksen SR, Epstein DR. Efficacy of an insomnia intervention on fatigue, mood and quality of life in breast cancer survivors. J Adv Nurs 2008; 61:664–675.
51. National Commission on Sleep Disorders Research. Wake up America: A National Sleep Alert, Vol 1. Executive Summary and Executive Report of National Commission of Sleep Disorders Research. Washington, D.C.: U.S. Government Printing Office, 1993.
52. Leger D. The cost of sleep related accidents: a report for the national commission of sleep disorders research. Sleep 1994; 17:84–93.
53. Stoller MK. Economic effects of insomnia. Clin Ther 1994; 16:873–897.
54. Walsh JK, Engelhardt CL. The direct economic costs of insomnia in the United State for 1995. Sleep 1999; 22(suppl 2):S386–S393.
55. Leger D, Levy E, Paillard M. The direct costs of insomnia in France. Sleep 1999; 22(suppl 2):S394–S401.
56. Ozminkowski RJ, Wang S, Walsh JK. The direct and indirect costs of untreated insomnia in adults in the United States. Sleep 2007; 30(3):263–273.
57. Godet-Cayré V, Pelletier-Fleury N, Le Vaillant M, et al. Insomnia and absenteeism at work. Who pays the cost? Sleep 2006; 29(2):179–184.
58. Idzikowski C. Impact of insomnia on health-related quality of life. Pharmacoeconomics 1996; 10(suppl 1):15–24.
59. Iliescu EA, Coo H, McMurray MH, et al. Quality of sleep and health-related quality of life in haemodialysis patients. Nephrol Dial Transplant 2003; 18:126–132.
60. Leger D, Janus C, Pellois A, et al. Sleep, morning alertness and quality of life in subjects treated with zopiclone and in good sleepers. Study comparing 167 patients and 381 good sleepers. Eur Psychiatry 1995; 10(suppl 3):99–102.
61. Smith IE, Shneerson JM. Is the SF-36 sensitive to sleep disruption? A study in subjects with sleep apnoea. J Sleep Res 1995; 4:183–188.
62. Zammitt GK, Weiner J, Damato N, et al. Quality of life in people with insomnia. Sleep 1999; 22:S379–S385.
63. Russel IT. The SF-36 health survey questionnaire: an outcome measure suitable for routine use in the NHS. Br Med J 1993; 306:1440–1444.
64. Leger D, Scheuermaier K, Philip P, et al. SF-36: evaluation of quality of life in severe and mild insomniacs compared with good sleepers. Psychosom Med 2001; 63:49–55.
65. Schubert CR, Cruickshanks KJ, Dalton DS, et al. Prevalence of sleep problems and quality of life in an older population. Sleep 2002; 25:889–893.
66. Pilowski I, Cettenden I, Townley M. Sleep disturbance in pain clinic patients. Pain 1985; 23:27–33.
67. Stark D, Kiely M, Smith A, et al. Anxiety disorders in cancer patients: their nature, associations and quality of life. J Clin Oncol 2002; 20:3137–3148.
68. Lindley C, Vasa S, Sawyer WT, et al. Quality of life and preferences for treatment following systemic adjuvant therapy for early-stage breast cancer. J Clin Oncol 1998; 16:1380–1387.
69. Caap-Ahlgren M, Dehlin O. Insomnia and depressive symptoms in patients with Parkinson disease. Relationship to health-related quality of life. An interview study of patients living at home. Arch Gerontol Geriatr 2001; 32:23–33.
70. Molnar MZ, Novak M, Szeifert L, et al. Restless legs syndrome, insomnia, and quality of life after renal transplantation. J Psychosom Res 2007; 63:591–597.
71. Krystal AD, Thakur M, Roth T. Sleep disturbance in psychiatric disorders: effects on function and quality of life in mood disorders, alcoholism, and schizophrenia. Ann Clin Psychiatry 2008; 20:39–46.
72. Nokes KM, Kendrew J. Correlates of sleep quality in persons with HIV disease. J Assoc Nurses AIDS Care 2001; 12:17–22.
73. Goldenberg F, Hindmarch J, Joyce CRB,et al. Zopiclone, sleep and health related quality of life. Hum Psychopharmacol 1994; 9:245–252.
74. Walsh JK, Krystal AD, Amato DA, et al. Nightly treatment of primary insomnia with eszopiclone for six months: effect on sleep, quality of life, and work limitations. Sleep 2007; 30(8):959–968.
75. Baca E, Estivill E, Hernandez B, et al.; on behalf of Castivil group. Quality of life in insomnia: influence of zolpidem. J Sleep Res 2002; 11(suppl 1):10.
76. Quesnel C, Savard J, Simard S, et al. Efficacy of cognitive–behavioral therapy for insomnia in women treated for nonmetastatic breast cancer. J Consult Clin Psychol 2003; 71:189–200.
77. Dixon S, Morgan K, Mathers N, et al. Impact of cognitive behavior therapy on health-related quality of life among adult hypnotic users with chronic insomnia. Behav Sleep Med 2006; 4(2):71–84.
78. Leger D, Scheuermaier K, Raffray T, et al. HD-16: a new quality of life instrument specifically designed for insomnia. Sleep Med 2005; 6:191–198.

4 Insomnia as a Risk Factor in Disease

Wilfred R. Pigeon

Sleep and Neurophysiology Research Lab, University of Rochester Medical Center, Rochester, New York, U.S.A.

INTRODUCTION

As reviewed in the prior two chapters, insomnia can have a variety of daytime consequences for the individual as well as present a considerable socioeconomic burden to society. As a disease entity, insomnia also exists as an independent risk factor for psychiatric and medical illness, compounding its consequences.

In this chapter, we will review the evidence that insomnia is "something that increases a person's chances of developing a disease." This most common definition of risk factor will be expanded to also include something that increases the chances for diminished treatment response or in the case of adequate treatment response, increases relapse rates. It is important to note that several definitions of the term risk factor exist and that the reader is often left to determine what definition authors have in mind (if any). For that reason we also follow a definition proffered by Beck (1) that additionally defines a risk factor as being part of the casual chain, thus requiring temporal evidence, which can only be derived from longitudinal studies. In the insomnia literature, there is a good deal of cross sectional data linking insomnia to a variety of disease entities, which will be reviewed. Such studies, however, will be considered as evidence that insomnia is a risk indicator that Burt (2) has defined as a probable or putative risk factor.

Another matter of definition arises when reviewing the broad insomnia literature. Namely, insomnia is not measured or defined in a consistent manner across studies. This is especially true for data drawn from epidemiologic and community samples, but is also found in studies in which sleep was not among the primary outcomes. Typically such investigations report on single item measures of sleep complaints either developed for the study or embedded within other instruments. For instance, the Hamilton Rating Scale for Depression (3) has three items, one each pertaining to early, middle, and late night insomnia. Until recently, this item approach to sleep or insomnia assessment had not been validated, but Manber et al. (4) have now shown that, at least in a depressed sample, such approaches can be validated against the assessment of insomnia via daily sleep diaries traditionally used by sleep researchers. This sleep outcome has been called variably "insomnia" or "sleep disturbance." The latter term has some merit when the sleep items are few and very broad (e.g., one item that asks for a rating of sleep quality). This chapter has adopted a convention of using the term "insomnia" in cases where there are not validated measures of insomnia, but the sleep items are consistent with insomnia.

INSOMNIA AS A RISK FACTOR IN PSYCHIATRIC ILLNESS

In the psychiatric domain, there is a preponderance of data to suggest that insomnia is a risk factor for new onset and recurrent major depressive disorder (MDD) (5). Less data are available for the anxiety disorders, although insomnia is equally or more prevalent in anxiety, as compared to mood disorders (6–9). As in the depression literature, available data suggest that subjects with insomnia are more likely to have an anxiety disorder than those without insomnia (10).

Insomnia and Depression

Again, the largest body of evidence for a relationship between psychiatric illness and sleep disturbances exists for the association between depression and insomnia. Both disorders are highly prevalent and frequently co-occur in all age ranges and especially in older cohorts (11,12). In the vast majority of these studies both female gender and increased age are associated with higher prevalence rates. Cross sectional data allow not only for prevalence rate estimates for each disorder, but also an estimate of how often the disorders co-occur. Longitudinal studies meanwhile allow for the direct assessment of risk factors.

Table 1 Prevalence Rates of Insomnia and Depression

Study	Sample type (size)	Sleep measures	Depressed (%)	Insomnia (%)	In depressed, % with insomnia	In insomnia, % with depression
Foley (119)	Epid (9282)	5 sleep items	20	28	49	34
Weyerer (117)	Comm (1536)	6 sleep items	7	16	47	24
Bixler (118)	Comm (1006)	5–6 sleep items	15	32	43	19
Mellinger (8)	Comm (3161)	2 sleep items	5	17	71	21
Ohayon (120)	Epid (5622)	DSM criteria	6	17	57	18
Stewart (6)	Epid (8580)	Clinical interview	3	5	40	21
Taylor (9)	Comm (772)	Sleep diaries	10	20	41	20
Ford (10)	Epid (7954)	2 sleep items	5	10	42	23
Hohagen (121)	PC (2512)	DSM criteria	7	19	52	18
Total *N*	40,425	Weighted averages	9	16	49	26

Abbreviations: Epid, epidemiologic sample; Comm, community-based sample; PC, primary care sample.

Prevalence Estimates for Insomnia and Depression

A number of community and epidemiologic studies have been conducted to determine the prevalence of both insomnia and depression. While both disorders are variably defined across studies, in general the prevalence of insomnia is approximately 16% and that of depression is approximately 9%. The estimates are lower in studies with more stringent criteria, approximately 10% and 5% for insomnia and depression, respectively. Table 1 summarizes data from nine such studies that also reported (or allowed the calculation of) the prevalence of depression in only those subjects deemed to have insomnia and conversely, the prevalence of insomnia in only those subjects deemed to be depressed.

For example, baseline estimates of prevalence rates from a study ($n = 7954$) based on the National Institute of Mental Health Epidemiologic Catchment Area data were 10% for insomnia and 5% for depression. Among those subjects with insomnia, 23% were depressed; among subjects with depression, 42% had insomnia (10). Stewart et al. applied more stringent diagnostic criteria than most prior studies to data from the Second National Survey of Psychiatric Morbidity conducted in the United Kingdom ($n = 8580$). Their prevalence rate estimates were 5% for insomnia and 3% for depression (6). Among those subjects with insomnia 21% were depressed, whereas among subjects with depression 40% had insomnia.

Overall, in a combined sample of 40,425 subjects, the prevalence of insomnia is nearly twice that of depression. Perhaps more interesting is that the likelihood of having insomnia in the context of depression is approximately twice that of having depression in the context of insomnia. Such data suggest that insomnia may be considered a risk indicator for depression.

Longitudinal Studies of Insomnia and Depression

A number of longitudinal studies provide additional insight into the relationship between insomnia and depression. One such study (13) sought to assess the course of depressive symptoms prior to a depressive episode by following patients with recurrent but remitted MDD for up to 42 weeks with weekly administration of the Beck Depression Inventory (14). Subjects who experienced a recurrence of depression were matched controls with no recurrence. Time series data showed that the nonrecurrent group exhibited an elevated, but stable, level of insomnia while the recurrent group exhibited an even higher level of sleep disturbance that began five weeks prior to recurrence. The insomnia symptom cluster was the most prominent depressive symptom cluster leading up to the depressive episode and reached its zenith at the week of recurrence. This suggests that insomnia is both a risk factor for and a prodromal sign of a recurrent depressive episode.

Most other longitudinal studies have assessed whether insomnia occurring at one or two time points predicts depression at the second time point. These include several studies assessing the onset of new depression over a one-year period. Two of these have found that insomnia posed an increased risk for the development of depression with odds ratios of 40 (CI: 19.8–80) and 5.4 (2.6–11.3) respectively (10,15), while Dryman and Eaton found an increased risk of depression [OR: 9.4(4.3–20.3)], but only in women (16).

While the above studies sampled populations of varying ages, others have focused on younger adults. In a study that began with college-aged men, insomnia in college conferred a relative risk of 2.0 (1.2–3.3) for developing depression at some point during the following 30 years (17). Breslau et al. (18) sampled 979 members of a health maintenance organization who were 21 to 30 years old at baseline assessment and reassessed three years later. At baseline, persons reporting two weeks or more of insomnia nearly every night at any point in their life were at increased risk of developing new onset depression by the three-year follow-up [OR: 2.4(1.2–4.8)] than those with no history of insomnia even after controlling for prior depressive symptoms.

In longitudinal studies performed in older cohorts, findings have been slightly mixed. One study limited by power, found that in 147 patients with no prior history of depression, the presence of persistent insomnia at baseline was associated with new onset depression one year later (but only in females) (19). In a study of 524 community-dwelling elders, insomnia at baseline and three years later was associated with depression at three years compared to those with no insomnia or those with insomnia at one time point (20). In a reanalysis of this data set including only subjects with activity limitations and no psychiatric morbidity at baseline, baseline insomnia was not associated with depression three years later (21). Roberts et al. (22) found that insomnia at baseline was associated with an increased risk of depression one year later [OR: 2.5(1.7–3.7)] and insomnia at both time points carried an eightfold risk, though other factors were more significant predictors. In older adults followed for 12 years (23), baseline insomnia was an independent predictor of depression at 12 years in women only [OR: 4.1(2.3–7.2)]. Brabbins (24) determined that in a sample of 771 elders, only initial insomnia (and not middle of the night or early morning awakening) that occurred at both baseline and three years was associated with the development of new depression at three years.

Finally, a meta-analysis of studies conducted in older adults found that sleep disturbance, with an odds ratio of 2.6, was second to recent bereavement (OR 3.3) as a risk factor for late-life depression (25). In summary, while there is a good body of evidence that suggest that both incident and persistent insomnia predict new onset depression, the findings are not unanimous, and insomnia is not the only significant risk factor. Taken as a whole these sets of longitudinal studies support the insomnia as one risk factor for developing depression.

As Table 1 shows, insomnia and depression do not always co-occur, nor does one necessarily presage the other across all cases. As is the case for any risk factor, insomnia is neither a necessary condition for nor the sole pathway to depression, but it does, in fact, appear to be part of the casual chain for many individuals. Two recent publications further this case with respect to depression. Buysse et al. (26) were able to assess insomnia and depression from an epidemiologic study in Zurich that included 6 time points over a 20-year span. In their analyses, the presence of insomnia absent depression at each time point was strongly associated with the presence of co-occurring insomnia and depression at the subsequent time point. A similar finding occurred with respect to the presence of depression absent insomnia, though the findings for insomnia were more robust. Departing from the epidemiologic data, Pigeon et al. assessed insomnia in the context of a depression treatment trial of 1801 older adults in primary care settings (26,27). They found that patients with insomnia that persisted across a baseline and three-month assessment had a diminished treatment response at 6 and 12 months compared to patients with insomnia at one or neither of the baseline and two-month time points. This expands the notion of insomnia as a risk factor for depression to include comorbid insomnia as a risk factor for unremitting depression.

While it is not the case that a putative risk factor must be demonstrated to improve a disease entity when it is removed, there are emerging data in this regard for insomnia in the context of depression. Two uncontrolled studies have shown that patients presenting with stringent definitions of insomnia and depression who completed a course of cognitive-behavioral therapy for insomnia had improvements in both sleep and depression (28,29). In addition two randomized, controlled trials have shown that treating insomnia and depression simultaneously has a greater impact on both conditions than when treating the depression alone. One of these trials found that patients treated concomitantly with fluoxetine and eszopiclone exhibited less illness severity over the course of an eight-week intervention and a faster time to recovery than subjects treated with fluoxetine only (30) and the other that escitalopram and cognitive-behavioral therapy for insomnia produced a higher rate of remission for depression and insomnia than escitalopram alone (31). This set of studies supports the assertion that insomnia is a modifiable risk factor for depression.

Insomnia in Other Mood Disorders and Related Conditions

Bipolar disorders must include at least one episode of mania to meet symptom criteria and are far less prevalent than depressive disorders. Insomnia and/or sleep deprivation is often cited by patients and practitioners as a precursor to manic episodes, though the empirical data are relatively sparse in this area. There are nearly as many reviews on this topic as there are well-designed studies and the reader is referred to these excellent reviews and theoretical discussions (32–34). As Jackson (34) reports, five retrospective studies indicate that patients identify sleep disturbance as a top prodromal sign of a manic episode, but not bipolar depression. As summarized by Harvey (32) four studies have assessed sleep and bipolar symptoms prospectively on a daily basis and found relationships between poor sleep and next-day worsening of manic or depressive symptoms (though whether mania or depression was correlated with sleep varied by study). These are limited data on which to call insomnia a risk factor for bipolar disorder or for a manic episode, so that the field awaits more in the way of prospective data. This would be important given the widespread belief that sleep disturbance is indeed a harbinger of particularly a manic episode, but may lend itself to preventive intervention.

Complicated Grief Disorder is not a mood disorder per se, but is included in this section. It occurs as a reaction to bereavement, the loss of a loved one by death. Between 10% to 20% of persons experiencing bereavement have a complicated grief reaction (35). Current nosologies do not include insomnia as a symptom, although sleep interference is included as one of seven symptom criteria for a proposed diagnostic entity (36). Given that approximately 75% of all deaths occur in persons ≥ 65 years old, bereavements, like insomnia, increase across the lifespan (37) and may have some relationship to sleep. A prospective PSG study comparing 27 nondepressed elders with spousal bereavement to matched nonbereaved elders found the only difference in groups to be elevated phasic REM activity and a slight decrement in slow wave sleep in the bereaved group (38). In a meta-analytic review of studies in community-dwelling elders, Cole and Dendukuri (25) determined that recent bereavement was the biggest risk factor for depression. Across a number of smaller studies, sleep disturbance in the form of difficulty sleeping and/or insomnia has been reported in one-third to one-half of subjects with bereavement (36,39–43) and the level of sleep disturbance was higher than in that of control groups without bereavement (41–43). There is no data to suggest, however, that insomnia represents a risk factor for complicated grief following bereavement.

Suicide and suicidality may also be associated with insomnia. An early mention of this association appeared in an article titled "Insomnia and Suicide" in a 1914 issue of *The Lancet* (44). In it, C Ernest Pronger writes "For a long time past newspaper reports of suicide, associated with insomnia, have attracted my attention..." and goes on to note how assessing and potentially treating insomnia might prevent many calamities. Sadly, it has taken some time to take up this call. Recent work includes a cross sectional study of 165 hospitalized suicide attempters in which the vast majority endorsed one or more sleep complaints, with difficulty initiating sleep the most commonly endorsed symptom (73%), but nightmares were the only independent predictor of suicidality (45). Similarly, in 176 outpatients regression analyses revealed that insomnia and nightmare symptoms were associated with both depressive symptoms and suicidality, but after controlling for depressive symptoms, only nightmares were associated with suicidality (46). Insomnia has also been found to be associated with suicidal thoughts in a sample of outpatient chronic pain patients (47).

In a cross sectional study of 1362 high school students in China, both shorter sleep duration and the presence of nightmares were significantly associated with reporting suicidality (48). In one of two prospective studies, Bernert collected data from 14,456 community elders over a 10-year period during which time 21 individuals died by suicide. When matched to 20 randomly selected controls, disturbances in sleep consistent with insomnia and independent of depression predicted an increased risk for eventual death by suicide (49). Goldstein et al. (50) assessed sleep disturbances in 140 adolescent suicide victims and 131 controls with a psychological autopsy protocol and semistructured psychiatric interview, respectively. Suicide completers had higher rates of overall sleep disturbance, insomnia, and hypersomnia compared to controls within the last week after controlling for affective disorders. These data suggest that insomnia is a risk indicator for suicidality with some evidence that it is a risk factor for suicide.

Insomnia and Anxiety Disorders

Although sleep disturbances are more prevalent in anxiety disorders than they are in mood disorders, far less research has been conducted in these areas with the possible exception of posttraumatic stress disorder (PTSD). The Ford and Kamerow (10) catchment area study reported that 24% of respondents with insomnia had an anxiety disorder and were six times more likely to have an anxiety disorder than those without insomnia. Others have found anxiety disorders in general population samples to be equally or more prevalent than depression in their respective insomnia subsamples (6–9).

Insomnia and Posttraumatic Stress Disorder

Sleep disturbances are a common feature of PTSD in both the general population (51) and in combat veterans (52). Interestingly, while nightmares have historically been considered the hallmark of PTSD, insomnia is actually a more prevalent symptom. This has been shown in an epidemiologic survey of the general population as well as in a clinical sample seeking treatment for insomnia (51,53). In an assessment of the National Vietnam Veterans Readjustment Study database (52), Nelylan found that insomnia was more frequent than nightmares in both combat veterans with PTSD (90.7% vs. 52.4%) and combat veterans without PTSD (62.5% vs. 4.8%). While these findings speak about the specificity of nightmares for PTSD, they also underscore the extremely high prevalence of insomnia in trauma-exposed populations of 60% to 90%. There remains considerable debate, and little data to come to a consensus, on whether insomnia represents a risk factor for the development of PTSD. Harvey and Bryant found that 72% of civilians experiencing a sleep disturbance within one month of their trauma went on to develop PTSD (54). In what may be some of the only other prospective assessments of sleep acutely following trauma (but prior to the development of PTSD), Mellman et al. have shown that the nature of dream content (55) and disturbances in REM sleep (56) predict PTSD outcome.

Most of the work in PTSD and sleep has focused on characterizing the sleep of trauma survivors. Therefore, while insomnia can be considered a risk indicator it remains to be shown whether it is a risk factor. Nonetheless it remains the case that insomnia is a prevalent residual symptom following otherwise successful treatment of PTSD (53) and that a handful of studies with stringent definitions of insomnia have shown that cognitive-behavioral interventions specifically tailored to the sleep of PTSD populations have met with some success (57–60).

Other Anxiety Disorders

There is a relative paucity of sleep data in generalized anxiety disorder (GAD), which is surprising given that sleep disturbance is one of the six DSM symptom criteria for its diagnosis, two additional symptoms (irritability and fatigue) are often associated with insomnia, and both GAD and insomnia tend to present with features of hyperarousal (61–63). In a report of 141 patients presenting to an insomnia clinic, GAD was the most common co-occurring psychiatric disorder (7). Breslau et al. (18) reported cross sectional data from their large sample ($n = 1007$) indicating that in the 167 respondents with insomnia, 36% had at least one anxiety disorder as opposed to 19% in those with no insomnia. In the insomnia sample, the disorder specific occurrences reported were: GAD 8%, panic disorder 6%, obsessive–compulsive disorder 5%, and phobia 25%.

Substance Abuse Disorders

Substance abuse occurs in approximately twice as many individuals with insomnia as compared to those without insomnia (10,15,18). In a sample of 172 alcoholics admitted to inpatient treatment, patients with insomnia were more likely to report frequent alcohol use for sleep than those without insomnia (55% vs. 28%) (64).

Anecdotal reports also suggest that particularly in patients acutely recovering from alcoholism, sleeping problems lead to relapse. This has been borne out in one study, where insomnia and fragmented sleep were found to predict relapse in 20 abstinent alcoholics (65). In another sample of 74 recently abstinent alcoholics, 60% with baseline insomnia versus 30% without baseline insomnia relapsed to any use of alcohol within five months (64). Brower et al. (66) also recently completed a small randomized controlled trial of gabapentin in 21 patients with active alcoholism and comorbid insomnia. Albeit a limited sample size, those in the treatment arm had a reduced time to relapse.

These data indicate that insomnia is a risk indicator for the development of alcoholism; there is not enough data to posit such an assertion in other forms of substance abuse. The data also suggest that insomnia represents a risk factor for relapse in alcohol dependence.

INSOMNIA AS A RISK FACTOR IN MEDICAL ILLNESS

In the medical domain there are a series of studies that suggest that poor sleep is a risk factor for increased mortality, especially in the elderly (e.g., 24,67–69). Insomnia and/or short sleep duration are also associated with increased mortality (70,71). In general, data with respect to specific medical illnesses are less substantial than in the psychiatric domain.

Insomnia and Chronic Pain

Approximately 50% patients with diverse chronic pain conditions complain of significant sleep disturbance, with some investigations finding sleep disturbance as high as 70% to 88% (72–75). The directionality of this relationship is largely untested however. One exception comes from Affleck et al. (76) who analyzed 30 consecutive days worth of daily sleep and pain diaries from fibromyalgia patients and found that pain and sleep had a bidirectional influence on each other. Experimental data in animals and humans suggest that sleep disruption or deprivation (not insomnia) increases various types of pain sensitivity (77–79) or can produce or worsen pain (80–82). As in some of the psychiatric literature, there are also some studies demonstrating that treating insomnia in the context of chronic pain can improve insomnia (83) or both conditions (84,85). The available data, therefore, while strongly implicating insomnia as a risk indicator does not speak about the issue of risk factor directly.

Insomnia and Other Medical Conditions

A number of cross sectional studies have implicated sleep disturbance in conditions such as gastrointestinal distress (86), recovery from and physical function and emotional well-being after cardiac surgery (87–91), and Type II diabetes and glucose homeostasis dysregulation (prediabetic syndromes) (92–94). There are also some longitudinal epidemiologic studies that have assessed the relationship of insomnia to hypertension and cardiovascular disease. Suka et al. used an annual health examination database of a Japanese telecommunication company and followed 4794 men from a baseline assessment for up to four years or until they developed hypertension (95). After adjusting for potential confounding factors, persistent complaints of difficulty initiating sleep and difficulty maintaining sleep were significantly associated with a significant increased risk of hypertension with OR 1.96 (1.42–2.70) and OR 1.88 (1.45–2.45), respectively. Phillips and Manino (96) used 8757 participants without hypertension and 11,863 without cardiovascular disease from the Atherosclerosis Risk in Communities Study and followed them from a baseline assessment to the development of disease or up to six years. Either difficulty falling asleep or waking up repeatedly predicted a slight increased risk of hypertension [OR 1.2(1.03–1.3)] and endorsement of these two symptoms plus awaking tired or fatigued increased risk of cardiovascular disease [OR 1.5(1.1–2.0)]. In a subsequent analysis of this data set comparing single item sleep disturbances at Year 5 to subsequent hypertension incidence at Year 11, these authors did not find any single item measure of insomnia to be associated with subsequent incident hypertension (97). The above studies represent the first set of evidence that favor insomnia as a risk factor in these conditions, but negative findings have been reported.

Insomnia and Immune Function

To date, the association between immunity and sleep has been evaluated primarily in terms of whether plasma levels of either NK cells or sleep-related cytokines vary with sleep, sleep loss, sleep deprivation, or with clinical diagnosis (i.e., insomnia) (98–104). As reviewed by Krueger et al. (101), numerous cytokines appear to have some relation to sleep. A small number of studies have found that insomnia (as compared to good sleep) tends to be associated with altered innate immunity. In general, insomnia is associated with decreased NK activity (105,106), and a shift in the circadian distribution of IL-6 and TNF-α from the night to the daytime (107), despite higher evening levels of Il-6 (107). Only one study has found that immune alterations are correlated with self-report or PSG measures of disturbed sleep. Burgos et al. (108) found in patients with insomnia that IL-6 secretion is inversely correlated with self-reported sleep quality and PSG-measured SWS minutes. While intriguing none of these data point to insomnia as a possible risk factor for subsequent disease.

Data from three adaptive immune system studies (as opposed to the innate immunity studies above) are also suggestive. In a companion study to a clinical trail of an experimental avian influenza vaccine (109), 46 patients receiving the active vaccine were assessed with the Pittsburgh Sleep Quality Index (PSQI) (110). Compared to vaccine responders, the nonresponders had higher PSQI scores, poorer sleep efficiency, and shorter sleep duration. Cohen et al. (111), in a study of 276 healthy adults, sought to assess whether social ties were related to susceptibility to the common cold. All participants were infected with a live rhinovirus and the development and severity of common cold symptoms were assessed. While the primary hypothesis was borne out (greater social ties were protective against the development of cold symptoms), several potential variables were found to moderate the relationship, including decreased self-reported sleep efficiency. In a follow-up study designed to further test this association in 153 participants, these authors found that sleep durations under seven hours and sleep efficiency under 92% immediately preceding exposure to a rhinovirus were each associated with significantly higher rates of infection (112). Thus, preliminary data exist demonstrates that insomnia is a risk factor for infectious disease.

SUMMARY AND CONCLUSION

Insomnia is highly prevalent across a wide range of psychiatric and medical conditions with considerable evidence that it is a risk indicator for the majority of these conditions. Moreover, insomnia represents a risk factor for the development of highly prevalent disorders ranging from mood and anxiety disorders to chronic pain and hypertension as well as for all cause mortality and suicide. Finally, for many of these conditions, insomnia also represents a risk factor for relapse or delayed recovery.

Authors who have been calling for an end to the notion of insomnia as a secondary disorder (see for example, 113–116) have considerable evidence to draw upon to make their case. The task now falls to the sleep community to continue its efforts to identify and possibly treat insomnia across these many disease states.

REFERENCES

1. Beck JD. Risk revisited. Community Dent Oral Epidemiol 1998; 26(4):220–225.
2. Burt BA. Risk factors, risk markers, and risk indicators. Community Dent Oral Epidemiol 1998; 26(4):219.
3. Hamilton M. Development of a rating scale for primary depressive illness. Br J Soc Clin Psychol 1967; 6:278–296.
4. Manber R, Blasey C, Arnow B, et al. Assessing insomnia severity in depression: comparison of depression rating scales and sleep diaries. J Psychiatr Res 2005; 39(5):481–488.
5. Pigeon W, Perlis ML. Insomnia and depression: birds of a feather? Int J Sleep Disord 2007; 1(3): 82–91.
6. Stewart R, Besset A, Bebbington P, et al. Insomnia comorbidity and impact and hypnotic use by age group in a national survey population aged 16 to 74 years. Sleep 2006; 29(11):1391–1397.
7. Mahendran R, Subramaniam M, Chan YM. Psychiatric morbidity of patients referred to an insomnia clinic. Singapore Med J 2007; 48(2):163–165.
8. Mellinger GD, Balter MB, Uhlenhuth EH. Insomnia and its treatment: prevalence and correlates. Arch Gen Psychiatry 1985; 42(3):225–232.
9. Taylor DJ, Lichstein KL, Durrence HH, et al. Epidemiology of insomnia, depression, and anxiety. Sleep 2005; 28(11):1457–1464.

10. Ford DE, Kamerow DB. Epidemiologic study of sleep disturbances and psychiatric disorders. An opportunity for prevention? JAMA 1989; 262(11):1479–1484.
11. Benca R. Mood disorders. In: Kryger M, Roth T, Dement W, eds. Principles and Practice of Sleep Disorders Medicine. Philadelphia: W.B. Saunders Company, 2005:1311–1326.
12. Tsuno N, Besset A, Ritchie K. Sleep and depression. J Clin Psychiatry 2005; 66(10):1254–1269.
13. Perlis ML, Buysse D, Giles DE, et al. Sleep disturbance may be a prodromal symptom of depression. J Affect Disord 1997; 42(2):209–212.
14. Beck AT, Steer RA, Garbin MG. Psychometric properties of the Beck depression inventory—25 years of evaluation. Clin Psychol Rev 1988; 8(1):77–100.
15. Weissman MM, Greenwald S, Nino-Murcia G, et al. The morbidity of insomnia uncomplicated by psychiatric disorders. Gen Hosp Psychiatry 1997; 19(4):245–250.
16. Dryman A, Eaton WW. Affective symptoms associated with the onset of major depression in the community: findings from the US National Institute of Mental Health Epidemiologic Catchment Area Program. Acta Psychiatr Scand 1991; 84(1):1–5.
17. Chang PP, Ford DE, Mead LA, et al. Insomnia in young men and subsequent depression. The Johns Hopkins Precursors Study. Am J Epidemiol 1997; 146(2):105–114.
18. Breslau N, Roth T, Rosenthal L, et al. Sleep disturbance and psychiatric disorders: a longitudinal epidemiological study of young adults. Biol Psychiatry 1996; 39(6):411–418.
19. Perlis M, Smith LJ, Lyness JM, et al. Insomnia as a risk factor for onset of depression in the elderly. Behav Sleep Med 2006; 4(2):104–113.
20. Livingston G, Blizard B, Mann A. Does sleep disturbance predict depression in elderly people? A study in inner London. Br J Gen Pract 1993; 43(376):445–448.
21. Livingston G, Watkin V, Milne B, et al. Who becomes depressed? The Islington community study of older people. J Affect Disord 2000; 58(2):125–133.
22. Roberts RE, Shema SJ, Kaplan GA, et al. Sleep complaints and depression in an aging cohort: a prospective perspective. Am J Psychiatry 2000; 157(1):81–88.
23. Mallon L, Broman JE, Hetta J. Relationship between insomnia, depression, and mortality: a 12-year follow-up of older adults in the community. Int Psychogeriatr 2000; 12(3):295–306.
24. Brabbins CJ, Dewey ME, Copeland JR, et al. Insomnia in the elderly: prevalence, gender differences and relationships with morbidity and mortality. Int J Geriatr Psychiatry 1993; 8(6):473–480.
25. Cole MG, Dendukuri N. Risk factors for depression among elderly community subjects: a systematic review and meta-analysis. Am J Psychiatry 2003; 160(6):1147–1156.
26. Buysse DJ, Angst J, Gamma A, et al. Prevalence, course, and comorbidity of insomnia and depression in young adults. Sleep 2008; 31(4):473–480.
27. Pigeon WR, Hegel MT, Unutzer J, et al. Is insomnia a perpetuating factor for late-life depression in the IMPACT cohort? Sleep 2008; 31(4):481–488.
28. Morawetz D. Behavioral self-help treatment for insomnia: a controlled evaluation. Behav Ther 1989; 20:365–379.
29. Taylor DJ, Lichstein K, Weinstock J, et al. A pilot study of cognitive-behavioral therapy of insomnia in people with mild depression. Behav Ther 2007; 38:49–57.
30. Fava M, McCall WV, Krystal A, et al. Eszopiclone co-administered with fluoxetine in patients with insomnia coexisting with major depressive disorder. Biol Psychiatry 2006; 59(11):1052–1060.
31. Manber R, Edinger JD, Gress JL, et al. Cognitive behavioral therapy for insomnia enhances depression outcome in patients with comorbid major depressive disorder and insomnia. Sleep 2008; 31(4):489–495.
32. Harvey AG. Sleep and circadian rhythms in bipolar disorder: seeking synchrony, harmony, and regulation. Am J Psychiatry 2008; 165(7):820–829.
33. Plante DT, Winkelman JW. Sleep disturbance in bipolar disorder: therapeutic implications. Am J Psychiatry 2008; 165(7):830–843.
34. Jackson A, Cavanagh J, Scott J. A systematic review of manic and depressive prodromes. J Affect Disord 2003; 74(3):209–217.
35. Prigerson HG. When the path of adjustment leads to a dead-end. Bereavement Care 2004; 23:38–40.
36. Horowitz MJ, Siegel B, Holen A, et al. Diagnostic criteria for complicated grief disorder. Am J Psychiatry 1997; 154(7):904–910.
37. Hamilton BE, Minino AM, Martin JA, et al. Annual summary of vital statistics: 2005. Pediatrics 2007; 119(2):345–360.
38. Reynolds CF, Hoch CC, Buysse DJ, et al. Sleep after spousal bereavement—a study of recovery from stress. Biol Psychiatry 1993; 34(11):791–797.
39. Prigerson HG, Frank E, Kasl SV, et al. Complicated grief and bereavement-related depression as distinct disorders: preliminary empirical validation in elderly bereaved spouses. Am J Psychiatry 1995; 152(1):22–30.

40. Germain A, Caroff K, Buysse DJ, et al. Sleep quality in complicated grief. J Trauma Stress 2005; 18(4):343–346.
41. Richardson SJ, Lund DA, Caserta MS, et al. Sleep patterns in older bereaved spouses. Omega-J Death Dying 2003; 47(4):361–383.
42. Valdimarsdottir U, Helgason AR, Furst CJ, et al. Long-term effects of widowhood after terminal cancer: a Swedish nationwide follow-up. Scand J Public Health 2003; 31(1):31–36.
43. Beem EE, Maes S, Cleiren M, et al. Psychological functioning of recently bereaved middle-aged women: the first 13 months. Psychol Rep 2000; 87(1):243–254.
44. Pronger CE. Insomnia and suicide. Lancet 1914; 184:1356–1359.
45. Sjostrom N, Waern M, Hetta J. Nightmares and sleep disturbances in relation to suicidality in suicide attempters. Sleep 2007; 30(1):91–95.
46. Bernert RA, Joiner TE, Cukrowicz KC, et al. Suicidality and sleep disturbances. Sleep 2005; 28(9):1135–1141.
47. Smith MT, Perlis ML, Haythornthwaite JA. Suicidal ideation in outpatients with chronic musculoskeletal pain—an exploratory study of the role of sleep onset insomnia and pain intensity. Clin J Pain 2004; 20(2):111–118.
48. Liu XC. Sleep and adolescent suicidal behavior. Sleep 2004; 27(7):1351–1358.
49. Bernert R, Turvey C, Conwell Y, et al. Sleep disturbance as a unique risk factor for completed suicide. Sleep 2007; 30:A334.
50. Goldstein TR, Bridge JA, Brent DA. Sleep disturbance preceding completed suicide in adolescents. J Consult Clin Psychol 2008; 76(1):84–91.
51. Ohayon MM, Shapiro CM. Sleep disturbances and psychiatric disorders associated with posttraumatic stress disorder in the general population. Compr Psychiatry 2000; 41(6):469–478.
52. Neylan TC, Marmar CR, Metzler TJ, et al. Sleep disturbances in the Vietnam generation: findings from a nationally representative sample of male Vietnam veterans. Am J Psychiatry 1998; 155(7): 929–933.
53. Zayfert C, Deviva JC. Residual insomnia following cognitive behavioral therapy for PTSD. J Trauma Stress 2004; 17(1):69–73.
54. Harvey AG, Bryant RA. The relationship between acute stress disorder and posttraumatic stress disorder: a prospective evaluation of motor vehicle accident survivors. J Consult Clin Psychol 1998; 66(3):507–512.
55. Mellman TA, David D, Bustamante V, et al. Dreams in the acute aftermath of trauma and their relationship to PTSD. J Trauma Stress 2001; 14(1):241–247.
56. Mellman TA, Pigeon WR, Nowell PD, et al. Relationships between REM sleep findings and PTSD symptoms during the early aftermath of trauma. J Trauma Stress 2007; 20(5):893–901.
57. Krakow BJ, Melendrez DC, Johnston LG, et al. Sleep Dynamic Therapy for Cerro Grande Fire evacuees with posttraumatic stress symptoms: a preliminary report. J Clin Psychiatry 2002; 63(8): 673–684.
58. Krakow B, Johnston L, Melendrez D, et al. An open-label trial of evidence-based cognitive behavior therapy for nightmares and insomnia in crime victims with PTSD. Am J Psychiatry 2001; 158(12):2043–2047.
59. Deviva JC, Zayfert C, Pigeon WR, et al. Treatment of residual insomnia after CBT for PTSD: case studies. J Trauma Stress 2005; 18(2):155–159.
60. Germain A, Shear MK, Hall M, et al. Effects of a brief behavioral treatment for PTSD-related sleep disturbances: a pilot study. Behav Res Ther 2007; 45(3):627–632.
61. Saletu-Zyhlarz G, Saletu B, Anderer P, et al. Nonorganic insomnia in generalized anxiety disorder. 1. Controlled studies on sleep, awakening and daytime vigilance utilizing polysomnography and EEG mapping. Neuropsychobiology 1997; 36(3):117–129.
62. Saletu B, Anderer P, Brandstatter N, et al. Insomnia in generalized anxiety disorder: polysomnographic, psychometric and clinical investigations before, during, and after therapy with a long- versus a short-half-life benzodiazepine (Quazepam versus Triazolam). Neuropsychobiology 1994; 29:69–90.
63. Fuller KH, Waters WF, Binks PG, et al. Generalized anxiety and sleep architecture: a polysomnographic investigation. Sleep 1997; 20(5):370–376.
64. Brower KJ, Aldrich MS, Robinson EAR,et al. Insomnia, self-medication, and relapse to alcoholism. Am J Psychiatry 2001; 158(3):399–404.
65. Drummond SP, Gillin JC, Smith TL, et al. The sleep of abstinent pure primary alcoholic patients: natural course and relationship to relapse. Alcohol Clin Exp Res 1998; 22(8):1796–1802.
66. Brower KJ, Kim HM, Strobbe S, et al. Randomized double-blind pilot trial of gabapentin versus placebo to treat alcohol dependence and comorbid insomnia. Alcohol Clin Exp Res 2008; 32(8):1429–1438.

67. Dew MA, Reynolds CF, Buysse DJ, et al. Electroencephalographic sleep profiles during depression. Effects of episode duration and other clinical and psychosocial factors in older adults. Arch Gen Psychiatry 1996; 53(2):148–156.
68. Kripke DF. Mortality risk of major depression. Am J Psychiatry 1995; 152(6):962.
69. Althuis MD, Fredman L, Langenberg PW, et al. The relationship between insomnia and mortality among community-dwelling older women. J Am Geriatr Soc 1998; 46:1270–1273.
70. Kripke DF, Simons RN, Garfinkel L, et al. Short and long sleep and sleeping pills: is increased mortality associated? Arch Gen Psychiatry 1979; 36:103–116.
71. Dew MA, Hoch CC, Buysse DJ, et al. Healthy older adults' sleep predicts all-cause mortality at 4 to 19 years of follow-up. Psychosom Med 2003; 65(1):63–73.
72. Atkinson JH, Ancoli-Israel S, Slater MA, et al. Subjective sleep disturbance in chronic back pain. Clin J Pain 1988; 65(2):225–232.
73. Morin C, Gibson D, Wade J. Self-reported sleep and mood disturbance in chronic pain patients. Clin J Pain 1998; 14(4):311–314.
74. Pilowsky I, Crettenden I, Townley M. Sleep disturbance in pain clinic patients. Pain 1985; 23(1):27–33.
75. Smith MT, Perlis ML, Smith MS, et al. Sleep quality and presleep arousal in chronic pain. J Behav Med 2000; 23(1):1–13.
76. Affleck G, Urrows S, Tennen H, et al. Sequential daily relations of sleep, pain intensity, and attention to pain among women with fibromyalgia. Pain 1996; 68:363–368.
77. Onen SH, Alloui A, Gross A, et al. The effects of total sleep deprivation, selective sleep interruption and sleep recovery on pain tolerance thresholds in healthy subjects. J Sleep Res 2001; 10(1): 35–42.
78. Onen SH, Alloui A, Jourdan D, et al. Effects of rapid eye movement (REM) sleep deprivation, selective sleep interruption, and sleep recovery on pain tolerance thresholds in healthy subjects. Brain Res 2001; 900:261–267.
79. Hicks RA, Coleman DD, Ferrante F, et al. Pain thresholds in rats during recovery from REM sleep deprivation. Percept Mot Skills 1979; 48(3, pt 1):687–690.
80. Moldofsky H, Scarisbrick P. Induction of neurasthenic musculoskeletal pain syndrome by selective sleep stage deprivation. Psychosom Med 1976; 38(1):35–44.
81. Lentz MJ, Landis CA, Rothermel J, et al. Effects of selective slow wave sleep disruption on musculoskeletal pain and fatigue in middle aged women. J Rheumatol 1999; 26(7):1586–1592.
82. Older SA, Battafarano DF, Danning CL, et al. The effects of delta wave sleep interruption on pain thresholds and fibromyalgia-like symptoms in healthy subjects; correlations with insulin-like growth factor I. J Rheumatol 1998; 25(6):1180–1186.
83. Currie SR, Wilson KG, Pontefract AJ, et al. Cognitive-behavioral treatment of insomnia secondary to chronic pain. J Consult Clin Psychol 2000; 68(3):407–416.
84. Edinger JD, Wohlgemuth WK, Krystal AD, et al. Behavioral insomnia therapy for fibromyalgia patients—a randomized clinical trial. Arch Intern Med 2005; 165(21):2527–2535.
85. Pigeon W, Jungquist C, Matteson S, et al. Pain, sleep and mood outcomes in chronic pain patients following cognitive behavioral therapy for insomnia. Sleep 2007; 30:A255–A256.
86. Kupperman M, Lubeck DP, Mazonson PD. Sleep problems and their correlates in a working population. J Gen Intern Med 1995; 10:25–32.
87. Redeker NS, Ruggiero JS, Hedges C. Sleep is related to physical function and emotional well-being after cardiac surgery. Nurs Res 2004; 53(3):154–162.
88. Redeker NS. Why is sleep relevant to cardiovascular disease? J Cardiovasc Nurs 2002; 17(1):v–ix.
89. Jenkins CD, Stanton BA, Jono RT. Quantifying and predicting recovery after heart surgery. Psychosom Med 1994; 56(3):203–212.
90. Jenkins CD. Psychosocial risk factors for coronary heart disease. Acta Med Scand Suppl 1982; 660:123–136.
91. Schwartz S, McDowell AW, Cole SR, et al. Insomnia and heart disease: a review of epidemiologic studies. J Psychosom Res 1999; 47(4):313–333.
92. Mander B, Colecchia E, Spiegel K, et al. Short sleep: a risk factor for insulin resistance and obesity. Diabetes 2001; 50:A45.
93. Ryden AM, Knutson KL, Mander BA, et al. Association between sleep quality and glycemic control in type 2 diabetic African-American women. Diabetes 2002; 51:A620.
94. Ryder AM, Knutson KL, Mander BA, et al. Sleep in Type II diabetes: a survey study. Sleep 2002; 25:A105–A106.
95. Suka M, Yoshida K, Sugimori H. Persistent insomnia is a predictor of hypertension in Japanese male workers. J Occup Health 2003; 45(6):344–350.
96. Phillips B, Mannino D. Do insomnia complaints cause hypertension or cardiovascular disease? J Clin Sleep Med 2007; 3(5):489–494.

97. Phillips B, Buzkova P, Enright P. Insomnia did not predict incident hypertension in older adults in the cardiovascular health study. Sleep 2009; 32(1):65–72.
98. Vgontzas AN, Zoumakis E, Bixler EO, et al. Adverse effects of modest sleep restriction on sleepiness, performance, and inflammatory cytokines. J Clin Endocrinol Metab 2004; 89(5):2119–2126.
99. Dinges DF, Douglas SD, Hamarman S, et al. Sleep deprivation and human immune function. Adv Neuroimmunol 1995; 5(2):97–110.
100. Krueger JM, Toth LA, Floyd R, et al. Sleep, microbes and cytokines. Neuroimmunomodulation 1994; 1(2):100–109.
101. Krueger JM, Obal FJ, Fang J, et al. The role of cytokines in physiological sleep regulation. Ann N Y Acad Sci 2001; 933:211–221.
102. Opp MR. Cytokines and sleep: the first hundred years. Brain Behav Immun 2004; 18(4):295–297.
103. Opp MR, Toth LA. Neural-immune interactions in the regulation of sleep. Front Biosci 2003; 8:d768–d779.
104. Irwin M. Effects of sleep and sleep loss on immunity and cytokines. Brain Behav Immun 2002; 16(5):503–512.
105. Cover H, Irwin M. Immunity and depression: insomnia, retardation, and reduction of natural killer cell activity. J Behav Med 1994; 17(2):217–223.
106. Irwin M, McClintick J, Costlow C, et al. Partial night sleep deprivation reduces natural killer and cellular immune responses in humans. FASEB J 1996; 10(5):643–653.
107. Vgontzas AN, Zoumakis M, Papanicolaou DA, et al. Chronic insomnia is associated with a shift of interleukin-6 and tumor necrosis factor secretion from nighttime to daytime. Metabolism 2002; 51(7):887–892.
108. Burgos I, RIchter L, Klein T, et al. Increased nocturnal interleukin-6 excretion in patients with primary insomnia: a pilot study. Brain Behav Immun 2006; 20(3):246–253.
109. Pigeon WR, Duberstein P, Tang W, Moynihan J. The association of poor sleep to immunogenicity following an avian influenza vaccine in healthy older adults. Paper presented at: Psychoneuroimmunology Research Society Meeting; May 29, 2008; Madison, WI.
110. Buysee DJ, Reynolds CF III, Monk TH, et al. The Pittsburgh Sleep Quality Index: a new instrument for psychiatric practice and research. Psychiatry Res 1989; 28(2):193–213.
111. Cohen S, Doyle WJ, Skoner DP, et al. Social ties and susceptibility to the common cold. JAMA 1997; 277(24):1940–1944.
112. Cohen S, Doyle WJ, Alper CM, et al. Sleep habits and susceptibility to the common cold. Arch Intern Med 2009; 169(1):62–67.
113. Lichstein KL, McCrae CS, Wilson NM. Secondary insomnia: diagnostic issues, cognitive-behavioral treatment and future directions. In: Perlis M, Lichstein KL, eds. Treating Sleep Disorders: Principles and Practice of Behavioral Sleep Medicine. New York: John Wiley & Sons, Inc., 2003:286–304.
114. Pigeon WR, Perlis ML. The long-term management of chronic insomnia: recommendations for primary care physicians. INSOM 2005;(5):4–9.
115. Smith MT, Huang MI, Manber R. Cognitive behavior therapy for chronic insomnia occurring within the context of medical and psychiatric disorders. Clin Psychol Rev 2005; 25(5):559–611.
116. Turek FW. Insomnia and depression: if it looks and walks like a duck. Sleep 2005; 28(11):1362–1363.
117. Weyerer S, Dilling H. Prevalence and treatment of insomnia in the community: results from the upper Bavarian Field Study. Sleep 1991; 14(5):392–398.
118. Bixler EO, Kales A, Soldatos CR, et al. Prevalence of sleep disorders in the Los Angeles metropolitan area. Am J Psychiatry 1979; 136:1257–1262.
119. Foley DJ, Monjan AA, Brown SL, et al. Sleep complaints among elderly persons: an epidemiologic study of three communities. Sleep 1995; 18(6):425–432.
120. Ohayon M. Epidemiological study on insomnia in the general population. Sleep 1996; 19(3 Suppl):S7–S15.
121. Hohagen F, Kappler C, Schramm E, et al. Sleep onset insomnia, sleep maintaining insomnia and insomnia with early morning awakening–temporal stability of subtypes in a longitudinal study on general practice attenders. Sleep 1994; 17(6):551–554.

5 Psychological Models of Insomnia

Lisa S. Talbot and Allison G. Harvey

Department of Psychology, University of California, Berkeley, California, U.S.A.

The critical role of psychological processes in the cause and/or maintenance of insomnia has received considerable attention over the past four decades. In this chapter, we begin by describing an influential overarching psychological theory, the three-P model. We then move on to review several of the behavioral, cognitive, and hybrid models in chronological order.

A range of psychological processes may contribute to insomnia, including behavior, cognition, affect, and personality. As will become evident, the bulk of the excellent work completed thus far has targeted the behavioral and/or cognitive types of explanation. These theories vary across a number of dimensions. First, several of the theories attempt to capture the entire life course of the disorder, from its inception to its most chronic form, while others take a narrower focus on just the maintaining or perpetuating factors. The former tend to be more general and the latter tend to be more detailed or specific. Second, some of the theories examine several types of explanation (e.g., the hybrid models) while others take on the task of delving into the detail of one type of explanation. Other psychological processes, such as affect and personality traits, may also be relevant but have been understudied. We will return to this topic later in this chapter.

THREE P-MODEL

The three-P model, also referred to as the three-factor or Spielman model, is a diathesis-stress theory that includes predisposing, precipitating, and perpetuating factors (1,2). The predisposing factors can be biological (e.g., regularly elevated cortisol), psychological (e.g., tendency to worry), or social (e.g., work schedule incompatible with sleep schedule). These factors represent a vulnerability for insomnia. Precipitating factors, such as stressful life events, trigger the acute onset of insomnia. The influence of precipitating factors diminishes over time. Perpetuating factors, such as maladaptive coping skills or an extension of time in bed, contribute to the acute insomnia developing into a chronic or longer term disorder. As the perpetuating factors serve to maintain the insomnia, they are typically the targets of treatment. Importantly, the model has been refined such that the three types of factors are dynamic over time (3). For example, predisposing factors are not necessarily viewed as constant vulnerabilities in the refined model (Fig. 1).

The unique feature of this model is that it provides a framework across types of explanation; that is, this model is relevant to biological, cognitive, social, and other types of explanation. However, in the early discussions of the model the behavioral processes were emphasized. In particular, an important perpetuating factor was identified as extending sleep opportunity, or lengthening the time in bed by going to bed earlier or getting up later. In this conceptualization, this behavior results in a discrepancy between time in bed and ability to sleep. This theory has resulted in a well-established therapy according to American Psychological Association criteria (4), known as sleep restriction (5), as described in chapter 25.

STIMULUS CONTROL MODEL

The stimulus control model was proposed by Bootzin (6). It is founded upon the conditioning principle that a stimulus can elicit a variety of responses; the particular response elicited depends on the conditioning history. Bootzin's theory is that insomnia occurs when sleep stimuli, either temporal (e.g., bedtime) or environmental (e.g., bed or bedroom), are no longer specifically paired with sleep, but instead have become paired with numerous other activities (e.g., reading, working, being awake and anxious about not sleeping, etc.). That is, a conditioning history in which the bed/bedroom was continually paired with nonsleep activities

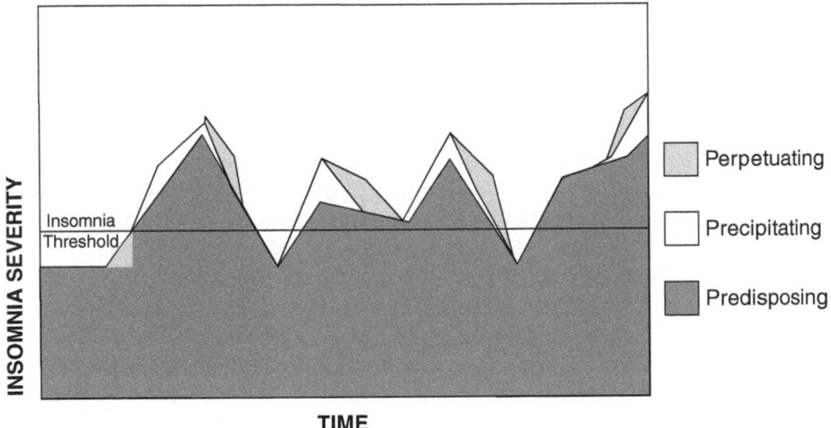

Figure 1 Characteristics contributing to insomnia over time. *Source*: Adapted from Ref. 3.

leads to a new association of the bed/bedroom with not sleeping. In this model, individuals' attempts to cope with insomnia may maintain and actually exacerbate the disorder through strengthening such maladaptive associations. For example, an individual with insomnia may lie in bed awake for long periods of time, believing it is better to get rest. Or the individual may get up and do work in the bedroom when sleep is elusive. In both cases, the behavior results in a lower likelihood that the sleep stimuli of the bed/bedroom will elicit the desired response of falling asleep. The intervention arising from this theory is another that meets the American Psychological Association criteria for a well-validated treatment (4), as described in chapter 24.

HYBRID COGNITIVE-BEHAVIORAL MODEL (MORIN)

Morin's hybrid cognitive-behavioral model of insomnia (7) is an integrative model that incorporates individual, temporal, and environmental variables. A central factor of this model is hyperarousal. The hyperarousal can be cognitive affective, behavioral, or physiological. Conditioning can exacerbate arousal; for example, after sleeping poorly for several consecutive nights, an individual may begin to associate temporal (e.g., bedtime) or contextual (e.g., bedroom) stimuli with the responses of worry and fear of poor sleep—both of which are arousing. Such conditioning may occur at different rates among individuals, likely dependent on such factors as predisposition to insomnia and current daytime problems (e.g., interpersonal conflict).

In this model, individuals' sleeplessness leads to worry and rumination, along with misperceptions of sleep (e.g., distortions in how much time the individual believes he/she was awake during the night). Morin's model stipulates daytime consequences including fatigue and mood disturbance, which then trigger further worry and other negative cognitions about sleep. These negative cognitions play an important role in insomnia; for example, they may consist of unhelpful beliefs about sleep (i.e., if I don't get eight hours of sleep, I cannot function the next day). Such negative cognitions lead to emotional distress, which further exacerbates the insomnia. The result of this cycle of conditioning, arousal, worry and rumination, misperception, and daytime consequences is a sense of learned helplessness. The individual comes to believe that the insomnia is uncontrollable and unpredictable.

According to this model, to attempt to cope with insomnia, individuals develop maladaptive sleep habits such as excessive time in bed or daytime napping, which contribute to the maintenance of insomnia through preventing the development of a regular sleep–wake rhythm. Thus, in this model hyperarousal often serves as a trigger, but a multitude of factors such as maladaptive sleep habits or negative cognitions perpetuate the negative cycle. It is important to note that the consequences of sleeplessness can also serve as a further trigger for the cycle; that is, there is a bidirectional relationship among the variables. This theory has resulted in a form of cognitive-behavior therapy (7) that was manualized, tested, and shown to be an empirically supported treatment according to American Psychological Association criteria (4).

HYBRID COGNITIVE-BEHAVIORAL MODEL (LUNDH AND BROMAN)

Based on a detailed review of the existing empirical literature, Lundh and Broman (8) propose that there are two different categories of psychological processes involved in insomnia: (*i*) processes that *interfere* with sleep (e.g., cognitive, emotional, and physiological arousal, which may be due to stressful events or emotional conflicts, and may be moderated by various personality variables such as arousability, neuroticism, etc.) are referred to as *sleep-interfering processes;* and (*ii*) processes that make the individual perceive or *interpret* his or her sleep patterns in a distorted or otherwise dysfunctional manner (e.g., misperceptions of sleep, dysfunctional beliefs about sleep quantity requirements and consequences of not meeting these requirements, dysfunctional beliefs about natural variations in sleep, misattribution of negative aspects of daily functioning to poor sleep, attentional biases, etc.) are referred to as *sleep-interpreting processes.*

The central tenet of Lundh and Broman's model is that insomnia is the result of various combinations, and interactions, of sleep-interfering and sleep-interpreting processes. These two kinds of processes have a bidirectional relationship. For example, sleep-interfering arousal can lead to increasingly negative interpretations of sleep difficulties. Similarly, negative sleep-interpreting processes (dysfunctional beliefs about need to sleep, worries about sleep, rumination about causes and effects of poor sleep, etc.) can contribute to increases in sleep-interfering arousal.

Lundh and Broman argue that it is important to distinguish between these two types of processes as they may require different forms of treatment. In some cases, sleep-interfering processes may dominate and the treatment should focus on these (e.g., by emotional processing, training in relaxation or mindfulness skills, or stimulus control and sleep restriction techniques); in other cases sleep-interpreting processes may dominate, which require cognitive methods. In still other cases, both kinds of processes may be equally involved, causing various kinds of vicious cycles between cognition, behavior, and sleep-interfering arousal, and requiring both kinds of treatment approaches.

NEUROCOGNITIVE MODEL

The neurocognitive model (9) extends behavioral models by explicitly allowing for the possibility that conditioned *arousal* may act as a maintaining factor in insomnia. In this model, arousal includes somatic, cognitive, and cortical arousal. Somatic arousal corresponds to measures of metabolic rate, cognitive arousal typically refers to mental constructs like worry rumination, and cortical arousal refers to the level of cortical activation [primarily electroencephalography (EEG) activity, though cortical arousal may also include all CNS arousal]. Cortical arousal is hypothesized to occur as a result of classical conditioning and can lead to abnormal levels of sensory and information processing and long-term memory formation.

In this model, the cortical arousal phenomena become linked to sleep continuity disturbance and/or sleep state misperception (i.e., the individual judging that he was awake for a longer duration than actually occurred). In particular, enhanced sensory processing around sleep onset and during NREM sleep is thought to make the individual vulnerable to environmental stimuli (e.g., a noise outside on the street) interfering with sleep initiation and/or maintenance. Enhanced information processing (detection of, and discrimination between, stimuli and the formation of a short-term memory of the stimulating event) during NREM sleep may blur the distinction between sleep and wakefulness. That is, one cue for "knowing" that one is asleep is the lack of awareness for events occurring during sleep. Enhanced information processing may therefore account for the tendency in insomnia to judge PSG sleep as wakefulness (i.e., sleep state misperception). Finally, enhanced long-term memory (e.g., recollection of a stimulating event hours after its occurrence) around sleep onset and during NREM sleep may interfere with the subjective experience of sleep initiation and duration. Typically individuals cannot recall information from periods immediately prior to sleep, during sleep, or during brief arousals from sleep. An enhanced ability to encode and retrieve information in insomnia would thus be expected to influence judgments about sleep latency, wakefulness after sleep onset, and sleep duration.

PSYCHOBIOLOGICAL INHIBITION MODEL

Espie's psychobiological inhibition model of insomnia (10) includes psychological (cognitive and emotional), physiological, and environmental arousal in the maintenance of insomnia and proposes that insomnia results from chronic inhibition of homeostatic and circadian processes. This model of insomnia differs from many others in that the starting point is good sleep instead of pathology. Espie posits that in good sleepers homeostatic and circadian processes are involuntary and naturally default to good sleep. To maintain the automaticity and plasticity of these processes in good sleep, however, several critical component processes must occur, including sleep-related stimulus control (e.g., regular sleep habits), daytime facilitation of nighttime sleep (e.g., effective coping skills), sleep-related physiological dearousal, and sleep-related cognitive dearousal.

According to this model, insomnia results when there is a failure of these automated sleep activation and maintenance processes. In particular, inhibitory feedback from one or more of the psychobiological processes disrupts the automaticity and plasticity of the system and thus prevents normal sleep. For example, the automaticity of the process of sleep stimulus control would be weakened if an individual developed a conditioned association of sleep-incompatible activities (e.g., watching TV) with the bedroom environment. Another feature of this model is that it accounts for the contribution of daytime factors; for example, disturbed daytime affect could undermine cognitive and behavioral preparation for sleep.

Recently this model has been extended. Espie et al. (11) have proposed the importance of an attention–intention–effort pathway to explain how insomnia develops and to describe the critical factors that maintain it. Again, good sleep is considered to be a relatively automatic process, but this automaticity can be inhibited by attempts to control the process including three overlapping stages: (*i*) selective attention to sleep, (*ii*) explicit intention to sleep, and (*iii*) effort to sleep. In the first stage, selectively "attending" to sleep involves shifting attentional focus to sleep-salient stimuli, such as monitoring for signs inconsistent with sleep (12). The second part of the pathway, explicitly "intending" to sleep, is explained in part by examining the contrast whereby individuals who are good sleepers typically passively abandon wakefulness and fall into sleep, whereas individuals with insomnia try to initiate sleep, such as through thought control. This explicit intention—or the planning mode—is dysfunctional in that it inhibits normal dearousal, and thus the intention paradoxically inhibits sleep. The final stage is a further development of intention, whereby sleep "effort"—or the performing mode—includes two related processes: (*i*) direct (i.e., trying to force sleep to come) and (*ii*) indirect (i.e., increasing sleep opportunity, such as going to bed earlier). This final stage further inhibits sleep–wake automaticity.

In sum, this model starts with an assumption of good sleep and posits that in insomnia the automaticity of good sleep is interrupted via the attention, intention, and effort maintaining processes. The role of the attention–intention–effort pathway in this model suggests that cognitive-behavioral interventions that target and modify these processes may reduce insomnia and restore normal sleep.

COGNITIVE MODEL

According to Harvey's cognitive model of insomnia, insomnia is maintained by a cascade of cognitive processes that operate at night *and* during the day. The five key cognitive processes that comprise the cascade are worry (accompanied by arousal and distress), selective attention and monitoring, misperception of sleep and daytime deficits, unhelpful beliefs, and counterproductive safety behaviors (13). Two assumptions are made. First, the cognitive processes that are proposed to operate at night apply equally to difficulty getting to sleep at the beginning of the night and to difficulty getting back to sleep after waking during the night and to waking too early in the morning. Second, the maintaining processes described can "kick in" at any point in the model and as a consequence of either daytime or nighttime experiences.

This cognitive model suggests that worry in *the night* activates the sympathetic nervous system thereby triggering physiological arousal and distress. This combination of worry, arousal, and distress plunges the individual into an anxiety state (10). Research in cognitive psychology indicates that when one is anxious the range of stimuli in the environment that is attended to narrows (14) and attention is preferentially directed toward potential threats (15). On this basis the model suggests that the anxious state leads people with insomnia to narrow their attention and selectively attend to or monitor for sleep-related threats that might be internal stimuli (e.g., bodily sensations) and/or external stimuli (e.g., clock). As monitoring for threat increases the chance of detecting random and meaningless cues that can then be misinterpreted (16) and the aroused state means that there is likely to be an abundance of body sensations present to be detected, monitoring is likely to provide further cause for worry. Hence, a vicious cycle is established.

This model suggests that this cycle may help explain the robust finding that some individuals with insomnia overestimate the extent to which their sleep is inadequate. For example, in the time perception literature time seems longer when the number of units of information processed per unit of time increases (17). Hence, worry may distort the perception of how long it is taking to get to sleep (18). Monitoring increases the chance of detecting random and meaningless cues. These may then be misinterpreted as indicative of threat (16,19) that, in turn, contributes to misperception of sleep and/or daytime functioning. Of course, if an individual perceives they have not slept adequately a further cause for worry is established, thus fuelling the vicious cycle.

It is proposed that there are two additional exacerbating processes operating at night. First, unhelpful beliefs about sleep are likely to exacerbate worry (7). Second, in an attempt to cope with the escalating anxiety caused by the processes described, individuals with insomnia often make use of safety behaviors (20), such as drinking alcohol to reduce anxiety and promote sleep onset. A safety behavior is an overt or covert action that is adopted to avoid feared outcomes. The problem is that these behaviors (*i*) prevent the person experiencing disconfirmation of their unrealistic beliefs and (*ii*) may make the feared outcome more likely to occur (20).

The same cognitive processes are suggested to be operating during *the day*. For example, people with insomnia often worry during the day that they have not obtained sufficient sleep. This worry, in turn, triggers arousal and distress, selective attention and monitoring for sleep-related threats, misperception and the use of counterproductive safety behaviors. Each of these processes serves to maintain the insomnia. In addition, worry, arousal, and distress are likely to interfere with satisfying and effective daytime performance. Further, the use of safety behaviors can contribute to distress and worsening of sleep, as well as preventing disconfirmation of unhelpful beliefs.

It is suggested that these processes culminate in a *real sleep deficit*. Three points are relevant here. First, when an individual suffers from a real sleep deficit it is conceived to be the product of escalating anxiety that is not conducive to sleep onset (10) nor to effective daytime performance (21). Second, misperception of sleep and a real sleep deficit can coexist. An individual may report sleeping only two hours on a night but on polysomnography is shown to have slept for four hours. In this example, the individual is misperceiving his sleep *and* suffering from a serious real sleep deficit. Third, for the occasional individual with insomnia who *thinks* he is not getting enough sleep but, in reality, is sleeping sufficiently (sleep state misperception), the cognitive model suggests that such individuals will be at grave risk of getting trapped into becoming progressively more absorbed by and anxious about their sleep problem. The unfortunate consequence of this is that they are at high risk of developing a real sleep deficit. The process of empirically validating predictions from this model is ongoing (see Ref. 22 for a summary of evidence to date) and a treatment derived from the model has preliminary support in an open trial (23).

UNDERSTUDIED PSYCHOLOGICAL PROCESSES: AFFECT AND PERSONALITY

Within the psychological level of explanation for causal and maintaining factors in insomnia, the majority of the models reviewed have addressed behavioral and cognitive factors. However, it seems likely that other psychological processes, such as affect and personality, are also important.

The role of affect is increasingly recognized to be important across a number of psychiatric disorders (24). Following Gross (25), we use the term "affect" to include emotion (short-lived responses that involve changes in the behavioral, experiential, autonomic, and neuroendocrine systems), emotion episodes (emotions more extended in time and space), and mood (longer duration responses than emotions, more diffuse than emotions).

It is well established that insomnia is associated with psychiatric disorders characterized by affect regulation difficulties, such as depression, bipolar disorder, and anxiety disorders (26,27). However, there is minimal research on the role of presleep affect in insomnia. An interesting untested hypothesis is that individual differences in ability to downregulate affect could be a predisposing or perpetuating factor. One study that supports this hypothesis found that individuals with insomnia rated the impact of daily minor stressors and the intensity of major negative life events as higher than good sleepers (28). Furthermore, such individuals used more emotion-oriented coping strategies and had greater presleep arousal than good sleepers, while a path model indicated that emotion-focused coping indirectly negatively impacted sleep by increasing both the impact of stress and presleep cognitive arousal.

While in the previously paragraph we suggest that affect can negatively impact sleep, a further hypothesis is that the lack of sleep experienced by individuals with insomnia will adversely impact next-day affect. Accumulating evidence has begun to provide support for this possibility. For example, a number of investigators have examined daytime affect in individuals with insomnia. Buysse et al. (29) used ecological momentary assessment, a technique in which individuals report on their subjective experience in their natural context several times per day, to assess daytime symptoms in insomnia patients. Results demonstrated that individuals with insomnia endorsed lower positive moods and higher negative moods, including higher depression and anxiety scores, compared to good sleepers. Additionally, Riedel and Lichstein (30) reviewed studies examining daytime affective symptoms of insomnia. A small majority of studies utilizing three measures of affect (Beck Depression Inventory, the State-Trait Anxiety Inventory, and the Profile of Mood States) observed increases in depression and anxiety scores in individuals with insomnia.

A study by Yoo et al. (31) with healthy participants provides additional, though indirect, evidence for the possibility of insomnia affecting next-day affect. Healthy participants who were sleep deprived for 35 hours or who had slept normally completed an emotional stimulus viewing task (100 images varying in emotional intensity) in an event-related fMRI design. The two groups showed amygdala activation to negative picture stimuli. This was an anticipated result on the basis that the amygdala is involved in the generation of emotions and the development of emotional memories. However, relative to those who slept normally, those in the sleep deprived group exhibited more than 60% greater amygdala activity. Furthermore, this large increase was associated with a loss of activity in the medial prefrontal cortex (MPFC). The MPFC exerts top–down control on the limbic area (including the amygdala) and functions to modulate emotional responses so that they are appropriate for the context. Thus, this study suggests that sleep contributes to maintaining connectivity between the MPFC and amygdala, which is critical for responding appropriately to next-day emotional challenges.

Hence, the research to date provides initial support for the hypothesis that insomnia contributes to affective impairment and that affective impairment contributes to insomnia. However, affective theories of insomnia have not yet been developed. Future research testing the possibility that there may be a bidirectional relationship between affect and sleep may be a wise investment.

There is also limited research on the role of personality in insomnia. A few studies have found personality disturbances in individuals with insomnia, such as a higher score on the Neuroticism scale of the Eysenck Personality Questionnaire (e.g., Ref. 32) and an "abnormal" score on the Minnesota Multiphasic Personality Inventory (MMPI) (33–35). In particular, one study that used the MMPI found that individuals with insomnia demonstrated personality profiles suggestive of neurotic depression. Additionally, individuals with insomnia appeared to handle conflicts and stressors through internalizing emotions (as opposed to through irritability or hostility) (35). However, the research on this topic has been mostly correlational and thus the question remains as to whether personality characteristics predispose individuals to insomnia or result from insomnia.

CONTEXTUAL/ENVIRONMENTAL FACTORS

Context likely underlies the expression of and interaction between all the psychological factors we have discussed, including behavior, cognition, affect, and personality. The role of context, or environmental factors, is also understudied. Examples of potentially important contextual factors include bed partners who may interfere with each other's sleep through snoring, movement, or dyssynchronous bedtimes. Other contextual factors include the noise and safety levels of the environment that could lead to sleep disturbance and/or hypervigilance for threat. Increased use of technology and busier schedules may also impact insomnia through increased stress and poorer sleep habits.

CONCLUSION

A number of the important psychological models have been reviewed in this chapter, ranging from behavioral to cognitive to several hybrid cognitive-behavioral models. These substantial theoretical contributions have led to the development of numerous efficacious treatments (4), but more work remains. In particular, future research on the role of emotion, personality, and contextual factors could pave the way for even more successful treatments.

REFERENCES

1. Spielman AJ, Caruso LS, Glovinsky PB. A behavioral perspective on insomnia treatment. Psychiatr Clin North Am 1987; 10:541–553.
2. Spielman AJ. Assessment of insomnia. Clin Psychol Rev 1986; 6:11–25.
3. Glovinsky P, Spielman A. The insomnia answer: a personalized program for identifying and overcoming the three types of insomnia. New York: Penguin, 2006.
4. Morin CM, Bootzin RR, Buysse DJ, et al. Psychological and behavioral treatment of insomnia: an update of recent evidence (1998–2004). Sleep 2006; 29:1396–1406.
5. Spielman AJ, Saskin P, Thorpy MJ. Treatment of chronic insomnia by restriction of time in bed. Sleep 1987; 10:45–56.
6. Bootzin RR. Stimulus control treatment for insomnia. In: Proceedings of the American Psychological Association; 1972; Washington, D.C., 7:395–396.
7. Morin CM. Insomnia: Psychological Assessment and Management. New York: Guilford Press, 1993.
8. Lundh L-G, Broman J-E. Insomnia as an interaction between sleep-interfering and sleep-interpreting processes. J Psychosom Res 2000; 49:299–310.
9. Perlis ML, Giles DE, Mendelson WB, et al. Psychophysiological insomnia: the behavioural model and a neurocognitive perspective. J Sleep Res 1997; 6:179–188.
10. Espie CA. Insomnia: conceptual issues in the development, persistence, and treatment of sleep disorder in adults. Annu Rev Psychol 2002; 53:215–243.
11. Espie CA, Broomfield NM, MacMahon KM, et al. The attention-intention-effort pathway in the development of psychophysiologic insomnia: a theoretical review. Sleep Med Rev 2006; 10:215–245.
12. Semler CN, Harvey AG. Monitoring of sleep-related threat in primary insomnia: development and validation of the sleep associated monitoring inventory (SAMI). Psychosom Med 2004; 66:242–250.
13. Harvey AG. A cognitive model of insomnia. Behav Res Ther 2002; 40:869–894.
14. Easterbrook JA. The effect of emotion on cue utilization and the organization of behavior. Psychol Rev 1959; 66:183–201.
15. Dalgleish T, Watts FN. Biases of attention and memory in disorders of anxiety and depression. Clin Psychol Rev 1990; 10:589–604.
16. Clark DM. Anxiety disorders: why they persist and how to treat them. Behav Res Ther 1999; 37(suppl 1):S5–S27.
17. Thomas EA, Cantor NE. On the duality of simultaneous time and size perception. Percept Psychophys 1975; 18:44–48.
18. Borkovec TD. Insomnia. J Consult Clin Psychol 1982; 50:880–895.
19. Clark DM, Salkovskis PM, Ost L-G, et al. Misinterpretation of body sensations in panic disorder. J Consult Clin Psychol 1997; 65:203–213.
20. Salkovskis PM. The importance of behaviour in the maintenance of anxiety and panic: a cognitive account. Behav Psychother 1991; 19:6–19.
21. Eysenck MW. Attention and Arousal, Cognition and Performance. Berlin/New York: Springer-Verlag, 1982.
22. Harvey AG. A cognitive theory of and therapy for chronic insomnia. J Cogn Psychother Int Q 2005; 19:41–60.
23. Harvey AG. An open trial of cognitive therapy for insomnia. Behav Res Ther 2007; 45:2491–2501.
24. Rottenberg J, Johnson SL. Emotion and Psychopathology: Bridging Affective and Clinical Science. Washington, DC: American Psychological Association, 2007.
25. Gross JJ. The emerging field of emotion regulation: an integrative review. Rev Gen Psychol 1998; 2:271–299.

26. Benca RM, Obermeyer WH, Thisted RA, et al. Sleep and psychiatric disorders: a meta-analysis. Arch Gen Psychiatry 1992; 49:651–668.
27. Harvey AG. Sleep and circadian rhythms in bipolar disorder: seeking synchrony, harmony, and regulation. Am J Psychiatry 2008; 165:820–829.
28. Morin CM, Rodrigue S, Ivers H. Role of stress, arousal, and coping skills in primary insomnia. Psychosom Med 2003; 65:259–267.
29. Buysse DJ, Thompson W, Scott J, et al. Daytime symptoms in primary insomnia: a prospective analysis using ecological momentary assessment. Sleep Med 2007; 8:198–208.
30. Riedel BW, Lichstein KL. Insomnia and daytime functioning. Sleep Med Rev 2000; 4:277–298.
31. Yoo S, Gujar N, Hu P, et al. The human emotional brain without sleep—a prefrontal amygdala disconnect. Curr Biol 2007; 17:877–878.
32. Adam K, Tomeny M, Oswald I. Physiological and psychological differences between good and poor sleepers. J Psychiatr Res 1986; 20:301–316.
33. Monroe LJ. Psychological and physiological differences between good and poor sleepers. J Abnorm Psychol 1967; 72:255–264.
34. Schneider-Helmert D. Twenty-four-hour sleep-wake function and personality patterns in chronic insomniacs and healthy controls. Sleep 1987; 10:452–462.
35. Kales A, Caldwell AB, Soldatos CR, et al. Biopsychobehavioral correlates of insomnia. II. Pattern specificity and consistency with the Minnesota Multiphasic Personality Inventory. Psychosom Med 1983; 45:341–356.

6 Sleep EEG in Patients with Primary Insomnia

Michael Perlis and Phil Gehrman
Department of Psychiatry, University of Pennsylvania, Philadelphia, Pennsylvania, U.S.A.

Mario Terzano
Department of Neurology, University of Parma, Parma, Italy

Kimberly Cote
Department of Psychology, Brock University, St. Catharines, Ontario, Canada

Dieter Riemann
Center for Sleep Research and Sleep Medicine, Department of Psychiatry, Freiburg University, Freiburg, Germany

INTRODUCTION

With the advent of the electroencephalographic study of sleep (1–3) and the more comprehensive methodology of polysomnography (4), the era of the objective assessment of sleep had arrived. Along with this technology, came the promise that sleep related complaints could be accounted for by abnormal physiologic function during sleep. That is, it was believed that the simultaneous and long duration monitoring of sleep continuity and sleep architecture along with pulmonary, cardiac, motor, and cortical function would reveal the abnormalities that account for sleep initiation and maintenance problems, the report of shallow and/or fragmented and/or nonrestorative sleep, and/or the diurnal complaints of sleepiness and fatigue. To a large extent this promise was realized for the complaint of shallow and/or fragmented and/or nonrestorative sleep, and/or the diurnal complaints of pathologic sleepiness. The polysomnographic study of sleep revealed that these complaints were, in large measure, directly related to sleep disordered breathing. The promise, however, was not realized for the complaint of insomnia (sleep initiation and maintenance problems). In fact, the very effort to objectively measure sleep continuity disturbance[1] raised more questions than it answered. That is, the objective assessment of sleep with electroencephalography brought into sharp resolution that remarkable discrepancies existed between the subjective and objective measure of sleep latency, wake after sleep onset, number of awakenings, and total sleep time (4,5). Further, no evidence was obtained for physiologic abnormalities that clearly accounted for difficulty initiating or maintaining sleep (e.g., abnormal REM pressure, slow wave sleep deficiency, sleep onset related central apneic events, sleep induced cardiac or CNS irregularities, etc.). At best some of these factors were found to be indicative of "Secondary Insomnia" and particularly the sleep of patients with major depression (6,7).

The lack of obvious abnormalities resulted in a new program of research, one that was focused on the effort to document that physiologic and/or cognitive hyperarousal is pathognomic for primary insomnia[2]. This program of research yielded a variety of findings and theories, all of which provide partial support for the "hyperarousal hypotheses" (8). Interestingly, these efforts also gave rise to a fundamentally new concept with respect to the etiology and pathophysiology of insomnia—the concept that the primary defect in primary insomnia may be less related to "hyperarousal" and more related to "the failure to inhibit wakefulness" (9).

[1] Sleep Continuity refers to the collection of variables that correspond to sleep initiation and maintenance, including Sleep Latency (SL), Wake After Sleep Onset (WASO), Number of Awakenings (NWAK), and Total Sleep Time (TST). While the term is not formally part of the sleep lexicon, it has the heuristic value of being a global term whose meaning may be contrasted with the class of variables that correspond to "Sleep Architecture".

[2] For the purposes of this chapter, the term "primary insomnia" is meant to be synonymous with psychophysiologic insomnia.

In this chapter, information will be provided regarding the findings from all of the EEG based technologies including those from Polysomnography (PSG), Quantitative Electroencephalography (QEEG), Cyclic Alternating Patterns analysis (CAPs) and Event-Related Potentials (ERPs).

EEG SLEEP CONTINUITY MEASURES

When assessed with the sleep EEG, patients with primary insomnia, on average, do exhibit problems with initiating and maintaining sleep. The sleep continuity abnormalities, however, are generally less severe than when assessed by self report (4,5,10–19). These incongruities appear to various extents in at least two forms of primary insomnia including both psychophysiologic insomnia and paradoxical insomnia (formerly referred to as sleep state misperception insomnia) but may or may not be characteristic of "secondary insomnia" [c.f. Perlis 2000 (19)]. These "subjective-objective" discrepancies, it should also be noted, occur for when subjects are queried about their state of consciousness when awakened from polysomnographically defined sleep.

Subjective vs. PSG Measures of Sleep Continuity

As noted above, patients with primary insomnia tend to overestimate how long it takes them to fall asleep and the amount of time that they are awake over the course of the night when compared with objective assessments. Good sleepers tend to estimate correctly how long it takes them to fall asleep, and if a trend is evident, they tend to overestimate the amount of sleep they obtain. Both patients with insomnia and good sleepers, when compared to polysomnographic measures, tend to underestimate number of awakenings or number of nocturnal arousals. This last finding may be an artifact of the manner in which sleep is scored. Most laboratories score in 30-second epochs and thus intervals as brief as 16 seconds may be categorized as wakefulness and/or as separate bouts of wakefulness. Such extremely brief awakenings may not be recalled by either good sleepers or patients with insomnia (20,21) and/or in the case of patients with insomnia may be perceived as continuous wakefulness. Figure 1 depicts "subjective-objective" discrepancies as they occur in patients with primary insomnia, insomnia comorbid with Depression, and in Good sleeper subjects (19,22).

The Perception of PSG Sleep

When awakened from polysomnographically verified sleep, patients with primary insomnia more frequently report having been awake than good sleeper subjects (11,23–25). On average, the patient with insomnia tends to identify PSG sleep as wakefulness 73% of the time. Good sleepers identify PSG sleep as wakefulness between 45% and 50% of the time. These kinds of findings vary as a function of number of sleep study nights, sleep stage from which the subject is awakened, and the manner in which the subject is awakened. The discrepancy between PSG sleep and subjective impression, however, is most evident for awakenings that occur shortly after sleep onset(s) (26).

EEG SLEEP AND SLEEP ARCHITECTURE

While there is a long standing tradition of research regarding sleep architectural abnormalities in psychiatry illness, especially major depression, there is remarkably little work on such abnormalities as they occur with primary insomnia. In the case of major depression, where there are hundreds of studies over thousands of subjects, there appears to be a reasonably reliable constellation of sleep architectural abnormalities including short REM Latency, a prolonged first REM period, increased REM Density, increased REM percent, and diminished slow wave sleep (SWS) (7).

The dearth of PSG studies in primary insomnia is partly related to at least three factors. First, insomnia's characterization as only a "symptom" discouraged the effort to characterize it as a unique disease state. Second, studies conducted prior to 1990 (prior to the publication of the ICSD or the DSM-IV) relied on definitions of insomnia that were nonstandard and study protocols that did not have exclusions for medical and psychiatric illnesses and/or medications known to affect PSG sleep. As a result, the findings were mixed, and when trends were available, they were remarkably like those seen with major depression.

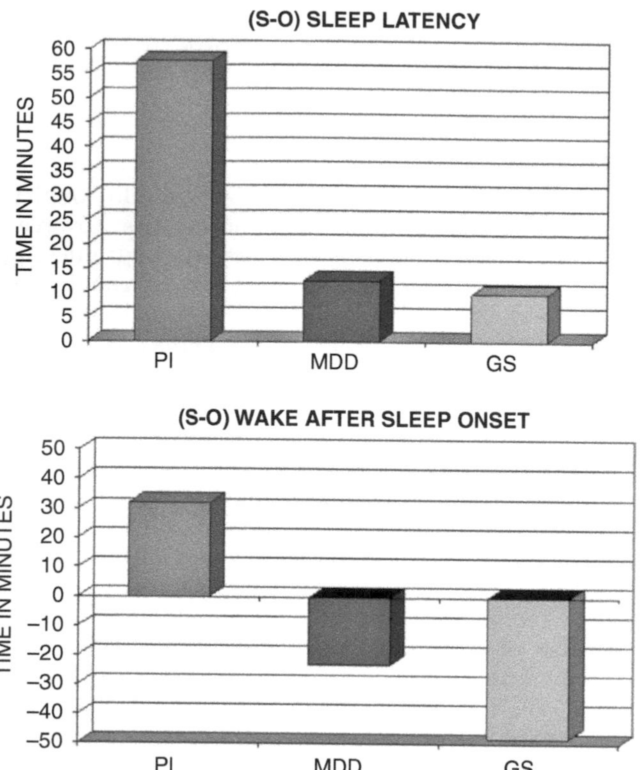

Figure 1 In both figures, time in minutes are difference scores between the group average subjective values and the objective values. For example, if subjective SL = 90 and the objective SL = 30 then the difference score if 60 minutes. Accordingly, these difference scores represent the absolute magnitude of the "sub-ob discrepancies" as seen in PI, MDD and GS subjects.

Third, insomnia's characterization, prior to and after 1990, as a disorder of initiation and maintenance of sleep (DIMS) came with the suggestion that sleep continuity disturbance was the (vs. a) defining attribute of insomnia and thus many PSG studies of insomnia simply did not contain sleep architecture data.

With these caveats in mind, the PSG findings in insomnia from 1975 to 1989 insomnia were characterized by Benca and colleagues in 1992 (7). This metaanalytic study summarized the results from 25 investigations in patients with insomnia. The findings for patients with insomnia, and nine other psychiatric patient classifications, were expressed as whether they significant differed from values calculated for healthy good sleepers. The results from this study suggested that patients with insomnia exhibit reduced SWS%. REM% and REM latency were found to be within normal limits. Data for stage 1 and stage 2 were not reported.

In order to assess whether these results are also typical of a more modern cohort, a set of 17 studies from 1994 to the present was reviewed. All the studies included in this review (1) used ICSD or DSM-IV definitions of insomnia, (2) reported one or more sleep architectural findings, and (3) indicated that patients were medication free at the time of study. Most of the studies for this review had small samples although there were two investigations with samples of 100 or more subjects (27,28). Table 1 provides a list of these studies, their findings, and study related information. The sleep architecture findings are summarized below by stage of sleep.

Stage 1%: One study reported a statistical tendency ($p < 0.10$) for stage 1% to be increased in patients with primary insomnia as compared to good sleepers (28). Fifteen studies report no difference and one study does not provide data (29).

Table 1 Sleep Architecture Findings in Primary Insomnia

Authors	Sample	STG1	STG2	SWS	REM	RL	Date	Citation
Lichstein et al.	20	—	—	—	—		1994	Sleep 17: 693–402
Bonnet & Arand	10	—	↓	—	↓	(↑)	1995	Sleep 18: 581–588
Lamarche & Ogilvie	6	—	—	—	—	—	1997	Sleep 20: 724–733
Dorsey & Bootzin	18	—	—	—	—	—	1997	Biol Psychiatry 41: 209–216
Edinger et al. Crenshaw & Edinger	32	—		—		—	1997	Sleep 20: 1119–1126 Physiology & Behavior 66: 485–492
Stepanski et al.	10	—	—	—	—	—	2000	Sleep 23: 1–5
Edinger et al.	31			↓			2000	Physiology & Behavior 70: 127–134
Rosa & Bonnet	121	—	—	—	—	—	2000	Psychosom Med 62: 474–482
Edinger et al.	35	—	—	—	—	—	2001	Sleep 24: 761–770
Riemann et al.	10	—	—	—	—	—	2002	Psychiat Res 113: 11–27
Means et al.	52	—	—	—	—		2003	Sleep Med 4: 285–296
Bastein et al.	20	—	—				2003	J Psychosom Res 54: 39–49
Backhaus et al.	16	—	—	↓	—	—	2006	Biol Psychiat
Burgos et al.	11	—	—	—	—	—	2006	Brain Behav Immun 20: 246–253
Orff et al.	32	—	—	—	—		2007	Sleep 30: 1205–1211
Bastien et al.	15	—	—	—	↓		2008	Sleep 31: 887–898
Feige et al.	100	(↑)	—	—	↓	—	2008	J Sleep Res 17: 180–190
# supportive studies		1	1	2	3	1		

Stage 2: One study reported differences for this stage of sleep. Bonnet & Arand (1995) (30) found that patients with insomnia exhibited a slight decrease in stage 2 percent. Fourteen studies report no difference and two studies do not provide these data (29,31).

SWS: Two studies describe a reduction of SWS percent in insomniacs compared to controls (29,32). Fourteen studies report no difference and one study did not provide these data (33).

REM: Three studies described significantly reduced REM sleep percent in insomnia (28,30,34). Eleven studies report no difference and three studies do not provide these data (29,31,33).

REM latency: One study described a statistical tendency for REM latency to be prolonged in patients with insomnia (30). Seven studies report no difference (27–29,31,32,35–37) and nine studies do not provide these data.

Apart from naturalistic studies, there are two investigations that probe the issue of SWS deficiency and/or sleep homeostasis dysregulation as it occurs in patients with insomnia in response to sleep deprivation. Besset and colleagues (38) conducted a study in which patients with primary insomnia were subjected to a partial sleep deprivation protocol (three hour sleep) and then allowed a recovery sleep period of 10 hour on the following night. Both the PI and GS subjects exhibited increase in total sleep time and SWS percent. When compared to good sleepers, the patients with PI exhibited a smaller increase in total sleep time (although a comparable percent) and a smaller increase in SWS minutes (although a comparable percent). Stepanski et al. (2000) (39) found that patients with primary insomnia, when sleep deprived for approximately 36 hours, exhibited larger increases in total sleep time, but a smaller percentage increase in SWS than good sleepers.

In sum, the most conservative interpretation of the findings to date is that patients with insomnia do not exhibit reliably altered sleep architecture. If trends exist, they do so as cohort effects or relative to probative conditions. With respect to cohort effects, the earlier generation of studies tended to show reduced slow wave sleep percent as a feature of insomnia while the later generation studies tend to show reduced REM percent. With respect to probative conditions, there is mixed evidence that patients with insomnia exhibit a reduced capacity to generate SWS in response to sleep loss. Given these findings, clearly further research is needed where such studies may benefit by having large samples, the use of both absolute and percent time (differences may exist for the former where they do not for the latter), the application of quantitative electroencephalographic techniques to quantify SWS activity, and/or the use of challenge paradigms to resolve underlying abnormalities.

QUANTITATIVE ELECTROENCEPHALOGRAPHY

Quantitative electroencephalography (QEEG) refers to a group of mathematical techniques used for detecting periodicities within time series data. The techniques include, but are not limited to, power spectral analysis (PSA) and digital period analysis (DPA). As employed within electroencephalography, the technique is used to deconstruct complex waveforms into their constituent frequencies. In the case of PSA, quantification is accomplished by determining the amount of voltage that occurs per bin and/or prespecified bandwidth. This technique and related techniques have been extensively used to quantify delta frequency EEG in good sleepers (during normal sleep or manipulations like constant routine schedules or sleep deprivation). The technique has also been used to quantify high frequency EEG activity in the 14 to 45 Hz range in both good sleepers and in patients with insomnia.

High frequency EEG was first observed in the waking state by Berger in 1937. He hypothesized that such activity, observed during mental arithmetic, must be a "material concomitant of mental processes" (40). In the last two decades, there has been substantial work indicating that during wakefulness high frequency EEG activity in the beta (14–35 Hz) and gamma (35–45 Hz) ranges is associated with attention in animals [e.g., (41,42)] and with attention, perception, and, more generally, cognitive function in humans (43–58).

Recently, eight investigations have demonstrated that patients with insomnia exhibit an unusual amount of beta EEG activity during polysomnographically-monitored sleep (59–66). The majority of the investigations found that the increase in beta activity was apparent in patients with insomnia compared to good sleeper controls for time period's at/around sleep onset and/or during NREM sleep. These findings were based on (1) EEG measurements from central sites using monopolar or bipolar measures that included C3, Cz or C4, and O2, (2) relative, as opposed to absolute, measures of power density, and (3) definitions of beta activity ranging from 14 to 32 Hz. Three studies provided evidence that increased beta activity during sleep occurs specifically in association with primary, as opposed to secondary, insomnia (63,64,66). Two studies provided data to suggest that patients with insomnia also have more beta activity during REM sleep (60,61). One study indicated that beta activity varies with clinical course given nonpharmacological interventions (65). The most recent study of high frequency EEG activity in patients with insomnia suggests that women with primary insomnia, but not men, showed increased high-frequency and low-frequency EEG activity during NREM sleep compared to good sleepers. Figure 2 represents the all night distribution of delta and beta activity in good sleepers and in patients with primary insomnia.

While the data acquired from this measurement strategy appear to support the perspective that cortical arousal may be a biomarker for insomnia (and this is theoretically appealing to the extent that the increased occurrence of beta and gamma activity is thought to be permissive of increased sensory and information processing), the lack of replication across large scale contemporary investigations (e.g., 67) and unpublished studies (Buysse D, personal communication, 2005; Perlis M, personal communication, 2005) suggests that this approach has some limitations. In our hands, the occurrence of beta and gamma activity varies not only with trait considerations (diagnostic category) but also appears to be mediated/moderated by a variety of factors including:

- Whether or not the patient experiences a first night effect or a reverse-first night effect (a precedent also exists in the published literature) (e.g., 68)
- Whether or not the patient experiences a good night's sleep in relation to the amount of prior sleep loss or amount of prior wakefulness (i.e., increased homeostatic pressure for sleep)
- The extent to which circadian dysrhythmia contributes to the insomnia (e.g., delayed sleep phase syndrome subjects would be expected to show more beta/gamma activity when attempting to sleep in a nonpreferred sleep phase)

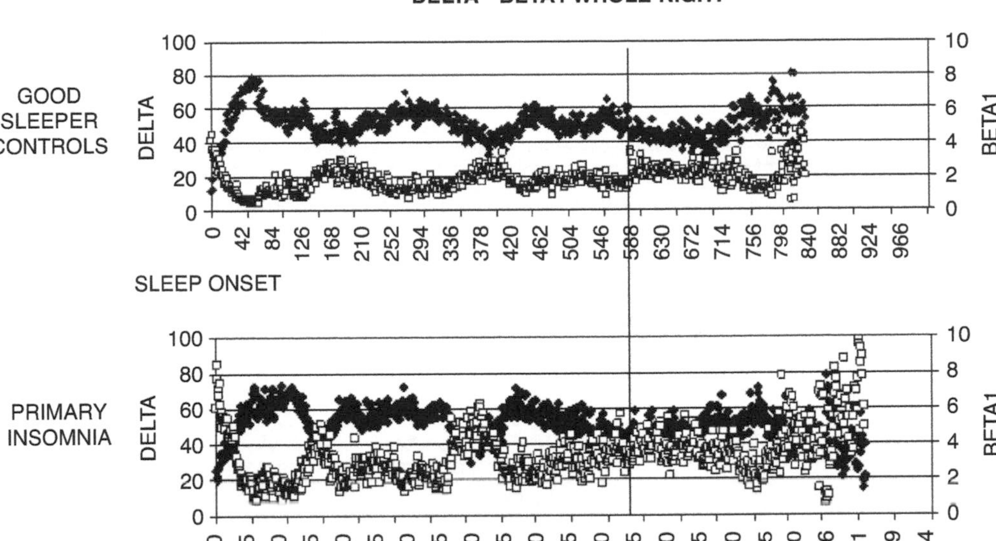

Figure 2 In both figures, (1) the left and right ordinates represent relative power [e.g., (beta power/total power)], (2) the abscissa represents time (from sleep onset, in 30 second increments, to sleep offset), (3) the black boxes represent delta power and the white boxes represent beta power, (4) the data are average plots for nine individuals per group.

- Technical considerations regarding how the EEG signals are acquired (e.g., signals transmitted over long cable runs may significantly alter the power spectrum)
- Ambient noise in the recording/sleep environment (e.g., sound, light, temperature, etc.)

The extent to which one or more of these factors obscure simple group contrasts underscores the need to identify a biomarker, probe, or challenge paradigm that provides for stable group characterizations of the phenomena that contribute to the occurrence of and/or severity of insomnia.

CYCLIC ALTERNATING PATTERN

The cyclic alternating pattern (CAP) is a periodic EEG activity of sleep that occurs spontaneously throughout NREM sleep (69,70). CAP is characterized by repetitive slow (high amplitude bursts) and fast EEG transients that are distinct from background EEG activity and recur at up to one minute intervals (see Figure 3 for examples of NCAP and CAP). CAPs occur following cerebral activation (phase A) and cerebral deactivation (phase B). A CAP cycle is composed of a phase A and the following phase B. Two or more CAP cycles constitute a CAP sequence. CAP sequences have no upper limits either on overall duration or on the number of CAP cycles. CAP sequences, during the A Phase, may be further categorized into subtypes (71): A1 which is represented by EEG synchrony; A2 which is a mixed signal (slow and fast rhythms); and A3 which is largely low voltage fast frequency signal. CAP sequences, as opposed to NCAP, are thought to be indicative of unstable sleep (72). NCAP and CAP sequences are illustrated below.

CAP sequences can be identified by computer assisted devices. In brief, the metrics of the PSG derived CAP analysis is based on the quantification of CAP time (the time duration of all CAP sequences) and CAP rate (the ratio between CAP time and NREM sleep time). To date, CAP rate has been show to be correlated with self-reported sleep quality [in both good sleepers (73) and in patients with insomnia] and with treatment outcome (74).

In the case of good sleepers (74), it was found that auditory stimulation across four sound intensities (white noise at 45 dBA, 55 dBA, 65 dBA and 75 dBA) resulted in a linear increase in CAP rate and these changes were significantly correlated with self reported sleep quality.

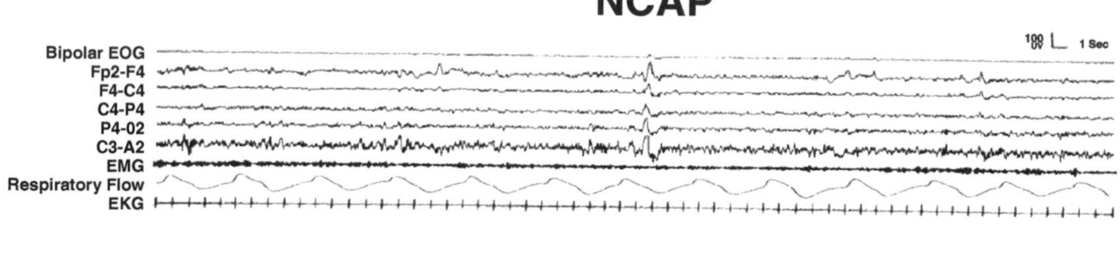

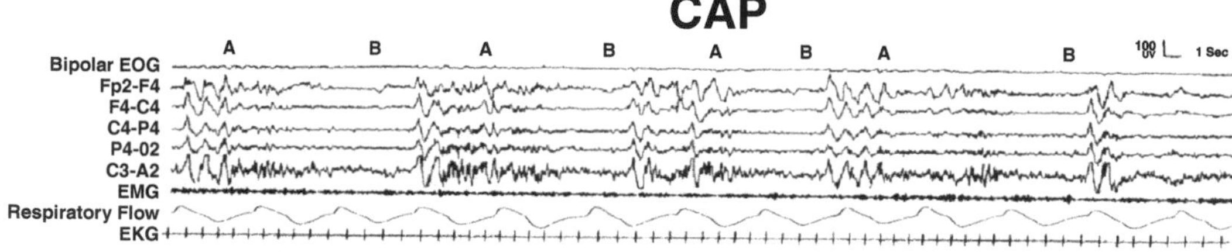

Figure 3 The letter designations "A" and "B" represent phase A and B CAPS. Fp2-F4, F4-C4, C4-P4, P4–02, are bipolar EEG derivations. C3-A2 is a monopolar derivation (typically used for sleep scoring) EMG is mentalis electromyogram EKG is an electrocardiograph tracing.

In the case of patients with insomnia (74), it was found that, under placebo conditions, patients exhibited a significantly higher CAP rate than did controls (evident for subtypes A1 and A2 but not A3). Treatment with several medications [zolpidem (10 mg), triazolam (0.25 mg), zopiclone (7.5 mg), brotizolam (0.25 mg)] significantly reduced CAP rates, although only for subtypes A1 and A2 (74). Finally, sleep quality was significantly improved by the use of hypnotics, and improved sleep quality was significantly correlated with CAP rate.

These data suggest that "hyperarousal" within NREM sleep can be assessed in terms of CAP rate and that the association of CAP rate with sleep quality suggests that this form of arousal during sleep (or processes associated with this form of arousal) may undermine sleep's capacity to be restorative.

EVENT-RELATED POTENTIALS (ERPs)

ERPs are EEG-based brain potentials that occur in response to sensory stimulation and represent the timing and extent of information processing. (75,76) They provide information on how quickly a stimulus is identified and encoded and the degree of attentional resources allocated to processing. ERPs vary predictably with changes in arousal and attention, (77) and have been well described in healthy good sleepers. They have been used as an index of attention during alert and drowsy wakefulness, at sleep onset and during sleep (77–81).

The most common ERP paradigm applied in sleep research is the auditory odd-ball task, where a rare 'deviant' tone is presented at random in a train of frequently occurring 'standard' tone pips (75). EEG is then averaged over numerous trials for each stimulus category and the ERP emerges as a series of peaks and troughs in a waveform which represent the brain's processing of the stimuli. ERPs elicited in this task between 50 and 350+ ms are most sensitive to changes in arousal and attention (77,82). The earliest peaks, N1 and P2, are elicited by both standard and deviant stimuli. N1 is a negative peak around 80 to 120 ms that represents early sensory processing such as encoding (75,76,82). P2 is a positive wave around 175 to 225 ms, which is thought to index the degree to which stimuli are inhibited or blocked (83). P300 is a large amplitude positive wave, which peaks around 300 ms when the target stimulus has been detected (84). The parietal maximum P300 wave generally reflects conscious detection of the target and stimulus discrimination. One variation of the oddball task involves stimuli that are presented rapidly. This elicits the mismatch negativity (MMN) waveform, which is thought to reflect automatic processing of stimulus change in a repetitive stimulus stream or attentional switching (85).

Based on ERP studies in good sleepers (77,80,81,85–94) one would expect signs of hyperarousal and/or deficits in inhibition in patients with insomnia to appear as larger N1, smaller P2, and larger P300 amplitudes in wakefulness. One would also expect N350 to be smaller in poor sleepers. Figure 4 represents the transition from wakefulness to sleep and the changes that one would expect in patients with chronic insomnia.

To date, there have been two types of studies applying ERPs to investigate the phenomena of insomnia: (1) a number of studies have examined information processing in patients with insomnia during wakefulness (95–99) (2) two studies have investigated ERPs at sleep onset or during early NREM sleep (34,100).

ERPs During Wakefulness

Early studies employing peak-to-peak measurement techniques reported equivocal results with respect to N1 and P2 amplitude to varying stimulus intensities (95,98). More recent studies employing baseline to peak measurement provide a clearer picture. Wang et al.(99) examined MMN during wakefulness while performing a distracter task in patients with insomnia and in good sleepers. Poor sleepers had larger amplitude MMN at frontal sites that was correlated with depression and impulsivity scores. These findings reflect hyperactivity in the patient group, which the authors suggested, was related to weak gating mechanisms.

Devoto et al. (96,97) proposed that waking hyperarousal may be more of a state-like phenomena which would only be associated with a relatively poor night of sleep. To test this, they investigated ERPs in the morning following a good and poor night of sleep in patients with primary insomnia compared to good sleepers (99). Insomnia patients had larger P300 amplitudes at Fz compared to good sleepers, but only following a poor night of sleep. Investigators interpreted the enhanced P300 as cortical hyperarousal, and speculated that it was also present in the pre-sleep and sleep period. As a follow-up, Devoto et al. (97) then repeated the study with ERP recordings in both the evening (30 min before bed) and morning (30 min after awakening) for one week at home (96). They again found that P300 at Fz was enhanced in the poor sleeper group compared to good sleepers, for the worst but not best night of the week. The authors concluded that hyperarousal varies night to night with quality of sleep, and that it begins in the pre-sleep period. In a commentary, Colrain (101) pointed out the preliminary nature of these data because of the small sample and effect sizes, and the atypical frontal distribution of the peak.

Taken together, the studies during wakefulness suggest that there is evidence of hyperarousal or enhanced information processing and attention during wakefulness in patients with insomnia. Given the paucity of research in this area, the preliminary nature of many of these reports, and the disparate methodology, it would be appropriate to further investigate waking ERPs in order to determine when hyperarousal is present in wakefulness (e.g., only the pre-sleep onset period or all day; only surrounding subjectively bad nights or as a trait-like phenomena; or only in some subtypes of insomnia).

ERPs at Sleep Onset and/or During Early NREM Sleep

There are only two published reports which have applied ERPs to the problem of insomnia by investigating the period of time in which they report their sleep difficulties (34,100). Yang and Lo (100) examined the first five-minute of stage 2 sleep and found that patients with insomnia had larger N1 and smaller P2 amplitudes to deviant tones, and smaller N350 amplitude to standard tones (100). These differences, which were not evident for whole night averages, were taken to mean that there is an enhancement in attention and a reduction in the inhibitory process at sleep onset. Although these findings are consistent with a view of hyperarousal, some caution should be taken in interpretation because the sleep onset period itself was not examined (i.e., the transition from wake to stage 1 to stage 2), ERPs were averaged from a brief five-minute period, and K-complexes were not removed from the averages. Moreover, since N1 and P2 changes were only noted for the rare deviant stimuli, replication is needed to establish reliability of findings.

Bastien and colleagues investigated good sleepers and patients with psychophysiological insomnia who had either sleep onset and/or sleep maintenance complaints (34). Waking ERPs were recorded during evening and morning over four nights, whereas ERPs during sleep onset

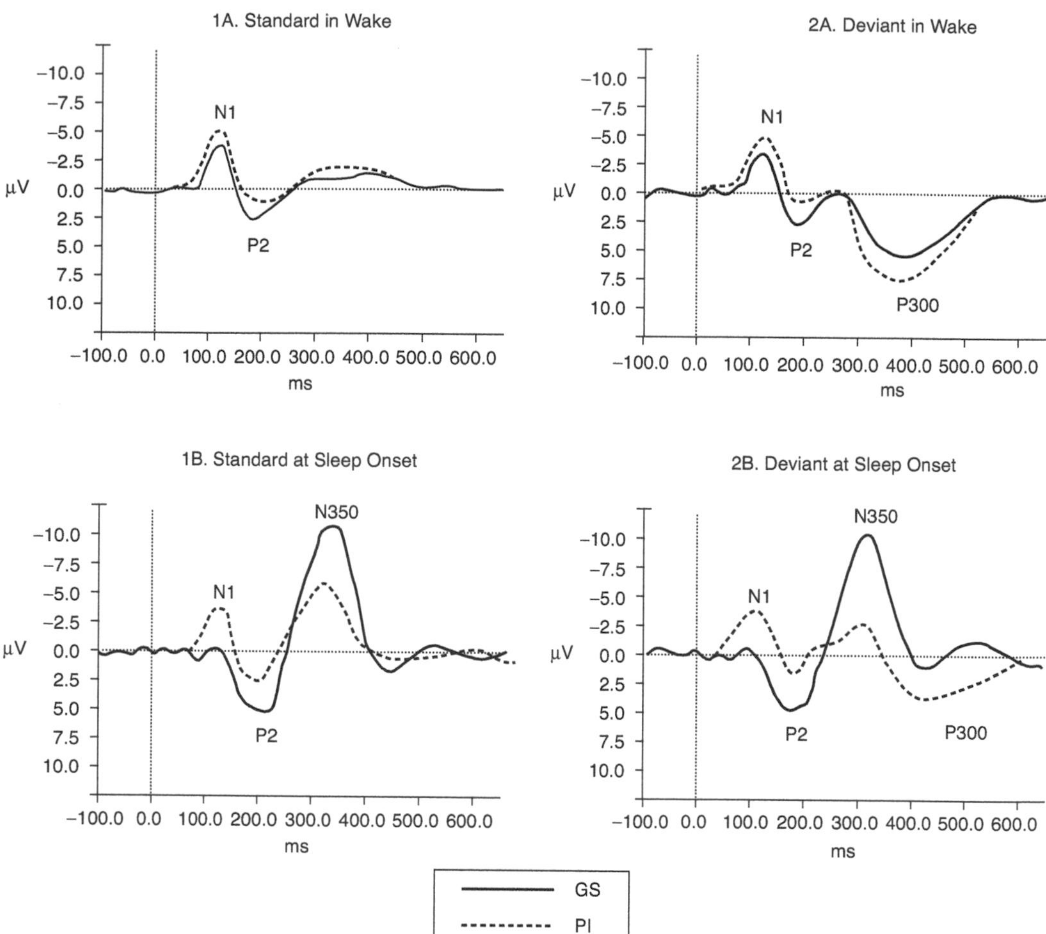

Figure 4 Theoretical ERP waveforms following standard and deviant stimuli in good sleepers (GS) and patients with primary insomnia (PI) in an alert waking state (1A and 2A) and at sleep onset (1B and 2B). Panel 1A: In attentive wakefulness, GS have a large N1 and a small P2 peak. PIs should have a larger N1 and smaller P2 depicting heightened attention. PIs may also show the sleep-related N350 reflecting sleepiness. Panel 1B: At sleep onset in GS, N1 decreases to baseline while P2 increases in amplitude reflecting that attention is disengaged. For PIs, it is expected that N1 might remain large and P2 small (similar to wakefulness) reflecting failure to inhibit. Research shows a smaller N350 emerging at sleep onset in PIs compared to controls, reflecting a failure of sleep inhibition processes. Panel 2A: N1 and P2 appear similar following the standard and deviant stimuli in GS, but it is possible that early sensory processing of the deviant may differ for PIs. In GS, the large P300 reflects conscious detection of the deviant in waking-attend conditions. Waking P300 has been reported by Devoto et al to be larger in amplitude for PIs compared to GS reflecting hyperarousal. Panel 2B: In GS, P300 is diminished at sleep onset (i.e., present in stage 1 when there is a behavioral response but absent in stage 2). For PIs, it is theorized that P300 may be larger in early or late stage 1 or remain present in stage 2 sleep.

were investigated during a single night. Participants were instructed to ignore tones in a classic oddball paradigm. In-wake, N1 to the standard tone was larger for patients than controls on the fourth night at Pz, and larger on the fourth morning at both Cz and Pz sites. There were no P2 or P300 differences. These data are in agreement with some previous reports of increased N1 in wakefulness reflecting hyperarousal and attentiveness (98,100). To examine the sleep onset period, ERPs were averaged to stimuli presented from lights out to any sign of stage 2 sleep, and the K-complexes were appropriately excluded from averages. The authors observed that N350 was smaller in patients with insomnia compared to good sleepers at sleep onset, which reflects a failure of the inhibition processes needed to initiate sleep. In addition, the authors observed a smaller N1 to standards at Cz, and a larger P2 to deviants at Pz in patients with insomnia compared to good sleepers. These results are contrary to what would be expected based on selective attention research, (77) and what has been found to date with waking ERPs in patients with insomnia. Replication is necessary given that only a single sleep onset period was observed, ERPs were collapsed across wake and stage 1, and results were not consistent at all sites or apparent in both categories of stimuli.

The data from these two reports of ERPs at sleep onset and during early NREM sleep are in agreement in some respects, but not others. It is thus important that this area be pursued through further study. It is necessary that researchers collect enough ERP trials for reliable averaging (e.g., through more stimuli delivered, and more subjects or multiple nights). The findings on N350 are most compelling to date; N350 may be a sensitive metric of deficits in information processing associated with sleep initiation problems in particular. It will also be important to carefully select patient samples, by ensuring they do not have comorbid medical conditions and by systematically investigating differences between qualitatively different types of insomnia (e.g., sleep onset versus maintenance complaints). Finally, the sleep period itself needs to be more systematically investigated, particularly for those with sleep maintenance complaints, to investigate information processing in NREM stages at various times of night and in REM sleep periods.

CONCLUDING COMMENTS

In many ways, the assessment of the sleep EEG in primary insomnia is in its infancy. This is ironic in that that insomnia is likely to be the oldest established diagnostic entity of the various sleep disorders and it was likely the first to be studied with most, if not all, EEG techniques. This said, it is an inescapable fact that each methodological approach has been applied to the problem of insomnia in only a few dedicated studies where each of the studies are generally on very small samples. Thus, at this point in time, it is difficult to definitively say whether subjects with primary insomnia reliably exhibit any form of abnormal sleep EEG and it is nearly impossible to make claims about how the types (e.g., psychophysiologic, paradoxical, idiopathic insomnia) subtypes (i.e., initial, middle, late or mixed insomnia) or the comorbid insomnias (insomnia comorbid with psychiatric or medical illnesses) are similar to, or different from, primary insomnia on EEG measures.

At the present time, the following claims can be made, albeit tentatively

- Sleep continuity disturbance as measured by PSG tends to be more normal than is measured by self-report. This suggests that there is a tendency to report more insomnia severity than exists or that patients are reporting phenomena that are not properly assessed by polysomnography (102).
- Sleep architecture does not appear reliably altered in patients with primary insomnia, and to the extent that trends are evident they exist as modest alterations to SWS and REM sleep. This suggests that systems that are responsible for the regulation of these forms of sleep are not related to sleep induction and maintenance. This said it seems likely that SWS (as it related to sleep homeostasis) would be altered in insomnia (103). Resolution of effects within this domain may require more than naturalistic studies but instead challenge paradigms that use sleep deprivation, pharmacologic probes or treatment as ways of assessing the functioning of these systems.
- QEEG abnormalities have been reported where the primary finding is in terms of elevated beta/gamma frequency activity around sleep onset and during NREM sleep (104). These findings have been interpreted as supporting that hyperarousal is a primary etiologic factor in insomnia.
- CAP irregularities have been shown to be correlated with self-reported sleep quality and to be associated with treatment outcome. These findings have been interpreted as supporting that hyperarousal is a primary etiologic factor in insomnia.
- ERP activity appears to be altered in patients with insomnia. As compared to healthy controls, patients with primary insomnia (during sleep onset and/or early NREM sleep) tend to exhibit larger N1 and smaller P2 amplitudes to deviant tones, and smaller N350 amplitudes to standard tones. These findings suggest that insomnia (around sleep onset and during NREM sleep) is characterized by both elevated CNS activation and by an attenuation of the processes that serve to inhibit sensory and information processing.

Given the tenuousness of the present sleep EEG findings, further studies are clearly indicated. The problem with the "call" for further research is that there is a fundamental disagreement about whether insomnia merits targeted research. The lack of merit owes to a variety of factors including (1) the widespread belief that insomnia is only a symptom; and (2) that insomnia, when considered a primary disorder, does not have significant medical, psychiatric, personal or social consequences.

The former is a conceptual issue that has been under siege from within the sleep community for nearly a decade (105,106). At present it is commonly held (within the sleep community) that insomnia is disorder which, when it occurs with other medical and/or psychiatric illness, is best characterized as a comorbid disorder. This change in perspective, which has yet to gain wide spread acceptance outside the sleep community, carries with it the implication that further research is warranted and likely to be fruitful with respect to the delineation of specific biological correlates.

The latter is an empirical issue. That is, there needs to be enough research that demonstrates the medical, psychiatric, personal or social effects of insomnia to persuade the larger science and medical communities of the importance of conducting the research needed to reach a detailed consensus view on the pathophysiology of insomnia based on sleep EEG techniques as well as other approaches ranging from animal models to functional and anatomical imaging for both global and regional activation in human subjects (107–109) and the profiling of specific neurotransmitter system activity (110).

REFERENCES

1. Davis H, Davis PA, Loomis AL, et al. Human brain potentials during the onset of sleep. Neurophysiol 1937; 1:24–38.
2. Dement WC, Kleitman N. Cyclic variations in EEG during sleep and their relation to eye movements, body motility and dreaming. Neurophysiology 1957; 9:673–690.
3. Rechtschaffen A, Kales A. A Manual of Standardized Terminology, Techniques and Scoring System for Sleep Stages of Human Subjects. Washington, D.C.: U.S. Government Printing Office, 1968.
4. Carskadon M, Rechtschaffen A. Monitoring and staging human sleep. In: Kryger MH, Roth T, Dement WC, eds. Principles and Practice of Sleep Medicine. Philadelphia, PA: Elsevier-Saunders, 2006: 665–682
5. Monroe LJ. Psychological and physiological differences between good and poor sleepers. J Abnorm Psychol 1967; 72:255–264.
6. Reynolds CF, Kupfer DJ. Sleep research in affective illness: State of the art circa 1987. [Review]. Sleep 1987; 10:199–215.
7. Benca RM, Obermeyer WH, Thisted RA, et al. Sleep and psychiatric disorders: A meta-analysis. Arch Gen Psychiatry 1992; 49:651–668.
8. Perlis ML, Pigeon W, Smith MT. Etiology and pathophysiology of insomnia. In: Kryger M, Roth T, Dement W, eds. Principles and Practice of Sleep Medicine, 4th Edn. Philadelphia, PA: W.B. Saunders Company, 2005:714–725.
9. Espie CA, Broomfield NM, MacMahon KMA, et al. The attention-intention-effort pathway in the development of Psychophysiologic Insomnia: An invited theoretical review. Sleep Med Rev 2006; 10:215–245.
10. Edinger JD, Fins A. The distribution and clinical significance of sleep time misperceptions among insomniacs. Sleep 1995; 18:232–239.
11. Coates T, Killen J, Silberman S, et al. Cognitive activity, sleep disturbance, and stage specific differences between recorded and reported sleep. Psychophysiology 1983; 20:243.
12. Coates TJ, Killen J, George J, et al. Estimating sleep parameters: A multitrait-multimethod analysis. J Consult Clin Psychol 1982; 50:345–352.
13. Monroe L, Marks P. MMPI differences between adolescent poor and good sleepers. J Consult Clin Psychol 1977; 45:151–152.
14. Lutz T, Roth T, Kramer M, et al. The relationship between objective and subjective evaluations of sleep in insomniacs. Sleep Res 1977; 6:178.
15. Frankel BL, Coursey R, Buchbinder R, et al. Recorded and reported sleep in primary chronic insomnia. Arch Gen Psuchiatry 1976; 33:615–623.
16. Rechtschaffen A, Monroe L. Laboratory studies of insomnia. In: Kales A, ed. Sleep: Physiology and Pathology. Philadelphia, PA: J.B. Lippincott Company, 1969:158–169.

17. Mercer JD, Bootzin RR, Lack LC. Insomniacs' perception of wake instead of sleep. Sleep 2002; 25: 564–571.
18. Bixler E, Kales A, Leo I, et al. A comparison of subjective estimates and objective sleep laboratory findings in insomnia patients. Sleep Res 1973; 2:143.
19. Perlis ML, Smith MT, Orff HJ, et al. Beta/Gamma EEG activity in patients with primary and secondary insomnia and good sleeper controls. Sleep 2001; 24:110–117.
20. Koukkou M, Lehmann D. EEG and memory storage experiments with humans. Electroencephalogr Clin Neurophysiol 1968; 25:455–462.
21. Koukkou M, Lehmann D. Human learning and EEG analysis in sleep experiments. In: Jovanovic, UJ, ed. The Nature of Sleep. Stuttgart, Germany: Fisher Corporation, 1973:146–149.
22. Perlis ML, Kehr EL, Smith MT, et al. Temporal and stagewise distribution of high frequency EEG activity in patients with primary and secondary insomnia and in good sleeper controls. J Sleep Res 2001; 10:93–104.
23. Mendelson W, Martin J, Stephens H, et al. Effects of flurazapam on sleep, arousal threshold, and perception of being asleep. Psychopharmacology (Berl) 1988; 95:258–262.
24. Mendelson WB, James SP, Garnett D, et al. A psychophysiological study of insomnia. Psychiatry Res 1986; 19:267–284.
25. Borkovec T, Lane T, van Oot P. Phenomenology of sleep among insomniacs and good sleepers: Wakefulness experience when corticallsy asleep. J Abnorm Psychol 1981; 90:607–609.
26. Mendelson WB. Effects of flurazepam and zolpidem on the perception of sleep in normal volunteers. Sleep 1995; 18:88–91.
27. Rosa RR, Bonnet MH. Reported chronic insomnia is independent of poor sleep as measured by electroencephalography. Psychosom Med 2000; 62:474–482.
28. Feige B, Al Shajlawi A, Nissen C, et al. Does REM sleep contribute to subjective wake time in primary insomnia? A comparison of polysomnographic and subjective sleep in 100 patients. J Sleep Res 2008; 17:180–190.
29. Edinger JD, Glenn DM, Bastian LA, et al. Slow-wave sleep and waking cognitive performance II: Findings among middle-aged adults with and without insomnia complaints. Physiol Behav 2000; 70:127–134.
30. Bonnet MH, Arand DL. 24-Hour metabolic rate in insomniacs and matched normal sleepers. Sleep 1995; 18:581–588.
31. Edinger JD, Radtke RA, Wohlgemuth WK, et al. The efficacy of cognitive-behavioral therapy for sleep-maintenance insomnia. Sleep Res 1997; 26:357.
32. Backhaus J, Junghanns K, Born J, et al. Impaired declarative memory consolidation during sleep in patients with primary insomnia: Influence of sleep architecture and nocturnal cortisol release. Biol Psychiatry 2006; 60:1324–1330.
33. Bastien CH, Fortier-Brochu E, Rioux I, et al. Cognative Performance and Sleep Quality in the Elderly Suffering From Chronic Insomnia Relationship Between Objective and Subjective Measures. J Psychosom Res 2003; 54(1):39–49.
34. Bastien CH, St Jean G, Morin CM, et al. Chronic psychophysiological insomnia: Hyperarousal and/or inhibition deficits? An ERPs investigation. Sleep 2008; 31:887–898.
35. Riemann D, Klein T, Rodenbeck A, et al. Nocturnal cortisol and melatonin secretion in primary insomnia. Psychiatry Res 2002; 113:17–27.
36. Burgos I, Richter L, Klein T, et al. Increased nocturnal Interleukin-6 excetion in patients with primary insomnia: A pilot study. Brain Behav Immun 2006; 20:246–253.
37. Riemann D, Klein T, Rodenbeck A, et al. Nocturnal cortisol and melatonin secretion in primary insomnia. Psychiatry Res 2002; 113:17–27.
38. Besset A, Villemin E, Tafti M, et al. Homeostatic process and sleep spindles in patients with sleep-maintenance insomnia: Effect of partial (21 h) sleep deprivation. Electroencephalogr Clin Neurophysiol 1998; 107:122–132.
39. Stepanski E, Zorick F, Roehrs T, et al. Effects of sleep deprivation on daytime sleepiness in primary insomnia. Sleep 2000; 23:215–219.
40. Pantev C, Makeig S, Hoke M, et al. Human auditory evoked gamma-band magnetic fields. Proc Natl Acad Sci U S A 1991; 88:8996–9000.
41. Bouyer JJ, Montaron MF, Rougeul A. Fast fronto-parietal rhythms during combined focused attentive behavior and immobility in cat: Cortical and thalamic localizations. Electroencephalogr Clin Neurophysiol 1981; 51:244–252.
42. Rougeul A, Bouyer JJ, Dedet JJ, et al. Fast somato-parietal rhythms during combined focal attention and immobility in baboon and squirrel monkey. Electroencephalogr Clin Neurophysiol 1979; 46: 310–319.

43. Basar-Eroglu C, Struber D, Schurmann M, et al. Gamma-band responses in the brain: A short review of psychophysiological correlates and functional significance. [Review] [69 refs]. Int J Psychophysiol 1996; 24:101–112.
44. Galambos R, Makeig S, Talmachoff PJ. A 40-Hz auditory potential recorded from the human scalp. Proc Natl Acad Sci U S A 1981; 78:2643–2647.
45. Goertz R, Jokeit H, Kuchler E. Event related dynamics of 40 Hz electroencephalogram during visual discrimination task. Int J Neurosci 1994; 79:267–273.
46. Joliot M, Ribary U, Llinas R. Human oscillatory brain activity near 40 Hz coexists with cognitive temporal binding. Proc Natl Acad Sci U S A 1994; 91:11748–11751.
47. Leung LS. Generation of theta and gamma rhythms in the hippocampus. Neurosci Biobehav Rev 1998; 22:275–290.
48. Llinas R, Ribary U. Coherent 40-Hz oscillation characterizes dream state in humans. Proc Natl Acad Sci U S A 1993; 90:2078–2081.
49. Loring DW, Ford M, Sheer D. Laterality of 40 Hz EEG and EMG during cognitive performance. Psychophysiology 1984; 21:34–38.
50. Lutzenberger W, Pulvermuller F, Birbaumer N. Words and pseudowords elicit distinct paterns of 30-Hz EEG responses in humans. Neurosci Lett 1994; 176:115–118.
51. Lutzenberger W, Pulvermuller F, Elbert T, et al. Visual stimulation alters local 40-Hz responses in humans: An EEG-study. Neurosci Lett 1995; 183:39–42.
52. Makeig S, Inlow M. Lapses in alertness: Coherence of fluctuations in performance and EEG spectrum. Electroencephalogr Clin Neurophysiol 1993; 86:23–35.
53. Pantev C. Evoked and induced gamma-band activity of the human cortex. Brain Topogr 1995; 7: 321–330.
54. Pfurtscheller G, Neuper C, Kalcher J. 40-Hz oscillations during motor behavior in man. Neurosci Lett 1993; 164:179–182.
55. Pulvermuller F, Lutzenberger W, Preissl H, et al. Spectral responses in the gamma-band: Physiological signs of higher cognitive processes? Neuroreport 1995; 6:2059–2064.
56. Sheer D. Focused arousal and 40 Hz EEG. In: Knight R, Bakker D, eds. The Neuropsychology of Learning Disorders. Baltimore, MD: University Press, 1976:71–87.
57. Spydell J, Sheer D. Effect of problem solving on right and left hemisphere 40 Hz EEG activity. Psychophysiology 1982; 19:420–425.
58. Tiitinen H, Sinkkonen J, Reinikainen K, et al. Selective attention enhances the auditory 40-Hz transient response in humans. Nature 1993; 364:59–60.
59. Buysse DJ, Germain A, Hall ML, et al. EEG spectral analysis in primary insomnia: NREM period effects and sex differences. Sleep 2008; 31:1673–1682.
60. Freedman R. EEG power in sleep onset insomnia. Electroencephalogr Clin Neurophysiol 1986; 63: 408–413.
61. Merica H, Blois R, Gaillard JM. Spectral characteristics of sleep EEG in chronic insomnia. Eur J Neurosci 1998; 10:1826–1834.
62. Merica H, Gaillard JM. The EEG of the sleep onset period in insomnia: A discriminant analysis. Physiol Behav 1992; 52:199–204.
63. Lamarche CH, Ogilvie RD. Electrophysiological changes during the sleep onset period of psychophysiological insomniacs, psychiatric insomniacs, and normal sleepers. Sleep 1997; 20:724–733.
64. Nofzinger EA, Nowell PD, Buysee DJ, et al. Towards a Neurobiology of Sleep Disturbance in Primary Insomnia and Depression: A Comparison of Subjective, Visually Scored, Period Amplitude, and Power Spectral Density Sleep Measures. Sleep 1999; 22(supp 1):S99.
65. Jacobs GD, Benson H, Friedman R. Home-based central nervous system assessment of a multifactor behavioral intervention for chronic sleep-onset insomnia. Behav Ther 1993; 24:159–174.
66. Perlis ML, Andrews PJ, Orff HJ, et al. Fast frequency EEG activity in patients with insomnia and in good sleeper controls. Sleep 2000; 23 Supplemental #1:A5.
67. Bastien CH, LeBlanc M, Carrier J, et al. Sleep EEG power spectra, insomnia, and chronic use of benzodiazepines. Sleep 2003; 26:313–317.
68. Curcio G, Ferrara M, Piergianni A, et al. Paradoxes of the first-night effect: A quantitative analysis of antero-posterior EEG topography. Clin Neurophysiol 2004; 115:1178–1188.
69. Terzano MG, Mancia D, Salati MR, et al. The cyclic alternating pattern as a physiologic component of normal NREM sleep. Sleep 1985; 8:137–145.
70. Terzano MG, Parrino L. The cyclic alternating pattern (CAP) in human sleep. In: Guilleminault C, ed. Sleep and its Disorders. Handbook of Clinical Neurophysiology. 2005:79–93.
71. Halasz P, Terzano M, Parrino L, et al. The nature of arousal in sleep. J Sleep Res 2004; 13:1–23.
72. Terzano MG, Parrino L, Smerieri A, et al. Atlas, rules, and recording techniques for the scoring of cyclic alternating pattern (CAP) in human sleep. Sleep Med 2002; 3:187–199.

73. Terzano MG, Parrino L, Fioriti G, et al. Modifications of sleep structure induced by increasing levels of acoustic perturbation in normal subjects. Electroencephalogr Clin Neurophysiol 1990; 76:29–38.
74. Terzano MG, Parrino L, Spaggiari MC, et al. CAP variables and arousals as sleep electroencephalogram markers for primary insomnia. Clin Neurophysiol 2003; 114:1715–1723.
75. Handy T. Event-related potentials: A methods handbook. Cambridge: MA: MIT Press.
76. Picton TW, Lins OG, Scherg M. The recording and analysis of event-related potentials. In: Boller F, Grafman J, eds. Handbook of Neuropsychology vol. 10. Amsterdam: Elsevier. 1995:3–73.
77. Muller-Gass A, Campbell K. Event-related potential measures of the inhibition of information processing: I. Selective attention in the waking state. Int J Psychophysiol 2002; 46:177–195.
78. Cote KA. Probing awareness during sleep with the auditory odd-ball paradigm. Int J Psychophysiol 2002; 46:227–241.
79. Bastuji H, Garcia-Larrea L. Evoked potentials as a tool for the investigation of human sleep. Sleep Med Rev 1999; 3:23–45.
80. Campbell K, Bell I, Bastien C. Evoked potential measures of information processing during natural sleep. In: Broughton RJ, Ogilvie RD, eds. Sleep, Arousal, & Performance. Boston: Birkhauser, 1992: 88–116.
81. Campbell KB, Colrain IM. Event-related potential measures of the inhibition of information processing: II: The sleep onset period. Int J Psychophysiol 2002; 46:197–214.
82. Naatanen R. The Role of Attention in Auditory Information-Processing As Revealed by Event-Related Potentials and Other Brain Measures of Cognitive Function. Behav Brain Sci 1990; 13:201–232.
83. Crowley K, Colrain I. A review of the evidence for the P2 being an independent component process: age, sleep and modality. Clin Neurophysiol 2004; 115:732–744.
84. Picton TW. The P300 wave of the human event-related potential. J Clin Neurophysiol 1992; 9:456–479.
85. Atienza M, Cantero JL, Dominguez-Marin E. Mismatch negativity (MMN): An objective measure of sensory memory and long-lasting memories during sleep. Int J Psychophysiol 2002; 46:215–225.
86. Campbell K. Event-related potential measures of information processing during sleep. Int J Psychophysiol 2002; 46:159–162.
87. Cote KA, De Lugt DR, Campbell KB. Changes in the scalp topography of event-related potentials and behavioral responses during the sleep onset period. Psychophysiology 2002; 39:29–37.
88. Campbell KB, Colrain I. Event-related potential measure on the inhibition of information processing: II. The sleep onset period. Int J Psychophysiol 2002; 46:197–214.
89. Harsh J, Voss U, Hull J, et al. ERP and behavioral changes during the wake/sleep transition. Psychophysiology 1994; 31:244–252.
90. Ogilvie RD, Simons IA, Kuderian RH, et al. Behavioral, event-related potential, and EEG/FFT changes at sleep onset. Psychophysiology 1991; 28:54–64.
91. Hull J, Harsh J. P300 and sleep-related positive waveforms (P220, P450, and P900) have different determinants. J Sleep Res 2001; 10:9–17.
92. Colrain IM. The K-complex: A 7-decade history. Sleep 2005; 28:255–273.
93. Cote KA, Etienne L, Campbell KB. Neurophysiological evidence for the detection of external stimuli during sleep. Sleep 2001; 24:791–803.
94. Perrin F, Garcia-Larrea L, Mauguiere F, et al. A differential brain response to the subject's own name persists during sleep. Clin Neurophysiol 1999; 110:2153–2164.
95. Coursey RD. Personality measures and evoked responses in chronic insomniacs. J Abnorm Psychol 1975; 84:239–249.
96. Devoto A, Violani C, Lucidi F, et al. P300 amplitude in subjects with primary insomnia is modulated by their sleep quality. J Psychosom Res 2003; 54:3–10.
97. Devoto A, Manganelli S, Lucidi F, et al. Quality of sleep and P300 amplitude in primary insomnia: A preliminary study. Sleep 2005; 28:859–863.
98. Regenstein QR, Dambrosia J, Hallett M, et al. Daytime alertness in patients with primary insomnia. Am J Psychiatry 1993; 150:1529–1534.
99. Wang W, Zhu SZ, Pan LC, et al. Mismatch negativity and personality traits in chronic primary insomnia. Funct Neurol 2001; 16:3–10.
100. Yang CM, Lo HS. ERP evidence of enhanced excitatory and reduced inhibitory processes of auditory stimuli durina sleep in patients with primary insomnia. Sleep 2007; 30:585–592.
101. Colrain IM. P300 and the daytime consequences of disturbed nocturnal sleep: Easy to measure but difficult to interpret. Sleep 2005; 28:790–792.
102. Perlis ML, Giles DE, Mendelson WB, et al. Psychophysiological insomnia: The behavioural model and a neurocognitive perspective. J Sleep Res 1997; 6:179–188.
103. Pigeon WR, Perlis ML. Sleep homeostasis in primary insomnia. Sleep Med Rev 2006; 10:247–254.
104. Perlis ML, Merica H, Smith MT, et al. Beta EEG activity and insomnia. Sleep Med Rev 2001; 5:365–376.
105. Lichstein KL. Secondary insomnia: A myth dismissed. Sleep Med Rev 2006; 10:3–5.

106. McCrae CS, Lichstein KL. Secondary insomnia: Diagnostic challenges and intervention opportunities. Sleep Med Rev 2001; 5:47–61.
107. Nofzinger EA, Buysse DJ, Germain A, et al. Functional neuroimaging evidence for hyperarousal in insomnia. Am J Psychiatry 2004; 161:2126–2129.
108. Smith MT, Perlis ML, Chengazi VU, et al. Neuroimaging of NREM sleep in primary insomnia: A Tc-99-HMPAO single photon emission computed tomography study. Sleep 2002; 25:325–335.
109. Drummond SP, Smith MT, Orff HJ, et al. Functional imaging of the sleeping brain: Review of findings and implications for the study of insomnia. Sleep Med Rev 2004; 8:227–242.
110. Winkelman JW, Buxton OM, Jensen JE, et al. Reduced brain GABA in primary insomnia: Preliminary data from 4 T proton magnetic resonance spectroscopy (1 H-MRS). Sleep 2008; 31:1499–1506.

7 Neurobiological Disturbances in Insomnia: Clinical Utility of Objective Measures of Sleep

Slobodanka Pejovic and Alexandros N. Vgontzas

Sleep Research and Treatment Center, Department of Psychiatry, Penn State University College of Medicine, Hershey, Pennsylvania, U.S.A.

INTRODUCTION

Insomnia is, by far, the most commonly encountered sleep disorder in medical practice. Its prevalence varies considerably based on the definition used. While one-fourth to one-third of the general population reports a complaint of difficulty falling and/or staying asleep, about 10% present chronic complaints and seek medical help for insomnia (1–11). However, insomnia has always been and still is an underrecognized and therefore undertreated problem, since about 60% of the people suffering from insomnia never discuss their sleeping difficulties with their physicians (12,13).

Relatively little is known about the mechanisms, causes, clinical course, and consequences of this highly prevalent chronic condition (14). Insomnia occurs more frequently in women as well as in middle aged and older adults. Many studies have established that insomnia is highly comorbid with psychiatric disorders and is a risk factor for the development of depression, anxiety, and suicide (14,15). However, despite the evidence that insomnia has significant public health implications, including impaired occupational performance, increased absenteeism at work, higher health care costs, and decreased quality of life, there is a paucity of data linking chronic insomnia with significant medical morbidity, for example, cardiovascular disorders. This paucity may in part be due to our limited understanding of its neurobiology.

NEUROBIOLOGY OF INSOMNIA: THE HYPERAROUSAL MODEL

Early studies from the 1970s pointed to the presence of increased physiological activation in insomnia patients before and during sleep (16). At about the same time, it was reported that insomnia is associated with depression, anxiety, rumination, and inhibition of emotions (16). These findings from biological and psychometric studies led to the formulation of the hypothesis that insomnia is a disorder of physiologic and emotional arousal. These early studies have been enhanced by more recent studies that evaluated various aspects of neurobiology in insomnia patients and suggest that insomnia is a disorder of hyperarousal present through 24-hour sleep/wake cycle rather than a disorder of sleep loss. In this section, we will review data suggesting that hyperarousal may be a core neurobiological mechanism of chronic insomnia and its degree is associated with objective measures of sleep.

AUTONOMIC CHANGES IN INSOMNIA

An early study comparing "good" and "poor" sleepers showed that the poor sleepers' rectal temperature and peripheral vasoconstriction were elevated during a 30-minute presleep period as well as during sleep. Also, during sleep poor sleepers had more body movements and higher skin resistance compared to controls (17). In two other early studies, insomniacs were found to have higher levels of muscle tension compared to controls, as measured by frontalis EMG activity before sleep (18,19). Additionally, insomnia patients had lower levels of finger temperature than controls prior to sleep; this is consistent with the inverse relationship between core body temperature and distal peripheral temperature (18,20). Furthermore, a more recent study investigating core body temperature in aged insomniacs in comparison to controls showed increased core body temperature prior to their habitual sleep onset time at home that persisted during the wakeful constant routine night until early in the morning (21). Finally, in a group of insomnia patients with polysomnographically verified sleep disturbance, a significantly increased pupil size was observed compared to controls indicative of sympathetic system activation (22).

In contrast, two other studies, in which diagnosis of insomnia was based on subjective measures only, showed opposite results, that is, decreased pupil size (23,24). Overall, these studies show that poor sleepers, particularly those with objective sleep disturbance, exhibit increased levels of autonomic system activity compared to good sleepers before and during sleep.

HEART RATE

Heart rate variability is under the control of the sympathetic nervous system activity and represents another measure of physiologic arousal in humans. An early study by Monroe (17) showed significantly increased heart rate 30 minutes before sleep in insomniacs as compared to normal sleepers. During sleep, their heart rate was slightly, but not significantly, faster. Similarly, in another study insomniacs were found to have increased heart rate prior to sleep, but these differences were not present during sleep (18). In contrast to these early studies, two more recent studies found significant changes in nocturnal heart rate and heart rate variability when comparing insomnia patients who also met objective criteria of sleep disturbance to normal sleepers (25,26). Specifically, in a 36-hour laboratory study, sleep and EKG measures were evaluated in insomnia patients and age-, gender-, and BMI (body mass index)-matched controls. Heart period was decreased, that is, heart rate was increased, and heart rate variability was decreased in all sleep stages in insomniacs as compared to good sleepers. Furthermore, spectral analysis of heart rate variability revealed significant increase in low frequency reflecting sympathetic system activity and decrease in high-frequency power reflecting parasympathetic system activity in insomniacs as compared to controls. Those changes were present across all sleep stages. The authors concluded that chronic insomniacs could be at higher risk for the development of disorders associated with increased sympathetic system, such as coronary artery disease (25). The other study assessed heart rate in chronic insomnia patients with objective sleep disturbance and normal sleepers before sleep, during sleep, and in response to acute stress (i.e., stressful performance task given in the morning after a night of sleep recording) (26). Nocturnal heart rate was significantly higher in insomniacs. The morning after no difference was found in heart rate between the two groups, but there was a significant increase in heart rate during the stressful performance task. The lack of significant increase in nocturnal heart rate in insomnia groups in two early studies may be due to the fact that insomnia was defined only subjectively in contrast to the two recent studies, in which insomniacs met both subjective and objective polysomnographic criteria.

METABOLIC FUNCTION

Whole Body Metabolic Rate

Two recent studies by Bonnet and Arand investigated whole body metabolic rate in insomnia patients by measuring overall oxygen consumption (VO_2), which is considered an index of whole body metabolic rate. In a study that assessed whole body VO_2 for 36 hours in insomnia patients with polysomnographically documented sleep disturbance, VO_2 was constantly elevated at all measurement points in insomnia patients as compared to carefully matched controls (Fig. 1) (27). The nocturnal increase remained significant even after eliminating from the data set metabolic values from periods during the night that contained wake time or arousals. The authors concluded that the chronic insomnia patients may suffer from a more general disorder of hyperarousal that may be responsible for their daytime symptoms as well as poor nighttime sleep. Another study assessed whole body VO_2 in patients with "sleep state misperception" ("paradoxical insomnia"), a condition in which patients perceive their sleep as poor but whose polysomnographic parameters do not significantly differ from those of matched controls (28). Whole body metabolic rate over the 24-hour period as measured by VO_2 was significantly increased in "sleep state misperception insomnia patients" compared to controls but to a lesser degree compared to insomnia patients with polysomnographically documented sleep disturbance (27,28). Additionally, in experimentally induced insomnia, by using 400 mg of caffeine three times a day for seven consecutive days young healthy adults exhibited increased whole body metabolic rate, reduced total sleep time and sleep efficiency, and increased wake time after sleep onset, sleep latency, and MSLT values (29). Collectively, these studies yield the

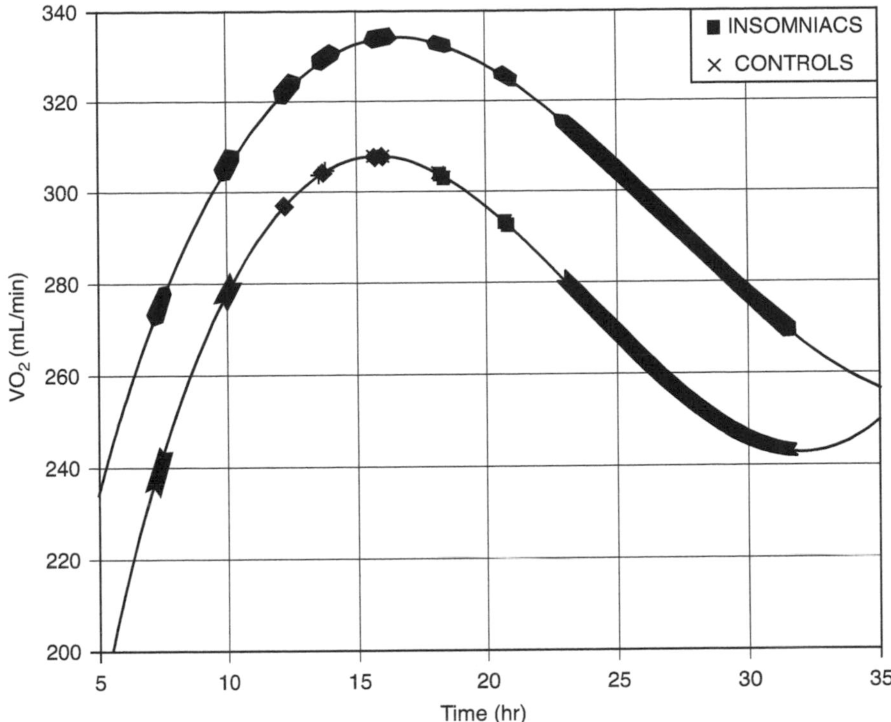

Figure 1 Average best fit VO_2 in groups of insomnia patients and normal controls as a function of time of day. The data represent averaged best fit third degree polynomials. A marker has been added at the right and left margin of both lines to indicate the group. The average $t = 13.10$, $P < 0.0001$.

conclusion that increased whole body metabolic rate is primarily present in insomnia patients with objective short sleep duration.

Brain Metabolic Activity

Recently, functional neuroimaging techniques have been used to assess cerebral glucose metabolism and changes in brain neurochemistry in different brain regions during sleep and wakefulness in insomnia patients and healthy controls. In a study that compared PET imaging data obtained from insomnia patients and healthy controls during wakefulness as well as during nonrapid eye movement (NREM) sleep states, the patients showed significantly greater cerebral glucose metabolism during NREM sleep and while awake (30). Additionally, insomnia patients had a smaller decline in relative glucose metabolism from waking to sleep states in regions that promote wakefulness, that is, ascending reticular activating system, hypothalamus and thalamus, and reduced relative glucose metabolism in the prefrontal cortex during wakefulness. The authors concluded that disturbed sleep in insomnia patients is associated with greater brain metabolism and that inability to fall asleep may be related to failure of arousal mechanisms to decrease in activity from waking to sleep states. In another study, using PET imaging technique, the same authors investigated the NREM sleep-related cerebral metabolic correlates of sleep disturbance as measured by wake time after sleep onset (WTASO) in patients with primary insomnia. Both objective and subjective WTASO were positively correlated with relative metabolism in pontine tegmentum and in thalamocortical networks and this may be the result of increased activity in arousal systems (31). Finally, a recent study reported a 30% reduction of GABA in insomnia patients as compared to controls and a significant negative correlation between GABA levels and WTASO in insomnia patients after adjusting for age, BMI, and gender (32).

NEUROENDOCRINE CHANGES IN INSOMNIA

Hypothalamic–Pituitary–Adrenal Axis

Stress has been associated with the activation of the hypothalamic–pituitary–adrenal (HPA) axis, while corticotrophin-releasing hormone (CRH) and cortisol, products of the hypothalamus and the adrenals, respectively, are known to cause arousal and sleeplessness in humans and animals. On the other hand, sleep, and particularly deep sleep, has an inhibitory effect on the stress system, including its two major components, the HPA axis and the sympathetic system (33).

In the past, few studies have assessed cortisol levels in insomnia patients and their results were inconsistent. Two reported no difference between good and poor sleepers in urinary 24-hour cortisol or 17-hydroxysteroid (17-OHCS) excretion (34,35), whereas a third reported a significantly higher 24-hour rate of urinary free 11-hydroxycorticosteroid (11-OHCS) excretion in young adult poor sleepers as compared to young adult normal sleepers (36).

More recently, in a preliminary study that investigated the possible association between chronic insomnia and the activity of the stress system, mean 24-hour urinary free cortisol (UFC) levels, although within the normal range, were correlated positively with indices of sleep disturbance, that is, total wake time (TWT) (37). In a following controlled study that tested 24-hour serial adrenocorticotropic hormone (ACTH) and cortisol level in young adult insomnia patients and age- and BMI-matched healthy controls, ACTH and cortisol were significantly higher in insomniacs (Fig. 2) (38). Within the 24-hour period the strongest elevations were observed in the evening and during the first half of the night. Furthermore, within the group of insomnia patients, the subgroup with high degree of objective sleep disturbance [percent of total sleep time (%TST) <70] had higher amount of cortisol compared to the subgroup with low degree of sleep disturbance (Fig. 3). Finally, pulsatile analysis revealed a significantly higher number of ACTH and cortisol pulses in insomnia patients as compared to normal sleepers, while cosinor analysis indicated a significant circadian rhythm without differences in the temporal pattern of ACTH and cortisol secretion between the two groups. Hence, this study suggests that insomnia is associated with an overall 24-hour increase in ACTH and cortisol secretion, which nonetheless retains a normal circadian pattern. Based on these two studies the authors concluded that in chronic insomnia (*i*) the activity of the stress system is directly proportional to the degree of objective sleep disturbance and (*ii*) polysomnographic measures can provide a reliable index of the biological impact and severity of chronic insomnia (37,38). Similarly, a recent study assessing plasma cortisol levels in patients with severe chronic primary insomnia found that evening and nocturnal cortisol levels were significantly increased in insomnia patients as compared to controls (39). Finally, a study that investigated the effects of the tricyclic antidepressant doxepin on nocturnal sleep and plasma cortisol levels in patients with primary insomnia showed that doxepin improved sleep and reduced mean cortisol levels suggesting that beneficial effects of the medication are at least partially mediated by the normalization of the HPA axis (40).

Contrary to the above findings, two studies found no increase in cortisol secretion in insomnia patients. It appears that the difference between these two groups of studies is the degree of polysomnographically documented sleep disturbance. For example, in a study by Rodenbeck et al. (39) the correlation between area under the curve (AUC) of cortisol and percentage sleep efficiency was 0.91 suggesting that high cortisol levels are present in insomnia patients with an objective short sleep duration. In contrast, in a study by Riemann et al. (41), in which no cortisol differences were observed between insomnia patients and controls, the objective sleep of insomniacs was very similar to that of controls, that is, sleep efficiency of 88.2% versus 88.6%. Furthermore, in a study that applied constant routine conditions, all indices of physiological arousal were increased but not to a significant degree due to lack of power and uncareful selection of controls (42,43). Interestingly, in this study a visual inspection of cortisol data suggested an elevation of cortisol values of 15% to 20% in the insomnia group, a difference similar to that reported in a study by Vgontzas et al. and is considered of clinical significance (37,42).

Similar findings have been reported in a community sample investigating evening and morning saliva cortisol levels in 393 children of ages 5 through 11 (44). A univariate analysis controlling for BMI percentile, age, and gender demonstrated significantly higher morning

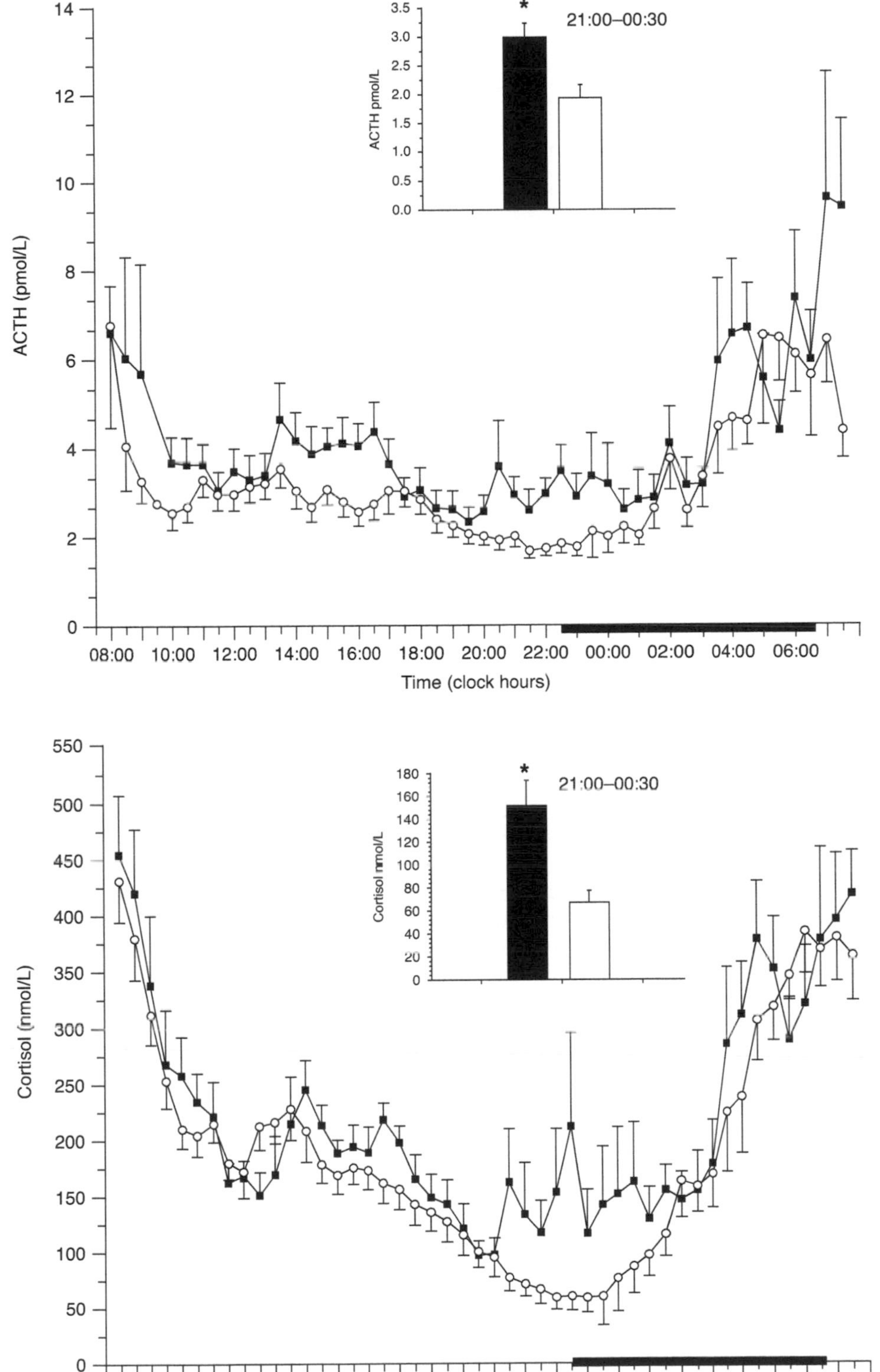

Figure 2 The 24-hour plasma ACTH (*top*) and cortisol (*bottom*) concentrations in insomnia patients (■) and controls (○). The thick black line on the abscissa indicates the sleep-recording period. Error bar indicates SE, $^*P < 0.01$.

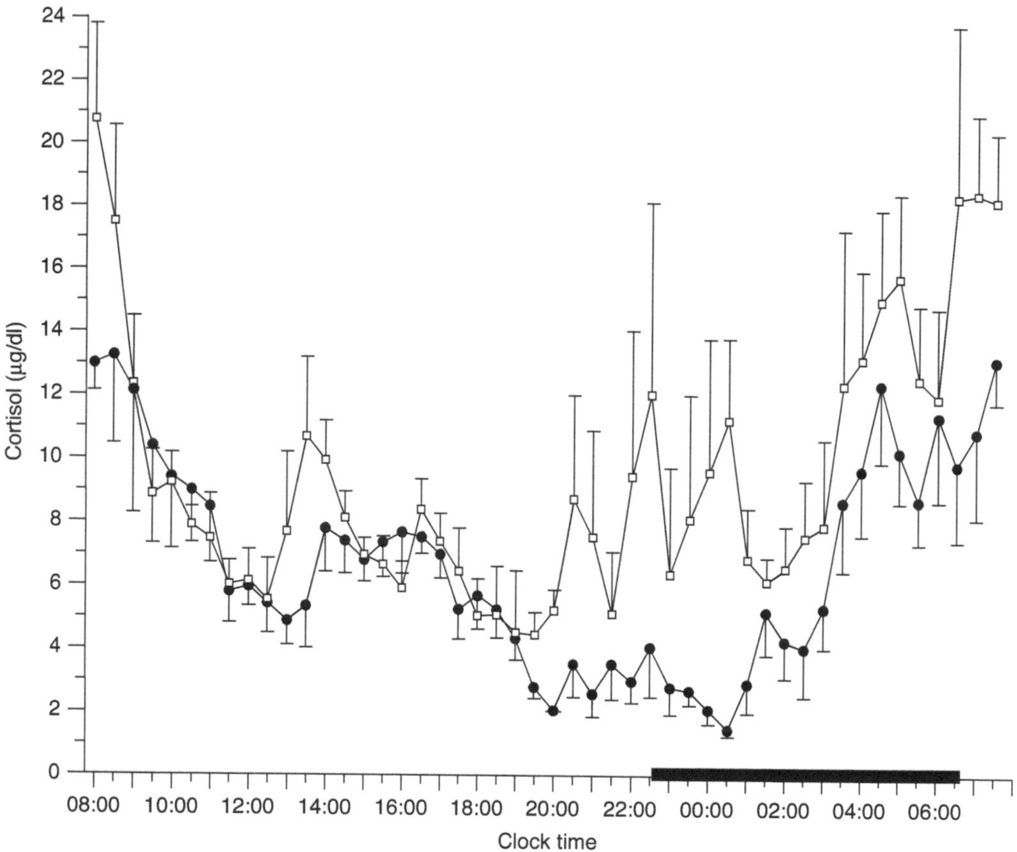

Figure 3 The 24-hour circadian secretory pattern of cortisol in insomnia patients with low TST (□) and high (●) TST. The thick black line on the abscissa indicates the sleep-recording period. Error bar indicates SE, $^*P < 0.05$.

levels of cortisol in the insomnia group with objective low sleep efficiency than in both the control group and insomnia group without objective low sleep efficiency. Evening cortisol levels were also significantly higher in the insomnia group with objective low sleep efficiency than in the insomnia group without objective low sleep efficiency. It appears that childhood insomnia combined with objective low sleep efficiency is associated with high cortisol levels.

The findings of the 24-hour HPA axis activation in primary insomnia are consistent with a disorder of central nervous system hyperarousal rather than one of sleep loss, which is usually associated with no change or a decrease in cortisol secretion. Most of the studies investigating the effects of sleep loss on cortisol secretion have found no change or decrease in the secretion of cortisol after sleep deprivation. On the other hand, in studies that reported significant increase of cortisol in the evening following the night of sleep loss, sleep deprivation was associated with rather stressful experimental conditions, that is, lying in bed in a dimly lit room and receiving calories through an IV catheter (45–51). Also, the higher evening cortisol levels reported in studies where sleep was curtailed at the beginning of the night may represent a change of the 24-hour secretory pattern, for example, a shift of the nadir point of cortisol secretion later at night.

Catecholamines

Sympathetic system activation results in the release of norepinephrine from sympathetic nerve terminals and in the secretion of epinephrine from the adrenals.

In an early study that investigated urinary epinephrine levels in middle-aged good and poor sleepers no significant difference was found, although there was a trend toward higher epinephrine levels in poor sleepers (35).

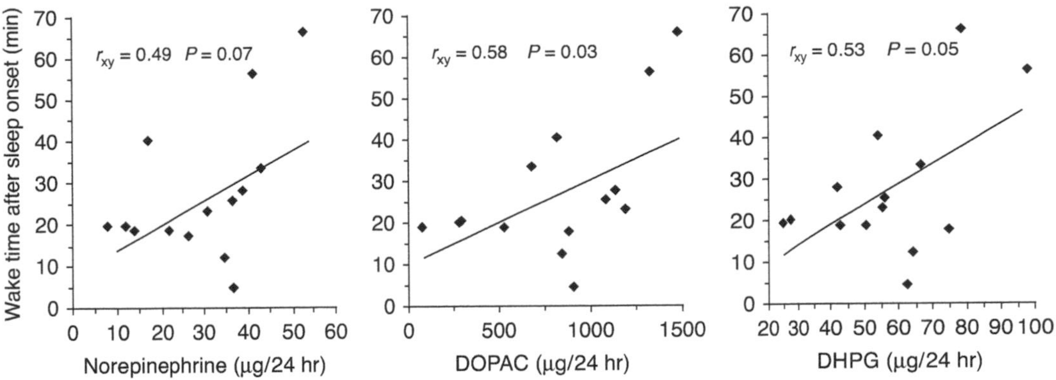

Figure 4 Correlation between wake time after sleep onset with 24-hour urinary NE, DHPG, and DOPAC.

About 10 years ago, Vgontzas et al. (37) in a preliminary study in young chronic insomnia patients correlated 24-hour catecholamines levels with polysomnographic measures of sleep architecture and continuity. Catecholamine metabolites, DHPG (dihydroxyphenylglycol), and DOPAC (3,4-dihydroxyphenylacetic acid) were positively correlated with percentage stage 1 (%ST1) sleep and WTASO, while norepinephrine tended to be significantly positively associated with %ST1 and WTASO and negatively associated with percentage slow wave sleep (%SWS) (Fig. 4). In the same study, growth hormone (GH) was detectable in a small percent of the participants suggesting that GH axis may be suppressed in chronic insomniacs. These findings were further supported by a controlled study, which found that circulating levels of norepinephrine during the nocturnal period were elevated in patients with primary insomnia compared to patients with major depression and normal controls (52). Additionally, sleep efficiency was negatively correlated with norepinephrine levels in insomnia patients but not in the controls or depressives. Those findings together indicate that sympathetic nervous system activity as measured by cathecholamines levels is increased in chronic insomnia patients with objective sleep disturbance.

Finally, based on the previous reports that insomnia with objective short sleep duration is associated with hypercortisolemia, increased catecholaminergic activity, and increased autonomic activity (e.g., increased heart rate and 24-hour metabolic rate and impaired heart rate variability), a recent study examined the relationship between insomnia and hypertension in a large general population sample using objective measures of sleep, that is, polysomnography (53). After controlling for age, gender, race, BMI, diabetes, smoking, alcohol use, depression, and sleep disordered breathing, chronic insomnia with objective short sleep duration was found to be associated with a high risk for hypertension suggesting that objective measures of sleep duration of insomnia may serve as clinically useful predictors of the medical severity of chronic insomnia.

IMMUNE SYSTEM CHANGES IN INSOMNIA

Proinflammatory Cytokines in Insomnia

Proinflammatory cytokines, interleukin-6 (IL-6) and tumor necrosis factor α (TNF α), are considered to induce sleepiness and fatigue (48,54–57). Insomnia patients frequently report daytime fatigue and sleepiness, poor concentration, and inattention (16). In a study in which a potential role of IL-6 and TNFα secretion in mediating daytime fatigue was investigated, 24-hour plasma levels of IL-6 and TNFα were compared between insomnia patients and normal sleepers (58). Although mean 24-hour circulating levels of cytokines were not different between the two groups, IL-6 levels were elevated significantly in insomnia patients compared to controls in the mid-afternoon and evening presleep period (5–11 p.m.). Furthermore, cosinor analysis of IL-6 levels showed a significant shift of the peak secretion from nighttime to evening in the insomnia group (Fig. 5). Moreover, the characteristic circadian TNFα secretion with a peak close to the sleep offset, which was found in the normal sleepers, was not present in the insomnia patients,

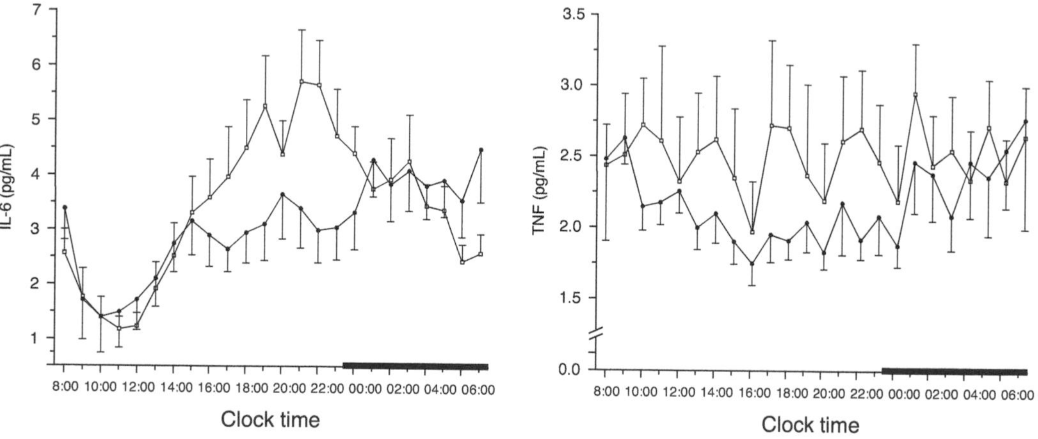

Figure 5 The 24-hour circadian secretory pattern of IL-6 (left) and TNFα (right) in insomnia patients (□) and controls (●). The thick black line on the abscissa indicates the sleep-recording period. Error bar indicates SE, $^*P < 0.05$.

whereas their TNFα secretion was characterized by a regular 4-hour rhythm, a pattern that was not present in the normal sleepers group. Based on these findings, the authors concluded that chronic insomnia is associated with a shift of IL-6 and TNFα secretion from nighttime to daytime, which may explain the daytime fatigue and performance decrements associated with this disorder. Another recent study of IL-6 secretion in chronic insomnia patients of wide age range showed a significant increase in nocturnal IL-6 levels in insomnia patients compared to controls (59).

Cytokine secretion is elevated in disorders of "true" excessive daytime sleepiness defined by falling asleep quickly in objective daytime sleep testing [multiple sleep latency test (MSLT)], that is, sleep apnea and narcolepsy, and in healthy individuals experiencing daytime sleepiness secondary to acute and short-term total or partial sleep loss. Cytokine peripheral levels are also elevated in insomnia patients who experience "fatigue" but not true "sleepiness," that is, not falling asleep quickly in objective daytime sleep testing (48,49,54,56,60,61). What modulates the effect of cytokines so that in one instance they are associated with true "sleepiness" and in another with "fatigue"? Based on accumulated evidence, we proposed that it is the interaction of cytokines and cortisol secretion that determines sleepiness versus fatigue (61). Specifically, the hypersecretion and/or circadian alteration of the cytokines secretion associated with an HPA axis activation may explain the fatigue and poor sleep associated with insomnia (38,58). In contrast, hypersecretion and/or circadian alteration of the cytokines that is not associated with HPA axis activation, that is, sleep deprivation in normal sleepers, may explain their true sleepiness and poor sleep (48,49,58,62).

HORMONAL CHANGES ASSOCIATED WITH MIDDLE AGE AND MENOPAUSE INCREASE VULNERABILITY TO INSOMNIA

The role of psychological characteristics, such as certain personality traits and inadequate coping mechanisms, as vulnerability factors increasing the susceptibility for insomnia is well-documented. However, our knowledge on physiologic changes that may predispose to insomnia is very limited. The prevalence of insomnia increases during middle and old age. Up to 40% of the general population reports difficulties in falling or staying asleep in middle age in contrast to about 20% of young subjects (16). It has been assumed that this increase is a result of increasing prevalence of comorbid psychiatric and medical conditions. Recently, studies have suggested that physiologic factors, such as age-related sleep changes, can also increase the vulnerability to insomnia. In order to investigate if middle age is associated with increased sensitivity to the sleep-disturbing effects of the HPA axis, a recent study examined the effects of exogenous administration of CRH, a hormone with an arousing/waking effect, in middle aged vs. young men. Although both middle aged and young men responded with similar elevations of ACTH and cortisol, wakefulness increased significantly only in the middle-aged group (63). This increase was more pronounced during the first half of the night. Moreover, CRH administration caused a significant reduction of SWS only in the middle-aged group. These findings suggest that middle-aged men as compared with the young are more vulnerable to the arousing effects of CRH. Therefore, the increased prevalence of insomnia in middle age may be the result of deteriorating sleep mechanisms associated with increased sensitivity to arousal-producing stress hormones, such as CRH and cortisol, rather than to increased life stresses during this period. This suggests that a middle-aged individual compared with a young individual is at a significantly higher risk of developing insomnia when faced with equivalent stressors.

Disturbed sleep also is a common complaint of women entering the menopause phase of life. A recent study investigating the objective sleep patterns associated with menopause and hormonal replacement therapy (HRT) in a large population sample found that the objective sleep of postmenopausal women without HRT was worse than that of men matched for age and postmenopausal women on HRT (64). Specifically, menopause appears to have a negative effect on sleep latency (SL) and SWS, that is, postmenopausal women without HRT had a longer SL and less SWS than women on HRT and compared with men. SL was not significantly different between premenopausal women and men as well as between menopausal women with HRT and men. However, postmenopausal women without HRT had significantly longer SL compared to men and compared to women with HRT. Furthermore, postmenopausal women without HRT were less likely to have SWS compared to those with HRT. These objective findings are consistent with the complaint of poor sleep in some postmenopausal women as well as the symptomatic relief reported by those on HRT (65–72). These data are also consistent with early epidemiological findings from a large community cohort in which there was a greater increase of prevalence of insomnia in women compared to men in middle age, a difference that could not be explained by changes in the prevalence of psychiatric disorders such as depression or anxiety (73).

CONCLUSION

Consistent data from numerous biological studies conducted over the 30-year period and assessing different physiological domains including autonomic nervous system status, heart rate, sympathetic system and HPA axis activity, whole body and brain metabolic rate, and immune system basal activity suggest that (*i*) insomnia is a disorder of physiologic hyperarousal present throughout 24-hour sleep–wake cycle and (*ii*) insomnia and sleep loss are two distinct states. Central nervous system hyperarousal, either as preexisting and/or induced by psychiatric pathology and worsened by stressful events, as well as aging- and menopause-related physiological decline of sleep mechanisms appears to be at the core of this common sleep disorder. Finally, there is emerging evidence that the levels of physiologic hyperarousal are directly related to the degree of polysomnographically documented sleep disturbance in insomnia patients, suggesting that objective measures of sleep duration in insomnia may be a useful marker of the biological severity of the disorder.

ACKNOWLEDGMENTS

We thank Barbara Green for overall preparation of the manuscript and Athanasia F. Vgontzas for editing of the manuscript.

REFERENCES

1. National Center for Health Statistics (U.S.). Division of Health Examination Statistics. Selected Symptoms of Psychological Distress. Rockville, MD: U.S. Health Services and Mental Health Administration, 1970.
2. Karacan I, Thornby JI, Anch M, et al. Prevalence of sleep disturbances in a primarily urban Florida county. Arch Gen Psychiatry 1976; 10(5):239–244.
3. Bixler EO, Kales A, Soldatos CR, et al. Prevalence of sleep disorders in the Los Angeles metropolitan area. Am J Psychiatry 1979; 136(10):1257–1262.
4. Mellinger GD, Balter MB, Uhlenhuth EH. Insomnia and its treatment. Prevalence and correlates. Arch Gen Psychiatry 1985; 42(3):225–232.

5. Klink M, Quan SF. Prevalence of reported sleep disturbances in a general adult population and their relationship to obstructive airways diseases. Chest 1987; 91(4):540–546.
6. Klink M, Quan SF, Kaltenborn WT, et al. Risk factors associated with complaints of insomnia in a general adult population. Arch Intern Med 1992; 152(8):1634–1637.
7. Dodge R, Cline MG, Quan SF. The natural history of insomnia and its relationship to respiratory symptoms. Arch Intern Med 1995; 155(16):1797–1800.
8. Foley DJ, Monjan AA, Brown SL, et al. Sleep complaints among elderly persons: an epidemiologic study of three communities. Sleep 1995; 18(6):425–432.
9. U.S. Department of Health and Human Services (DHHS). National Center for Health Statistics. Third National Health and Nutrition Examination Survey: 1988–1994. NHANES III laboratory data file. Hyattsville, MD: Centers for Disease Control and Prevention, 1996.
10. Ancoli-Israel S, Roth T. Characteristics of insomnia in the United States: results of the 1991 National Sleep Foundation Survey. I. Sleep 1999; 22(2):S347–S353.
11. Ford DE, Kamerow DB. Epidemiologic study of sleep disturbances and psychiatric disorders. JAMA 1989; 262(11):1479–1484.
12. Cortoos A, Verstraeten E, Cluydts R. Neurophysiological aspects of primary insomnia: implications for its treatment. Sleep Med Rev 2006; 10(4):255–266.
13. Ohayon MM. Prevalence of DSM-IV diagnostic criteria of insomnia: distinguishing insomnia related to mental disorders from sleep disorders. J Psychiatr Res 1997; 31(3):333–346.
14. National Institutes of Health. NIH state of the science statement on manifestations and management of chronic insomnia in adults. J Clin Sleep Med 2005; 1(4):412–421.
15. Basta M, Chrousos GP, Vela-Bueno A, et al. Chronic insomnia and the stress system. Sleep Med Clin 2007; 2(2):279–291.
16. Kales A, Kales J. Evaluation and Treatment of Insomnia. New York: Oxford University Press, 1984.
17. Monroe LJ. Psychological and physiological differences between good and poor sleepers. J Abnorm Psychol 1967; 72(3):255–264.
18. Freedman RR, Sattler HL. Physiological and psychological factors in sleep-onset insomnia. J Abnorm Psychol 1982; 91(5):380–389.
19. Haynes SN, Follingstad DR, McGowan WT. Insomnia: sleep patterns and anxiety level. J Psychosom Res 1974; 18(2):69–74.
20. Krauchi K, Wirz-Justice A. Circadian rhythm of heat production, heart rate, and skin and core temperature unmasking conditions in men. Am J Physiol 1994; 267(3, pt 2), R819–R829.
21. Lushington K, Dawson D, Lack L. Core body temperature is elevated during constant wakefulness in elderly poor sleepers. Sleep 2000; 23(4):1–7.
22. Lichstein K, Johnson RS. Pupillometric discrimination of insomniacs. Behav Res Ther 1994; 32(1):123–129.
23. Lichstein K, Johnson RS, Sen Gupta S,et al. Are insomniacs sleepy during the day? A pupillometric assessment. Behav Res Ther 1992; 30(3):283–292.
24. Lichstein K, Wilson NM, Noe SL, et al. Daytime sleepiness in insomnia: behavioral, biological and subjective indices. Sleep 1994; 17(8):693–702.
25. Bonnet MH, Arand DL. Heart rate variability in insomniacs and matched normal sleepers. Psychosom Med 1998; 60(5):610–615.
26. Stepanski E, Glinn M, Zorick F, et al. Heart rate changes in chronic insomnia. Stress Med 1994; 10(4):261–266.
27. Bonnet MH, Arand DL. 24-hour metabolic rate in insomniacs and matched normal sleepers. Sleep 1995; 18(7):581–588.
28. Bonnet MH, Arand DL. Physiological activation in patients with sleep state misperception. Psychosom Med 1997; 59(5):533–540.
29. Bonnet MH, Arand DL. Caffeine use as a model of acute and chronic insomnia. Sleep 1992; 15(6):526–536.
30. Nofzinger EA, Buysse DJ, Germain A, et al. Functional neuroimaging evidence for hyperarousal in insomnia. Am J Psychiatry 2004; 161(11):2126–2128.
31. Nofzinger EA, Nissen C, Germain A, et al. Regional cerebral metabolic correlates of WASO during NREM sleep in insomnia. J Clin Sleep Med 2006; 2(3):316–322.
32. Winkelman JW, Buxton OM, Jensen JE, et al. Reduced brain GABA in primary insomnia: preliminary data from 4 T proton magnetic resonance spectroscopy (1 H-MRS). Sleep 2008; 311(11):1499–1506.
33. Vgontzas AN, Chrousos GP. Sleep, the hypothalamic-pituitary-adrenal axis, and cytokines: multiple interactions and disturbances in sleep disorders. Endocrinol Metab Clin North Am 2002; 31(1): 15–36.
34. Frankel BL, Buchbinder R, Coursey RD, et al. Sleep patterns and psychological test characteristics of chronic primary insomnia. Sleep Res 1973; 2:149.

35. Adam K, Tomeny M, Oswald I. Physiological and psychological differences between good and poor sleepers. J Psychiatr Res 1986; 20(4):301–316.
36. Johns MW, Gay TJ, Masterton JP, et al. Relationship between sleep habits, adrenocortical activity and personality. Psychosom Med 1971; 33(6):499–508.
37. Vgontzas AN, Tsigos C, Bixler EO, et al. Chronic insomnia and activity of the stress system: a preliminary study. J Psychosom Res 1998; 45(1):21–31.
38. Vgontzas AN, Bixler EO, Lin HM, et al. Chronic insomnia is associated with nyctohemeral activation of the hypothalamic-pituitary–adrenal axis: clinical implications. J Clin Endocrinol Metab 2001; 86(8):3787–3794.
39. Rodenbeck A, Huether G, Ruether E, et al. Interactions between evening and nocturnal cortisol secretion and sleep parameters in patients with severe chronic primary insomnia. Neurosci Lett 2002; 324(2):163–459.
40. Rodenbeck A, Cohrs S, Jordan W, et al. The sleep-improving effects of doxepin are paralleled by a normalized plasma cortisol secretion in primary insomnia. Psychopharmacology 2003; 170(4): 423–428.
41. Riemann D, Klein T, Rodenbeck A, et al. Nocturnal cortisol and melatonin secretion in primary insomnia. Psychiatry Res 2002; 113(1–2):17–27.
42. Varkevisser M, Van Dongen HP, Kerkhof GA. Physiologic indexes in chronic insomnia during a constant routine: evidence for general hyperarousal? Sleep 2005; 28(12):1588–1596.
43. Bonnet MH. Hyperarousal as the basis for insomnia: effect size and significance. Sleep 2005; 28(12):1500–1501.
44. Bixler EO, Tsaoussoglou M, Calhoun S, et al. Insomnia with low sleep efficiency is associated with high salivary cortisol levels in children. Sleep 2008; 31:A143.
45. Moldofsky H, Lue FA, Davidson JR, et al. Effects of sleep deprivation on human immune functions. FASEB J 1989; 3(8):1927–1977.
46. Scheen AJ, Byrne MM, Plat L, et al. Relationships between sleep quality and glucose regulation in normal humans. Am J Physiol 1997; 271(2, pt 1):E261–E270.
47. Brun J, Chambe G, Khalfallah Y, et al. Effect of modafinil on plasma melatonin, cortisol and growth hormone rhythms, rectal temperature and performance in healthy subjects during 36 h sleep deprivation. J Sleep Res 1998; 7(2):105–114.
48. Vgontzas AN, Zoumakis E, Bixler EO, et al. Adverse effects of modest sleep restriction on sleepiness, performance, and inflammatory cytokines. J Clin Endocrinol Metab 2004; 89(5):2119–2126.
49. Vgontzas AN, Mastorakos G, Bixler EO, et al. Sleep deprivation effects on the activity of hypothalamic–pituitary-adrenal and growth axes: potential clinical implications. Clin Endocrinol (Oxf) 1999; 51(2):205–215.
50. Leproult R, Copinschi C, Buxton O, et al. Sleep loss results in an elevation of cortisol levels the next evening. Sleep 1997; 20(10):865–870.
51. Spiegel K, Lerpoult R, Van Cauter E. Impact of sleep debt on metabolic and endocrine function. Lancet 1999; 354(9188):1435–1439.
52. Irwin M, Clark C, Kennedy B, et al. Nocturnal catecholamines and immune function in insomniacs, depressed patients, and controls subjects. Brain Behav Immun 2003; 17(5):365–372.
53. Vgontzas AN, Liao D, Bixler EO, et al. Insomnia with objective short sleep duration is associated with a high risk for hypertension. Sleep 2009; 32(4):491–497.
54. Vgontzas AN, Papanicolaou DA, Bixler EO, et al. Elevation of plasma cytokines in disorders of excessive daytime sleepiness: role of sleep disturbance and obesity. J Clinc Endocrinol Metab 1997; 82(5):1313–1316.
55. Vgontzas AN, Papanicolaou DA, Bixler EO, et al. Sleep apnea and daytime sleepiness and fatigue: relations with visceral obesity, insulin resistance, and hypercytokinemia. J Clin Endocrinol Metab 2000; 85(3):1151–1158.
56. Vgontzas AN, Papanicolaou DA, Bixler EO, et al. Circadian interleukin-6 secretion and quantity and depth of sleep. J Clin Endocrinol Metab 1999; 84(8):2603–2607.
57. Chrousos GP. The hypothalamic-pituitary-adrenal axis in immune-mediated inflammation. N Engl J Med 1995; 332(2):1351–1362.
58. Vgontzas AN, Zoumakis E, Papanicolaou DA, et al. Chronic insomnia is associated with a shift of interleukin-6 and tumor necrosis factor secretion from nighttime to daytime. Metabolism 2002; 51(7):887–892.
59. Burgos I, Richter L, Klein T, et al. Increased nocturnal interleukin-6 excretion in patients with primary insomnia: a pilot study. Brain Behav Immun 2006; 20(3):246–253.
60. Shearer WT, Reuben JM, Mullington JM, et al. Soluble TNF-alpha receptor 1 and IL-6 plasma levels in humans subjected to the sleep deprivation model of spaceflight. J Allergy Clin Immunol 2001; 107(1):165–170.

61. Vgontzas AN, Bixler EO, Lin HM, et al. IL-6 and its circadian secretion in humans. Neuroimmunomodulation 2005; 12 (3):131–140.
62. Stepanski E, Zorick F, Roehrs T, et al. Daytime alertness in patients with chronic insomnia compared to asymptomatic controls subjects. Sleep 1988; 1(1):54–60.
63. Vgontzas AN, Bixler EO, Wittman AM, et al. Middle-aged men show higher sensitivity of sleep to the arousing effects of corticotrophin-releasing hormone that young men: clinical implications. J Clin Endocrinol Metab 2001; 86(4):1489–1495.
64. Bixler EO, Papaliaga MN, Vgontzas AN,et al. Women sleep objectively better than men and the sleep of young women is more resilient to external stressors: effects of age and menopause. J Sleep Res 2009; 18(2):221–228.
65. Young T, Rabago D, Zgierska A, et al. Objective and subjective sleep quality in premenopausal, perimenopausal, and postmenopausal women in the Wisconsin Sleep Cohort Study. Sleep 2003; 26(6):667–672.
66. Kuh DL, Wadsworth M, Hardy R. Women's health in midlife: the influence of the menopause, social factors and health in earlier life. Br J Obstet Gynaecol 1997; 104(8):923–933.
67. Matthews KA, Wing RR, Kuller LH, et al. Influences of natural menopause on psychological characteristics and symptoms of middle-aged healthy women. J Consult Clin Psychol 1990; 58:345–351.
68. Kravitz HM, Ganz P, Bromberger J, et al. Sleep difficulty in women at midlife: a community survey of sleep and the menopausal transition. Menopause 2003; 10(1):19–28.
69. Thomson J, Oswald I. Effect of oestrogen on the sleep, mood, and anxiety of menopausal women. Br Med J 1977; 2(6098):1317–1319.
70. Scharf MB, McDannold MD, Stover R, et al. Effects of estrogen replacement therapy on rates of cyclic alternating patterns of hot-flush events during sleep in postmenopausal women: a pilot study. Clin Ther 1997; 19(2):304–311.
71. Schiff I, Regestein Q, Tulchinsky D, et al. Effects of estrogens on sleep and psychological state of hypogonadal women. JAMA 1979; 242(22):2405–2407.
72. Hays J, Ockene J, Brunner R, et al. Women's Health Initiative Investigators. Effects of estrogen plus progestin on health-related quality of life. N Engl J Med 2003; 348(19):1839–1854.
73. Lugaresi E, Cirignotta F, Zucconi M, et al. Good and poor sleepers: an epidemiological survey of the San Marino population. In: Guilleminault C, Lugaresi E, eds. Sleep/Wake Disorders: Natural History, Epidemiology, and Long-Term Evolution. New York: Raven Press, 1983:1–12.

8 Brain Imaging in Insomnia

Eric A. Nofzinger

Sleep Neuroimaging Research Program, University of Pittsburgh School of Medicine, Pittsburgh, Pennsylvania, U.S.A.

INTRODUCTION

Clinically, insomnia patients describe overactive minds that do not turn off at night to allow them to sleep. This chapter will review brain imaging studies that comment on whether or not there is abnormal brain function in insomnia patients that may in some way relate to their difficulty sleeping. Interpretations will be aided by review of relevant preclinical studies of the neurobiology of sleep and recent neuroimaging studies in healthy humans across the sleep/wake cycle. The organization of this paper will follow a systems neuroscience view of a hierarchical arousal network in the central nervous system. Abnormalities in any component of this interactive system may produce insomnia complaints. Finally, evidence will be presented as to the location where interventions may impact on regional brain function in insomnia patients.

BRAINSTEM, HYPOTHALAMUS, AND BASAL FOREBRAIN

Preclinical research has identified the basic, or most primitive, circuits in the brain that are responsible for promoting arousal (1,2). A major component of this network is the brainstem reticular core, a diffuse network of predominantly glutamatergic long-projecting neurons and a smaller collection of presumed local circuit GABA neurons. Additional components include a collection of nuclei in the brainstem tegmentum dorsal to the reticular formation that include cholinergic and monoaminergic (serotonergic, noradrenergic, and dopaminergic) neurons. These nuclei send rostral projections that are parallel and interconnected with those of the brainstem reticular core. Cholinergic nuclei are also clustered rostrally in the basal forebrain including septal nuclei and the diagonal band of Broca. Recent attention has focused on the hypothalamus playing a significant role in arousal and in homeostasis. Specifically, the tuberomamillary histaminergic neurons and the perifornical hypocretin neurons in the posterior hypothalamus have extensive interconnections and interactions with the basic arousal systems.

Human sleep neuroimaging studies in healthy subjects support the involvement of these basic arousal networks in NREM sleep. Blood flow has been shown to negatively correlate with the presence of NREM sleep in the pontine reticular formation (3–5) and in the basal forebrain/hypothalamus (3,5). Reduction of activity in this network from waking to sleep is consistent with their role in promoting arousal and potentially in initiating sleep.

Human sleep neuroimaging studies in insomnia subjects support the involvement of these basic arousal networks in disturbances in NREM sleep (6). Nofzinger et al. investigated the neurobiological basis of poor sleep in insomnia. Insomnia patients and healthy subjects completed regional cerebral glucose metabolic assessments during both waking and NREM sleep using [^{18}F]fluoro-2-deoxy-D-glucose (FDG) positron emission tomography (PET). Healthy subjects reported better sleep quality than did insomnia subjects. The two groups did not differ on any measure of visually scored or automated measure of sleep. A group × state interaction analysis confirmed that insomnia subjects showed a smaller decrease than did healthy subjects in relative metabolism from waking to NREM sleep in the brainstem reticular core and in the hypothalamus. This study supports the concept that persistent activity in this basic arousal network may be responsible for impaired objective and subjective sleep in insomnia patients.

In terms of interventions, the mechanism of action of sedative hypnotics may be primarily on these basic arousal systems. For example, Kajimura et al. (7) assessed regional cerebral blood flow during NREM sleep in response to triazolam, a short acting benzodiazepine sedative hypnotic. They found that blood flow in the basal forebrain was lower during NREM sleep following triazolam administration than following placebo.

A recent study aimed to determine if eszopiclone, a nonbenzodiazepine cyclopyrrolone, reversed the pattern of brainstem, hypothalamus, and basal forebrain abnormalities found in insomnia patients (8). In this study, 106 subjects were screened, 23 received in person assessments and 12 met DSM-IV criteria for primary insomnia. Of these, 8 subjects (4 women/4 men, mean age + s.d. = 35 + 13 years) completed two weeks eszopiclone 3 mg qhs open label treatment. Pre and posttreatment assessments included sleep diary, three nights of polysomnography, and waking and NREM sleep [^{18}F]-FDG PET scans. Paired *t*-tests were performed on subjective and EEG sleep data. Voxel-based repeated measures ANCOVA (group = pre vs. post, repeated measure = regional cerebral metabolism in waking and sleep, covarying for global metabolism) were performed on cerebral metabolic data. From pre to posttreatment, insomnia patients showed improvements in all subjective measures of sleep, sleep quality, mood, and next morning alertness [e.g., Pittsburgh Sleep Quality Index Total = 11.9 + 2.5 pre vs. 7.5 + 2.3 posttreatment, paired $t(7) = 3.86$, $P = 0.006$]. Patients showed increases in stage 2 sleep and REM latency and decreases in stage delta sleep from pre to posttreatment. Brain imaging analyses showed that the reduction in relative metabolism in an arousal network from waking to NREM sleep was greater following eszopiclone treatment than before. Specific regions included the pontine reticular formation and ascended into the midbrain, subthalamic nucleus, culmen of the cerebellum, and thalamus. Related neocortical areas showing this interaction included the orbitofrontal cortex, superior temporal lobe, right paracentral lobule of the posterior medial frontal lobe, right precuneus, dorsal cingulate gyrus, and portions of the frontal lobe. Comparisons involving only sleep, but not wake, revealed similar regions of posttreatment reductions in relative metabolism. These results demonstrate that eszopiclone reverses a pattern of central nervous system hyperarousal in insomnia patients. This effect is most pronounced during NREM sleep, at a time when the concentration of eszopiclone in the brain, when given prior to sleep, should be highest. The inhibitory actions of eszopiclone, and likely similar nonbenzodiazepine sedative hypnotics and potentially the benzodiazepine sedative hypnotics, then, that are likely responsible for the sedating properties of these medications, appear to be largely on a CNS arousal neural network within sleep that includes the pontine and midbrain reticular activating system.

LIMBIC AND PARALIMBIC SYSTEM

Behaviorally, maintaining an alert brain serves broader functions than a simple homeostatic one related to sleep at night. It allows an individual to adapt in an efficient manner to a variety of salient events in real time while awake. Importantly, the basic biology of arousal can be modified by neural systems that regulate emotional and goal-directed behavior. These systems may play an important role in modulating or perpetuating the increased arousal of insomnia patients. This is especially true given the significant epidemiologic and neurobiological overlaps between insomnia and mental disorders.

The results of preclinical, healthy human, and depressed human neuroimaging studies support the importance of two neural systems in emotional behavior (9). A more ventrally located system, with important contributions from the amygdala, has been shown to be fundamental to the initial experience of emotions and to the automatic generation of emotional responses. The function of this system is a reactive one in response to emotional stimuli. Other structures related to this system include the anterior insula, ventral striatum, and ventral regions of the anterior cingulate cortex and ventral prefrontal cortex. A more dorsally located system, with important contributions from the dorsolateral prefrontal cortex, has been shown to be fundamental to the conscious, planned regulation of emotional behavior in light of future behavior. The function of this system is one of planning behavior in response to emotional stimuli. Other structures related to this system include the hippocampus and dorsal regions of the anterior cingulate cortex. A primary structure in the ventral system is the amygdala. It has been shown to participate in the sensory component of emotional behavior and in the initial organization of a reactive emotional response. In humans, the amygdala shows increased activation in response to a variety of emotional stimuli including fearful (10), and sad (11) faces, threatening words (12), and fearful vocalizations (13). A reactive "motor" role for the amygdala includes the recruitment and coordinating of cortical arousal and vigilant attention for optimizing sensory and perceptual processing of stimuli associated with underdetermined contingencies (14).

Recent work shows that the amygdala is anatomically connected with and functionally modulates effects on the brainstem centers involved in arousal and sleep regulation (15,16). Similarly, other components of the ventral emotional system such as the ventral striatum, the subgenual anterior cingulate cortex, and the ventromedial prefrontal cortex are known to have both anatomical and functional relationships with brainstem centers thought to play a role in behavioral state regulation in addition to the primary roles they each play in cortical arousal (17,18).

Human sleep neuroimaging studies support a role for the ventral emotional system in sleep processes. Blood flow has been shown to negatively correlate with the presence of NREM sleep in the anterior cingulate (3–5), the amygdala (5), and in the orbitofrontal cortex (3–5). These changes suggest that components of the ventral emotion system play a role in modulating sleep or in the manifestation of sleep. Declining function in the amygdala raises the possibility that this structure modulates activity in core structures involved in regulating arousal.

Human sleep neuroimaging studies support the role for components of the ventral emotion system in pathological sleep associated with both depression and insomnia. Nofzinger et al. (19) used [^{18}F]-FDG PET to define regional cerebral correlates of arousal in NREM sleep in 9 healthy and 12 depressed patients. They assessed EEG power in the beta high frequency spectrum as a measure of cortical arousal. They then correlated beta power with metabolism in NREM sleep. They found that beta power negatively correlated with sleep quality. Further, beta power positively correlated with ventromedial prefrontal cortex metabolism in both group of depressed and healthy subjects. They concluded that elevated function in the ventromedial prefrontal cortex, an area associated with obsessive behavior and anatomically linked with brainstem and hypothalamic arousal centers, may contribute to dysfunctional arousal. Nofzinger et al. (6) investigated the neurobiological basis of poor sleep in insomnia. Insomnia patients and healthy subjects completed regional cerebral glucose metabolic assessments during both waking and NREM sleep using [^{18}F]-FDG PET. Healthy subjects reported better sleep quality than did insomnia subjects. A group × state interaction analysis confirmed that insomnia subjects showed a smaller decrease than did healthy subjects in relative metabolism from waking to NREM sleep in the insular cortex, amygdala, hippocampus, anterior cingulate, and medial prefrontal cortices. This study supports the notion that persistent overactivity in a limbic/paralimbic level of the arousal system contributes to the nonrestorative sleep in insomnia patients.

Pharmacotherapy for insomnia may have some of its mechanism of action on these limbic and paralimbic structures, especially the psychotropic medications. When Kajimura et al. (7) assessed regional cerebral blood flow during NREM sleep in response to triazolam, they also found that blood flow in the amygdaloid complexes, in addition to basal forebrain, was lower than following placebo. While not always consistent, several neuroimaging studies show that serotonergic antidepressants tend to lower, or inhibit, brain function (blood flow or metabolism) in ventral limbic and paralimbic cortex including the amygdala (20,21), perhaps via actions on 5-HT1 postsynaptic receptors given their high density in these areas (22). Inhibiting hyperarousal in this limbic/paralimbic emotional neural network could benefit insomnia patients.

Recent studies have focused on the role of sleep in memory consolidation utilizing both cognitive neuroscience and brain imaging of the hippocampus. Nissen et al. (23) compared sleep-related consolidation of procedural memory in seven patients with primary insomnia and seven healthy controls. Performance on a mirror tracing task was measured before and after sleep. Performance in the mirror tracing task before sleep did not differ between the groups. Both groups performed significantly better in the recall condition after sleep. Healthy controls showed an improvement of 42.8% ± 5.8% in the mirror tracing draw time, whereas patients with insomnia showed an improvement of 20.4% ± 14.8% (multivariate analyses of variance test session × group interaction: $F_{3,10} = 10.9$, $P = 0.002$). These preliminary findings support the view that sleep-associated consolidation of procedural memories may be impaired in patients with primary insomnia.

Another study focused on morphology of the hippocampus in insomnia patients (24). Morphometric analysis of magnetic resonance imaging brain scans was used to investigate possible neuroanatomic differences between patients with primary insomnia compared to good sleepers. MRI images (1.5 Tesla) of the brain were obtained from insomnia patients and good sleepers. MRI scans were analyzed bilaterally by manual morphometry for different brain areas including hippocampus, amygdala, anterior cingulate, orbitofrontal and dorsolateral prefrontal cortex. Patients with primary insomnia demonstrated significantly reduced hippocampal volumes bilaterally compared to the good sleepers. None of the other regions of interest analyzed revealed differences between the two groups. While replication of the findings in larger samples is needed to confirm the validity of the data, these pilot data raise the possibility that chronic insomnia is associated with alterations in brain structure. The integration of structural, neuropsychological, neuroendocrine, and polysomnographic studies is necessary to further assess the relationships between insomnia and brain function and structure.

THALAMUS AND NEOCORTEX

In many respects, maintaining efficient thalamocortical activity during waking could be conceptualized as a primary function of sleep. The best way for the neocortex to maintain adequate daytime function is for an individual to sleep well at night. At the macroscopic level, sleep has been shown to discharge a wake-dependent sleep drive as measured by EEG spectral power in the delta frequency band. At the molecular and neuronal levels, hypothetical functions of sleep include the restoration of brain energy metabolism through the replenishment of brain glycogen stores that are depleted during wakefulness (25) and the downscaling of synapses that have been potentiated during waking brain function (26). These restorative components of sleep are recognized to have regional selectivity. Slow wave sleep rhythms have both thalamic and cortical components (27). Decreases in brain activity from waking to NREM sleep are most pronounced in frontoparietal cortex. An anterior dominance of EEG spectral power in the delta EEG spectral power range has been reported (28). A frontal predominance for the increase in delta power following sleep loss has also been reported (29). This region of cortex plays a prominent role in waking executive functions that are preferentially impaired following sleep deprivation (30). These sleep deprivation-induced cognitive impairments have been related to declines in frontal metabolism after sleep loss (31). Further, recent topographic EEG studies during NREM sleep before and after training on a task revealed slow wave activity increases in regions of cortex known to involve the task (32). Evidence such as this suggests that NREM sleep is important for prefrontal cortex function. As such, the alterations in NREM sleep in insomnia patients may relate to alterations in prefrontal cortex function.

Prefrontal cortex function may play a role in insomnia in several respects. As noted above, there are significant epidemiologic links between insomnia and disorders of emotion. The dorsolateral prefrontal cortex (DLPFC) is a primary structure in the dorsal emotional neural system. This structure has been shown to play an important role in executive function, including selective attention, planning, and effortful regulation of affective states (9). The DLPFC maintains the representation of goals and the means to achieve them. It sends bias signals to other areas of the brain to facilitate the expression of task-appropriate responses in the face of competition with other responses (33). Davidson et al. has emphasized the importance of left-lateralized PFC regions in approach-related appetitive goals and the right in behavioral inhibition and vigilant attention (14). The DLPFC is not only responsible for recruiting or inhibiting limbic regions as appropriate to performing tasks (e.g., Davidson et al.) (34) but appears to be modulated by early limbic processing (35). A related component of the dorsal emotional system is the dorsal anterior cingulate cortex (9). This region has been associated with conflict monitoring (e.g., it is particularly active during conditions when one must arbitrate quickly between two likely responses) (36). Given its role in the executive aspects of emotional behavior, an abnormal increase in vigilant functions of the prefrontal cortex function could lead to insomnia, whereas deficient executive behavior could be a consequence of inadequate sleep resulting from insomnia.

Functional neuroimaging studies have revealed reliable global decreases in cerebral metabolism or blood flow from waking to NREM sleep (e.g., Nofzinger et al.) (37). Regionally, studies across several laboratories and using various imaging methods have demonstrated that between waking and NREM sleep there are relative reductions in activity in heteromodal association cortex in the frontal, parietal, and temporal lobes as well as in the thalamus. Sleep deprivation (31) is associated with global declines in absolute cerebral metabolism. Regionally, these declines are most notable in frontoparietal cortex and in the thalamus. Alertness and cognitive performance on a sleep deprivation-sensitive serial addition/subtraction test declined in association with the sleep deprivation-associated regional deactivations. These studies demonstrate that reductions in global brain function and especially in prefrontal cortex function are important for the restorative function of sleep. Inadequate sleep in insomniacs may lead to a deficit in prefrontal cortex function.

Nofzinger et al. (6) investigated regional cerebral glucose metabolism in insomnia patients and healthy subjects during both waking and NREM sleep using [^{18}F]-FDG PET. Insomnia subjects scored worse on measures of daytime concentration and fatigue consistent with prefrontal cortex impairment. Insomnia patients showed increased global cerebral glucose metabolism during sleep and wakefulness suggesting an increased vigilant or attentive function of the neocortex consistent with hyperarousal. A group × state interaction analysis confirmed that insomnia subjects showed a smaller decrease than did healthy subjects in relative metabolism from waking to NREM sleep in the thalamus, the anterior cingulate, and medial prefrontal cortices suggesting a persistence of thalamocortical arousal even within sleep in insomnia patients. While awake, in relation to healthy subjects, insomnia subjects showed relative hypometabolism in a broad region of the frontal cortex bilaterally, left hemispheric superior temporal, parietal and occipital cortices, and the thalamus. Their daytime fatigue may reflect decreased activity in prefrontal cortex that results from inefficient sleep.

Several interventions may alter activity in the prefrontal cortex in a beneficial manner for insomnia patients. For example, Lou et al. (38), assessed regional brain function associated with Yoga Nidra, a meditative state in which there is a loss of conscious control and an increased awareness of sensory experience. In their study, they found reduced blood flow during meditation in an attentional network that included the DLPFC and anterior cingulate cortex, as well as increased blood flow in posterior sensory and associative cortex associated with visual imagery. Cognitive approaches to the treatment of insomnia may have similar mechanisms of action in prefrontal areas. Serotonergically active antidepressants also increase brain function (blood flow or metabolism) in dorsal paralimbic and DLPFC (21,39). Increasing activity in prefrontal cortex may reverse prefrontal deficits in insomnia patients leading to improved daytime cognitive function. Alternatively, further increasing an already metabolically overactive prefrontal cortex may increase attentive and vigilant functions, thereby producing further insomnia, a not uncommon side effect of SSRI therapy in either depressed or insomnia patients.

A recent study documented prefrontal hypoactivation in insomnia as predicted from the background review above. Although subjective complaints about daytime cognitive functioning are an essential symptom of chronic insomnia, abnormalities in functional brain activation have not previously been investigated. This study investigated functional brain activation differences as a possible result of chronic insomnia, and the reversibility of these differences after nonmedicated sleep therapy. Twenty-one insomniacs and 12 carefully matched controls underwent functional magnetic resonance imaging (fMRI) scanning during the performance of a category and a letter fluency task. Insomniacs were randomly assigned to either a six-week period of nonpharmacological sleep therapy or a wait list period, after which fMRI scanning was repeated using parallel tasks. Task-related brain activation and number of generated words were considered as outcome measures. Compared to controls, insomnia patients showed hypoactivation of the medial and inferior prefrontal cortical areas (Brodmann Area 9, 44, 45), which recovered after sleep therapy but not after a wait list period. These studies support the hypothesis that insomnia interferes in a reversible fashion with activation of the prefrontal cortical system during daytime task performance.

SUMMARY

Cerebral metabolic studies, in light of preclinical work, suggest that there are hierarchical levels of arousal that may be disturbed in insomnia. Further, interventions may have their effects at different levels of a hierarchical arousal neural network. Additional work is needed to clarify the degree to which alterations in these levels of arousal distinguish insomnia patients from other sleep disorders, or the degree to which distinct levels may be disturbed in individual patients. Additional work is also needed to match interventions for the treatment of insomnia with the levels of arousal that are unique to the individual patient.

REFERENCES

1. Jones B. Anatomy and neurophysiology. In: Opp M, ed. SRS Basics of Sleep Guide. Westchester, IL: Sleep Research Society, 2005.
2. Henriksen S. Stimulants. In: Opp M, ed. SRS Basics of Sleep Guide. Westchester, IL: Sleep Research Society, 2005.
3. Braun AR, Balkin TJ, Wesenten NJ, et al. Regional cerebral blood flow throughout the sleep-wake cycle. An H2(15)O PET study. Brain 1997; 120:1173–1197.
4. Hofle N, Paus T, Reutens D, et al. Regional cerebral blood flow changes as a function of delta and spindle activity during slow wave sleep in humans. J Neurosci 1997; 17:4800–4808.
5. Maquet P, Degueldre C, Delfiore G, et al. Functional neuroanatomy of human slow wave sleep. J Neurosci 1997; 17:2807–2812.
6. Nofzinger EA, Buysse DJ, Germain A, et al. Functional neuroimaging evidence for hyperarousal in insomnia. Am J Psychiatry 2004; 161:2126–2131.
7. Kajimura N, Nishikawa M, Uchiyama M, et al. Deactivation by benzodiazepine of the basal forebrain and amygdala in normal humans during sleep: a placebo-controlled [^{15}O]H_2O PET study. Am J Psychiatry 2004; 161:748–751.
8. Nofzinger EA, Buysse D, Moul D, et al. Eszopiclone reverses brain hyperarousal in insomnia: evidence from [18]-FDG PET. Sleep 2008; 31:A232.
9. Phillips ML, Drevets WC, Rauch SL, et al. Neurobiology of emotion perception I: the neural basis of normal emotion perception. Biol Psychiatry 2003; 54:504–514.
10. Wright CI, Fishcer H, Whalen PJ, et al. Differential prefrontal cortex and amygdala habituation to repeatedly presented emotional stimuli. Neuroreport 2001; 12:379–383.
11. Blair RJR, Morris JS, Frith CD, et al. Neural responses to sad and angry expressions. Brain 1999; 122:883–893.
12. Isenberg N, Silbersweig D, Engelien A, et al. Linguistic threat activates the human amygdala. Proc Natl Acad Sci U S A 1999; 96:10456–10459.
13. Phillips ML, Young AW, Scott SK, et al. Neural responses to facial and vocal expressions of fear and disgust. Proc R Soc Lond B Biol Sci 1998; 265:1809–1817.
14. Davidson RJ, Kabat-Zinn J, Schumacher J, et al. Alterations in brain and immune function produced by mindfulness meditation. Psychosom Med 2003; 65:564–570.
15. Morrison AR, Sanford LD, Ross RJ. Initiation of rapid eye movement sleep: beyond the brainstem. In: Mallick BN, Inoue S, eds. Rapid Eye Movement Sleep. New York: Marcel Dekker, 1999.
16. Sanford LD, Ross RJ, Morrison AR. Serotonergic mechanisms in the amygdala terminate REM sleep. Sleep Res 1995; 24:54
17. Semba K. The mesopontine cholinergic system: a dual role in REM sleep and wakefulness. In: Lydic R, Baghdoyan HA, eds. Handbook of Behavioral State Control: Cellular and Molecular Mechanisms. Boca Raton, FL: CRC Press, 1999:161–180.
18. Sherin JE, Elmquist JK, Torrealba F, et al. Innervation of histaminergic tuberomammillary neurons by GABAergic and galaninergic neurons in the ventrolateral preoptic nucleus of the rat. J Neurosci 1998; 18:4705–4721.
19. Nofzinger EA, Price JC, Meltzer CC, et al. Towards a neurobiology of dysfunctional arousal in depression: the relationship between beta EEG power and regional cerebral glucose metabolism during NREM sleep. Psychiatry Res 2000; 98:71–91.
20. Mayberg HS, Brannan SK, Tekell JL, et al. Regional metabolic effects of fluoxetine in major depression: serial changes and relationship to clinical response. Biol Psychiatry 2000; 48:830–843.
21. Buchsbaum MS, Wu J, Siegel BV, et al. Effect of sertraline on regional metabolic rate in patients with affective disorder. Biol Psychiatry 1997; 41:15–22.
22. Tsukada H, Kakiuchi T, Nishiyama S, et al. Effects of aging on 5-HT(1A) receptors and their functional response to 5-HT(1A) agonist in the living brain: PET study with [carbonyl-(11)C]WAY-100635 in conscious monkeys. Synapse 2001; 42:242–251.
23. Nissen C, Kloepfer C, Nofzinger EA, et al. Impaired sleep-associated memory consolidation in primary insomnia. Sleep 2006; 29:1068–1073.
24. Riemann D, Voderholzer U, Spiegelhalder K, et al. Chronic insomnia and MRI-measured hippocampal volumes: a pilot study. Sleep 2007; 30:955–958.
25. Benington JH, Heller HC. Restoration of brain energy-metabolism as the function of sleep. Prog Neurobiol 1995; 45:347–360.
26. Tononi G, Cirelli C. Sleep and synaptic homeostasis: a hypothesis. Brain Res Bull 2003; 62:143–150.
27. Steriade M, Amzica F. Coalescence of sleep rhythms and their chronology in corticothalamic networks. Sleep Res Online 1998; 1:1–10.
28. Werth E, Achermann P, Borbely AA. Brain topography of the human sleep EEG: antero-posterior shifts of spectral power. Neuroreport 1996; 8:123–127.

29. Cajochen C, Foy R, Dijk D-J. Frontal predominance of a relative increase in sleep delta and theta EEG activity after sleep loss in humans. Sleep Res Online 1999; 2:65–69.
30. Harrison Y, Horne JA. The impact of sleep deprivation on decision making: a review. J Exp Psychol Appl 2000; 6:236–249.
31. Thomas M, Sing H, Belenky G, et al. Neural basis of alertness and cognitive performance impairments during sleepiness. I. Effects of 24h of sleep deprivation on waking human regional brain activity. J Sleep Res 2000; 9:335–352.
32. Huber R, Ghilardi MF, Massimini M, et al. Local sleep and learning. Nature 2004; 430:78–81.
33. Miller EK, Cohen JD. An integrative theory of prefrontal cortex function. Annu Rev Neurosci 2001; 24:167–202.
34. Davidson RJ, Jackson DC, Kalin NH. Emotion, plasticity, context, and regulation: perspectives from affective neuroscience. Psychol Bull 2000; 126:890–909.
35. Perez-Jaranay JM, Vives F. Electrophysiological study of the response of medial prefrontal cortex neurons to stimulation of the basolateral nucleus of the amygdala in the rat. Brain Res 1991; 564: 97–101.
36. Botvinick M, Nystrom LE, Fissell K, et al. Conflict monitoring versus selection-for-action in anterior cingulate cortex. Nature 1999; 402:179–181.
37. Nofzinger EA, Buysse DJ, Miewald JM, et al. Human regional cerebral glucose metabolism during non-rapid eye movement sleep in relation to waking. Brain 2002; 125:1105–1115.
38. Lou HC, Kjaer TW, Friberg L, et al. A ^{15}O H_2O PET study of meditation and the resting state of normal consciousness. Hum Brain Mapp 1999; 7:98–105.
39. Mayberg HS, Brannan SK, Tekell JL, et al. Regional metabolic effects of fluoxetine in major depression: serial changes and relationship to clinical response. Biol Psychiatry 2000; 48:830–843.

9 History Taking in Insomnia

Karl Doghramji

Jefferson Sleep Disorders Center and the Department of Psychiatry and Human Behavior, Thomas Jefferson University, Philadelphia, Pennsylvania, U.S.A.

Scott E. Cologne

American Sleep Medicine, St. Louis, Missouri, U.S.A.

INTRODUCTION

A comprehensive history is the cornerstone of the evaluation process in insomnia. This fact deserves special emphasis in the case of insomnia, since less than half of primary care physicians obtain a sleep history despite being confronted with a complaint of insomnia (1). In this chapter, we will assume that an insomnia complaint has already been established; nevertheless, it is noteworthy that only a minority of insomnia complaints are actually captured during patient–physician encounters. Even severe insomnia remains undetected by physicians in 60% of cases (2,3). Therefore, active inquiry about sleep disturbances is especially important since 70% of insomnia sufferers do not raise the problem with their physicians (4).

The history should be explored in a systematic fashion. Although a variety of formulations have been described in the history-taking process, empirical studies of the optimal method are lacking (5).

THE PRIMARY COMPLAINT

The complaint may involve difficulty in initiating sleep, multiple nocturnal awakenings, difficulty in reinitiating sleep, early morning awakening, or a combination of these. The nature of symptoms can change with the progression of time as a complaint of initial insomnia, for example, progresses into a sleep maintenance difficulty. In one study, the nature of symptoms changed in over half of patients with insomnia over the course of four months (2).

The onset and duration of the difficulty should be carefully assessed. Acute bouts of insomnia are commonly experienced, yet long lasting insomnias are presumed to be of greater clinical relevance since they may pose a greater risk for daytime consequences. Such distinctions have not, however, been subjected to empirical validation. Additionally, a State-of-the-Science conference held in 2005 underscored the variability in the definitions of acute and chronic insomnia, with minimum durations for chronic insomnia ranging from 30 days to as long as 6 months (6). Most cases of insomnia are chronic by the time of presentation; in a survey of community dwellers, the history of insomnia spanned 9.3 to 13 years (7).

The temporal pattern of insomnia can also be relevant. Insomnia tends to recur episodically over time; hence, the frequency and duration of episodes should be assessed. The frequency of nights affected per week during each episode can also indicate degree of severity. In the national sample described above, 36% of 1000 adults reported a current sleep problem, of which 27% indicated that sleep problems occurred occasionally and 9% reported difficulty sleeping on a frequent basis; insomnia episodes typically lasted 4.7 days. Those with chronic insomnia reported that sleep problems affected over half of the nights in an average month (16.4 days).

Events or circumstances that may have precipitated the insomnia, such as the occurrence of a medical or psychiatric illness, job loss, or shift work, should be identified. Subsequent complications, such as poor sleep hygiene practices and development of anticipatory anxiety regarding sleep, may have perpetuated the difficulty. From the standpoint of future treatment, it is useful to understand the type of interventions that have already been attempted and the effectiveness and side effects of each of these.

SLEEP PATTERNS

The list below summarizes critical elements of the sleep/wake history

1. Bedtime
2. Sleep latency
3. Nocturnal awakenings; number and duration
4. Final morning awakening
5. Out-of-bed time
6. Number, time, and duration of daytime naps
7. Levels of sleepiness and fatigue as the day progresses

Characteristic disturbances in these areas can point to certain circadian rhythm disturbances such as delayed sleep phase syndrome and sleep hygiene impairments such as spending excessive time in bed while awake, among others. It is also useful to ascertain each of these parameters not only for the "average" day, but also for a sequence of days, as such a temporal record can demonstrate variability in sleep patterns over time that can, in turn, contribute to poor sleep. The assessment of variability between workdays/schooldays, weekends, and vacations can be useful. Poor sleepers characteristically do not maintain rigorous sleep/wake schedules. Identification and correction of this variability is a primary element of sleep hygiene education and other cognitive-behavioral techniques.

DAYTIME SYMPTOMS, HABITS, AND BEHAVIORS

Insomnia is associated with a variety of daytime symptoms (see chapter 3 for a detailed discussion of daytime symptoms). Typically, their severity covaries with the perceived degree of impairment in nocturnal sleep. However, in some patients, the degree of abnormality in sleep latency or maintenance may be modest, yet the patient may complain that sleep is unproductive and nonrestorative. It is, therefore, important to independently explore daytime symptoms. In order to understand their nature and magnitude, it is useful to initially ask the patient to elaborate on these symptoms in an open-ended fashion, and to follow-up with specific questions regarding each area of concern. Insomnia patients more frequently report a variety of psychological symptoms during the day, including feeling depressed, hopeless, helpless, worried, tense, anxious, irritable, lonely, and lacking in self confidence, than do controls (8). They report feeling tired and sleepy. They also report cognitive difficulties such as memory impairment, difficulty with focusing and attention, and mental slowing. They suffer from impairments in reaction time (9). They report decrements in coping, accomplishing tasks, mood, personal relationships, and family and social life (4). Many report work-related impairments (10). Sleep difficulties are associated with traffic accidents (11).

Daytime behaviors can modulate sleep patterns. Those that are relevant include the amount and timing of exercise, as intense exercise too close to bedtime can disrupt sleep (12). Long periods of bed rest, inactivity, and excessive napping can foment circadian rhythm disturbances. Exposure to bright light can be helpful in establishing circadian cycling and, conversely, lack of sufficient light exposure can disrupt sleep. Frequent travel and shift work can disrupt sleep and contribute to daytime sleepiness. It is useful to understand the patient's preferred social and occupational activities, as this information can be helpful in devising a daily structure that promotes consistent sleep scheduling.

SLEEP-RELATED BEHAVIORS AND HABITS

The behaviors in which the patient engages during the few hours prior to bedtime, during bedtime hours, and just after morning awakening can modulate the degree of sleep difficulty, and, in some cases, cause it. These include the consumption of caffeine and alcohol prior to bedtime; smoking; eating large meals or excessive fluid intake within three hours of bedtime; exercising within three hours of bedtime; utilizing the bed for nonsleep activities such as work, telephone conversations, or the internet; working and conducting other emotionally taxing activities up to the point of bedtime, without a transitional "down" time; clock watching prior to falling asleep or during nocturnal awakenings; exposure to bright light prior to bedtime or following nocturnal awakenings; excessive worrying at bedtime; keeping the bedroom too hot or too cold; exposure to noise from external sources such as cars and airplanes or from internal sources such as family members or a television set; and being disturbed by the movements of a bed partner. Aerobic exercise increases body temperature, which may contribute to reduced sleep propensity in the immediate postexercise period. This is followed by a drop within four to six hours which, in turn, can promote sleep continuity (13). Certain behaviors are compensatory and intended to address the sleep difficulty, but have a detrimental effect nevertheless. These include strategies for catching up on lost sleep such as going to bed too early and staying in bed for extended periods of time after awakening. A similar strategy includes staying in bed for extended periods of time after nocturnal awakenings.

SYMPTOMS OF COMORBID DISORDERS

Insomnia is often comorbid with other psychiatric, medical, and neurological conditions. Therefore, it is often helpful to inquire about certain symptoms that may indicate the presence of comorbid disorders as a contributing factor to the insomnia complaint. An exhaustive list of the disorders and their symptoms is beyond the scope of this chapter, and readers are referred to chapters 14 to 17 on comorbid insomnias. In Table 1, we refer to specific disorders and symptoms that occur primarily during, or surrounding, sleep. For many of these symptoms, interviewing a bed partner can be highly productive, as bed partners are typically more aware of symptoms that arise while the patient is asleep.

Table 1 Symptoms of Specific Selected Sleep Disorders

Sleep disorder	Symptoms
Obstructive sleep apnea syndrome	Snoring Breathing pauses during sleep Choking Gasping Morning dry mouth Morning headaches
Restless legs syndrome	Irresistible urge to move the extremities Limb paresthesia Onset of symptoms during periods of rest and in the evening or at bedtime Relief of symptoms with movement
Periodic limb movement disorder	Twitching and repetitive movements of the extremities during sleep or just prior to falling asleep
Congestive heart failure	Paroxysmal nocturnal dyspnea Orthopnea
Chronic obstructive pulmonary disease	Dyspnea
Pain from various disorders	Pain
Gastroesophageal reflux	Epigastric pain or burning Laryngospasm Acid taste in mouth Sudden nocturnal awakenings
Prostatic hypertrophy	Frequent nocturia
Nocturnal seizures	Thrashing in bed Loss of bladder or bowel control
Nocturnal panic attacks	Sudden surges of anxiety Tachycardia Diaphoresis Choking Laryngospasm
Posttraumatic stress disorder	Vivid dreams and nightmares Recurring dreams
Major depression	Depressed mood Anhedonia
Attention deficit hyperactivity disorder	Excessive physical activity and shifting attention
Psychophysiological insomnia	"Trying" to fall asleep

MEDICATIONS

A history of current and prior medications is always of relevance. The list should include not only prescribed medications, but also over-the-counter agents, nutraceuticals, herbals substances, dietary supplements, and even foods. Their effects, side effects, dosages or quantities, and timing of administration should be recorded. Allergies to medications should also be recorded. The effects of psychotropic and pain medications on sleep are reviewed in chapters 13 and 14 of this book.

SUBSTANCES

It is useful to determine the type and extent of use of various substances. Chronic and excessive use may lead to substance use disorders, including abuse or dependence. The effects of substances on sleep are reviewed in chapter 16 of this book. Of particular relevance are stimulants such as caffeine, amphetamines, and cocaine. Sedatives such as alcohol, at low dosages, can help with sleep initiation, yet chronic and excessive use may lead to disturbed sleep and the complaint of insomnia (14,15).

PAST MEDICAL, PSYCHIATRIC, AND SURGICAL HISTORY

Comorbid disorders should be reviewed, along with their dates of onset, types of treatment, and results of treatment. Surgeries and hospitalizations should also be evaluated. Major disorders can affect sleep by virtue of their psychological impact such as anxiety and depression, through pain and discomfort, as well as by direct effects on sleep and wakefulness. For a review of these disorders and their effects on sleep, please see chapters 13–16.

FAMILY HISTORY

Certain sleep disorders have a hereditary component. In the case of restless legs syndrome, 50% of primary cases have a positive family history (16). Other comorbid disorders such as obstructive sleep apnea may demonstrate familial predisposition by virtue of inherited metabolic or anatomical conditions. Fatal familial insomnia is a relatively rare disorder in which family history is clearly key.

SOCIAL AND OCCUPATIONAL HISTORY

Disruption in interpersonal relationships, family, job, and hobbies can cause anxiety, leading to insomnia. Such stresses, especially job loss, can also lead to insomnia by causing erratic sleep/wake hours.

PRIOR MEDICAL DOCUMENTS

Prior polysomnographic studies and other laboratory tests are especially relevant to the evaluation and should be carefully reviewed as part of the overall assessment.

CONCLUSIONS

A thorough history provides the clinician with critical information for the formulation of a differential diagnosis and establishes the foundation for therapy. As already indicated, approaches to the clinical history have not been subjected to empirical validation and, indeed, it is difficult to imagine how a single process might apply to all clinicians and patients. However, this chapter has provided a framework upon which the history-taking process can be organized. Therefore, we recommend that clinicians tailor the guidelines and principles that have been provided to develop history-taking strategies that are most appropriate for their work styles and patient types in the evaluation of insomnia.

REFERENCES

1. Everitt DE, Avom J, Baker MW. Clinical decision making in the evaluation and treatment of insomnia. Am J Med 1990; 89(3):357–362.
2. Hohagen F, Rink K, Kappler C, et al. Prevalence and treatment of insomnia in general practice: a longitudinal study. Eur Arch Psychiatry Clin Neurosci 1993; 242(6):329–336.

3. Schramm E, Hohagen F, Kappler C, et al. Mental comorbidity of chronic insomnia in general practice attenders using DSM-III-R. Acta Psychiatr Scand 1995; 91(1):10–17.
4. Gallup Organization.Sleep in America. Princeton, NJ: Gallup Organization, 1995.
5. Sateia M, Doghramji K, Hauri P, et al. Evaluation of chronic insomnia. Sleep 2000; 23(2):1–66.
6. Anonymous. National Institutes of Health State of the Science Conference Statement. Manifestations and management of chronic insomnia in adults June 13–15, 2005. Sleep 2005; 28:1049–1057.
7. Ancoli-Israel S, Roth T. Characteristics of insomnia in the United States: results of the 1991 National Sleep Foundation Survey. I. Sleep 1999; 22(suppl 2):S347–S353.
8. Kales JD, Kales A, Bixler EO, et al., Biopsychobehavioral correlates of insomnia, V: clinical characteristics and behavioral correlates. Am J Psychiatry 1984; 141(11):1371–1376.
9. Edinger JD, Means MK, Carney CE, et al. Psychomotor performance deficits and their relation to prior nights' sleep among individuals with primary insomnia. Sleep 2008; 31(5):599–607.
10. Kupperman M, Lubeck DP, Mazonson PD, et al. Sleep problems and their correlates in a working population. J Gen Intern Med 1995; 10:25–32.
11. Stutts JC, Wilkins JW, Osbert JS, et al. Driver risk factors for sleep-related crashes. Accid Anal Prev 2003; 35:321–331.
12. Stepanski EJ, Wyatt JK. Use of sleep hygiene in the treatment of insomnia. Sleep Med Rev 2003; 7(3):215–225.
13. Horne JA, Staff LH. Exercise and sleep: body heating effects. Sleep 1983; 6(1):36–46.
14. Roehrs T, Roth T. Sleep, sleepiness and alcohol use. Alcohol Res Health 2001; 25(2):101–109.
15. Brower KJ. Alcohol's effects on sleep in alcoholics. Alcohol Res Health 2001; 25(2):110–125.
16. Montplaisir J, Allen R, Walters A, et al. Restless legs syndrome and periodic limb movements in sleep. In: Kryger M, Roth T, Dement W, eds. Principles and Practice of Sleep Medicine. 4th ed. Philadelphia: Elsevier, 2005:839–852.

10 Evaluation Instruments and Methodology

Anne Germain
Department of Psychiatry, University of Pittsburgh School of Medicine, Pittsburgh, Pennsylvania, U.S.A.

Douglas E. Moul
Department of Psychiatry, Louisiana State University at Shreveport School of Medicine, Shreveport, Louisiana, U.S.A.

INTRODUCTION

Epidemiological studies (1,2) have shown that the most prevalent form of insomnia occurs concurrently with other medical, psychiatric, or sleep disorders. For researchers studying the psychophysiological and neurobiological mechanisms underlying insomnia, however, primary insomnia offers the advantages of being uncomplicated by other conditions. While not entirely homogenous, primary insomnia also offers the advantage of providing a group of relatively uncomplicated patients to evaluate treatment efficacy in clinical trials. Nevertheless, the differential diagnosis and evaluation of insomnia in epidemiological and treatment effectiveness studies require similar measurement approaches for insomnia and relevant domains, to thoroughly characterize the populations of interest. While most insomnia measurement scales and methods described here are derived from instruments developed to study primary insomnia, the goal of capturing insomnia as a distinct and addressable measurement problem remains the same, irrespective of the cause of insomnia. In this chapter, we discuss evaluation measures and methods that have been widely used, and that are validated, reliable, and/or recommended by expert consensus on insomnia measurements (3). These methods are amenable to different purposes for the evaluation of insomnia: clinical evaluation, research assessments, and epidemiological studies. As such, we first discuss the requirements and constraints of these three contexts in relation to the evaluation of insomnia. Selected measures of insomnia reviewed here include clinician-administered scales, self-report questionnaires, sleep diaries, and actigraphy. Polysomnography (PSG) has been used widely as a screening method to rule out other sleep disorders that may masquerade as insomnia (e.g., sleep apnea, periodic leg movement disorder), as a quantitative measurement of sleep disturbances, and as an objective outcome measure in treatment efficacy studies. However, PSG is not a clinically recommended measurement method to diagnose insomnia (4). Additionally, PSG does not quantify all features of insomnia, which also include sleep dissatisfaction, daytime impairments, and related symptoms. These latter daytime symptoms may partially explain the modest relationships between subjective and objective sleep measures in patients with sleep disorders (5).

In addition to assessing the nighttime features and daytime symptoms of insomnia, measuring insomnia requires the evaluation of exclusionary criteria of insomnia. Therefore, measures that do not assess insomnia are also required to enhance the ability to discriminate insomnia from other sleep or psychiatric disorders, and to determine whether insomnia is present in a primary or comorbid form.

MEASUREMENT OF INSOMNIA IN CLINICAL, RESEARCH, AND EPIDEMIOLOGICAL STUDIES

The needs and constraints of insomnia measurement vary depending on the requirements of a given application. For the clinician, primary tasks in responding to a patient's complaint of insomnia are to establish a provisional diagnosis, identify differential diagnoses, initiate treatment(s), and monitor outcomes. For the most part, provisional and differential diagnoses are best accomplished through clinical interviewing conducted by an expert clinician. Self-report questionnaires, actigraphy, and sleep diaries can be helpful in increasing the efficiency of obtaining an accurate diagnosis. Some questionnaires focus on psychological difficulties common among insomnia patients, and may aid in differential diagnoses, especially in distinguishing primary insomnia from a comorbid insomnia related to depression or other psychiatric disorders. If the goal is to derive a "caseness" decision for screening purposes, then some questionnaires with clinical cut-off scores may assist with population-level management efforts. Outcome measurement is an additional area where questionnaires may help both the clinician and the patient measure progress with treatment.

For the clinical researcher, self-report instruments, actigraphy, and PSG can document the relative success of treatments of insomnia. Detailed clinical interviews to accurately select research participants are essential in obtaining replicable and robust findings. For research methods and instruments, reliability, validity, precision, and sensitivity to change are highly desirable, since these instrument characteristics decrease the number of subjects needed to convincingly answer a research question. An additional task for research is theory testing. To test theories, the items in questionnaires need to relate directly to the concepts proposed in a theory of insomnia onset, maintenance, or therapy. For example, if a theory proposes that particularly anxious thoughts contribute to sustaining insomnia, then the theory-related questionnaire should ask about the presence and frequency of these thoughts.

Two differing types of epidemiological studies also guide choices of questionnaire. For analytic epidemiological studies, the goal is to pursue causal theories of insomnia by assessing potential risk factors. For such analytic studies, questionnaires for primary insomnia need to be quite detailed and elaborate, since primary insomnia is a diagnosis of exclusion. Similarly, risk factors also need to be queried with high specificity, so that the relationships derived in the statistical analysis are not susceptible to measurement errors and biases. The second kind of epidemiological study is largely descriptive. For such an effort, the main goal of measurement is to estimate the population burden of chronic insomnia. Here it may be possible to use one of the instruments listed below to derive some estimate of prevalence. This kind of description will be helpful to health policy planners and services researchers in planning for health resource utilization.

MEASURES OF INSOMNIA

Clinician-Administered Scales for Insomnia

As described in the previous chapter, the use of unstructured yet detailed clinical interviews combined with a thorough review of sleep history is widely used for diagnosis and screening for insomnia in clinical and research contexts. Semistructured interviews are used in-house by research teams and by clinicians to standardize evaluation procedures, but the reliability of these in-house measures has not been thoroughly assessed and the measures are typically not widely distributed. Structured interviews are available (6,7) but not easily accessible (8), nor have they been updated with recent nosologies for insomnia disorders (6). Currently, a reliable clinician-administered gold standard measure for insomnia remains to be developed and validated.

Self-Report Questionnaires

Whether they are used alone or in conjunction with clinical assessment measures and methods, self-report questionnaires of insomnia are by far the most common method for assessing insomnia in clinical, research, and epidemiological contexts. There are numerous insomnia scales or single-item measures that have been developed and used across different types of studies (9). Some self-report instruments are specifically designed to assess the frequency and/or severity of sleep and wake symptoms of insomnia. Since instruments vary in their popularity, format, ease of scoring, and psychometrics, clinicians and researchers can make the best choices when considering instruments' characteristics in relation to their specific measurement goals and target populations. Other more global assessments of sleep quality and sleep patterns have been widely used in clinical, research, and epidemiological sleep studies, and are also described here. These instruments may have a role in settings where the population studied contains a variety of sleep disturbances other than chronic insomnia.

The *Insomnia Severity Index* (ISI) (10,11) is a seven-item questionnaire that assesses subjective severity of insomnia symptoms, degree of satisfaction with sleep, nature and salience of daytime impairments, and concerns caused by the sleep difficulties. Each item is rated on a

0 to 4 point scale. A cut-off score of 14 has been shown to optimize sensitivity and specificity. Scores from zero to seven reflect no clinically significant insomnia; scores from 8 to 14 reflect subthreshold insomnia; scores from 15 to 21 reflect clinically significant insomnia of moderate severity; and scores from 22 to 28 reflect clinically significant, severe insomnia. The ISI is considered to be one of the best standards for evaluation of treatment efficacy in clinical research (3). Because of its brevity, the ISI can also be comfortably included in large epidemiological studies. Drawbacks of the ISI include its lack of items specifically focusing on nighttime symptoms and its dependence on the cognitive theory of insomnia. The ISI has not yet been studied with Item Response Theory (IRT) methods.

The *Spielman Insomnia Symptom Questionnaire* (12) contains 13 100-mm visual analog scales evaluating the frequency of some nighttime features of insomnia, daytime consequences, and behavior characteristics of insomnia. The questionnaire items are addressed using a visual analog scale that ranges from "never" at the far left side of the scale (0 mm) to "always" at the far right (100 mm). The individual items refer to symptoms and events during the week prior to completing the questionnaire. The total questionnaire score is the average of the 13-item scores measured as the distance in millimeters from 0 to 100 on each scale. It has been used in clinical trials, but has not been studied psychometrically in relation to depression, anxiety, or fatigue scales. It has a Cronbach's alpha of 0.92, based on data studying the Pittsburgh Insomnia Rating Scale (PIRS) (5). Clinical cut-off scores have not been determined.

The *Pittsburgh Insomnia Rating Scale, 20-item version* (PIRS-20) (13,14) is derived from the original 65-item version of the PIRS. From the original study of insomnia patients and control subjects, these 20 items were selected based on both their classical and item response characteristics, to include daytime and nighttime items, excluding the influence of depressive or anxiety symptomatology. The PIRS-20 focuses on sleep and wake symptoms as they occurred in the week prior to completion of the instrument. It does not discriminate between primary or comorbid insomnia. The PIRS-20 assesses the intensity of distress related to 12 nighttime and daytime symptoms of insomnia on a 0 (not at all bothered) to 3 (severely bothered) scale; four items on quantitative sleep parameters (e.g., sleep latency, sleep durations) also scored on a 0 to 3 scale, and four items evaluating quality, regularity, and depth of sleep on a 0 (excellent) to 3 (poor) scale. The total score is the simple sum of the item scores, which provides an index of insomnia severity. A score higher than 20 (out of a maximum of 60) appears to be a useful cut-off for clinical insomnia (15). The PIRS-20 has a Cronbach's alpha of 0.95, and has a test–retest reliability of 0.92. It responds robustly to clinical change (6). Of note, two items of the PIRS-20, items #9 (*lack of energy because of poor sleep*) and #18 (*satisfaction with your sleep*) comprise the PIRS-2, which can serve as an ultrashort severity questionnaire for screening or epidemiological purposes. On the PIRS-2, a score equal to or higher than 2 (out of maximum of 6) may serve as an index of clinically meaningful insomnia. The PIRS-20 was designed as a comparatively theory-neutral instrument for scaling insomnia severity.

The *Athens Insomnia Scale* (AIS) (16) is an instrument for measuring insomnia based on the diagnostic criteria of the International Classification of Diseases, 10th Edition (17). The AIS refers to symptoms as they occurred in the past month. It has five-item and eight-item versions, with scores being the simple sum of the item scores. It contains eight items that ask about daytime and nighttime symptoms, but without containing items that ask about specific time lengths associated with sleep. A cut-off score of 6 on the AIS can serve as a clinical case definition for chronic insomnia. The Cronbach's alpha of the five- and seven-item versions is 0.87 and 0.89, respectively (16). Its test–retest reliability was 0.89 at a one-week interval. The AIS has not been evaluated for its correlation against dimensions of depression, anxiety, or fatigue scaling, but has served well as an outcome measure.

In most epidemiological studies, insomnia is more common among women than men, particularly during and after the perimenopausal transition. As part of the Women's Health Initiative (WHI), researchers utilized the five-item *Women's Health Initiative Insomnia Rating Scale* in a very large sample of middle-aged women (18,19). The period covered by the rating scale is the four weeks preceding the completion of the questionnaire, and the score is a simple sum of item scores. Fatigue items were selected out of the questionnaire. This questionnaire correlated only 0.21 with the Center for Epidemiology Studies Depression scale (20). Clinical cut-offs were not described but the scale did serve as a useful outcome measure of sleep quality in a trial of hormone replacement in perimenopausal women. This instrument appears to be valid for middle-aged women, but has not been studied for use in evaluating men's symptoms.

Other self-report questionnaires have been widely used and have proven informative in clinical, research, and epidemiological studies of insomnia. While the following scales do not exclusively focus on insomnia, they have high predictive power and/or provide relevant information in the evaluation and treatment of insomnia. Among these, the *Pittsburgh Sleep Quality Index* (21) is the best known and most widely translated into other languages. It is a 19-item self-report measure that assesses seven components of sleep quality (i.e., subjective sleep quality, sleep latency, duration, efficiency, disturbances, use of sleep medication, and daytime dysfunction). Each component is rated on a 0 to 3 scale referring to the composite score derived from the frequency of each disturbance, where 0 = not in the past month, and 3 = three or more times a week, with a global score range from 0 to 21. A cut-off score of 5 has been shown to discriminate between good and bad sleepers. The PSQI has acceptable internal consistency (Cronbach's alpha = 0.83) and test–retest reliability ($r = 0.85$).

As part of the psychometrics effort in the *Medical Outcomes Survey*, from which the 36-item short form (SF-36) was developed, Hayes and Stewart (8,9) developed a 12-item questionnaire designed to measure sleep/wake functioning in large populations. This measure asks about symptoms in the past month. The scoring algorithm is complicated, but readily available (10). This scale has been well studied psychometrically. It was constructed with several sleep/wake domains considered. Minimum Cronbach's alpha estimates for its four sleep disturbance items were 0.80; that for two-item sleep adequacy scaling was 0.76, and that for daytime somnolence was 0.63. It includes two time period items, as well as several items related to sleep disordered breathing. It has not been examined in relation to correlations against anxiety, depression, or fatigue symptoms. Clinical cut-off scores have not been described.

The *Sleep Hygiene Awareness and Practices Scale* (22) is a 32-item questionnaire that evaluates the knowledge and practice of behaviors that promote or interfere with sleep and can contribute to perpetuation of insomnia. The frequency of individual habits and behaviors is rated for an average number of days during one week. The disruptive effects of these habits and behaviors are also rated on a scale from 1 (very beneficial for sleep) to 7 (very disruptive for sleep). However, psychometric performance of this instrument is not known, and has not been tested in anxious or depressed samples. Clinical cut-off scores are not described.

The *Dysfunctional Attitudes and Beliefs About Sleep* questionnaire (DBAS) (11,23,24) can be used to evaluate cognitions and beliefs about sleep that may contribute to poor sleep habits and/or bedtime and daytime worries about insomnia. This instrument has been shown to be sensitive to treatment-related improvements in sleep and insomnia (25). Two forms exist: the long, 30-item version (11), and the short, 10-item version (23,24). Items of the DBAS assess the degree to which one disagrees or agrees with statements related to the causes and consequences of sleep disruption using 100-mm visual analog scales. Scores on both versions are highly correlated, and both versions have acceptable internal consistency coefficients (11,23,24). Scores are sensitive to treatment-related improvements in sleep and insomnia symptoms. Although scores discriminate among patients with insomnia and good sleepers, cut-off scores are not provided.

Finally, one of the NIH Roadmap Initiatives, called the Patient-Reported Outcomes Management Information System (26) (http://www.nihpromis.org/default.aspx), focuses on patient-reported outcomes (PROs). The effort includes development of a sleep–wake functioning item bank. Using item response theory techniques, separate short form questionnaires for sleep and wake functioning have been developed for use alongside the other instruments within the PROMIS family (Global Health, Fatigue, Pain, Emotional Distress, Physical Function, among others). These forms are now available on the PROMIS website (http://www.nihpromis.org/default.aspx), which also provides item parameters for use by clinicians and researchers who may wish to use the functionality of this internet-based system of measurement. Further work is ongoing for the refinement of these items and their associated short forms. The Cronbach's alpha values for the sleep and wake disturbance item banks are 0.97 and 0.95, respectively. Individual items have been calibrated for their IRT indications in great detail, and have been inspected for differential item response functioning. While the PROMIS sleep–wake scales do not specifically focus on insomnia symptoms, they nevertheless provide a psychometrically advanced brief measure of sleep and wake function that can easily be translated into clinical, research, and epidemiological contexts.

Sleep Diaries

Sleep diaries are a widely used method to gather nightly information on sleep–wake timing, patterns, and sleep disturbances prospectively over one or two weeks. Because of the prospective nature of data collected with sleep diaries, recall bias is minimized compared to retrospective clinical interviews or self-report questionnaires. Sleep diaries also provide more information regarding night-to-night variability compared to PSG recordings that can only be practically collected over two nights. Sleep diaries typically collect information about quantitative sleep parameters, including sleep latency, number and duration of nocturnal awakenings, sleep timing, and total sleep time, and qualitative assessments of sleep quality and feelings upon awakenings. Many sleep diaries also include items aimed at gathering information of daytime habits and behaviors that can influence sleep and wake functions, such as napping or use of alcohol, stimulants, or medications.

Sleep diaries can be useful for screening purposes, but are a complementary piece of information necessary for diagnostic purposes. For clinical and research purposes, sleep diaries provide valuable longitudinal data that have been shown to closely correlate with PSG sleep measures (27,28), and that are sensitive to change related to pharmacological and behavioral insomnia treatments (12,29).

Numerous sleep diary formats have been used, but sleep diaries do not have an established form that has been validated or standardized for use across clinical or research settings. Nevertheless, they are typically of two common formats: the graphic format [Fig. 1A] and the text format [Fig. 1B]. These sleep diaries are typically distributed and used in pencil-and-paper formats, which do not allow for verification that the diary was indeed completed at the expected time of day, every day. The use of electronic versions of sleep diaries using handheld computers, web-based dairies, and interactive voice response systems eliminates such undesirable retrospective reporting.

Actigraphy

Actigraphs are wrist bracelets worn on the nondominant hand that record objective rest and activity patterns continuously for several consecutives days and nights, with minimal interference with one's daily and nightly routines. The bracelet detects and stores the number of movements per one-minute epoch. The rest–activity patterns are then downloaded and used as proxies for episodes or sleep and wakefulness. Algorithms code and classify the actigraphic data collected to derive estimates of sleep latency, total sleep time, wake time after sleep onset, and sleep fragmentation. Actigraphy is cost-effective (3,4,30–33). While actigraphy has been used in insomnia research, for example (30,33–35), its use in clinical practice remains controversial. Actigraphy can be used as a screening measure, and can complement clinical evaluation. However, actigraphy is neither sufficient nor necessary for either diagnostic purposes or mechanistic studies of insomnia. It is practical for use in monitoring adherence and for monitoring and displaying treatment-related changes in sleep.

Assessing Other Domains Relevant to Insomnia

As previously mentioned, evaluating and accurately characterizing the nature of insomnia complaints and daytime features requires evaluation of other relevant domains.

Medical history reviews and physical examinations should be included in research and clinical settings for accurate screening, diagnosis, and treatment planning. Other sleep disorders can also present as, or co-occur with, insomnia. Obstructive sleep apnea (OSA), restless legs syndrome, periodic leg movement disorder, and circadian disorders are all commonly described as insomnia by patients and research participants. Several self-report questionnaires can be used to estimate the likelihood of OSA using severity of daytime sleepiness, such as with the Epworth Sleepiness Scale (36,37), or a combination of predictive factors for OSA as with the Multivariate Apnea Index (38). Fatigue is another important domain that can be evaluated and quantified using self-report questionnaires such as the Multidimensional Fatigue Inventory (39), or Fatigue Severity Scale (40).

SLEEP DIARY Name:

		Noon	p.m. Afternoon								Evening			Midnight	a.m. Morning											Sleep Quality
	Date	12	1	2	3	4	5	6	7	8	9	10	11	12	1	2	3	4	5	6	7	8	9	10	11	
M																										
T																										
W																										
Th																										
F																										
Sa																										
Su																										
M																										
T																										
W																										
Th																										
F																										
Sa																										
Su																										

Instructions: Use the symbols below to indicate your sleep times in the grid. Rate your sleep quality each night from 0 (poor) to 10 (excellent).

↓ = Go to bed

↑ = Get out of bed

↔ = Actual sleep

Comments

The Pittsburgh Sleep Diary

SLEEP DIARY **BEDTIME** **KEEP BY BED**

Please fill out this part of the diary last thing at night.

day -------------- date ----------------------

Today, when did you have: (if none, write 'none')

breakfast --------------

lunch -----------------

dinner -----------------

How many of the following did you have in each time period? *(if none, leave blank)*

	before or with breakfast	after breakfast before/with lunch	after lunch before/with dinner	after dinner
caffeinated drinks	---------	------------	----------	---------
alcoholic drinks	---------	------------	----------	---------
cigarettes	---------	------------	----------	---------
cigars/pipes/plugs (of chewing tobacco)	---------	------------	----------	---------

Which drugs and medications did you take today? *(prescribed & over the counter)*

name	time	dose
----------------------	------------	------------------
----------------------	------------	------------------
----------------------	------------	------------------
----------------------	------------	------------------

What exercise did you take today? (if none, check here) ☐

start ---------- end ------------ type -------------------------

start ---------- end ------------ type -------------------------

How many daytime naps did you take today? (if none, write 0) --------
give times for each:

start ---------- end ---------- start --------- end ----------

SLEEP DIARY **WAKETIME** **KEEP BY BED**

Please fill out this part of the diary first thing in the morning:

day -------------- date ----------------------

went to bed last night at -----------------

lights out at -----------------

minutes untill fell asleep -----------------

finally woke at -----------------

Awakened by *(check one)*:

alarm clock/radio ☐

someone whom I asked to wake me ☐

noises ☐

just woke ☐

After falling asleep, woke up this many times during the night (circle)
0 1 2 3 4 5 or more

total number of minutes awake -------

– woke to use bathroom (circle # times)
0 1 2 3 4 5 or more

– awakened by noises/child/bedpartner (circle # times)
0 1 2 3 4 5 or more

– awakened due to discomfort or physical complaint (circle # times)
0 1 2 3 4 5 or more

– just woke (circle # times)
0 1 2 3 4 5 or more

Ratings (place a mark somewhere along the line):

Sleep Quality:
very bad ________________________________ very good

Mood on Final Wakening:
very tense ________________________________ very calm

Alertness on Final Wakening:
very sleepy ________________________________ very alert

Figure 1 Sleep diaries. (**A**) Graphic sleep diary. Patients/participants are asked to indicate time in and out of bed by arrows pointing down and up, respectively, and to mark time spent asleep during the night or during the day by side arrows pointing to the start and end time of sleep. Hours of the day and night are provided at the top of the chart. Sleep quality using a 10-point Likert scale can also be logged. (**B**) Pittsburgh (text) sleep dairy. The bedtime section is completed in the evening, prior to bed time, and collects information about daytime habits and behaviors that can influence sleep. The morning wake time section is completed upon awakening in the morning and inquires about timing of bed time and wake time, sleep latency, number and duration of nocturnal awakenings, and feelings upon final awakening. *Source*: From Ref. 51.

Finally, evaluating psychiatric health and psychiatric symptoms is an important component of the measurement of insomnia. Unstructured clinical interviews or clinician-administered scales such as the Structured Clinical Diagnostic Interview for DSM-IV (SCID) (41) and the Hamilton Rating Scale for Depression (42) or for Anxiety (43) are highly recommended (3) and necessary in treatment efficacy and mechanistic studies. Self-report measures of depression and anxiety such as the Beck Depression Inventory (44–46), Inventory of Depressive Symptomatology (47), Beck Anxiety Inventory (48), and the Spielberger State-Trait Anxiety Inventory (49) can provide screening information regarding conditions comorbid with insomnia and contribute to refining intervention plans or clinical referrals.

METHODOLOGICAL ISSUES

In selecting instruments for use in the clinic or in research studies, it is important to select ones that are best suited to the precise measurement goals of the effort and the expected case prevalence in the studied population. No single instrument is appropriate for all applications. If the measurement goal is to find as many cases as possible, then an instrument with a high sensitivity (# of cases/# test-positives) will be best. If the goal is to be sure that the identified cases really are true cases, then an instrument with a high specificity (# of noncases/# test-negatives) will be better. However, before deciding on the basis of sensitivity and specificity alone, consideration of the expected population prevalence in the setting of measurement should also be modeled with the sensitivities and specificities. With very high prevalence, it may not be especially informative to use any questionnaire, since virtually everyone will be a case. With very low prevalence, most of the test-positives will turn out to be false positives. Calculating the positive and negative predictive values will be helpful.

If the measurement goal is mainly to scale the severity of symptoms, then other considerations come into play. An ideal scale will behave like a thermometer, where only one dimension of phenomenology is measured and accuracy is uniform at each point along the scale. Often, semantically based scales have mixtures of dimensions. For example, people often think of depression and insomnia together. However, when measuring symptoms of depression and insomnia, it is best to have one scale for sad mood, another for insomnia, and as little correlation between the two scales as possible. Separating symptom dimensions avoids confounding one's measurements. Accuracy of measurement can also present difficulty. In traditional severity scales, the estimate of severity is the sum of the item scores in the scale. This method, using what are called short forms, works reasonably well, but may not afford the greatest accuracy of measurement. A newer general method, IRT, estimates severity as a point along a latent dimension of severity. This estimator makes the most use of each item's semantic severity to the respondent. For example, the PIRS item "Your satisfaction with your sleep" is less severe than the item "Lack of energy because of poor sleep." Judging how strongly a person endorses the second item even when first is strongly endorsed provides greater measurement accuracy than the summary score from the two items. Based on this principle, it is possible to use a computer algorithm to estimate symptom severity using only a few items, rather than deploying an entire short form. This method is called "computer-adapted testing," and is likely to be increasingly used as more is learned about the item characteristics of sleep-related symptom questions in population studies.

CONCLUSION

Insomnia is a prevalent complaint, whether primary or comorbid with other psychiatric, medical, or sleep disorders. The evaluation of both primary and comorbid insomnia requires capturing both the nighttime symptoms and the daytime consequences of insomnia, whether the context is clinical, experimental, or epidemiological in nature. The evaluation of insomnia also necessitates the evaluation of other sleep disorders, psychiatric symptoms, and medical conditions that can be comorbid to or a risk factor for insomnia. Unstructured and structured clinician-administered interviews, self-report measures, actigraphy, and sleep diaries are diverse assessment methods and tools that complement each other, and provide a comprehensive assessment of nighttime and daytime symptoms of insomnia. Not all measures, however, are amenable to all research contexts. For example, sleep dairies may be required for clinical trials, but may be difficult to implement in epidemiological studies.

The assessment and measurement of insomnia requires further empirical validation work in different areas. There is a clear need for developing and validating a reliable clinician-administered gold standard for the assessment of insomnia that closely parallels the diagnostic criteria for insomnia. Guidelines and recommendations for the selection of self-report measures are available (3,50), and a combination of tools is often necessary to fully cover the different domains of insomnia symptoms and related impairments and distress. Sleep diaries are also numerous, but the need to achieve consensus on the most effective format and content items has not yet been addressed. Actigraphy provides the advantages of allowing for objective measurements over extended periods with minimal burden to the participant, but data collection parameters and sleep–wake scoring algorithms vary widely, and few have been validated against PSG or sleep diary measures in patients with insomnia.

In summary, the selection of tools to assess insomnia in a given context (e.g., experimental mechanistic study vs. clinical trial vs. epidemiological population study) will be strongly guided by the research aims to be achieved and by the feasibility of using different measurement methods. The growing use of advanced measurement methods, such as computerized adaptive testing, can increase the sensitivity, specificity, and practicality of insomnia measurements and provide tools that enhance comparability of findings across study contexts and across populations.

REFERENCES

1. Ohayon MM, Roth T. Place of chronic insomnia in the course of depressive and anxiety disorders. J Psychiatr Res 2003; 37:9–15.
2. Ohayon MM. Prevalence of DSM-IV diagnostic criteria of insomnia: distinguishing insomnia related to mental disorders from sleep disorders. J Psychiatr Res 1997; 31(3):333–346.
3. Buysse DJ, Ancoli-Israel S, Edinger JD, et al. Recommendations for a standard research assessment of insomnia. Sleep 2006; 29(9):1155–1173.
4. Chesson A, Hartse K, Anderson WM, et al. Practice parameters for the evaluation of chronic insomnia. An American Academy of Sleep Medicine report. Standards of Practice Committee of the American Academy of Sleep Medicine. Sleep 2000; 23(2):237–241.
5. Edinger JD, Fins AI, Glenn DM, et al. Insomnia and the eye of the beholder: are there clinical markers of objective sleep disturbances among adults with and without insomnia complaints? J Consult Clin Psychol 2000; 68(4):586–593.
6. Schramm E, Hohagen F, Grasshoff U, et al. Test-retest reliability and validity of a structured interview for sleep disorders according to DSM-III-R(SIS-D). Am J Psychiatry 1993; 150(6):867–872.
7. Ohayon MM, Guilleminault C, Zulley J, et al. Validation of the sleep-EVAL system against clinical assessments of sleep disorders and polysomnographic data. Sleep 1999; 22(7):925–930.
8. Ohayon MM, Guilleminault C, Priest RG. Night terrors, sleepwalking, and confusional arousals in the general population: their frequency and relationship to other sleep and mental disorders. J Clin Psychiatry 1999; 60(4):268–276.
9. Moul DE, Hall M, Pilkonis PA, et al. Self-report measures of insomnia adults: rationales, choices, and needs. Sleep Med Rev 2004; 8:177–198.
10. Bastien CH, Vallieres A, Morin CM. Validation of the Insomnia Severity Index as an outcome measure for insomnia research. Sleep Med 2001; 2:297–307.
11. Morin CM. Insomnia: Psychological Assessment and Management. New York/London: The Guilford Press, 1993.
12. Spielman AJ, Saskin P, Thorpy MJ. Treatment of chronic insomnia by restriction of time in bed. Sleep 1987; 10:45–56.
13. Moul D, Mai E, Miewald J, et al. Psychometric study of the Pittsburgh Insomnia Rating Scale (PIRS) in an initial calibration sample [Abstract]. Sleep 2007; 30(suppl):A343.
14. Moul DE, Pilkonis PA, Miewald JM, et al. Preliminary study of the test-retest reliability and concurrent validities of the Pittsburgh Insomnia Rating Scale (PIRS) [Abstract]. Sleep 2002; 25(suppl):A246–A247.
15. Moul DE, Mai E, Miewald J, et al. Psychometric study of the Pittsburgh Insomnia Rating Scale (PIRS) in an initial calibration sample [Abstract]. Sleep 2007; 30(suppl):A343.
16. Soldatos CR, Dikeos DG, Paparrigopoulos TJ. Athens Insomnia Scale: validation of an instrument based on ICD-10 criteria. J Psychosom Res 2000; 48(6):555–560.
17. World Health Organization.International Statistical Classification of Diseases and Related Health Problems—10th revision. 10th revision ed. Geneva: World Health Organization, 1992.
18. Levine DW, Kaplan RM, Kripke DF, et al. Factor structure and measurement invariance of the Women's Health Initiative Insomnia Rating Scale. Psychol Assess 2003; 15(2):123–136.
19. Levine DW, Kripke DF, Kaplan RM, et al. Reliability and validity of the Women's Health Initiative Insomnia Rating Scale. Psychol Assess 2003; 15(2):137–148.

20. Radloff LS. The CES-D scale: a self-report depression scale for research in the general population. Appl Psychol Meas 1977; 1(3):385–401.
21. Buysse DJ, Reynolds CF, Monk TH, et al. The Pittsburgh Sleep Quality Index: a new instrument for psychiatric practice and research. Psychiatry Res 1989; 28:193–213.
22. Lacks P, Rotert M. Knowledge and practice of sleep hygiene techniques in insomniacs and good sleepers. Behav Res Ther 1986; 24(3):365–368.
23. Espie CA, Inglis SJ, Harvey L, et al. Insomniacs' attributions: psychometric properties of the Dysfunctional Beliefs and Attitudes about Sleep Scale and the Sleep Disturbance Questionnaire. J Psychosom Res 2000; 48(2):141–148.
24. Edinger JD, Wohlgemuth WK. Psychometric comparisons of the standard and abbreviated DBAS-10 versions of the dysfunctional beliefs and attitudes about sleep questionnaire. Sleep Med 2001; 2(6):493–500.
25. Edinger JD, Wohlgemuth WK, Radtke RA, et al. Does cognitive-behavioral insomnia therapy alter dysfunctional beliefs about sleep? Sleep 2001; 24(5):591–599.
26. Cella D, Yount S, Rothrock N, et al. The Patient-Reported Outcomes Measurement Information System (PROMIS): progress of an NIH Roadmap cooperative group during its first two years. Med Care 2007; 45(5, suppl 1):S3–S11.
27. Coates TJ, Killen JD, George J, et al. Estimating sleep parameters: a multitrait–multimethod analysis. J Consult Clin Psychol 1982; 50(3):345–352.
28. Riedel BW, Lichstein KL. Objective sleep measures and subjective sleep satisfaction: how do older adults with insomnia define a good night's sleep? Psychol Aging 1998; 13(1):159–163.
29. Krystal AD, Walsh JK, Laska E, et al. Sustained efficacy of eszopiclone over 6 months of nightly treatment: results of a randomized, double-blind, placebo-controlled study in adults with chronic insomnia. Sleep 2003; 26(7):793–799.
30. Lichstein KL, Stone KC, Donaldson J, et al. Actigraphy validation with insomnia. Sleep 2006; 29(2):232–239.
31. Morgenthaler T, Alessi C, Friedman L, et al. Practice parameters for the use of actigraphy in the assessment of sleep and sleep disorders: an update for 2007. Sleep 2007; 30(4):519–529.
32. Sadeh A, Hauri PJ, Kripke DF, et al. The role of actigraphy in the evaluation of sleep disorders. Sleep 1995; 18(4):288–302.
33. Verbeek I, Arends J, Declerck G, et al. Wrist actigraphy in comparison with polysomnography and subjective evaluation in insomnia. Sleep-Wake Res Neth 1994; 5:163–169.
34. Hauri PJ, Wisbey J. Wrist actigraphy in insomnia. Sleep 1992; 15(4):293–301.
35. Vallieres A, Morin CM. Actigraphy in the assessment of insomnia. Sleep 2003; 26(7):902–906.
36. Johns MW. Reliability and factor analysis of the Epworth Sleepiness Scale. Sleep 1992; 15(4): 376–381.
37. Johns MW. A new method for measuring daytime sleepiness: the Epworth Sleepiness Scale. Sleep 1991; 14(6):540–545.
38. Maislin G, Pack AI, Kribbs NB et al. A survey screen for prediction of apnea. Sleep 1995; 18(3):158–166.
39. Smets EMA, Garssen B, Bonke B, et al. The Multidimensional Fatigue Inventory (MFI) psychometric qualities of an instrument to assess fatigue. J Psychosom Res 1995; 39:315–325.
40. Krupp LB, LaRocca NG, Muir-Nash J, et al. The fatigue severity scale. Application to patients with multiple sclerosis and systemic lupus erythematosus. Arch Neurol 1989; 46(10):1121–1123.
41. First M, Spitzer RL, Gibbon M, et al. Structured Clinical Interview for DSM-IV Axis II Personality Disorders (SCID-II), Version 2.0. Version 2.0 ed. New York: New York State Psychiatric Institute, 1994.
42. Hamilton M. A rating scale for depression. J Neurol Neurosurg Psychiatry 1960; 23:56–62.
43. Hamilton M. The assessment of anxiety states by rating. Br J Med Psychol 1959; 32:50–55.
44. Beck AT, Steer RA. Manual for Beck Depression Inventory. San Antonio, TX: Psychological Corporation, 1987.
45. Beck AT, Ward CH, Mendelson M, et al. An inventory for measuring depression. Arch Gen Psychiatry 1961; 4:561–571.
46. Beck AT, Steer RA, Brown GK. Manual for Beck Depression Inventory II (BDI-II). San Antonio, TX: Psychology Corporation, 1996.
47. Rush AJ, Gullion CM, Basco MR, et al. The Inventory of Depressive Symptomatology (IDS): psychometric properties. Psychol Med 1996; 26(3):477–486.
48. Beck AT, Epstein N, Brown G, et al. An inventory for measuring clinical anxiety: psychometric properties. J Consult Clin Psychol 1988; 56:893–897.
49. Spielberger CD. State-Trait Anxiety Inventory for Adults. Palo Alto, CA: Consulting Psychologists Press, Inc., 1968.
50. Moul DE, Buysse DJ. Evaluation of insomnia. In: Lee-Chiong TL, ed. Sleep: A Comprehensive Handbook. Hoboken, NJ: John Wiley and Sons, Inc., 2006:117–123.
51. Monk TH, Reynolds CF, Kupfer DJ, et al. The Pittsburgh Sleep Diary. J Sleep Res 1994; 3:111–120.

11 Insomnia Diagnosis and Classification

Daniel J. Buysse

Neuroscience Clinical and Translational Research Center, University of Pittsburgh School of Medicine, Pittsburgh, Pennsylvania, U.S.A.

INTRODUCTION

Classification in medicine serves several purposes. In the clinical arena, disease classification is used to identify individuals with a consistent set of symptoms and signs. This permits conditions of a similar type or etiology to be recognized and discriminated from other conditions, and helps to guide therapeutic interventions. In serving these functions, classification provides a sort of "shorthand" for communication among professionals. Additionally, classification is important for administrative functions such as medical record-keeping and billing. Within the research arena, classification provides consistency in the identification of "cases" for scientific investigation into epidemiology, course, etiology, pathophysiology, and treatment. Ideally, the conceptualization and classification of disorders informs research into their etiology and treatment, and such research leads back to refinements of conceptualization and classification. Generalizations regarding etiology and treatment efficacy depend on reliable and valid diagnoses. In this chapter, we will briefly review some general aspects of disease classification, and present an overview regarding classification of insomnia, highlighting findings from empirical research studies.

Definitions

At the most basic clinical level, *symptoms* are defined as complaints or other subjective evidence presented by the patient. *Signs* are objective indicators of a health, illness, or functioning. Thus, "difficulty falling asleep" is a symptom; polysomnographic sleep latency value of 32 minutes is a sign. A *syndrome* is a characteristic set of symptoms and/or signs, which often follow a characteristic clinical course. An *illness* or *disorder* typically encompasses the elements of a syndrome, but also includes the connotation of suffering and a deviation from the normal state of function. Finally, the term *disease* includes all the elements of a syndrome, but also connotes a particular etiology. The etiology and pathophysiology of different diseases may vary widely. For instance, diseases may be defined in terms of morbid anatomy (e.g., mitral stenosis), cellular pathology (e.g., cancer), molecular pathology (e.g., porphyria) or an infectious agent (e.g., tuberculosis). A *diagnosis* is the determination of the nature of a case of illness or disorder, derived from the Latin verb meaning "to recognize". More commonly, diagnosis refers to the label placed on a specific case of disease, illness or disorder. A *nosology* is a classification system of diseases, an organizational structure comprising a set of specific diagnoses. Classification systems may use *categorical* or *dimensional* models of disorders and diseases, or some combination of the two (as is the case with sleep disorders classifications). A categorical model assumes that individuals with a disorder/disease differ in some fundamental, noncontinuous way from the remainder of the population, allowing a clean distinction between affected and unaffected individuals. In sleep medicine, narcolepsy is an example of a disease, which can be classified in categorical terms; an individual either has narcolepsy or does not. In dimensional disease models, affected and unaffected individuals are seen as coming from a single population, with affected individuals exceeding a specified threshold. In sleep medicine, sleep apnea is an example of a disorder based on a dimensional threshold.

According to these definitions, insomnia may best be seen as a symptom or a disorder rather than a true disease. Sometimes "insomnia" is used to refer to an isolated complaint (symptom); in other cases, it is used to indicate a disorder, i.e., a consistent set of symptoms and signs which causes distress or impairment, but for which no precise etiology has been defined. Whether as a symptom or disorder, insomnia is most often conceptualized in dimensional rather than categorical terms, which may help to explain why the percentage of affected individuals may vary from study to study, and why there is occasionally confusion as to whether an individual should be considered to have a disorder at all. However, the ultimate goal of classification, even in insomnia diagnosis, is to assign individuals to discrete diagnostic categories for purposes of clinical management or research investigation.

Finally, many disorders and diseases can have variable presentations of symptoms and signs. For some diseases, pathological structure is the only criterion; cancer is an example. For other diseases, even those with known pathophysiology, symptoms and signs can quite variable; systemic lupus erythematosus and multiple sclerosis are two common examples in which the pathophysiology is known, but specific manifestations vary considerably from one individual to another. Finally, disorders without established pathophysiology or etiology, defined by symptoms and signs alone, can be highly variable among individuals. For instance, two individuals who meet the criteria for major depressive disorder may have virtually no symptoms in common. Insomnia disorders encompass a similar wide degree of variability. For instance, the criteria for general insomnia disorder according to the International Classification of Sleep Disorders, Second Edition (ICSD-2) encompass individuals who present with sleep onset difficulty and irritability as well as individuals with nonrestorative sleep and daytime fatigue.

Key Attributes of Classification Systems

A classification system for insomnia diagnoses should possess several key attributes. First, the system should be reasonably easy to use. Complex diagnoses or classification systems are unlikely to be widely used, even if they accurately describe disorders or diseases. Second, for administrative reasons, classifications for insomnia should conform to or be compatible with widely accepted disease classifications, such as the International Classification of Diseases and the International Classification of Functioning, Disability and Health. Third, classifications and diagnoses must have acceptable reliability, which refers to the extent to which diagnoses are reproducible, either among multiple raters (inter-rater reliability), within a single rater (intra-rater reliability) or across time (test-retest reliability). Third, classifications and diagnoses should have acceptable measures of validity, defined as the extent to which a diagnosis serves its purpose of case identification, clinical prediction, or communication. The goals of classification and diagnosis sometimes differ in clinical and research settings. In clinical settings, an important goal is to have diagnostic and descriptive coverage for all or most cases, leaving very few cases, which cannot be classified. As a result, optimal clinical categories are often fairly broad. Research applications often benefit from more narrow diagnostic categories to ensure homogenous samples for pathophysiological and treatment research. Thus, the goal of classification in clinical practice is to diagnosis and treat *patients*, whereas the goal of classification in research is often to study a specific *disease or disorder*.

Classification Systems for Insomnia

Multiple systems have been proposed for classifying insomnia symptoms and disorders, with changes over time that reflect the prevailing zeitgeists. Most important has been an evolution in thinking about insomnia with regard to its conceptualization as a symptom or a disorder, and with regard to the nature of causality. Some of the earliest classifications describe insomnia as a symptom, not a disorder (1,2). Clinicians were encouraged to identify the symptom of insomnia in order to identify and treat underlying causes, most often emotional distress or frank psychiatric disorders. The implication was that treating the underlying condition would lead to resolution of insomnia. However, establishing causality or even the temporal relationship between insomnia and other disorders can be difficult, imprecise, and ineffective (3,4). For instance, insomnia and fatigue are the most common residual symptoms of depression, (5) and even when painful medical conditions such as arthritis are identified and treated, insomnia may persist (6,7). Thus, more recent conceptualizations suggest that it may be more appropriate to think of insomnia as a disorder that is frequently comorbid with, rather than secondary to, other conditions. This view was emphasized in the 2005 NIH State of the Science Conference on insomnia (8).

Another common method of classifying insomnia, also exemplified by the 1983 NIH Consensus Conference on Insomnia, (1) was to classify insomnia by its duration: Transient, defined as less than two weeks; short-term, lasting for two to four weeks; and chronic, lasting greater than four weeks (1). This type of classification, however, is recognized as being an intermediate step toward more specific etiologically-based diagnoses, which often differ in their duration. For instance, transient insomnia complaints are often associated with situational, environmental, or medical stresses, and chronic insomnia is more often associated with psychiatric disorders, circadian rhythm disorders, or primary dysregulation of sleep-wake mechanisms. Duration-based insomnia disorders are to some extent recognized in more formal nosologies such as ICSD-2 in disorders such as adjustment sleep disorder, with a duration of less than three months, and idiopathic insomnia, with a lifelong course. Empirical evidence and epidemiological studies also address potential subtypes based on duration. A Gallup Poll conducted for the National Sleep Foundation suggested that approximately 30% of adults complained of transient, short-term, or recurrent insomnia, and 10% complained of chronic problems (9). The cross-sectional national Comorbidity Survey Replication study demonstrated a more bimodal distribution of insomnia duration, with approximately 20% of patients reporting symptoms of less than four weeks duration, and approximately 30% reporting symptoms for greater than one year (10). Some longitudinal studies suggest a continuum of insomnia duration, including occasional insomnia, repeated brief insomnia, and more persistent forms (11,12). Studies with follow-up intervals of one to three years suggest that insomnia symptoms persist in approximately 50% to 80% of individuals, depending on the definition of insomnia symptoms (13,14). Other data suggest that more severe forms of insomnia have greater chronicity. A three-year follow-up study demonstrated remission in approximately 40% of individuals with insomnia *symptoms*, whereas approximately 80% of individuals with insomnia *syndrome* had a chronic course (15). Data from the Wisconsin Sleep Cohort indicate that approximately two-third of individuals with insomnia symptoms have persistent symptoms at 3 and 10 year follow-up (16). Therefore, some empirical data support the distinction between duration-based insomnia subtypes. However, duration in itself provides little guidance in terms of appropriate interventions, but merely points toward likely contributing factors that can be specifically addressed.

Another common, but informal, method for classifying insomnia is by the specific symptom presentation: sleep onset insomnia, sleep maintenance insomnia, or nonrestorative sleep. Epidemiological and survey data demonstrate that sleep maintenance insomnia is consistently the most prevalent symptom, and early morning awakening the least common.(17) Moreover, symptom types vary with age, with sleep onset insomnia and nonrestorative sleep being relatively more common in younger adults, and sleep maintenance insomnia being more common with increasing age [e.g., (17,18)]. However, such studies also demonstrate the high rate of cooccurrence of individual symptoms, and the strong correlation between them. For instance, in the National Comorbidity Survey Replication, each of the symptoms correlated with each of the others with r values of 0.65 to 0.84 (10), and up to 80% of insomnia patients have more than one symptom when followed longitudinally (16). Moreover, longitudinal studies demonstrate that individuals' specific symptom type frequently changes over time (16,19). Insomnia symptom types may provide clues to specific contributing factors such as Restless Legs Syndrome or subclinical circadian phase delays (20) in individuals with sleep onset complaints. Symptom patterns are also considered in selecting specific treatments. For instance, a patient who presents with predominantly sleep onset complaints may be an appropriate candidate for a short-acting benzodiazepine receptor agonist, and a patient with predominantly sleep maintenance complaints may benefit from a longer-acting agent. However, because of the frequent cooccurrence of symptoms and their poor stability over time, symptom subtype does not appear to be an adequate basis for diagnostic classification. Formal diagnostic classifications for insomnia have been proposed as part of more comprehensive sleep disorders nosologies. These classifications distinguish different insomnia disorders on the basis of specific sleep symptoms, other clinical features (e.g., duration, polysomnographic features), and the presence or absence of other sleep, general medical, and psychiatric disorders. Table 1 outlines the major classification systems for sleep disorders used the past 30 years: the diagnostic classification of sleep and arousal disorders (DCSAD) (2); the international classification of sleep disorders (ICSD) (21,22); the International Classification of Sleep Disorders, 2nd Edition (ICSD-2) (23); the Diagnostic and Statistical Manual of Mental Disorders, Third Edition Revised (DSM-III-R) (24); and Fourth Edition (DSM-IV) (25); and the International Classification of Diseases, 9th Edition, Clinical Modification (ICD-9CM) (26) and 10th Edition (27). These classification systems differ substantially in terms of their

Table 1 Diagnostic Classifications for Sleep Disorders

Diagnostic Classification of Sleep and Arousal Disorders (DCSAD) (2)	International Classification of Sleep Disorders (ICSD) (21,22)	International Classification of Sleep Disorders, 2nd Edition (ICSD-2) (23)	Diagnostic and Statistical Manual of Mental Disorders, 3rd Edition Revised (DSM-III-R) (24)	Diagnostic and Statistical Manual of Mental Disorders, 4th Edition (DSM-IV) (25)	International Statistical Classification of Diseases and Related Health Problems, 9th Edition, Clinical Modification (ICD-9-CM) (26)	International Statistical Classification of Diseases and Related Health Problems, 10th Edition (ICD-10) (27)
• Disorders of Initiating and maintaining sleep (DIMS) • Disorders of excessive sleep (DOES) • Disorders of the sleep–wake schedule • Parasomnias	• Dyssomnias – Intrinsic – Extrinsic – Circadian rhythm sleep disorders • Parasomnias • Sleep disorders–associated with mental, neurologic, or medical disorders • Proposed sleep disorders	• Insomnia • Sleep-related breathing disorders • Hypersomnias of central origin • Circadian rhythm sleep disorders • Parasomnias • Sleep-related movement disorders • Isolated symptoms, apparently normal variants, and unresolved issues • Other sleep disorders	• Dyssomnias – Insomnia disorder – Hypersomnia disorder – Sleep–wake schedule disorder • Parasomnias	• Primary sleep disorders – Dyssomnias – Parasomnias • Sleep disorders related to another mental disorder • Sleep disorders due to medical disorder • Substance-induced sleep disorder	• Sleep disturbances (organic) • Specific disorders of sleep of nonorganic origin	• Sleep disorders (organic) • Sleep disorders due to emotional causes

organizational schemes, the number of specific diagnoses, and their reliance on specific criteria. An overview of these features is presented in Table 2. Specific insomnia diagnoses within each classification are outlined in Table 3.

The DCSAD, the first widely used classification of sleep disorders, includes four major categories of disorders: Disorders of Initiating and Maintaining Sleep (DIMS or insomnias), Disorders of Excessive Sleepiness (DOES or hypersomnias), Disorders of the Sleep/Wake Schedule, and Parasomnias. This classification is easy to use, given its symptom-based organization. The number of individual categories is large, and approximately 30 diagnoses could conceivably include a complaint of insomnia. The DCSAD provides useful clinical descriptions of each disorder. However, it also has some important limitations. First, specific clinical and polysomnographic criteria are not included, which necessitates considerable clinical judgment in establishing a diagnosis and is likely to decrease reliability. Second, the symptom-based approach makes sense clinically but leads to duplicate listings for a single disorder. For instance, periodic limb movement disorder can produce either insomnia or hypersomnia, so the diagnosis was listed twice in the classification, in both the DIMS and DOES sections.

The ICSD is a successor to the DCSAD, published in 1990. It differs from the DCSAD classification in two major ways. First, the organization of disorders is by presumed etiology rather than symptom presentation. Second, the ICSD includes specific clinical and polysomnographic criteria, severity ratings, and both "minimal" and "complete" diagnostic criteria for each disorder. The three major categories of sleep disorders in ICSD are dyssomnias, parasomnias, and secondary sleep disorders. *Dyssomnias* are disorders in which the major signs and symptoms relate to sleep and/or wakefulness. The dyssomnias are further subdivided into intrinsic dyssomnias, in which some abnormality of brain function is thought to underlie the symptoms and signs; extrinsic disorders, in which some external factor leads to the sleep complaint; and circadian rhythm sleep disorders, which are thought to result from abnormal entrainment or misalignment of the circadian system with external time cues. *Secondary sleep disorders* are those associated with, and presumed to be causally related to, mental, neurologic, and medical disorders. In contrast to dyssomnias, secondary sleep disorders occur within a context of broader set of symptoms and signs of the "primary" disorder. Of the 84 diagnoses in ICSD, approximately 43 may be associated with insomnia complaints, including those in Dyssomnia and Secondary Sleep Disorder categories. ICSD defines insomnia as in general as a "complaint of an insufficient amount of sleep or not feeling rested after the habitual sleep episode." Daytime symptoms associated with insomnia, such as restlessness, irritability, anxiety, fatigue, and tiredness, are described in the severity criteria, rather than in the insomnia disorders themselves.

Although the ICSD has several advantages compared DCSAD, it also has some limitations, many of which apply to other classifications as well. First, diagnoses are based largely upon expert opinion, although literature reviews were also used. Second, for most sleep disorders, the exact pathophysiology remains unknown, despite the broad pathophysiological orientation, which drives ICSD. Third, most specific diagnostic criteria in the ICSD have not been rigorously tested against alternative criteria, being based largely upon expert opinion. Fourth, there is some concern that the ICSD's large number of categories may represent a form of pseudo precision. For instance, Reynolds and colleagues (28) argued that sub-typing chronic insomnia into different disorders may be premature, given the uncertain validity of concepts such as sleep state misperception, environmental sleep disorder, and inadequate sleep hygiene. Finally, the specific diagnostic criteria for certain disorders have been questioned by expert interest groups within those areas. For instance, alternative criteria had been proposed for the diagnosis of restless leg syndrome and periodic limb movements, (29) sleep apnea syndromes, (30) and narcolepsy (31,32).

ICSD-2 was published in 2005. The framework of ICSD-2 departs substantially from ICSD in two major ways. First, ICSD-2 groups sleep disorders into eight major categories based on major symptom presentation and presumed etiology (Table 2). Insomnia is one of these categories, and 11 specific insomnia diagnoses are grouped in that section. Brief descriptions of these diagnoses are presented in Table 3. Second, ICSD-2 specifies general criteria for insomnia which apply to all diagnoses within the Insomnia section (Table 4). The important elements of this definition are (1) a sleep-related insomnia complaint; (2) adequate opportunity and circumstances to sleep, clearly demarcating insomnia from problems related to

Table 2 Diagnostic Classifications for Sleep Disorders

	DCSAD (2)	ICSD (21,22)	ICSD-2 (23)	DSM-III-R (24)	DSM-IV (25)	ICD-9-CM (26)	ICD-10 (27)
Derivation	Expert opinion	Expert opinion, literature reviews	Expert opinion, literature reviews	Expert opinion	Expert opinion, literature reviews	Expert opinion	Expert opinion
Major organizing feature	Symptoms	Presumed pathophysiology/ etiology	Symptoms, Presumed pathophysiology/ etiology	Symptoms	Presumed pathophysiology/ etiology	Presumed pathophysiology/ etiology	Presumed pathophysiology/ etiology
Breadth of categories	Narrow	Narrow	Narrow	Broad	Intermediate	Broad	Broad
Number of specific disorders	68	88	81	15	25	18	15
Polysomnographic criteria	No	Yes, for some disorders, but not insomnia	Yes, for some disorders, but not insomnia	No	No	No	No

Table 3 ICSD-2 Insomnia Disorders

Adjustment insomnia (acute insomnia)	• Insomnia temporally associated with an identifiable stressor • Sleep disturbance expected to resolve when the acute stressor resolves or when the individual adapts • Sleep disturbance lasts for less than three months
Psychophysiological insomnia	• Insomnia present for at least one month • Evidence of conditioned sleep difficulty and/or heightened arousal as indicated by one or more of the following: (1) Excessive focus on and heightened anxiety about sleep (2) Difficulty falling asleep in bed at desired bedtime or during planned naps, but not during monotonous activities when not intending to sleep (3) Sleep better away from home than at home (4) Mental arousal in bed (intrusive thoughts or inability to cease sleep-preventing mental activity) (5) Heightened somatic tension in bed, perceived inability to relax the body
Paradoxical insomnia	• Insomnia present for at least one month • One or more of the following: (1) Chronic pattern of little or no sleep most nights with rare nights of relatively normal amounts of sleep (2) Sleep-log data show an average sleep time well below normative values (3) Consistent marked mismatch between objective findings from polysomnography or actigraphy and subjective sleep estimates • At least one of the following: (1) Constant or near constant awareness of environmental stimuli throughout most nights (2) Conscious thoughts or rumination throughout most nights while maintaining a recumbent posture • Daytime impairment consistent with that reported by other insomnia subtypes, but much less severe than expected given the extreme level of sleep deprivation
Idiopathic insomnia	• Course of the disorder is chronic, as indicated by each of the following: (1) Onset during infancy or childhood (2) No identifiable precipitant or cause (3) Persistent course with no periods of sustained remission
Due to mental disorder	• Insomnia present for at least one month • Mental disorder has been diagnosed according to standard criteria • Insomnia is temporally associated with the mental disorder (may appear a few days or weeks before the emergence of the mental disorder) • Insomnia is more prominent than that typically associated with the mental disorders, as indicated by marked distress or an independent focus of treatment
Inadequate sleep hygiene	• Insomnia present for at least one month • Inadequate sleep hygiene practices indicated by at least one of the following: (1) Improper sleep scheduling (frequent daytime napping, highly variable bedtimes or rising times, excessive amounts of time in bed) (2) Use of alcohol, nicotine, or caffeine, especially in the period preceding bedtime (3) Mentally stimulating, physically activating, or emotionally upsetting activities too close to bedtime (4) Frequent use of the bed for activities other than sleep (5) Failure to maintain comfortable sleeping environment
Behavioral insomnia of childhood	• Sleep onset association type includes each of the following: (1) Falling asleep is an extended process that requires special conditions (2) Sleep onset associations are highly problematic or demanding (3) In the absence of the associated conditions, sleep onset is significantly delayed or sleep is otherwise disrupted (4) Nighttime awakenings require caregiver intervention for the child to return to sleep

Table 3 ICSD-2 Insomnia Disorders (*Continued*)

	• Limit-setting type includes each of the following: (1) Difficulty initiating or maintaining sleep (2) Stalls or refuses to go to bed at an appropriate time or refuses to return to bed following a nighttime awakening (3) Caregiver demonstrates insufficient or inappropriate limit setting to establish appropriate sleeping behavior in the child
Due to drug or substance	• Insomnia present for at least one month • One of the following applies (1) Current ongoing dependence on or abuse of a drug or substance known to have sleep-disruptive properties either during use or intoxication or withdrawal (2) Current ongoing use of or exposure to a medication, food, or toxin known to have sleep-disruptive properties in susceptible individuals • Insomnia temporally associated with the substance exposure, use or abuse, or acute withdrawal
Due to medical condition	• Insomnia is present for at least one month • Coexisting medical or physiologic condition known to disrupt sleep • Insomnia associated with the medical or physiologic condition (began near the time of onset, or with significant progression of the medical or physiologic condition and varies the severity of this condition)

Source: From Ref. 23.

behaviorally-induced insufficient sleep or environmental disturbance; and (3) the presence of at least one type of daytime impairment related to the sleep disturbance. The general criteria for insomnia were derived from Research Diagnostic Criteria for Insomnia, (33) discussed further below. The ICSD-2 general criterion for insomnia includes not only complaints of difficulty initiating or maintaining sleep, but also complaints of "sleep that is chronically nonrestorative or poor in quality." Nonrestorative sleep has traditionally been included among insomnia complaints, although significant uncertainty exists regarding whether this symptom is similar to other symptoms of chronic insomnia with regard to precursors, precipitants, pathology and associated factors.

The subtypes of insomnia and diagnostic criteria in ICSD-2 are similar to those in ICSD, with a few exceptions. The ICSD diagnosis of Sleep State Misperception is renamed Paradoxical Insomnia in ICSD-2. More importantly, the ICSD diagnoses related to childhood insomnia, i.e., Limit-setting Sleep Disorder and Sleep-onset Association Disorder, were merged into a single diagnosis in ICSD-2 called Behavioral Insomnia of Childhood. This diagnosis was moved from the ICSD section of Extrinsic Sleep Disorders to the ICSD-2 section of Insomnia. Finally, ICSD-2

Table 4 ICSD-2 General Insomnia Criteria

(A) A complaint of difficulty initiating sleep, difficulty maintaining sleep, or waking up too early or sleep that is chronically nonrestorative or poor in quality. In children, the sleep difficulty is often reported by the caretaker and may consist of observed bedtime resistance or inability to sleep independently.
(B) The above sleep difficulty occurs despite adequate opportunity and circumstances for sleep.
(C) At least one of the following forms of daytime impairment related to the nighttime sleep difficulty is reported by the patient:

(i) Fatigue or malaise
(ii) Attention, concentration, or memory impairment
(iii) Social or vocational dysfunction or poor school performance
(iv) Mood disturbance or irritability
(v) Daytime sleepiness
(vi) Motivation, energy, or initiative reduction
(vii) Proneness for errors or accidents at work or while driving
(viii) Tension, headaches, or gastrointestinal symptoms in response to sleep loss
(ix) Concerns or worries about sleep

Source: From Ref. 23.

brings the "secondary" insomnia disorders due to mental disorder, medical disorder, or substance abuse, into the insomnia section. Although ICSD-2 identifies insomnia disorders within a single section, clinicians must also be mindful of the fact that many, in fact most, other major sections within the nosology also contain diagnoses that may include an insomnia complaint as one element of the clinical presentation. For instance, insomnia complaints are ubiquitous in the circadian rhythm disorders and common among breathing and movement disorders as well. Even patients with narcolepsy often report insomnia, occasionally as a presenting complaint. Insomnia symptoms associated with these other major sleep disorders may coexist with major insomnia diagnoses (primary or comorbid), requiring that both disorders be targeted effectively in treatment.ICSD-2 employs the terminology of "insomnia due to. . ." in identifying what have historically been referred to as "secondary" insomnia conditions. As discussed above, current evidence suggests the importance of moving away from the concept of secondary insomnia and toward that of comorbid insomnia.

The DSM-III-R and DSM-IV were designed as classifications of mental disorders but also include sleep disorders sections. DSM-III-R includes two major sections of sleep disorders, *dyssomnias* and *parasomnias*. The dyssomnias include insomnia disorder, hypersomnia disorder, and other dyssomnias; within insomnia disorder are three subtypes, related to another mental disorder, related to a known organic factor, and primary insomnia. In DSM-IV, the major divisions of sleep disorders are arranged differently, and include a small number of additional categories. DSM-IV major divisions are *Primary Sleep Disorders,* which include dyssomnias and parasomnias; sleep disorders related to another mental disorder; sleep disorder due to a general medical disorder (including insomnia type); and substance-induced sleep disorder (including insomnia type). Thus, there is some homology between the organization of DSM-III-R and DCSAD, and between DSM-IV and ICSD. The main difference between the psychiatric and sleep medicine classifications is in the number of specific categories and the breadth of these diagnoses. For instance, DSM-IV includes only one diagnosis for chronic "primary" insomnia unrelated to mental, medical, or substance-induced sleep disorders (primary insomnia). This category subsumes more specific ICSD categories such as psychophysiological insomnia, inadequate sleep hygiene, idiopathic hypersomnia, adjustment sleep disorder, and environmental sleep disorder, both in theory and in practice (34). Like the ICSD, DSM-IV was derived from expert opinion and literature reviews, and the organization is based broadly on presumed pathophysiology. Also like ICSD, it includes clinical criteria, but unlike ICSD, it does not include specific polysomnographic criteria or severity descriptors. Although DSM-IV is appropriate for and appears to be well- accepted by the psychiatric community, it is not widely used by sleep disorders specialists.

ICD-9CM and ICD-10 include two broad categories of sleep disorders, those of *organic* origin, and those of *nonorganic origin (due to emotional causes)*. In ICD-10, *Organic sleep disorders* include insomnia, hypersomnia, circadian disorders, sleep apnea, and narcolepsy. *Sleep disorders due to emotional causes* include insomnia, hypersomnia, circadian rhythm disorders, sleepwalking, sleep terrors, and nightmares. Specific diagnostic descriptions are provided only for the nonorganic sleep disorders. The distinction between organic and nonorganic is largely arbitrary and may be difficult to operationalize in clinical practice. Therefore, ICD-9CM and ICD-10 are not widely used clinically for descriptive purposes. However, the diagnosis codes from ICD-9CM have been cross-referenced to ICSD, ICSD-2, and DSM-IV, and these codes are widely used for billing and records keeping purposes.

Although it was developed specifically as a research tool, the Research Diagnostic Criteria for Insomnia (RDC-I) (33) used a rigorous review process and consensus to evaluate reliability and validity data for various insomnia disorders. More than 400 published research studies of insomnia were examined to determine how often various criteria were used in the selection and characterization of study samples, and cross-referenced these actual study selection criteria against the specific DSM-IV or ICSD diagnosis which was said to be studied. For example, actual selection criteria included the use of specific insomnia diagnoses, insomnia duration, medical, psychiatric, and medication exclusions, self-reported symptoms, and polysomnographic findings. Based on this literature review and a consensus process, the work group developed research criteria for those diagnoses with the greatest empirical support. This led to the development of research diagnostic criteria for general insomnia disorder, nine specific insomnia disorders, and normal sleepers. The nine specific disorders include primary insomnia, insomnia due to a mental disorder, psychophysiological insomnia, paradoxical insomnia, idiopathic insomnia, insomnia related to periodic limb mvement disorder, insomnia related to sleep apnea, insomnia due to medical condition, and insomnia due to drug or substance. Note that these disorders include categories included in ICSD and in DSM-IV. Beyond the provision of specific diagnostic criteria, the rigorous process of the RDC-I influenced the development of insomnia disorder categories included in ICSD-2.

In summary, existing classifications for insomnia disorders show similarities and differences, and have their own strengths and weaknesses. The ICSD-2 is currently most widely used by sleep disorders specialists.

A survey conducted in 1996, prior to the introduction of ICSD-2, examined the use of various sleep disorders classifications in clinical practice (35). This survey indicated that 91.7% of participating sleep disorders centers used the ICSD for establishing clinical diagnoses, consistent with center accreditation standards at the time. However, clinicians rated the organizational structure of ICSD and DCSAD significantly more favorably than that of ICD-9 or DSM-IV, and DCSAD was ranked more favorably than ICSD. Thus, clinicians seemed to prefer the intuitive symptom-based structure of DCSAD. The "fit" of each classification to actual patients was also rated more highly for ICSD and DCSAD compared to ICD-9 and DSM-IV. In terms of "ease of use", clinicians rated the DCSAD as being simpler than ICSD. These data indicate that clinicians use the diagnostic classification systems available, but seem to find a symptom-based system easier to use. Although this survey preceded the introduction of ICSD-2, it is worth noting that the overall organization of ICSD-2, with six major diagnostic clusters, resembles the organization of DCSAD more than that of ICSD.

Reliability

Reliability is a measure of the extent to which diagnoses are reproducible across time (test-retest reliability), across multiple ratings by a single rater (intra-rater reliability), and among different raters (inter-rater reliability). Several sources of variance contribute to reduced reliability. First, test-retest reliability may be low because patients' actual clinical state may change from one time to another. Inter-rater reliability may be imperfect because the judgments of one clinician will not perfectly match those of another. In addition, both types of reliability may suffer from measurement error, either in the sensitivity of particular questions asked of a patient, or of physiological measures such as EEG sleep studies. Similarly, the interpretation of specific measurements may vary across raters and over time. Finally, the specific criteria used to establish a diagnosis may be imprecise. Table 5 summarizes data on inter-rater and test-retest reliability for insomnia diagnoses using various diagnostic criteria. The table illustrates that the total number of reliability studies and the total number of insomnia patients assessed has been small. The most rigorous work has been conducted with ICSD-2 and DSM-IV, although publication of peer-reviewed findings is pending at this time.

Although not a measure of reliability per se, one would expect similar patterns of insomnia diagnoses to be made at different sleep medicine centers. A field trial for DSM-IV examined diagnostic patterns in five sleep disorders centers found similar overall patterns of diagnoses, but significantly different relative frequencies for specific diagnoses (36). For instance, some sites made frequent diagnoses of insomnia related to another mental disorder, and very few

Table 5 Interrater Reliability and Convergent Validity for Insomnia Diagnoses

Reference	DSM-III-R/DSM-IV	ICSD	ICSD-2	Total number of subjects	Number of insomnia subjects
(37)	0.91[a]	–		68	54
(36)	0.35–0.56[a]	–		216	216
(38)	0.25[a]	0.22[a]		41	41
(39)	0.71[a]	0.68[a]		31	31
(40,41)	0.09–0.68[b]		0.15–0.68[b]	333	333

[a]Values reported are kappa values for interrater reliability.

[b]Values reported are correlation values for diagnostic ratings across pairs of raters. The reported range of values represents values for different specific diagnoses.

diagnoses of Primary Insomnia, whereas other sites had the opposite pattern. This study also examined diagnostic patterns of two different interviewers at each site, one a sleep specialist and one a nonsleep specialist clinician. The two types of interviewers had similar patterns of overall diagnoses, but nonspecialists tended to make more diagnoses of insomnia due to a medical condition, whereas sleep specialists tended to make more diagnoses such as delayed sleep phase syndrome.

Other studies have examined more traditional measures of inter-rater reliability. Schramm et al (37) used a structured diagnostic interview to establish DSM-III-R insomnia diagnoses in a sample of 68 patients with complaints of sleep disturbances. The overall kappa value for insomnia disorders was 0.91, indicating excellent inter-rater agreement. With regard to specific types of insomnia, kappa values ranged from 0.84 to 0.86 for insomnia related to a mental disorder, insomnia related to a known organic factor, and primary insomnia. Of note, the kappa for primary insomnia was derived from a total of only 10 cases, which again makes the reliability of this estimate uncertain.

The DSM-IV field trial included 216 patients clinically referred for a sleep disorder and evaluated by two interviewers, one an experienced sleep specialist and one a nonsleep specialist clinician. The two raters used their "usual clinical interview" to assess patients. Kappa values for the primary diagnosis ranged from 0.35 to 0.56 across the five sites, indicating only moderate diagnostic agreement. Kappa values for specific diagnoses were somewhat worse, ranging from 0.28 to 0.59 for primary insomnia and 0.34 to 0.60 for insomnia related to another mental disorder. The lower degree of inter-rater reliability in this study likely related to the use of clinical interviews, rather than structured interviews, and clinicians who varied in their sleep expertise. However, videotaped interviews for a subset of 41 patients were reviewed by sleep specialists at each of the five sites. The overall kappa value for DSM-IV and ICSD diagnoses ranged from 0.22 to 0.25, in the fair to poor range(38). Thus, it appears that different raters, even among sleep specialists, make use of clinical information in different ways to establish diagnoses.

Another small study (39) examined inter-rater agreement for DSM-III-R and ICSD diagnoses in 31 clinically referred patients with insomnia, with diagnoses based on clinical and polysomnographic information rather than direct interview with the patients. A kappa value of 0.71 was found for DSM-III-R diagnoses, and 0.68 for ICSD diagnoses, within the moderate to very good range of reliability.

No published studies have formally assessed the test-retest reliability of insomnia diagnoses. The study by Schramm and colleagues described above indicates that test-retest reliability was assessed, but the interval between interviews was only one to three days. In addition, this study combined elements of both a test-retest and inter-rater reliability study.

More recent preliminary data from a two-site study examined the reliability and validity of DSM-IV and ICSD-2 insomnia diagnoses in 333 patients.(40) Each patient was interviewed by six sleep specialists, using various combinations of clinical interview, structured interview, and PSG information. Inter-rater correlations for DSM-IV diagnoses were highest for disorders that might be considered secondary or comorbid forms of insomnia, such as alcohol-induced, insomnia related to another mental or medical disorder, breathing-related sleep disorder, and circadian rhythm sleep disorder, with inter-rater *r* values of approximately 0.40 to 0.70. DSM-IV primary insomnia and other forms of insomnia were least reliable, with *r* values of approximately 0.10 to 0.30. Among ICSD-2 diagnoses, highest reliability was associated with insomnia related to a mental or medical disorder, restless legs syndrome, idiopathic insomnia, delayed sleep phase syndrome, and obstructive sleep apnea (*r* values approximately 0.34–0.68); lowest reliability was seen for paradoxical insomnia. Some ICSD-2 insomnia diagnoses were never chosen. The authors conclude that reliability and validity of some, but not all, DSM-IV and ICSD-2 diagnoses was supported, and that the former nosology may have too few categories, and the latter too many. Further data from this study indicated that use of a structured diagnostic interview was associated with greater reliability against "gold standard" diagnoses than standard clinical interviews.(41)

In summary, available data suggest moderate inter-rater reliability for insomnia diagnoses using DSM-IV, ICSD, and ICSD-2 criteria. Test-retest reliability has yet to be adequately assessed. The finding of significant differences among sleep disorder centers and the diagnoses they establish, and the low rates of inter-rater agreement among sleep specialists at different sites, suggest that different investigators apply the diagnostic criteria for insomnia disorders in very different ways. Data from a small number of studies also suggest moderate improvements in reliability with the use of structured interview and/or PSG data.

Validity

Validity is a measure of the extent to which a diagnosis serves its purposes of case identification, clinical prediction, or communication. Several types of validity are commonly investigated. *Face validity* or *ecological validity* describes how reasonable a diagnosis is based on clinical experience; in other words, does the diagnosis make sense and reflect a condition seen in the real world? *Construct validity* refers to the degree to which a diagnosis (or other measurement scale) measures the theoretical, etiological, or pathological construct it is designed to measure, and is often inferred from discriminant and convergent validity. *Descriminant validity* relates to how well specific features discriminate one diagnosis from other diagnoses. *Convergent validity* refers to the degree to which one diagnosis or set of diagnostic criteria relates to similar diagnoses or criteria. *Predictive validity* assesses the degree to which a diagnosis corresponds with a particular natural history or treatment response.

A large number of studies have been reported which describe distinctive clinical features or polysomnographic features of one type of insomnia diagnosis compared to other insomnia diagnoses. For instance, traditional polysomnographic and clinical characteristics that distinguish "chronic insomnia" from the insomnia of depression (42,43) or "objective insomnia" from "subjective insomnia" (44,45) have been evaluated. Other analyses have demonstrated quantitative EEG sleep differences between subjects with psychophysiological insomnia, paradoxical insomnia, insomnia associated with depression, and good sleepers (46,47). Two studies have also demonstrated similarities and differences in the 24-hour metabolic rate patterns of psychophysological and paradoxical insomnia patients, both of whom differed from controls (48–50). However, confirmatory analyses and replications have been infrequently reported with all of these analyses. Likewise, the sensitivity, specificity, or receiver-operating characteristic curves of specific polysomnographic or clinical features have not been described for one subtype of insomnia versus another. By contrast, such studies have been conducted for measures such as reduced REM latency in depression (51,52). Perhaps partly as a result of infrequently-replicated findings, current clinical recommendations do not support the use of polysomnography for diagnosis in most patients with insomnia (53,54).

Another method of assessing construct validity is to determine how clinical and polysomnographic features empirically cluster, and to match such empirical clusters to clinical diagnoses. Hauri (55) reported a cluster analysis of psychological tests, clinical interview, and three nights of polysomnography in 89 insomnia patients and 10 controls compared to DCSAD diagnoses. Factor analysis identified 26 factors derived from these assessments, and subsequent cluster analysis provided empirical validation for the category of persistent psychophysiological insomnia, insomnia associated with affective disorder, and childhood onset (idiopathic) insomnia. However, six other clusters did not readily correspond to existing DCSAD diagnoses. A similar study used questionnaire data, polysomnographic data, and interview data to derive 15 factors in 113 insomnia patients and 39 healthy controls (39). The 14 empirically-identified clusters did not correspond strongly with either DSM-III-R or ICSD diagnoses. Caution is warranted given the small number of patients and controls relative to the large number of factors in both of these studies.

Construct validity, focusing on distinctions between primary insomnia and insomnia related to another mental disorder, was also addressed in the DSM-IV field trial described above (56). Clinicians were asked to rate factors they thought might contribute to the individual patients insomnia complaint regardless of diagnosis, then assigned a primary diagnosis and up to three secondary diagnoses for each patient. Patients with insomnia related to a mental disorder were identified as having less evidence of poor sleep hygiene and negative conditioning than patients with primary insomnia. Conversely, patients with primary insomnia were felt to have significantly less psychiatric disturbance contributing to their insomnia. These data support the distinction between the insomnia subtypes of primary and psychiatric insomnia, and suggest that additional criteria reflecting sleep hygiene and conditioning factors may help to improve the reliability of these diagnoses.

Clinicians also use diagnostic judgments to make treatment decisions. Further data from the DSM-IV field trial (38) showed that the pattern of diagnostic recommendations for different specific insomnia diagnoses do in fact differ in significant ways. Specifically, treatment recommendations for ICSD diagnoses of psychophysiological insomnia, delayed sleep phase syndrome, inadequate sleep hygiene, insomnia related to mood disorder, and obstructive sleep apnea syndrome have very distinct patterns of treatment recommendations. Treatment recommendations are not equivalent to treatment outcomes, but these data do provide some support for the notion that clinicians believe their diagnoses have predictive validity in the clinical setting.

Finally, the two-site study of DSM-IV and ICSD-2 diagnoses described above also addressed questions of convergent validity using multitrait/multi-method matrices based on the diagnoses of six raters (57). These analyses demonstrated strong validity indices for ICSD-2 idiopathic insomnia, moderate indices for psychophysiological insomnia, environmental sleep disorder, and inadequate sleep hygiene, and low indices for paradoxical insomnia. DSM-IV primary insomnia had lower validity indices than all ICSD-2 diagnoses except paradoxical insomnia. These findings suggest that specific diagnostic criteria may improve the reliability and validity of insomnia diagnoses, in contrast to the broad and nonspecific criteria used in DSM-IV primary insomnia.

Summary and Future Directions

Although insomnia has long been recognized as one of the fundamental forms of disordered sleep, approaches to its classification and diagnosis have varied considerably. The best current evidence suggests that insomnia is a disorder of brain function rather than a disease per se, and that it exists on a continuum of healthy to disordered sleep. Approaches to classification of insomnia have shifted over the past 30 to 40 years. Insomnia was long held to be exclusively a symptom of other underlying conditions, most often mental disorders. Subsequently, insomnia was conceptualized as existing in both primary and secondary forms. Most recently, as exemplified in the 2005 NIH State of The Science Conference, insomnia has been viewed as a disorder that is frequently comorbid with other conditions, but not necessarily caused by those conditions. This change in conceptualization has been mirrored to some extent by sleep disorder nosologies more than the past 30 years. During this time, considerable debate has continued regarding the issue of "lumping versus. splitting" insomnia disorders, about whether to include quantitative criteria in insomnia diagnoses, and about how to best define insomnia subtypes (e.g., by symptom presentation, duration, and/or presumed etiology).

Inter-rater reliability for insomnia diagnoses has generally been only fair to moderate for any of the diagnostic systems, although few published studies have been adequately powered to address this issue. Structured interviews improve diagnostic reliability. Although numerous studies have been published that lend support to the validity of insomnia as a disorder of sleep and arousal relative to "normal" sleep, few of these studies have been replicated, and no biological marker can be said to exist for insomnia. The best available evidence to support the validity of specific insomnia diagnoses is for idiopathic insomnia and comorbid insomnia, particularly insomnia comorbid with mental disorders. Both reliability and validity of insomnia diagnoses are improved with the inclusion of more specific diagnostic criteria; this observation may be useful as a way to increase the reliability of "primary" insomnia.

Clinicians should consider several additional factors when using any insomnia diagnostic system. While accurate diagnosis represents an important step in the assessment and management of the insomnia patient, it is not an end in itself. Most chronic insomnia is multifactorial in nature and some patients may satisfy criteria for more than one insomnia diagnosis. Moreover, a number will also satisfy criteria for other, noninsomnia diagnoses such as obstructive sleep apnea or a parasomnia. Therefore, it is essential that the clinician thinks in multifactorial terms and carefully consider the rich and complex interaction among various diagnoses and other contributing issues.

In the future, work on insomnia symptoms, pathophysiology, and biological markers will need to be conducted and replicated in much larger samples, and across multiple sites. Only studies of this sort can hope to identify reliable clinical and biological markers of insomnia. Insomnia classification will also be aided by the inclusion of genetic analyses in combination with careful clinical and physiological phenotyping. Such studies would also help to fulfill the goals of personalized medicine, by permitting an examination of treatment response in relation to carefully characterized patient phenotypes.

REFERENCES

1. National Institute of Mental Health. Consensus conference report: Drugs and insomnia—the use of medication to promote sleep. JAMA 1984; 251:2410–2414.
2. Association of Sleep Disorders Centers, Sleep Disorders Classification Committee, Roffwarg HP. Diagnostic classification of sleep and arousal disorders. Sleep 1979; 2:1–137.
3. McCrae CS, Lichstein KL. Secondary insomnia: Diagnostic challenges and intervention opportunities. Sleep Med Rev 2001; 5(1):47–61.
4. Harvey AG. Insomnia: Symptom or diagnosis? Clin Psychol Rev 2001; 21(7):1037–1059.
5. Nierenberg AA, Keefe BR, Leslie VC, et al. Residual symptoms in depressed patients who respond acutely to fluoxetine. J Clin Psychiatry 1999; 60(4):221–225.
6. Power JD, Perruccio AV, Badley EM. Pain as a mediator of sleep problems in arthritis and other chronic conditions. Arthritis Rheum 2005; 53(6):911–919.
7. Vitiello MV, Rybarczyk B, Von Korff M, et al. Cognitive behavioral therapy for insomnia improves sleep and decreases pain in older adults with co-morbid insomnia and osteoarthritis. J Clin Sleep Med 2009; 5(4):355–362.
8. National Institutes of Health. NIH State-of-the-Science Conference Statement on Manifestations and Management of Chronic Insomnia in Adults, Bethesda, MD, 2005:6–13.
9. National Sleep Foundation. Sleep in America: A National Survey of US Adults, 1991.
10. Roth T, Jaeger S, Jin R, et al. Sleep problems, comorbid mental disorders, and role functioning in the national comorbidity survey replication. Biol Psychiatry 2006; 60(12):1364–1371.
11. Angst J, Vollrath M, Koch R, et al. The Zurich Study: VII. Insomnia: Symptoms, classification and prevalence. Eur Arch Psychiatry Clin Neurosci 1989; 238:285–293.
12. Buysse DJ, Angst J, Gamma A, et al. Prevalence, course, and comorbidity of insomnia and depression in young adults. Sleep 2008; 31(4):473–480.
13. Dodge R, Cline MG, Quan SF. The natural history of insomnia and its relationship to respiratory symptoms. Arch Intern Med 1995; 155:1797–1800.
14. Foley DJ, Monjan A, Simonsick EM, et al. Incidence and remission of insomnia among elderly adults: An epidemiologic study of 6,800 persons over three years. Sleep 1999; 22(Suppl 2):S366–S372.
15. Morin CM, Belanger L, LeBlanc M, et al. The natural history of insomnia: A population-based 3-year longitudinal study. Arch Intern Med 2009; 169(5):447–453.
16. Buysse DJ, Finn L, Young T. Onset, remission, persistence, and consistency of insomnia symptoms over 10 years: Longitudinal results from the Wisconsin Sleep Cohort Study (WSCS). Sleep 2004; 27 [abstract Suppl]:A268.
17. Partinen M, Hublin C. Epidemiology of sleep disorders. In: Kryger M, Roth T, Dement W, eds. Principles and Practice of Sleep Medicine. 4th ed. Philadelphia, PA: Elsevier Saunders, 2005:626–647.
18. Lichstein KL, Durrence HH, Riedel BW, et al. Epidemiology of Sleep: Age, Gender, and Ethnicity. New Jersey: Lawrence Erlbaum Associates, Inc., 2004.
19. Hohagen F, Kappler C, Schramm E, et al. Sleep onset insomnia, sleep maintaining insomnia and insomnia with early morning awakening—temporal stability of subtypes in a longitudinal study on general practice attenders. Sleep 1994; 17(6):551–554.
20. Lack LC, Mercer JD, Wright H. Circadian rhythms of early morning awakening insomniacs. J Sleep Res 1996; 5(4):211–219.
21. American Sleep Disorders Association. International Classification of Sleep Disorders: Diagnostic and Coding Manual. Rochester, MN: American Sleep Disorders Association, 1990.
22. American Sleep Disorders Association. International Classification of Sleep Disorders, revised: Diagnostic and Coding Manual. Rochester, MN: American Sleep Disorders Association, 1997.
23. American Academy of Sleep Medicine. The International Classification of Sleep Disorders, Second Edition (ICSD-2): Diagnostic and Coding Manual. Second Edition 2005.
24. American Psychiatric Association. Diagnostic and Statistical Manual of Mental Disorders (DSM-III-R). 3rd ed. Washington, D.C.: American Psychiatric Association, 1987.
25. American Psychiatric Association. Diagnostic and Statistical Manual of Mental Disorders (DSM-IV). 4th ed. Washington, D.C.: American Psychiatric Association, 1994.
26. World Health Organization. Manual of the international classification of diseases, 9th revision, clinical modification (ICD-9-CM). Washington, DC: U.S. Government Printing Office, 1980.
27. World Health Organization. International statistical classification of diseases and related health problems, 10th revision (ICD-10). Geneva, Switzerland: World Health Organization, 1992.

28. Reynolds CF, Kupfer DJ, Buysse DJ, et al. Subtyping DSM-III-R primary insomnia: A literature review by the DSM-IV Work Group on sleep disorders. Am J Psychiatry 1991; 148(4):432–438.
29. Walters AS. The International Restless Legs Syndrome Study Group. Toward a better definition of the restless legs syndrome. Mov Disord 1995; 10(5):634–642.
30. American Sleep Disorders Association Task Force. The Chicago criteria for measurements, definitions, and severity ratings of sleep-related breathing disorders in adults. 1998; S1–S20..
31. Guilleminault C, Mignot E, Partinen M. Controversies in the diagnosis of narcolepsy. Sleep 1994; 17:S1–S6.
32. Bassetti C, Aldrich MS. Idiopathic hypersomnia—a series of 42 patients. Brain 1997; 120:1423–1435.
33. Edinger JD, Bonnet MH, Bootzin RR, et al. Derivation of research diagnostic criteria for insomnia: Report of an American Academy of Sleep Medicine Work Group. Sleep 2004; 27(8):1567–1596.
34. Buysse DJ, Reynolds CF, Kupfer DJ, et al. Clinical diagnoses in 216 insomnia patients using the International Classification of Sleep Disorders (ICSD), DSM-IV and ICD-10 categories: A report from the APA/NIMH DSM-IV field trial. Sleep 1994; 17(7):630–637.
35. Buysse DJ, Young T, Edinger JD, et al. Clinicans' use of the International Classification of Sleep Disorders: Results of a national survey. Sleep 2003; 26(1):48–51.
36. Buysse DJ, Reynolds CF, Hauri PJ, et al. Diagnostic concordance for DSM-IV sleep disorders: A report from the APA/NIMH DSM-IV field trial. Am J Psychiatry 1994; 151(9):1351–1360.
37. Schramm E, Hohagen F, Grasshoff U, et al. Test–retest reliability and validity of a structured interview for sleep disorders according to DSM-III-R(SIS-D). Am J Psychiatry 1993; 150(6):867–872.
38. Buysse DJ, Reynolds CF, Kupfer DJ, et al. Effects of diagnosis on treatment recommendations in chronic insomnia: A report from the APA/NIMH DSM-IV field trial. Sleep 1997; 20(7):542–552.
39. Edinger JD, Fins AI, Goeke JM, et al. The empirical identification of insomnia subtypes: A cluster analytic approach. Sleep 1996; 19(5):398–411.
40. Edinger JD, Wyatt JK, Olsen MK, et al. Comparative validity of the DSM-IV-TR and ICSD-2 insomnia nosologies: How many ways should we slice the insomnia pie? Sleep 2009; 32[Abstract Supplement]:A263.
41. Edinger JD, Wyatt JK, Olsen MK, et al. Reliability and validity of the Duke structured interview for sleep disorders for insomnia screening. Sleep 2009; 32[Abstract Supplement]:A265.
42. Gillin JC, Duncan W, Pettigrew KD, et al. Successful separation of depressed, normal, and insomniac subjects by EEG sleep data. Arch Gen Psychiatry 1979; 36:85–90.
43. Reynolds CF, Taska LS, Sewitch DE, et al. Persistent psychophysiologic insomnia: Preliminary Research Diagnostic Criteria and EEG sleep data. Am J Psychiatry 1984; 141(6):804–805.
44. Dorsey CM, Bootzin RR. Subjective and psychophysiologic insomnia: An examination of sleep tendency and personality. Biol Psychiatry 1997; 41:209–216.
45. Lichstein KL, Wilson NM, Noe SL, et al. Daytime sleepiness in insomnia: Behavioral, biological and subjective indices. Sleep 1994; 17(8):693–702.
46. Perlis ML, Smith MT, Andrews PJ, et al. Beta/gamma EEG activity in patients with primary and secondary insomnia and good sleeper controls. Sleep 2001; 24(1):110–117.
47. Krystal AD, Edinger JD, Wohlgemuth WK, et al. NREM sleep EEG frequency spectral correlates of sleep complaints in primary insomnia subtypes. Sleep 2002; 25(6):630–640.
48. Bonnet MH, Arand DL. 24-Hour metabolic rate in insomniacs and matched normal sleepers. Sleep 1995; 18(7):581–588.
49. Bonnet MH, Arand DL. Insomnia, metabolic rate and sleep restoration. J Intern Med 2003; 254(1): 23–31.
50. Bonnet MH, Arand DL. Physiological activation in patients with Sleep State Misperception. Psychosom Med 1997; 59(5):533–540.
51. Giles DE, Roffwarg HP, Rush AJ, et al. Age-adjusted threshold values for reduced REM latency in unipolar depression using ROC analysis. Biol Psychiatry 1990; 27:841–853.
52. Somoza E, Mossman D. Optimizing REM latency as a diagnostic test for depression using receiver operating characteristic analysis and information theory. Biol Psychiatry 1990; 27:990–1006.
53. Reite M, Buysse DJ, Reynolds CF, et al. The use of polysomnography in the evaluation of insomnia. Sleep 1995; 18(1):58–70.
54. Vgontzas AN, Kales A, Bixler EO, et al. Usefulness of polysomnographic studies in the differential diagnosis of insomnia. Int J Neurosci 1995; 82:47–60.
55. Hauri P. A cluster analysis of insomnia. Sleep 1983; 6:326–338.
56. Nowell PD, Buysse DJ, Reynolds CF, et al. Clinical factors contributing to the differential diagnosis of primary insomnia and insomnia related to mental disorders. Am J Psychiatry 1997; 154(10):1412–1416.
57. Carney CE, Edinger JD, Wyatt JK, et al. Should DSM-IV-TR primary insomnia be divided into specific subtypes? Sleep 2009; 32[abstract Suppl]:A264.

12 Clinical Assessment of Insomnia: Primary Insomnias

Rachel Manber
Psychiatry & Behavioral Sciences, Stanford, California, U.S.A.

Jason C. Ong
Department of Behavioral Sciences, Rush University Medical Center, Chicago, Illinois, U.S.A.

DEFINITION OF PRIMARY INSOMNIA

Primary insomnia is a diagnostic category in the psychiatric classification of the Diagnostic and Statistical Manual for Mental Disorders, Fourth Edition [DSM-IV (1)]. It is characterized by (a) difficulty initiating or maintaining sleep or nonrestorative sleep of at least one month duration that (b) causes significant distress or impairment in an important area of functioning and (c) does not occur exclusively in the context of another sleep disorder, or (d) mental disorder, and (e) is not due to the direct physiological effects of a substance. The American Academy of Sleep Medicine Work Group proposed a slightly refined Research Diagnostic Criteria (RDC) for primary insomnia (2). Under the RDC, an "*insomnia disorder*" that includes the presence of nocturnal symptoms and its associated waking complaints is distinguished from "*insomnia symptoms*," which include the nocturnal complaints only. As is true for the DSM-IV diagnosis, the RDC also requires that a primary insomnia disorder does not occur exclusively in the context of another medical, psychiatric or substance abuse disorder, or, if another disorder is present, the course of the insomnia disorder shows some independence from the temporal course of that disorder (2). This minor difference in criteria not withstanding, the diagnostic assessment of primary insomnia requires ascertaining the presence of an insomnia disorder and ruling out comorbidities that might be the primary reason for the reported sleep difficulties.

The epidemiology of insomnia is discussed in detail in chapter 2. Briefly, the prevalence of insomnia disorders is approximately 10%, with roughly 2:1 ratio of women to men (3–5). Epidemiological studies estimate the prevalence of primary insomnia at approximately 1% (3,4). Among individuals seen in sleep clinics with a complaint of insomnia, primary insomnia is diagnosed in approximately 25% (6,7). The prevalence of all insomnia disorders, including primary insomnia, increases with age.

Primary Insomnia Subtypes

The International Classification of Sleep Disorders, Second edition [ICSD-2 (8)] includes four adult diagnostic categories that can be considered subtypes of primary insomnia (2) and are therefore particularly relevant when assessing chronic insomnia. These include psychophysiological insomnia, paradoxical insomnia, idiopathic insomnia, and inadequate sleep hygiene.

Psychophysiological Insomnia

Psychophysiological insomnia is a primary insomnia subtype characterized by heightened sleep-related arousal or the presence of associations that are incompatible with sleep. According to the ICSD-2, the prevalence of psychophysiological insomnia is 12% to 15% among individuals presenting to a sleep center, regardless of chief complaint. Evidence for psychophysiological insomnia include any one of the following: (*i*) excessive focus on and heightened anxiety about sleep during the day (e.g., avoiding evening events for fear that such events might interfere with sleep, worrying about sleep during the day); (*ii*) relative ease of falling asleep during relatively monotonous activities (e.g., watching TV, reading, etc.) when not intending to sleep; (*iii*) ability to sleep better away from home than at home; (*iv*) intrusive thoughts in bed or inability to calm the mind; (*v*) heightened somatic tension in bed reflected by a perceived inability to relax the body. Sleep-related arousal that is prominent during the intended sleep period may be cognitive (e.g., racing thoughts or difficulty calming the mind when trying to sleep), emotional (anxiety or agitation while in bed or anticipatory anxiety prior to bedtime), and/or physiological (e.g., muscle tension). Sleep-related arousal can also be evidenced by excessive preoccupation with sleep during the day.

Paradoxical Insomnia

Paradoxical insomnia (formerly "sleep state misperception" or "subjective insomnia") is a subtype of primary insomnia characterized by a profound mismatch between subjective and objective sleep estimates. Evidence for paradoxical insomnia include any one of the following: (*i*) reporting a chronic pattern of little or no sleep most nights with rare nights during which relatively normal amounts of sleep are obtained; (*ii*) sleep log data during one or more weeks of monitoring show an average sleep time well below published age-adjusted normative values, often with no sleep at all for several nights per week. Typically there is an absence of daytime naps following such nights; (*iii*) a marked mismatch between objective findings from PSG or actigraphy and subjective sleep estimates. Patients with paradoxical insomnia report levels of daytime impairments that are similar to what is reported by other primary insomnia subtypes but much less severe than would be expected given the extreme level of sleep deprivation reported.

While there are no established criteria for a discrepancy threshold between subjective perception and objective findings, various definitions have been used in research. Krystal et al. defined paradoxical insomnia in patients with insomnia complaints based on PSG-defined total sleep time (TST) and sleep efficiency (SE) (9,10). The criteria were age dependent, taking into account shorter sleep durations in older adults. PSG sleep was deemed "normal" if TST was ≥6.5 hours. In those with TST between 6 and 6.5 hours, sleep was defined as "normal" based on their age. For those <60 years old, SE% had to be >85% and those ≥60, SE% had to be >80%. Individual differences in time estimates and the perception of sleep states (11) are at the core of a debate on the validity of paradoxical insomnia as a distinct diagnostic category. Those supporting the validity of the paradoxical insomnia diagnosis (12) claim that the underestimation of sleep time is unique to a subset of individuals with primary insomnia. Others claim that underestimation of sleep time is a generic characteristic of insomnia with some exhibiting larger discrepancy than others (13). According to the ICSD-2, the prevalence of paradoxical insomnia is less than 5% among individuals presenting to sleep centers, regardless of chief complaint. A survey of 11 sleep centers in the United States found that 9% of patients with insomnia received a diagnosis of subjective (now paradoxical) insomnia (6).

Idiopathic Insomnia

Idiopathic insomnia is a subtype of primary insomnia with an onset during infancy or childhood, no identifiable precipitating event, and a persistent course with no periods of sustained remission (8). The RDC specifies an onset prior to age 10 (2). According to the ICSD-2 the prevalence of idiopathic insomnia is less than 10% among individuals presenting to sleep centers, regardless of chief complaint. The diagnosis of idiopathic insomnia requires assessment of the age of onset of the first insomnia episode and its course. A typical statement volunteered by individuals with idiopathic insomnia is "I have always had problems sleeping."

The possibility that some cases of idiopathic insomnia might be related to a delayed sleep phase should be considered. Children with a delayed sleep phase might be predisposed to developing sleep onset difficulty because they are expected to sleep at times when their circadian clocks are generating strong activating signals. Early and repeated associations of efforts to sleep with heightened arousal may fuel a pattern of insomnia that persists into adulthood. As adults, these individuals might continue to express a preference for delayed sleep schedules but experience sleep difficulties even when allowed to choose their preferred sleep schedule, which precludes a diagnosis of delayed sleep phase syndrome. If their insomnia is primary, they will meet criteria for idiopathic insomnia. This suggests that a delayed sleep phase might constitute a predisposition for idiopathic insomnia. Though this possibility has not been directly tested, it is supported by evidence that children with ADHD and chronic sleep onset insomnia (> 1 year) have a delayed melatonin rhythm (14).

Inadequate Sleep Hygiene

Inadequate sleep hygiene is a primary insomnia subtype associated with at least one poor sleep hygiene practice that is not better explained by another sleep disorder (8). Sleep hygiene practices are sleep-related behaviors that have the potential to interfere with sleep. Although there is no agreement as to the specific behaviors that fall into this category, the core behaviors are those that are essential to the diagnosis of inadequate sleep hygiene disorder, which include irregular sleep schedule, frequent napping, spending excessive time in bed, consuming alcohol, nicotine, or caffeine in amounts or at times that will likely disrupt sleep, and routinely engaging in activating activities at bedtime (8). The RDC does not include a diagnostic category of inadequate sleep hygiene (2). Inadequate sleep hygiene practices are common in all forms of primary insomnia yet a diagnosis of inadequate sleep hygiene is merited only if the patient does not meet criteria for another ICSD-2 defined insomnia subtype. According to the ICSD-2, the prevalence of inadequate sleep hygiene is 5% to 10% among individuals presenting to sleep centers, regardless of chief complaint.

The assessment of sleep hygiene practices is essential for determining if inadequate sleep hygiene disorder is present. In addition, because poor sleep hygiene practices are common among patients with primary insomnia, information about sleep hygiene practices aids case conceptualization and identifies targets for intervention.

DIAGNOSTIC ASSESSMENT

Diagnostic assessment of primary insomnia is based primarily on a clinical interview. Sleep diaries and self-report questionnaires are often used to supplement the interview and are administered either before the initial interview to facilitate the intake evaluation or after the initial interview to clarify diagnostic issues that arise during the initial assessment (see chapter 11). Routine polysomnography is not indicated for the initial diagnosis of primary insomnia. Polysomnography is indicated when sleep disordered breathing or periodic limb movement disorder is suspected, when the diagnosis is uncertain, and when violent injurious behavior during sleep is present (15).

Diagnosis of Primary Insomnia

Figure 1 provides a schematic diagram of the algorithm for diagnostic assessment of primary insomnia. At the first level, the assessment is focused on determining if the complaint of insomnia is a symptom or a disorder. An insomnia symptom is a complaint of difficulty falling asleep, difficulty staying asleep, awakening too early, or nonrestorative sleep despite adequate opportunity and circumstance for sleep (16). A diagnosis of an insomnia disorder requires that the insomnia symptoms are also associated with significant waking distress or impairment, indicating that the nocturnal symptoms are clinically significant and merit clinical attention. Daytime symptoms of insomnia include preoccupation with sleep, mood disturbances, decreased vigor, impaired performance, and fatigue.

Once an insomnia disorder has been diagnosed, the next step is to ascertain duration of the current episode and determine if the disorder is primary; that is, the disorder is not related to another sleep, mental, or medical disorder or to substance use. Important sleep disorders that need to be ruled out include sleep disordered breathing, restless legs syndrome, a circadian rhythm disorder, or narcolepsy (a disorder of excessive daytime sleepiness that is often associated with disturbed sleep). A thorough evaluation of current medical and mental disorders is therefore essential for differential diagnosis of primary insomnia versus insomnia related to other disorders or substances. The most common medical disorders associated with poor sleep are those associated with dyspnea and those associated with pain (for a review see chapters 15 and 16). The most common psychiatric comorbidities are depressive illnesses, generalized anxiety disorder, and adjustment disorder with anxiety. When current comorbid conditions exist, the clinician should assess the temporal relationship between the insomnia disorder and the comorbid condition(s), both in terms of relative onset and in terms of changes in disease severity. Questionnaires quantifying depression and anxiety severity can complement the clinical assessment but are sometimes difficult to interpret in the context of an insomnia disorder. For example, an elevated score on a depression symptom severity questionnaire alone does not provide sufficient data to determine if a comorbid depressive disorder is present because

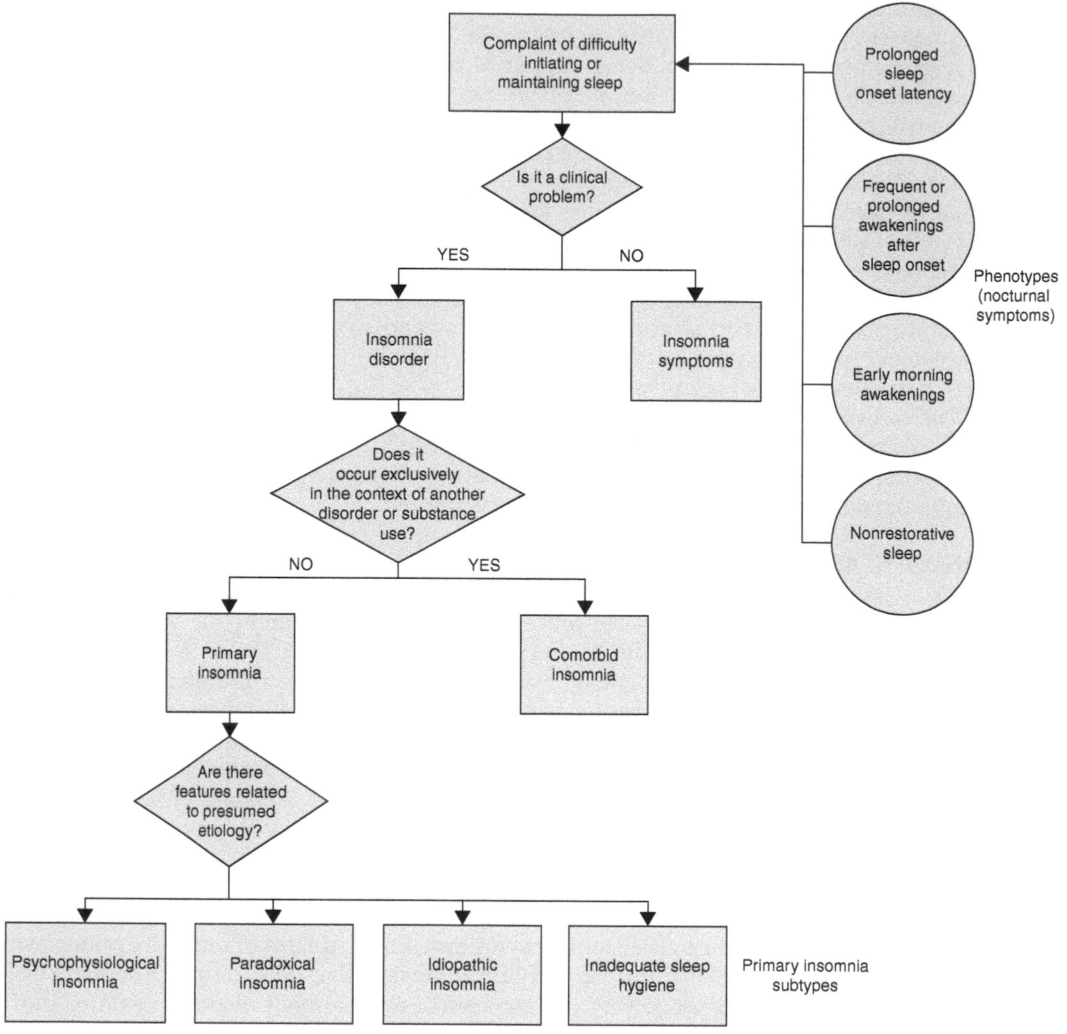

Figure 1 A schematic diagram for the diagnostic assessment of primary insomnia and its subtypes. This algorithm provides a general guideline for differential diagnosis of primary insomnia.

insomnia and depressive disorders share symptoms, such as poor sleep, poor concentration, and low energy.

Assessing Nocturnal Symptoms and Sleep-Related Behaviors

The initial focus of a diagnostic assessment is naturally on the presenting problem. Details about sleep onset latency, wake time after sleep onset, early morning awakening, estimated TST, and the refreshing value of sleep provide indications of the severity and specific nature of the presenting problem. This aspect of the assessment can be facilitated by administering sleep questionnaires and/or sleep diaries prior to the initial assessment visit. Both the self-report and the interview provide information about habitual sleep patterns. Specific aspects to assess are the habitual timing and variability of getting into and out of bed, lights out, and final awakening. These data together with the frequency and duration of daytime naps allow the clinician to ascertain if irregular sleep schedule and excessive time in bed are present. Both are relevant to the diagnosis of inadequate sleep hygiene and constitute important therapeutic targets for insomnia disorders. These data also inform the clinician to what extent circadian rhythm tendencies play a role in the patient's presentation (see section of circadian rhythm tendency below).

Table 1 A Chronological Assessment of Nocturnal and Daytime Symptoms of Insomnia

Time	Sample of interview questions	Targets for assessment
Presleep	What is your presleep routine? When is your last meal? When is your last alcoholic beverage? Do you engage in any self-soothing activities? When do you stop your work-related activities?	Presleep arousal, circadian factors, sleep hygiene
Bedtime	What time do you go to bed during the week and weekends? What goes on in your mind when you are not able to sleep? When do you take your sleep medication? Where do you do your work?	Conditioned arousal, behaviors associated with bedtime, sleep effort, pattern of medication use
Middle of the night	What do you do in the middle of the night when you cannot sleep? Do you look at the clock frequently throughout the night? Do you eat in the middle of the night?	Medications, reactions to nocturnal awakenings, strategies for going back to sleep, sleep hygiene
Morning/rise time	How difficult is it to wake-up and get out of bed in the morning? When do you get out of bed on the weekends?	Circadian factors, difficulty rising, early morning awakenings
Daytime	Do you take naps during the day? Have you made changes to your daytime activities following a night of poor sleep? Do you take any substances to help stay awake during the day?	Sleep-related cognitions, fatigue, sleepiness, napping behaviors, sleep hygiene

One practical way to gather these essential data is to ask the patient to describe in detail specific sleep-related behaviors in the chronological order they occur throughout the evening and night, starting with the presleep routines and progressing through the sleep period to the patient's morning rise time. Table 1 summarizes the type of information that can be obtained relative to this time line and how it pertains to case conceptualization, as discussed below. For better understanding of the patient's insomnia experience, the clinician should pay attention to and, if necessary, probe the patient's emotional reactions and behavioral responses in coping with insomnia. Knowledge of the patient's routine evening activities, particularly the hour or two before bedtime, allows the clinician to determine if activities at bedtime are likely to be interfering with sleep. This information is relevant to the diagnosis of inadequate sleep hygiene and it identifies specific sleep-interfering activities that need to be addressed in treatment.

Details about the consumption of substances, such as alcohol, nicotine, and caffeine should include the amount and timing of such consumption and their potential for disrupting sleep. The same holds true for prescription and over the counter medications and herbal preparations taken to promote sleep. Other behaviors that can interfere with sleep and should therefore be assessed include, clock watching (17), a sedentary lifestyle, and absence of sufficient stimulation during the day. The latter is particularly important to assess in institutional older adults.

Assessing Daytime Symptoms of Insomnia

Daytime symptoms of insomnia include fatigue or malaise, attention, concentration, or memory impairment, social or vocational dysfunction or poor school performance, mood disturbance or irritability, daytime sleepiness, motivation, energy, or initiative reduction, proneness for errors or accidents at work or while driving, tension, headache, or gastrointestinal symptoms, or concerns or worries about sleep (8). Nonrestorative sleep is associated with greater daytime impairment than other pure insomnia phenotypes (18,19). Table 1 includes information for assessing these daytime symptoms.

The distinction between sleepiness and fatigue is often not clear to insomnia patients. Patients tend to use the terms sleepiness and fatigue interchangeably. In the context of sleep medicine, sleepiness is usually defined as the propensity to sleep onset and fatigue as an index of low energy that may be influenced by psychological and physiological factors. Objectively measured daytime sleepiness using the Multiple Sleep Latency Test (MSLT) indicates that following habitual sleep, individuals with primary insomnia are not abnormally sleepy, with sleepiness scores comparable to that of good sleepers (20–22). Interestingly, when individuals with primary insomnia are sleep deprived to 80% of their habitual sleep time, objectively determined daytime sleepiness, as measured with the MSLT is increased (23).

Research suggests that the severity of reported daytime symptoms is impacted by the subjective perception of poor or insufficient sleep. Semler and Harvey manipulated the perception of sleep by providing individuals with primary insomnia "feedback" about the results of the actigraphic recording of their sleep in a random counter balanced fashion. Regardless of the actual observed sleep, participants reported more sleepiness during the day when they were told that they slept poorly on the previous night (24).

CASE CONCEPTUALIZATION

Beyond establishing a diagnosis of primary insomnia and its subtypes, the goal of the clinical assessment is reaching a case conceptualization and formulating a treatment plan. To that end the clinician considers etiological models and theories of insomnia while listening and inquiring for further information from the patient. We therefore present a prevailing model of insomnia, the diathesis-stress model, and the arousal/activation theories and discuss how to assess features relevant to these theories. We also discuss the relevance and assessment of circadian tendency and treatment history in primary insomnia.

A Diathesis-Stress Model of Insomnia

This model posits that insomnia emerges when a precipitating event is superimposed on premorbid predisposition and persists as a result of perpetuating factors (25). Predisposing factors may include psychologically based (e.g., personality traits) or biologically based (e.g., low parasympathetic tone) diathesis for insomnia. Precipitating factors include the triggers of an insomnia episode, such as psychosocial stressors or physical illness. About 75% of people with insomnia can identify a trigger of their insomnia, most commonly health issues and stress related to family or work situations (14). Perpetuating factors are maladaptive responses to disturbed sleep. They serve to maintain insomnia even after the resolution of the precipitating event and lead to a cyclical pattern of chronic insomnia. Examples of perpetuating factors are: extended time spent in bed, poor bedtime habits, compensatory daytime naps, increased sleep effort, and conditioning factors. This model is presumed to apply to the different insomnia subtypes and is not specific to primary insomnia.

It is therefore important to understand how these three processes are expressed in each individual patient. Information on precipitating factors can be gathered by inquiring about the circumstances surrounding the onset of the current episode of insomnia, including psychosocial stressors (e.g., going through a divorce, loss of a job) and change in health status (e.g., onset of thyroid disorder). These historical events provide insights into patients' stress reactivity and susceptibility to sleep disturbance. Understanding the context of the onset and precipitants of the insomnia episode can also facilitate communication with the patient when explaining the diathesis-stress model of insomnia at the onset of treatment and when discussing relapse prevention toward termination of treatment. The assessment of perpetuating factors typically focuses on the patient's reactions to the initial insomnia episode, including changes in sleep-related behaviors (such as staying in bed longer than before) and current sleep-interfering cognitions. Questions might include: What have you done to try to improve your sleep? What do you do in the middle of the night when you cannot sleep? How do you cope during the day? Are you trying to take naps? What goes on in your mind when you are not able to sleep? Have you made changes to your daytime activities following a night of poor sleep? Understanding factors that perpetuate sleep is particularly relevant in the context of psychological treatments as these factors are important therapeutic targets for cognitive-behavioral therapy of insomnia.

Cognitive and Emotional Arousal

Sleep-related cognitive and emotional arousal is a key feature of primary insomnia, regardless of subtypes. It is a diagnostic feature of one specific subtype of primary insomnia, psychophysiological insomnia, but it is frequently an associated feature across subtypes of primary insomnia. Compared with controls, individuals with primary insomnia have higher scores on trait arousability measures (26). Cognitive intrusions are also prominent among patients with insomnia disorders. Studies of analog and clinical samples conclude that sleep onset difficulties, particularly at the beginning of the night, are related to cognitive intrusions (27). These studies focused primarily on the period before initial sleep onset and concluded that, compared with good sleepers, intrusive thoughts are more prevalent in people with insomnia and their content is more laden with negative emotions, including rumination over the day's event, worrying about future events, and other anxious thoughts (for a review see Ref. 28). The intrusive thoughts may involve active problem solving, monitoring current sleep–wake state, or reacting to environmental stimuli (29). Two studies that examined cognitive activity in the middle of the night had similar findings (30,31). Thoughts about sleep and worries about the consequences of poor sleep are also common among patients with primary insomnia and often contribute to increased sleep effort (trying hard to sleep), which in turn perpetuates insomnia. The body of research on the role of cognition in insomnia has lead some to propose a cognitive model of insomnia (32) and others to examine mindfulness-based stress reduction as an intervention for insomnia aimed at reducing arousal and activation (33).

Assessment of sleep-related cognitions, most notably sleep effort, provides a window to the level of cognitive arousal experienced by the patient. While nondisturbed sleep occurs effortlessly, chronic insomnia is associated with increased sleep effort and increased preoccupation and apprehension related to obtaining optimal sleep, which increase arousal/activation and hinder sleep. During the interview the clinician should pay attention to overt and covert cognitions and behaviors that are manifestations of increased sleep effort. Attention should also be given to the coping strategies the patient uses, as many strategies serve to perpetuate insomnia either directly or by increasing cognitive arousal. To supplement the information about cognitive arousal that is obtained during the assessment interview one can use questionnaires developed to assess beliefs and attitudes about sleep, presleep cognition, and sleep effort that are discussed elsewhere in this book.

Cortical Arousal and Autonomic Activation

Individuals with primary insomnia have high cortical arousal and autonomic activation. Compared with controls, individuals with primary insomnia have higher cortical activity during non-REM sleep as indexed by EEG activity in the 14 to 45 Hz range Z range (34), higher 24-hour metabolic rate (21), higher metabolic activity during sleep in brain areas associated with activation (35), and higher sympathetic and lower parasympathetic tone as indexed by measures of heart rate variability (36). The latter was tested only in individuals with primary insomnia whose disturbed sleep was confirmed with polysomnography. Together these studies suggest increased arousal and activation at the cortical, autonomic, and cognitive levels among people with primary insomnia relative to normal sleepers. Using event-related potential methodology, a recent study provides additional support of the hyperarousal/hyperactivation theory of primary insomnia (37). This study found enhanced attention and reduction of the inhibitory process that normally facilitates sleep onset in the beginning part of sleep (37).

It is not entirely clear whether increased arousal or activation is the cause or consequence of having an insomnia disorder (28). A series of experiments conducted by Bonnet and Arandt support the causative theory. These researchers compared objective measures of daytime sleep propensity in subjects with primary insomnia and in research volunteers whose insomnia was induced by caffeine, people whose sleep was manipulated in the sleep laboratory to resemble sleep of yoked individuals with primary insomnia, and in healthy controls whose sleep was not manipulated. The results indicate that the sleep propensity of people with primary insomnia was similar to that of people with caffeine-induced insomnia and lower than the sleep propensity of those with laboratory-induced insomnia, who were, in turn, lower than normal controls (21,2338). Taken together these results were interpreted as evidence of a causative role of arousal in primary insomnia (21,23,38). These results also provide evidence that the daytime consequence of sleep disturbance associated with insomnia might be different from daytime sequelae of externally induced sleep deprivation of similar magnitude. Additional support for the contention that heightened arousal plays a causative role in insomnia comes from preliminary findings from a naturalistic follow-up after an open-label behavioral intervention for insomnia (39). The study found significantly greater presleep arousal and sleep effort at the end of treatment among participants who experienced at least one insomnia episode during the 12-month follow-up period than those who did not experience an insomnia episode during the follow-up period.

Circadian Contributions

Circadian factors are relevant to the presentation of primary insomnia both in terms of differential diagnosis and case conceptualization. For example, it has been suggested that individuals who present with sleep onset difficulties and no sleep maintenance problems have a delayed sleep phase. Their temperature rhythm markers were approximately 2.5 hours later than the respective phases of the good sleepers and their usual bedtimes fell within the "wake maintenance zone" (phases of the body's temperature rhythm during which sleep onset is seldom selected by free running subjects) of their temperature rhythm (40). However, the generalizability of this finding is not clear as this study did not report whether the participants with sleep onset difficulty met criteria for primary insomnia disorder or delayed sleep phase syndrome. The salient feature differentiating between insomnia and circadian rhythm sleep disorder, delayed type, is that in the latter case sleep initiation and maintenance are normal when sleep occurs during the patient's preferred time (8). It has also been suggested that individuals with primary insomnia presenting with early morning awakenings have a two to four hours advanced melatonin rhythm phases (41), and that this phase advance causes early arousal from sleep in these patients. The salient feature differentiating between insomnia and circadian rhythm sleep disorder, advanced type, is that in the latter case the patient typically experiences early evening sleepiness that is usually absent in primary insomnia (8).

In a clinical setting it is most practical to assess the patient's circadian tendencies either during the interview or by using validated questionnaires. In the absence of a full syndrome of delayed sleep phase, some patients with primary insomnia experience their best sleep during the second half of the night and report prolonged time to feel fully awake after rise time. These two symptoms suggest a natural evening chronotype that needs to be considered when recommending bedtime and rise time. Similarly, in the absence of a full syndrome of advanced sleep phase, some patients with primary insomnia present with an early bedtime, involuntary evening "naps," and very early wake-up times. Since comorbid psychiatric disorders that are associated with early morning awakening have been ruled out during the diagnostic portion of the assessment, these symptoms suggest a morning chronotype. Other circadian rhythm considerations concern irregular sleep schedules. The strength of the signal for optimal timing of sleep delivered by the suprachiasmatic nucleus is weakened when sleep–wake schedules change dramatically or frequently, as is the case in professions that require multiple shifts in time zones (e.g., airline industry and other jobs that require frequent changes in time zones) and in professions that involve varying shifts. Therefore, information about the patient's work schedule and travel patterns should be obtained.

Nocturnal Symptom Phenotypes

Classification of insomnia based on specific nocturnal symptoms [difficulty initiating sleep, difficulty maintaining sleep, waking up too early (early morning awakenings), or nonrestorative sleep] might be considered phenotyping of insomnia. Determining the specific primary insomnia phenotype might be relevant to pharmacological treatments of insomnia. For example, short acting hypotonic medications might not be ideal for individuals presenting with early morning awakening. However, the relevance of assessing phenotype for treatment matching has not been well studied. A few studies of cognitive-behavioral therapy for insomnia have targeted specific insomnia phenotypes. For example, Edinger et al., Morin et al., and Sivertsen et al. (42–44) focused on sleep maintenance insomnia and Jacobs et al. (45) targeted sleep onset insomnia. However, these studies did not modify CBT to specifically address the distinct phenotypes. Moreover, most studies demonstrate efficacy of CBT in samples consisting of mixed phenotypes, suggesting that phenotypes of insomnia might not be very relevant to cognitive-behavioral therapy for insomnia. Of note, however, is the possibility that the early morning awakening and nonrestorative sleep phenotypes might require specific modification of CBT or other specific treatment approaches. To the best of our knowledge no treatment outcome studies tested the efficacy of CBT or pharmacological treatments for these two insomnia phenotypes.

The distribution of the four phenotypes has been studied in epidemiological studies and surveys of the general population and clinic samples (46,47), but due to variations in nosology and study criteria specific findings for primary insomnia are unclear. Inference from these studies to primary insomnia cannot be made because the samples that were studied included individuals that did not meet criteria for an insomnia disorder and/or those whose insomnia disorder might be related to other medical or psychiatric conditions. The extant literature suggests that the pure early morning awakening phenotype is the least common among people with a probable insomnia disorder (4) and that the most common presentation in clinic samples (45,48) and in population surveys consists of more than one of the four nocturnal symptoms (4). One could infer from these studies that mixed symptoms are likely to be the most common presentation among individuals with primary insomnia. However, to the best of our knowledge, estimates of the symptom distribution among those who meet criteria for primary insomnia are lacking.

Nonrestorative sleep is the least studied nocturnal symptom of insomnia disorder. This nocturnal symptom is most commonly defined by reports of feeling unrefreshed upon awakening. Unlike sleep maintenance phenotype, whose prevalence increases with age, nonrestorative sleep is not associated with increasing age (6); it is more common among people younger than 55 years (18). Nonrestorative sleep has been studied mostly in individuals with medical disorders associated with fatigue, such as fibromyalgia, chronic fatigue, temporomandibular joint disorder, and irritable bowel syndrome (49) and in patients with other sleep disorders, such as sleep apnea (8). There is a fourfold increase in the prevalence of nonrestorative sleep among those with mood disorders (18). We were unable to find any study of nonrestorative sleep among individuals with primary insomnia and it is not clear if nonrestorative sleep exists in a pure form (i.e., without other nocturnal symptom) among individuals with primary insomnia (50).

Past and Present Treatments

Implementation and response to current and past treatments provide valuable information to the clinician, particularly when the patient reports past treatment failures. For pharmacological treatments, targets for assessment include the dose, frequency, and time of ingestion for all prescription medications and over-the-counter remedies taken to improve sleep. Is the medication taken on schedule or as needed? How does the patient decide if and when to take the medication or how much of the medication to take? This aspect of the assessment process is particularly relevant when making treatment choices. Response and side effects associated with past medications prescribed for sleep further inform a physician about the most appropriate next step in managing the patient with primary insomnia. For past pharmacological treatments these include the following: How well did the medication control the nocturnal symptoms of insomnia? Did efficacy remain optimal or diminish with continued use? How has the frequency and dose changed over time? Has morning sedation been a problem? What were the side effects? It is also important to evaluate psychological factors associated with medication use, such as ambivalence about using sleep medications and psychological dependence. These factors may complicate the presentation of patients with primary insomnia who still qualify for this diagnosis despite chronic nightly use of sleep medications.

Many insomnia patients are interested in nonpharmacological approaches to remedy their sleep problem and follow recommendations provided in books, magazines, and the internet. Relevant information about these previous attempts includes what was tried, how it was implemented, and the effectiveness of each strategy that was tried. Knowledge of these past experiences can help the insomnia therapist deliver some of the very same recommendations in a manner that is more likely to be adhered to and most likely to be effective. Patients presenting to a tertiary setting frequently report that they have tried "everything." Knowing specific details of previous approaches can inform the insomnia therapist of misunderstanding and adherence issues that have hindered response. For example, a patient might have gotten out of bed when unable to sleep, a component of stimulus control, but have done so expecting results on the first night, and since the procedure is rarely effective when used for a single night, has subsequently abandoned the practice. Using this information, the therapist can set more realistic expectations and encourage the patient to try implementing the full set of stimulus control instruction consistently for at least two weeks.

POLYSOMNOGRAPHIC FINDINGS

Comparisons of PSG-defined sleep parameters in primary insomnia relative to controls generally report minimal to modest differences. Average differences are less than 38 minutes for TST and less than 42 minutes for total wake time, with many studies detecting no significant difference (42). Individual differences in the perception of sleep states (11) might explain the inconsistency in the results from these, usually small, studies. In general, sleep time misperceptions are larger when subjective estimation of time awake after sleep onset is longer (51). Overestimation of time awake is associated with a complaint of nonrestorative sleep and the conviction that one's sleep difficulty is organically based (52). The severity of distress and daytime complaints of people with insomnia is not fully explained by the severity of the disruption in sleep.

Macro architecture of sleep in individuals with primary insomnia is only slightly different from that of good sleepers, with more time spent in stage 1 sleep, less time spent in stages 3 and 4, and more stage shifts (53). The micro architecture of sleep, as determined by spectral analyses of the EEG, reveals increases in fast frequency EEG (beta) among people with primary insomnia relative to controls (34). Krystal et al. found that individuals with paradoxical insomnia also have lower delta and greater alpha and sigma EEG activity during non-REM sleep than noninsomnia control subjects and that less delta EEG activity predicted greater deviation between subjective and PSG estimates of sleep time (2). These finding might suggest that the origins of the sleep complaints in patients with paradoxical insomnia are related to high cortical arousal during sleep (10,54).

Objectively defined sleep onset and sleep discontinuity parameters are not in high agreement with subjective recollections of sleep experiences provided by the patient. Only 12% of patients with insomnia (less than half of which were likely to have experienced primary insomnia) provide estimates of their TST that are congruent (off by no more that 15 minutes) relative to their PSG-defined TST (55). Approximately 44% had estimates that were lower than PSG TST by at least 60 minutes (55). Overestimation of sleep difficulties is common in all types of insomnia. It is more pronounced in people with paradoxical insomnia. For example, Edinger and Fins found that patients diagnosed with sleep state misperception (paradoxical insomnia) had actual (PSG defined) sleep times that were at least twice as large as their subjective time estimates, whereas those with psychophysiological insomnia or inadequate sleep hygiene estimated their sleep times more accurately, at a median of 88% of the objective (PSG) estimates (52).

MANAGEMENT OF PRIMARY INSOMNIA

Both pharmacological and nonpharmacological approaches are effective in the management of primary insomnia. Hypnotic medications are generally considered the pharmacological treatment of choice and cognitive-behavior therapy for insomnia (CBT-I) is the nonpharmacological treatment of choice. The preponderance of the evidence indicates that the two treatment modalities have comparable efficacy at the end of treatment and that the benefits of CBT-I are of greater long-term durability (43,44). (Please see the relevant chapters in part III of this book for a more through review of evidence.)

Most patients with primary insomnia are appropriate candidates for pharmacotherapy and for CBT-I. There is currently no information on how to best match patients to treatments and no conclusive evidence regarding the efficacy of specific treatments for insomnia phenotypes or subtypes. Patient preference often guides treatment but there has been little research on the impact of patient preference on outcome in primary insomnia. One study that evaluated treatment preference (CBT-I and pharmacological modalities) in a sample of patients that subsequently received group CBT-I found that it is more relevant to adherence to CBT-I than to outcome (56).

Beyond patient preference, the assessment provides useful information when considering treatments for primary insomnia. For example, in choosing the best pharmacological approach (e.g., short-acting vs. long-acting or controlled-release medication) to treat primary insomnia, the prescribing clinician should consider the average time spent in bed and the part of the night most affected (early middle, and/or late) as well as the pharmacokinetics of sleep inducing medications and over the counter preparations that the patient is using at the time of the assessment. The assessment also provides useful information when considering CBT-I. For example, habitual sleep times guide the initial time in bed prescription associated with sleep restriction. Evaluation of chronotypes can also help the insomnia therapist chose the optimal time in bed window. For example, the optimal bedtime for a patient who describes himself as a night owl will be later than what would be recommended for a patient who describes herself as a morning person. The information gathered in the assessment can aid in choosing the order and relative emphasis of the various CBT-I treatment components, allowing the therapist to work through compliance issues thus improving adherence with treatment recommendations.

CONCLUSION

The goal of this chapter was to provide an overview of the assessment process relevant to the diagnosis, case conceptualization, and treatment of the patient with primary insomnia. Evaluation of nonprimary forms of insomnia disorder necessitates additional assessments, discussed elsewhere in this book. However, the diathesis-stress model of insomnia applies to insomnia disorders other than primary insomnia, thus rendering much of the content of this chapter relevant to the assessment of other insomnia disorders.

REFERENCES

1. American Psychiatric Association. Diagnostic and Statistical Manual of Mental Disorders. 4th ed. Washington, DC: American Psychiatric Association, 1994.
2. Edinger JD, Bonnet MH, Bootzin RR, et al. Derivation of research diagnostic criteria for insomnia: report of an American Academy of Sleep Medicine Work Group. Sleep 2004; 27(8):1567–1596.
3. Ohayon MM. Prevalence of DSM-IV diagnostic criteria of insomnia: distinguishing insomnia related to mental disorders from sleep disorders. J Psychiatr Res 1997; 31(3):333–346.
4. Morin CM, LeBlanc M, Daley M, et al. Epidemiology of insomnia: prevalence, self-help treatments, consultations, and determinants of help-seeking behaviors. Sleep Med 2006; 7(2):123–130.
5. Ohayon MM, Caulet M, Priest RG, et al. DSM-IV and ICSD-90 insomnia symptoms and sleep dissatisfaction. Br J Psychiatry 1997; 171:382–388.
6. Coleman RM, Roffwarg HP, Kennedy SJ, et al. Sleep-wake disorders based on a polysomnographic diagnosis. A national cooperative study. JAMA 1982; 247(7):997–1003.
7. Buysse DJ, Reynolds CF III, Kupfer DJ, et al. Effects of diagnosis on treatment recommendations in chronic insomnia–a report from the APA/NIMH DSM-IV field trial. Sleep 1997; 20(7):542–552.
8. American Academy of Sleep Medicine. International Classification of Sleep Disorders. 2nd ed. Diagnostic and Coding Manual. Westchester, IL: American Academy of Sleep Medicine, 2005.
9. Edinger JD, Fins AI, Glenn DM, et al. Insomnia and the eye of the beholder: are there clinical markers of objective sleep disturbances among adults with and without insomnia complaints? J Consult Clin Psychol 2000; 68(4):586–593.
10. Krystal AD, Edinger JD, Wohlgemuth WK, et al. NREM sleep EEG frequency spectral correlates of sleep complaints in primary insomnia subtypes. Sleep 2002; 25(6):630–640.
11. Means MK, Edinger JD, Glenn DM, et al. Accuracy of sleep perceptions among insomnia sufferers and normal sleepers. Sleep Med 2003; 4(4):285–296.
12. Edinger JD, Krystal AD. Subtyping primary insomnia: is sleep state misperception a distinct clinical entity? Sleep Med Rev 2003; 7(3):203–214.
13. Trinder J. Subjective insomnia without objective findings: a pseudo diagnostic classification? Psychol Bull 1988; 103(1):87–94.
14. Bastien CH, Vallieres A, Morin CM. Precipitating factors of insomnia. Behav Sleep Med 2004; 2(1): 50–62.
15. Littner M, Hirshkowitz M, Kramer M, et al. Practice parameters for using polysomnography to evaluate insomnia: an update. Sleep 2003; 26(6):754–760.
16. Buysse DJ, Ancoli-Israel S, Edinger JD, et al. Recommendations for a standard research assessment of insomnia. Sleep 2006; 29(9):1155–1173.
17. Tang NK, Anne Schmidt D, Harvey AG. Sleeping with the enemy: clock monitoring in the maintenance of insomnia. J Behav Ther Exp Psychiatry 2007; 38(1):40–55.
18. Ohayon MM. Prevalence and correlates of nonrestorative sleep complaints. Arch Intern Med 2005; 165(1):35–41.

19. Roth T, Jaeger S, Jin R, et al. Sleep problems, comorbid mental disorders, and role functioning in the national comorbidity survey replication. Biol Psychiatry 2006; 60(12):1364–1371.
20. Stepanski E, Zorick F, Roehrs T, et al. Daytime alertness in patients with chronic insomnia compared with asymptomatic control subjects. Sleep 1988; 11(1):54–60.
21. Bonnet MH, Arand DL. 24-Hour metabolic rate in insomniacs and matched normal sleepers. Sleep 1995; 18(7):581–588.
22. Bonnet MH, Arand DL. Activity, arousal, and the MSLT in patients with insomnia. Sleep 2000; 23(2):205–212.
23. Bonnet MH, Arand DL. The consequences of a week of insomnia. II: patients with insomnia. Sleep 1998; 21(4):359–368.
24. Semler CN, Harvey AG. Misperception of sleep can adversely affect daytime functioning in insomnia. Behav Res Ther 2005; 43(7):843–856.
25. Spielman AJ, Caruso LS, Glovinsky PB. A behavioral perspective on insomnia treatment. Psychiatr Clin North Am 1987; 10(4):541–553.
26. Pavlova M, Berg O, Gleason R, et al. Self-reported hyperarousal traits among insomnia patients. J Psychosom Res 2001; 51(2):435–441.
27. Van Egeren L, Haynes SN, Franzen M, et al. Presleep cognitions and attributions in sleep-onset insomnia. J Behav Med 1983; 6(2):217–232.
28. Espie CA. Insomnia: conceptual issues in the development, persistence, and treatment of sleep disorder in adults. Annu Rev Psychol 2002; 53:215–243.
29. Wicklow A, Espie CA. Intrusive thoughts and their relationship to actigraphic measurement of sleep: towards a cognitive model of insomnia. Behav Res Ther 2000; 38(7):679–693.
30. Fichten CS, Creti L, Amsel R, et al. Poor sleepers who do not complain of insomnia: myths and realities about psychological and lifestyle characteristics of older good and poor sleepers. J Behav Med 1995; 18(2):189–223.
31. Borkovec TD, Lane TW, VanOot PH. Phenomenology of sleep among insomniacs and good sleepers: wakefulness experience when cortically asleep. J Abnorm Psychol 1981; 90(6):607–609.
32. Harvey AG. A cognitive model of insomnia. Behav Res Ther 2002; 40(8):869–893.
33. Ong JC, Shapiro SL, Manber R. Combining mindfulness meditation with cognitive-behavior therapy for insomnia: a treatment-development study. Behav Ther 2008; 39(2):171–182.
34. Perlis ML, Smith MT, Andrews PJ, et al. Beta/Gamma EEG activity in patients with primary and secondary insomnia and good sleeper controls. Sleep 2001; 24(1):110–117.
35. Nofzinger EA, Nissen C, Germain A, et al. Regional cerebral metabolic correlates of WASO during NREM sleep in insomnia. J Clin Sleep Med 2006; 2(3):316–322.
36. Bonnet MH, Arand DL. Heart rate variability in insomniacs and matched normal sleepers. Psychosom Med 1998; 60(5):610–615.
37. Yang CM, LO HS. ERP evidence of enhanced excitatory and reduced inhibitory processes of auditory stimuli during sleep in patients with primary insomnia. Sleep 2007; 30(5):585–592.
38. Bonnet MH, Arand DL. The consequences of a week of insomnia. Sleep 1996; 19(6):453–461.
39. Ong JC, Shapiro SL, Manber R. Mindfulness meditation and CBT for insomnia: a naturalistic 12-month follow-up. Explore: The Journal of Science and Healing 2009; 5:30–36.
40. Morris M, Lack L, Dawson D. Sleep-onset insomniacs have delayed temperature rhythms. Sleep 1990; 13(1):1–14.
41. Lack LC, Mercer JD, Wright H. Circadian rhythms of early morning awakening insomniacs. J Sleep Res 1996; 5(4):211–219.
42. Edinger JD, Glenn DM, Bastian LA, et al. Sleep in the laboratory and sleep at home II: comparisons of middle-aged insomnia sufferers and normal sleepers. Sleep 2001; 24(7):761–770.
43. Morin C, Colecchi C, Stone J, et al. Behavioral and pharmacological therapies for late-life insomnia: a randomized controlled trial. JAMA 1999; 281:991–999.
44. Sivertsen B, Omvik S, Pallesen S, et al. Cognitive behavioral therapy vs. zopiclone for treatment of chronic primary insomnia in older adults: a randomized controlled trial. JAMA 2006; 295(24):2851–2858.
45. Jacobs GD, Pace-Schott EF, Stickgold R, et al. Cognitive behavior therapy and pharmacotherapy for insomnia: a randomized controlled trial and direct comparison. Arch Intern Med 2004; 164(17):1888–1896.
46. Karacan I, Thornby JI, Anch M, et al. Prevalence of sleep disturbance in a primarily urban Florida County. Soc Sci Med 1976; 10(5):239–244.
47. Ohayon MM, Smirne S. Prevalence and consequences of insomnia disorders in the general population of Italy. Sleep Med 2002; 3(2):115–120.
48. Hryshko-Mullen AS, Broeckl LS, Haddock CK, et al. Behavioral treatment of insomnia: the Wilford Hall Insomnia Program. Mil Med 2000; 165(3):200–207.

49. Moldofsky H. Nonrestorative sleep, musculoskeletal pain, fatigue, and psychological distress in chronic fatigue syndrome, fibromyalgia, irritable bowel syndrome, temporal mandibular joint dysfunction disorders. In: Yehuda S, ed. Chronic Fatigue Syndrome. New York: Plenum Press, 1997:95–117.
50. Stone KC, Taylor DJ, McCrae CS, et al. Nonrestorative sleep. Sleep Med Rev 2008; 12(4): 275–288.
51. Vanable PA, Aikens JE, Tadimeti L, et al. Sleep latency and duration estimates among sleep disorder patients: variability as a function of sleep disorder diagnosis, sleep history, and psychological characteristics. Sleep 2000; 23(1):71–79.
52. Edinger JD, Fins AI. The distribution and clinical significance of sleep time misperceptions among insomniacs. Sleep 1995; 18(4):232–239.
53. Morin CM, Espie CA. Insomnia: A Clinical Guide to Assessment and Treatment. New York: Springer, 2004.
54. Bonnet MH, Arand DL. Physiological activation in patients with Sleep State Misperception. Psychosom Med 1997; 59(5):533–540.
55. Carskadon MA, Dement WC, Mitler MM, et al. Self-reports versus sleep laboratory findings in 122 drug-free subjects with complaints of chronic insomnia. Am J Psychiatry 1976; 133(12):1382–1388.
56. Vincent N, Lionberg C. Treatment preference and patient satisfaction in chronic insomnia. Sleep 2001; 24(4):411–417.

13 Clinical Assessment of Comorbid Insomnias: Insomnia in Psychiatric Disorders

Meredith E. Rumble and Ruth M. Benca
Department of Psychiatry, University of Wisconsin-Madison, Madison, Wisconsin, U.S.A.

INTRODUCTION

Insomnia and psychiatric disorders frequently occur together. Epidemiological studies have demonstrated that between approximately 25% and 50% of individuals with insomnia in the general population meet criteria for insomnia comorbid with a psychiatric disorder, including most commonly the psychiatric comorbidities of depressive disorders, anxiety disorders, and substance use disorders (1–3). Sleep difficulties are a common symptom of many psychiatric disorders and in some cases treatment of the psychiatric disorder may lead to improvement or resolution of the sleep difficulties. However, insomnia commonly persists despite treatment of the psychiatric illness (e.g., Ref. 4) and can cause significant distress to the patient as well as an adverse impact on the course of the psychiatric disorder.

Mounting evidence suggests a dynamic and potentially bidirectional relationship between insomnia and psychiatric disorders. For example, longitudinal research has demonstrated that individuals with insomnia but without a comorbid psychiatric illness at baseline are at a significantly higher risk for developing future depressive, anxiety, and substance abuse or dependence disorders (1,5–8). Not only is insomnia a risk factor for the onset of psychiatric disorders, but it has also been shown that insomnia can increase the risk for relapse and exacerbation of psychiatric symptoms. For example, individuals with residual insomnia symptoms after treatment for depression are at a higher risk of relapse of depression than those without residual insomnia (9). Conversely, treatment of insomnia may improve the course of a depressive episode; recent research has demonstrated how individuals with depression and insomnia who receive both general treatment for depression as well as insomnia-specific treatment (e.g., fluoxetine with eszopiclone or escitalopram with cognitive-behavioral therapy for insomnia) have significantly greater improvements in depressive symptoms than those who only receive general treatment for depression (10,11).

Given this dynamic relationship, it is essential to assess both insomnia and psychiatric symptomatology in patients with either an insomnia or psychiatric complaint so that appropriate treatment planning and implementation can occur. The focus of the current chapter is to provide recommendations regarding the assessment of insomnia comorbid with psychiatric issues. The first section of this chapter will discuss the assessment of psychiatric disorders commonly occurring with insomnia (i.e., depressive disorders, bipolar disorders, generalized anxiety disorder, panic disorder, posttraumatic stress disorder, and schizophrenia), including a description, associated sleep complaints, characteristic abnormalities detected in sleep electroencephalography (EEG), and possible screening measures for each psychiatric disorder. The second section will review the assessment of important factors commonly contributing to insomnia in patients with psychiatric disorders, including behavioral factors, the effects of psychotropic medications, and other sleep disorders. With the aim of promoting more standardized insomnia assessment in clinical practice and facilitating a connection between clinical and research settings, the standardized insomnia assessment recommendations for research developed by Buysse et al. (12) will be used as a guide whenever possible. Of note, assessment of insomnia related to substance issues is not covered in this chapter as this particular comorbidity is covered in chapter 16.

ASSESSMENT OF PSYCHIATRIC DISORDERS COMMONLY OCCURRING WITH INSOMNIA

Psychiatric disorders commonly associated with insomnia include depressive disorders, bipolar disorders, generalized anxiety disorder, panic disorder, posttraumatic stress disorder, and schizophrenia. Despite their high prevalence, psychiatric disorders often remain undiagnosed, untreated or undertreated in patients who present with insomnia (13). Factors that can contribute to the lack of diagnosis and treatment include: (a) attribution of psychiatric symptomatology to sleep problems (e.g., "If I could only sleep, then I would be fine."); (b) lack of physician training in psychiatric assessment; (c) insufficient time during clinic visits to assess psychiatric symptoms in busy clinical practices; and (d) limited reimbursement for assessment and treatment of psychiatric disorders.

Descriptions of the psychiatric disorders commonly occurring with insomnia are provided below. In addition, associated sleep complaints, characteristic abnormalities in sleep EEG, and suggested screening questions and measures to potentially identify patients at risk for specific psychiatric disorders are described below and summarized in Table 1. It should be noted that the basic sleep patterns outlined below, including both sleep complaints and objective abnormalities in sleep EGG, should not be used as definitive diagnostic markers. The sleep patterns described are not necessarily present in all individuals with a particular psychiatric

Table 1 Basic Sleep Patterns, Screening Questions, and Screening Questionnaires for Common Psychiatric Disorders Comorbid with Insomnia

Psychiatric comorbidity	Basic sleep patterns	Screening question(s)	Screening questionnaires
Depressive disorders	• Sleep continuity disturbances • REM sleep abnormalities • SWS deficits	• "Have you been feeling depressed or down?" • "Have you lost interest in things you usually enjoy?"	• Beck Depression Inventory II (17) • Inventory of Depressive Symptomatology Self-Report (18) • Geriatric Depression Scale (21)
Bipolar disorders	• Sleep continuity disturbances • REM sleep abnormalities • SWS deficits	• "Have you felt so high, 'hyper', or irritable that people told you that you were not your normal self?"	• Mood Disorders Questionnaire (23)
Generalized anxiety disorder	• Sleep continuity disturbances	• "Have you been anxious or worried?"	• State-Trait Anxiety Inventory, trait version (29) • Penn State Worry Questionnaire (30)
Panic disorder	• Sleep continuity disturbances • Nocturnal panic attacks with related fears of going to sleep	• "Have you ever had a panic attack when you suddenly felt anxious or experienced a lot of physical symptoms?"	• Brief Panic Disorder Screen (36)
Posttraumatic stress disorder	• Sleep continuity disturbances • REM sleep abnormalities • Nightmares/flashbacks with related fears of going to sleep	• "Have you experienced any traumas in your life?"	• Posttraumatic Stress Diagnostic Scale (42)
Schizophrenia	• Sleep continuity disturbances • NREM sleep spindle deficits in the vertex region	• If psychotic symptoms are observed and there is no diagnosis, an immediate referral for psychiatric assessment is recommended	• If psychotic symptoms are observed and there is no diagnosis, an immediate referral for psychiatric assessment is recommended

Abbreviations: REM, rapid eye movement; SWS, slow wave sleep; NREM, nonrapid eye movement.

diagnosis and similar sleep abnormalities may be seen in individuals without those disorders, including healthy, normal individuals. Likewise, the screening questions and measures outlined below should not be used to make specific diagnoses but instead to identify individuals at greater risk for particular psychiatric disorder. Further psychiatric assessment is recommended for any case where clinical suspicion for possible psychiatric disorder is increased based on clinical or objective sleep abnormalities and/or positive screening questionnaires.

When treating an individual with insomnia and a known psychiatric disorder, the screening measures outlined below can also be used to track psychiatric symptom severity along with insomnia symptom severity so that intervention can be better guided. For example, if increases and decreases in psychiatric and insomnia symptom severity seem to correspond, treatment could focus more prominently on the psychiatric disorder. Other the other hand, if insomnia symptom severity remains high in the context of low psychiatric symptom severity, treatment could center more on insomnia.

Depressive Disorders

Major depressive disorder is characterized by the presence of at least one major depressive episode (14). The starting criterion for a major depressive episode is the presence of depressed mood or anhedonia for two weeks or longer. Other symptoms include: (a) significant weight loss or weight gain, (b) insomnia or hypersomnia, (c) psychomotor agitation or retardation, (d) fatigue or loss of energy, (e) feelings of worthlessness or guilt, (f) decreased ability to concentrate, and (g) recurrent thoughts of death and suicide. Five or more symptoms must be present with at least one of these symptoms being depressed mood or anhedonia. Major depressive episodes also cause clinically significant distress or impaired social or occupational functioning. Dysthymic disorder is diagnosed in individuals with chronic depressive symptoms for at least two years who have significant impairment in functioning, but do not meet full criteria for a major depressive episode.

Basic Sleep Patterns

Patients who are depressed typically complain of insomnia, including difficulty falling asleep, difficulty staying asleep, early morning awakenings, nonrestorative sleep, and decreased amounts of sleep. A minority of patients report hypersomnia or increased sleepiness and/or sleep amounts, and some individuals with mood disorders may report periods of both insomnia and hypersomnia (5). Common polysomnographic abnormalities in individuals with depression include sleep continuity disturbances, such as prolonged latency to sleep onset, increased wakefulness during sleep, and early morning awakenings, resulting in decreased amounts of total sleep time and more fragmented sleep (15,16). One of the more specific changes in sleep architecture associated with depressive disorders is alteration in rapid eye movement (REM) sleep patterns. Reduced latency to REM sleep is the most commonly described alteration, but other findings include increased duration of the first REM sleep period, increased rapid eye movements during REM sleep periods, and increased percentage of REM sleep. Finally, individuals with depression also have deficits in slow wave sleep (SWS), including decreased total amounts of SWS, decreased proportion of SWS, and less SWS during the first nonrapid eye movement (NREM) sleep period (15,16).

Possible Screening Measures

Given the particularly strong association between insomnia and depressive disorders, all individuals with complaints of insomnia should be assessed for depression. There are two general screening questions that can be helpful as an initial assessment of depression: "Have you been feeling depressed or down?" and "Have you lost interest in things you usually enjoy?" Patients who endorse either of these symptoms should be assessed more carefully for depression.

There are also a number of validated self-report screening measures available to assess depressive symptoms in insomnia (12), including the Beck Depression Inventory II (BDI-II; 17) and the Inventory of Depressive Symptomatology Self-Report (IDS-SR; 18). The BDI-II is a 21-item self-report scale that reflects DSM-IV criteria and takes approximately 5 to 10 minutes to complete. Each item is rated on a 4-point scale ranging from 0 to 3 and summed into a single score ranging from 0 to 63. Severity of depression based on scores is as follows: 0–13 minimal, 14–19 mild, 20–28 moderate, and 29–63 severe. A cut-off score of 18 or higher yielded a sensitivity of 94% and a specificity of 92% when predicting a diagnosis of major depressive disorder as diagnosed by the Patient Health Questionnaire (PHQ, 19) in a sample of primary care patients (20).

The IDS-SR is a 30-item self-report scale that includes all DSM-IV symptom domains for a major depressive episode. This measure takes approximately 15 to 20 minutes to complete. Each item is rated on a 4-point scale ranging from 0 to 3 and summed into a single score ranging from 0 to 84. Depression severity ranges are as follows: 0 to 11 normal, 12 to 23 mildly ill, 24 to 36 moderately ill, 37 to 46 moderately to severely ill, and 47 to 84 severely ill. In a sample of outpatients with and without current symptomatic major depressive disorder as determined by diagnostic interview, a cut-off score of 18 or higher revealed a sensitivity of 100% and a specificity of 94% (18).

In comparison to the BDI-II, the IDS-SR is a longer measure that takes more time to complete; however, this measure also offers the benefits of assessment of a larger number of depressive symptoms, a wider score range, better detection of depression in less severely ill populations, and easy accessibility (www.ids-qids.org; 18). Furthermore, the IDS-SR has four items specifically assessing sleep compared to only one item on the BDI-II.

In addition to these two scales, the Geriatric Depression Scale (GDS; 21) may be helpful for assessment of depressive symptoms in older adults with insomnia (12). The GDS is a 30-item self-report scale and each item is answered by circling yes or no. Some of the items are reversed scored, and then the items are summed into a single score ranging from 0 to 30. In one of the original validation studies for the GDS, a cut-off score of 11 yielded a sensitivity rate of 84% and a specificity rate of 95% (22). There are two main benefits of using this measure for older adults. First, the GDS is in a simpler format with yes/no questions in comparison to items with 4-point scales. Second, the scale does not include physical symptoms that may mimic depressive symptoms in older adults, such as motor retardation, which could result from a chronic medical condition rather than depression.

Bipolar Disorders

Bipolar disorders are characterized by the occurrence of at least one manic or mixed episode (14). Criteria for diagnosis of a manic episode include abnormally elevated or irritable mood, lasting one week or longer, accompanied by three or more of the following symptoms (four or more if only irritable mood): (a) grandiosity, (b) decreased need for sleep (usually with significantly decreased amounts of total sleep), (c) talkativeness, (d) racing thoughts, (e) distractibility, (f) increased goal-directed activity, and (g) excessive involvement in pleasurable activities with potential for negative consequences. Mixed episodes are diagnosed when the patient meets criteria for both a manic episode and a depressive episode simultaneously. Both manic and mixed episodes cause clinically significant distress or impaired social or occupational functioning. Hypomanic episodes are of lesser severity and associated functional impairment.

Basic Sleep Patterns

Patients meeting criteria for bipolar disorder often report a decreased need for sleep during periods of mania or hypomania. These patients also commonly have insomnia complaints, including difficulty falling asleep, difficulty staying asleep, and nonrestorative sleep. As for polysomnographic abnormalities, individuals with bipolar disorder demonstrate similar patterns as individuals with depression, including sleep continuity disturbances, REM sleep abnormalities, and SWS deficits (15).

Possible Screening Measures

A standard screening question for mania is, "Have you felt so high, 'hyper', or irritable that people told you that you were not your normal self?" For patients in whom mania is suspected, one instrument that can be used to screen for manic and hypomanic symptoms is the Mood Disorders Questionnaire (MDQ; 23). The MDQ is a 13-item self-report scale with two additional items assessing whether any of the endorsed symptoms have occurred together and the degree of impairment associated with symptoms. The first 13 items are answered in a yes/no response format and scores range from 0 to 13. Using a cut-off of seven or more endorsed symptoms, one study demonstrated a sensitivity of 58% and a specificity of 93% in a primary care clinic sample with and without bipolar disorder as determined by a diagnostic interview (24). Using this same cut-off and similar methods, sensitivity was higher and specificity was lower (73% and 90%, respectively) in a psychiatric clinic sample (23).

Generalized Anxiety Disorder

Generalized anxiety disorder (GAD) is characterized by excessive and uncontrollable worry and anxiety about a number of events or activities (14). In addition, this worry and anxiety occurs most days for at least six months and is associated with three or more of the following symptoms: (a) restlessness, (b) increased fatigue, (c) difficulty concentrating, (d) irritability, (e) muscle tension, and (f) difficulty falling asleep, staying asleep, or nonrestorative sleep. GAD also causes clinically significant distress or impaired social or occupational functioning.

Basic Sleep Patterns

Individuals with GAD often report difficulty falling asleep and staying asleep (25). In addition, polysomnographic studies have shown a variety of sleep continuity disturbances, including prolonged sleep latency, decreased sleep efficiency, early morning awakenings, and decreased total sleep time (26–28). In contrast to those with mood disorders, individuals with GAD do not typically demonstrate changes in REM sleep patterns (15).

Possible Screening Measures

To screen for GAD, patients may be asked, "Have you been anxious or worried?" Self-report screening questionnaires assessing anxiety symptoms include the trait version of the State-Trait Anxiety Inventory (STAI-T; 29), which has been recommended for measuring anxiety in individuals with insomnia (12). The STAI-T is a 20-item self-report scale commonly used in insomnia research that measures feelings of anxiety (12). Individuals rate various anxious and nonanxious feeling states on a scale from 0 (not at all) to 3 (very much so). Some items are reverse scored, and then all items are summed into a single score ranging from 20 (mild) to 80 (severe) with no cut-off scores.

Although the STAI-T is used regularly in research setting to measure anxiety symptoms, more specific measures are available to assess possible GAD symptoms. One of these measures is the Penn State Worry Questionnaire (PSWQ; 30), a 16-item self-report scale that was designed to assess the frequency, excessiveness, and generalizability of worry (the main DSM-IV diagnostic criteria for GAD). Each item is rated on a 5-point scale ranging from 1 (not at all typical) to 5 (very typical), and the measure takes approximately five minutes to complete. Some items are reversed scored, and then all items are summed into a single score ranging from 16 to 80. Individuals with GAD usually have a score of 60 or higher. However, one study examining the screening utility of the PSWQ in a sample of individuals with and without GAD as determined by diagnostic interview found that a cut-off score of 45 provided the most optimization with a sensitivity of 99% and a specificity of 98% (31).

Panic Disorder

Patients with panic disorder experience repeated panic attacks, which are sudden occurrences of extreme anxiety accompanied by at least four of the following symptoms: palpitations, sweating, trembling, shortness of breath, choking, chest pain, nausea, dizziness, derealization or depersonalization, fear of losing control or dying, numbness or tingling, and chills or hot flushes (14). Agoraphobia, which is the fear of being in a place from which escape or help might not be possible should a panic attack ensue, often develops as a secondary feature. Panic attacks usually occur while awake, but may arise during sleep. Panic attacks occurring during sleep can be differentiated from night terrors since patients are usually awake and alert during panic attacks and remember them the next day, whereas they do not always fully awaken during a night terror or confusional arousal and are less likely to remember them. Night terrors are also more frequently associated with a frightening dream than are panic attacks.

Basic Sleep Patterns

Patients with panic disorder can have increased insomnia complaints. Some studies comparing objectively recorded sleep in patients with panic disorder to normal controls have demonstrated abnormalities related to decreased sleep continuity (32,33), including prolonged sleep latency and difficulties maintaining sleep. Patients with panic disorder also can develop fears of going to sleep due to anticipation of possible nocturnal panic attacks (34). Polysomnographic studies have demonstrated that nocturnal panic attacks most frequently occur when transitioning from stage 2 to SWS (35). Unlike patients with mood disorders, patients with panic disorder do not demonstrate REM sleep abnormalities.

Possible Screening Measures

A common screening question for panic disorder is, "Have you ever had a panic attack when you suddenly felt anxious or experienced a lot of physical symptoms?" The four-item version of the Anxiety Sensitivity Index (ASI), the Brief Panic Disorder Screen (BPDS), is a brief scale that assesses fear of anxiety-related bodily sensations or consequences (36) and can be used to screen for panic disorder. Each item on the four-item ASI is rated on a 5-point scale ranging from 0 to 4. All items are summed into a single score ranging from 0 to 16. In a sample of outpatients with anxiety disorders as determined by a diagnostic interview, a cut-off of 11 revealed a sensitivity of 78% and a specificity of 73% (36).

Posttraumatic Stress Disorder

Posttraumatic stress disorder (PTSD) develops in individuals who have experienced a traumatic event and is characterized by re-experiencing the event in flashbacks, intrusive recollections of the event, or recurrent dreams of the event (14). PTSD is also characterized by increased arousal and avoidance of stimuli associated with the trauma. Symptoms must be present longer than one month and cause clinically significant distress or impaired social or occupational functioning to meet diagnostic criteria for PTSD.

Basic Sleep Patterns

Patients with PTSD often complain of nightmares as well as difficulties initiating and maintaining sleep. The majority of polysomnographic research has demonstrated REM sleep abnormalities in PTSD patients, particularly disruption of REM sleep continuity and increased REM density (37–39). On the other hand, there have been mixed results for insomnia disturbances in that only some studies have demonstrated sleep initiation and maintenance difficulties (40,41).

Possible Screening Measures

When screening for PTSD, one frequently used question is, "Have you experienced any traumas in your lifetime?" As for screening questionnaires, the Posttraumatic Stress Diagnostic Scale (PDS; 42) is a 49-item self-report scale that assesses the severity of PTSD symptoms. This scale is divided into four parts. The first part assesses what types of traumas occurred in the person's life, and the second part has the patient identify the most bothersome trauma and when it occurred. The third part has patients rate the frequency of 17 PTSD symptoms on a 4-point scale ranging from 0 to 3. The final part assesses the degree to which PTSD symptoms impact functioning. In a psychiatric outpatient sample of individuals with and without PTSD as determined by diagnostic interview, Sheeran and Zimmerman (43) found that a simple cut-off score of 15 or higher on the third part of the questionnaire described above yielded a sensitivity of 89% and a specificity of 76%.

Schizophrenia

Schizophrenia is a chronic illness characterized by the presence of a constellation of symptoms that are associated with significant social or occupational dysfunction (14). The lifetime prevalence is 1% and death results from suicide in about 10% of cases. Positive symptoms include disorganization of speech and behavior, as well as psychotic features such as delusions and hallucinations. Negative symptoms consist of affective flattening, alogia (poverty of speech and its content), and avolition (decrease in goal-directed activity). Depressed mood, loss of interest or pleasure in normally pleasurable activities, anxiety, and irritability also may be present.

Basic Sleep Patterns

Patients with schizophrenia commonly will complain of sleep initiation or maintenance difficulties and poor sleep quality even when treated with antipsychotic medication (44,45). In addition, it is important to note that sleep difficulty in the context of discontinuation of antipsychotic medications is often an early symptom of relapse (46). Objective assessment of sleep demonstrates problems with sleep initiation and maintenance (47,48) as well as decreased REM sleep latency and SWS, but these findings are less consistent (47). Finally, using 256-electrode high-density EEG recording during sleep, a recent study found a significant deficit in NREM sleep spindles in the vertex region of the scalp in patients with schizophrenia when compared to both control participants and participants with a history of depression (49). Interestingly, a deficit in sleep spindles suggests a possible abnormality in the thalamic reticular nucleus and thalamocortical system, which, in turn, may represent a novel biological marker of schizophrenia.

Possible Screening Measures

Screening questionnaires are typically not used to identify patients at risk for schizophrenia, in contrast to mood and anxiety disorders, although several questionnaires are available to assess severity of symptomatology. Given the nature and severity of schizophrenia, however, the majority of standardized measures for schizophrenia, such as the Brief Psychiatric Rating Scale (50) or Positive and Negative Syndrome Scale (PANSS; 51), are designed to be given by mental health professionals trained in administering these instruments. Therefore, screening measures are more difficult to administer in nonmental health care settings. In the event that a patient presents with psychotic symptoms and does not currently have a psychotic disorder diagnosis, immediate referral to a mental health professional for further assessment is recommended.

ASSESSMENT OF FACTORS COMMONLY CONTRIBUTING TO INSOMNIA IN PATIENTS WITH PSYCHIATRIC DISORDERS

If a psychiatric disorder is present, that disorder should be treated to remission if possible, since sleep problems are generally worse in patients who are suffering from acute or inadequately treated episodes of illness. However, a thorough assessment of the sleep complaint is also warranted in the case of insomnia comorbid with psychiatric issues as even in remitted or optimally treated psychiatric patients insomnia frequently persists and can be a risk factor in relapse or exacerbation of the psychiatric illness. Particular factors that commonly contribute to insomnia in patients with psychiatric disorders include behavioral factors, the effects of psychotropic medications, and other sleep disorders. These factors should be of particular focus when assessing insomnia in this population. Each of these factors is discussed below, including recommendations for assessment and treatment, and is summarized in Table 2. Certainly, in addition to the factors discussed below, psychiatric disorder-specific factors that may be contributing to insomnia, such as nocturnal panic attacks in panic disorder, should be assessed and considered in the overall treatment plan.

Behavioral Factors

Behavioral factors are always important to assess in the context of insomnia. Furthermore, given that individuals with insomnia comorbid with depressive and/or anxiety disorders have been shown to report significantly higher levels of sleep-inhibitory behaviors (e.g., napping, smoking more than one pack of cigarettes a day, using caffeine within four hours of bedtime, and not relaxing prior to bedtime) than individuals with primary insomnia (52), assessment of behavioral factors in psychiatric patients with insomnia complaints is paramount. These patients often have a lack of daily structure, irregular bedtimes and wake-up times, and inconsistent patterns of activity and exercise. They also are prone to spend excessive amounts of time in bed sleeping and attempting to sleep. Finally, they frequently engage in daytime napping and accidental dozing, as well as use of caffeine, tobacco, alcohol, and/or recreational drugs. Collectively, these behaviors that commonly occur in reaction to both sleep loss and psychiatric symptoms can then perpetuate sleep difficulties through circadian disruption, homeostatic dysregulation, weakened associations between the bedroom and sleeping, and increased arousal. Furthermore, some of these behaviors, particularly daytime napping and accidental dozing, may be exacerbated by sedating psychiatric medications.

Table 2 Key Areas and Screening and Assessment/Treatment Recommendations for Factors Commonly Contributing to Insomnia in Patients with Psychiatric Disorders

Factors	Key areas	Screening recommendations	Assessment/treatment recommendations
Behavioral factors	• Lack of daily structure • Irregular sleep schedule • Lack of exercise • Excessive time in bed • Daytime napping • Accidental dozing • Substance use	• Patient's description of a typical day and night • Sleep Hygiene Practice Scale • Sleep logs • Activity logs • Actigraphy	• Cognitive-behavioral therapy for insomnia with an individual trained in behavioral techniques
Psychotropic medications	• Antidepressants • Antipsychotics • Stimulants	• Regular follow-up on sleep-related side effects when prescribing any of these medications	• Assess time of day medication is taken, dose and half-life • Consider alternative agents if possible
Primary sleep disorders	• OSA • PLMD • RLS • Delayed sleep phase	• OSA: screen for obesity, upper airway obstruction, snoring, witnessed apneas, poor sleep quality, and excessive daytime sleepiness • PLMD: screen for legs twitching or jerking at night • RLS: screen for uncomfortable or odd sensations in legs • Delayed sleep phase: sleep logs	• If OSA or PLMD suspected, referral for a diagnostic sleep study and consultation with sleep specialist • If RLS, referral to a sleep specialist for consultation • If delayed sleep phase, light therapy, chronotherapy, melatonin, and/or stimulus control

Abbreviations: OSA, obstructive sleep apnea; PLMD, periodic limb movement disorder; RLS, restless legs syndrome.

As part of the assessment, patients should describe a typical day and night. Questionnaires and/or daily monitoring with sleep logs and/or actigraphy can also provide information about sleep habits. The Sleep Hygiene Practice Scale (SHPS; 53), may be a particularly useful instrument for this population, which is especially prone to poor sleep hygiene. This measure has demonstrated good evidence of validity as it discriminates patients meeting criteria for insomnia from those who do not (52,53). Patients can engage in self-monitoring by completing sleep logs (e.g., 54) and/or activity logs (e.g., 55). An assessment of the 24-hour rest-activity pattern over days or weeks may also be assessed through the use of actigraphy devices, particularly if the patient's psychiatric issues significantly limit his or her ability to appropriately self-report sleep and waking patterns.

Patients who exhibit sleep-related behaviors that are counterproductive to promoting sleep (e.g., large amounts of time in bed awake, a variable sleep schedule, daytime napping or dozing, alcohol use to facilitate sleep) may benefit from cognitive-behavioral therapy for insomnia (CBT-I; see chapters 24–30). Several recent research studies have demonstrated the efficacy of CBT-I for insomnia comorbid with depression, showing not only improvements in sleep outcomes, but also improvements in depressive symptoms (11,56).

Effects of Psychotropic Medications

Psychopharmacological agents commonly used to treat psychiatric disorders, including antidepressants, antipsychotics, and stimulants, act on neurotransmitter systems involved in sleeping and waking, including 5-hydroxytryptamine, acetylcholine, dopamine, histamine, and norepinephrine. These various actions may result in improvement of insomnia, exacerbation of insomnia, and/or increased daytime sleepiness (57). The potential effects of different medications on sleep within each class are reviewed below. When evaluating the psychiatric patient with insomnia, it is important to consider the contribution of these medications to sleep complaints. The care provider should also verify that the patient is taking the medication at the appropriate time of day and at the appropriate dosage. If sleep-related side effects are clinically significant and timing and dosage have been optimized, it is recommended that other agents be tried whenever possible.

Antidepressants and Their Effects on Sleep

A majority of commonly prescribed antidepressants decrease sleep continuity. These include selective serotonin reuptake inhibitors (SSRIs) (e.g., fluoxetine, sertraline, paroxetine, citalopram), dual reuptake inhibitors (e.g., venlafaxine, duloxetine), buproprion, some tricyclics (e.g., imipramine, desipramine, and clomipramine), and monoamine oxidase inhibitors (58–60). In addition, SSRIs, venlafaxine, and particularly monoamine oxidase inhibitors have been shown to suppress REM sleep. REM sleep suppression is clinically important as patients can experience vivid dreams and nightmares (i.e., "REM sleep rebound") when discontinuing such medications abruptly or even simply missing a dose.

On the other hand, some antidepressants are sedating and are frequently used to treat insomnia comorbid with depression; these include trazodone, tricyclic antidepressants (e.g., amitriptyline, doxepin), mirtazapine, and nefazodone. However, sedating antidepressants often lead to increased daytime sleepiness because of their long half-lives. As noted above, tricyclic antidepressants suppress REM sleep (58,60) and thus cause REM sleep rebound and disrupted sleep on nights not taken.

Antipsychotics and Their Effects on Sleep

Antipsychotic medications are often sedating, and patients may be most bothered by this side effect (61). Typical antipsychotic agents that are high-milligram, low-potency agents, such as chlorpromazine and thioridazine, tend to produce greater sedation than low-milligram, high-potency agents, such as haloperidol and thiothixene (47). Newer atypical antipsychotics vary in the sedative effects, with clozapine and olanzapine being particularly sedating and aripiprazole and ziprasidone somewhat less so. In addition, newer atypical agents, such as clozapine and olanzapine, tend to enhance sleep continuity (57,62,63). Similarly, quetiapine has been shown to decrease sleep onset latency and waking time, increase total sleep time, and have no impact on SWS, REM sleep latency, or REM density (64); risperidone has been shown to decrease total wake time, improve sleep quality, and increase SWS (57,63). As a result, these medications are often administered at higher doses at bedtime to aid in sleep and minimize daytime sedation.

Stimulants and Their Effects on Sleep

Stimulants are increasingly used for attention deficit disorder/attention deficit hyperactivity disorder, depression, and fatigue (65). Not surprisingly, the effects of stimulants, such as methylphenidate, amphetamine, and modafinil, are decreased total sleep time, increased arousals, and suppressed REM sleep (65). In patients with significant insomnia who may require them for psychiatric reasons, these medications should be used in the lowest doses possible and dosing later in the day should be minimized or avoided if possible.

Other Sleep Disorders

When assessing insomnia in a patient with a known psychiatric illness, insomnia related to another primary sleep disorder should also be considered, particularly insomnia related to obstructive sleep apnea (OSA), sleep-related movement disorders, including periodic limb movement disorder (PLMD) and restless legs syndrome (RLS), or circadian rhythm disorders. Psychiatric medications may precipitate or exacerbate these disorders. If OSA or PLMD is suspected, a referral for a diagnostic sleep study is recommended. Patients with suspected RLS should be referred to a sleep specialist for consultation. Patients with circadian rhythm disorders may benefit from a referral to an individual trained in behavioral sleep medicine.

Obstructive Sleep Apnea

OSA is a common sleep disorder in which the upper airway collapses repeatedly during sleep causing pauses in breathing, arousals, and sleep fragmentation. OSA is associated with obesity and/or upper airway obstruction related to enlarged tonsils or other anatomic features, and individuals with OSA often complain of snoring, poor sleep quality, and excessive daytime sleepiness. Although OSA is more typically associated with excessive daytime sleepiness, OSA is also frequently comorbid with insomnia; about half of patients with OSA also complain of clinically meaningful insomnia (66). OSA can also be comorbid with psychiatric disorders; one study showed that almost one in five individuals with major depression had a breathing-related sleep disorder and approximately one in five with a breathing-related disorder had major depression (67). Overlapping symptoms among OSA, insomnia, depression, and other psychiatric disorders include fatigue, decreased attention/concentration, lack of motivation, and decreased enjoyment. Importantly, one must also consider how psychiatric medication can indirectly exacerbate OSA through weight gain (e.g., atypical antipsychotics, antidepressants, mood stabilizers) and muscle relaxation (e.g., benzodiazepines, barbiturates) (e.g., 68). Psychiatric patients with suspected OSA should not be given barbiturates, and sedating medications should be avoided or used with caution.

Sleep-Related Movement Disorders

Sleep-related movement disorders, including PLMD and RLS, are important to keep in mind when assessing insomnia within the context of a psychiatric disorder. PLMD is characterized by repeated contraction of the anterior tibialis muscles during sleep, resulting in leg movements, kicks, or twitches during sleep. If frequent or severe enough, they may lead to arousals and fragmented sleep. RLS is characterized by uncomfortable or odd sensations, mostly in the legs, that are accompanied by an urge to move. They tend to occur most commonly in the evening, when the patient is sitting or lying down, but may also occur at other times of day when the patient is sedentary. Furthermore, movement typically relieves these sensations temporarily. RLS is differentiated from akathisia, which is most commonly a side effect of neuroleptic antipsychotic medication, in that akathisia usually is experienced as restlessness throughout the body that does not demonstrate a circadian pattern or abate with movement (69). The presence of RLS and/or PLMD may prolong sleep onset latency or extend nocturnal awakenings.

Notably, many psychiatric medications can increase periodic limb movements (PLMs) and restless legs symptoms, including SSRIs, serotonin-norepinephrine reuptake inhibitors, and both typical and atypical antipsychotics. For example, a recent study found that approximately 9% of individuals experienced new onset or exacerbation of restless legs symptoms after starting newer antidepressants (e.g., SSRIs or dual reuptake inhibitors) (70). The pharmacological mechanisms thought to be associated with these symptoms are the reuptake inhibition of 5-hydroxytryptamine and dopamine antagonism. Agents such as buproprion, with significant dopaminergic activity, are thought to be less likely to exacerbate these symptoms (71,72).

Circadian Rhythm Disorders

Circadian rhythm disorders involve a mismatch between the 24-hour day and the endogenous circadian rhythm, which is generated by the master pacemaker within the suprachiasmatic nucleus of the hypothalamus. Various factors can entrain the human circadian rhythm, including light, melatonin, and social cues (e.g., mealtimes, start time for work). The most common circadian disorder is delayed sleep phase, which consists of profound insomnia at sleep initiation and then marked difficulty waking up in the morning. Delayed sleep phase occurs frequently in adolescents and young adults and is thought to be related to developmental changes in the circadian clock (73). Delayed sleep phase has also been observed to occur more frequently in mood disorder populations; several studies have suggested that patients with bipolar disorder may have greater rates of delayed sleep phase than individuals with schizophrenia or individuals without a psychiatric diagnosis, as seen by a significantly higher preference for "eveningness" and significantly delayed sleep times (74,75). If delayed sleep phase is suspected, it is recommend that patients engage in self-monitoring by completing sleep logs (e.g., 54) to confirm a regular pattern of extreme sleep initiation difficulties (e.g., several hours) and delayed wake-up times. Treatment for delayed sleep phase disorder includes morning bright light therapy for less significantly delayed sleep patterns and chronotherapy for more significantly delayed sleep patterns (76). Treatment may also include melatonin administration and/or other behavioral techniques, such as stimulus control therapy (77), if sleep-inhibitory behaviors are present (76).

SUMMARY

Insomnia and psychiatric disorders frequently occur together. Furthermore, mounting evidence has shown that insomnia is a risk factor for future onset and/or relapse and exacerbation of psychiatric disorders, particularly depression. Therefore, the assessment of both sleep and psychiatric symptomatology in individuals with either an insomnia or a psychiatric complaint is essential. Psychiatric disorders commonly occurring with insomnia include mood, anxiety, and psychotic disorders; these have effects on both subjective insomnia as well as affecting objective sleep EEG patterns. Screening questions and tools are often helpful to identify psychiatric disorders in patients with insomnia and to monitor the severity of psychiatric symptoms during the course of treatment. Other factors commonly contributing to insomnia in psychiatric patients include behavioral factors, the effects of psychotropic medications, and other sleep disorders. An understanding of the comorbidity between sleep and psychiatric disorders as well as ways to better screen, assess, and monitor both insomnia and psychiatric disorders should lead to more optimal management and outcome in insomnia patients.

REFERENCES

1. Ford DE, Kamerow DB. Epidemiologic study of sleep disturbances and psychiatric disorders. JAMA 1989; 262(11):1479–1484.
2. Ohayon MM. Prevalence of DSM-IV diagnostic criteria of insomnia: distinguishing insomnia related to mental disorders from sleep disorders. J Psychiatr Res 1997; 31(3):333–346.
3. Ohayon MM, Roth T. Place of chronic insomnia in the course of depressive and anxiety disorders. J Psychiatr Res 2003; 37:9–15.
4. Carney C, Segal Z, Edinger J, et al. A comparison of rates of residual symptoms following pharmacotherapy or cognitive-behavior therapy for major depressive disorder. J Clin Psychiatry 2008; 68:254–260.
5. Breslau N, Roth T, Rosenthal L, et al. Sleep disturbance and psychiatric disorders: a longitudinal epidemiological study of young adults. Biol Psychiatry 1996; 39:411–418.
6. Chang P, Ford D, Mead L, et al. Insomnia in young men and subsequent depression: The Johns Hopkins Precursor Study. Am J Epidemiol 1997; 146:105–114.
7. Johnson E, Roth T, Breslau N. The association of insomnia with anxiety disorder and depression: exploration of the direction of risk. J Psychiatr Res 2006; 40:700–708.
8. Weissman M, Greenwald S, Niño-Murcia G, et al. The morbidity of insomnia uncomplicated by psychiatric disorders. Gen Hosp Psychiatry 1997; 19:245–250.
9. Reynolds CF, Frank E, Houck P, et al. Which elderly patients with remitted depression remain well with continued interpersonal psychotherapy after discontinuation of antidepressant therapy? Am J Psychiatry 1997; 154:958–962.
10. Fava M, McCall V, Krystal A, et al. Eszopiclone co-administered with fluoxetine in patients with insomnia coexisting with major depressive disorder. Biol Psychiatry 2006; 59:1052–1060.
11. Manber R, Edinger J, Gress J, et al. Cognitive behavioral therapy for insomnia enhances depression outcome in patients with comorbid major depressive disorder and insomnia. Sleep 2008; 31:489–495.
12. Buysse DJ, Ancoli-Israel S, Edinger JD, et al. Recommendations for a standard research assessment of insomnia. Sleep 2006; 29(9):1155–1173.
13. Roth T. The relationship between psychiatric diseases and insomnia. Int J Clin Pract 2001; 116:3–8.
14. American Psychiatric Association. Diagnostic and Statistical Manual of Mental Disorders. 4th ed, text revision. Washington DC: American Psychiatric Association, 2001.
15. Benca R, Obermeyer W, Thisted R, et al. Sleep and psychiatric disorders. A meta-analysis. Arch Gen Psychiatry 1992; 49:651–670.
16. Kupfer D. Sleep research in depressive illness: clinical implications—a tasting menu. Biol Psychiatry 1995; 38:391–403.
17. Beck A, Steer R, Brown G. Beck Depression Inventory-II manual. San Antonio, TX: Psychological Corporation, 1996.

18. Rush A, Gullion B, Basco M, et al. The Inventory of Depressive Symptomatology (IDS): psychometric properties. Psychol Med 1996; 26:477–486.
19. Spitzer R, Kroenke K, Williams J. Validation and utility of a self-report version of the PRIME-MD: the PHQ primary care study. JAMA 1999; 282:1737–1744.
20. Arnau R, Meagher M, Norris M, et al. Psychometric evaluation of the Beck Depression Inventory-II with primary care patients. Health Psychol 2001; 20:112–119.
21. Yesavage J, Brink T, Rose T, et al. Development and validation of a geriatric depression screening scale: a preliminary report. J Psychiatr Res 1983; 17:37–49.
22. Brink T, Yesavage J, Lum O, et al. Screening tests for geriatric depression. Clin Gerontol 1982; 1:37–43.
23. Hirschfeld R, Williams J, Spitzer R, et al. Development and validation of a screening instrument for bipolar spectrum disorder: the Mood Disorder Questionnaire. Am J Psychiatry, 2000; 157:1873–1875.
24. Hirschfeld R, Cass A, Holt D, et al. Screening for bipolar disorder in patients treated for depression in a family medicine clinic. J Am Board Fam Med 2005; 18:233–239.
25. Belanger L, Morin C, Langlois F, et al. Insomnia and generalized anxiety disorder: effects of cognitive behavior therapy for GAD on insomnia symptoms. J Anxiety Disord 2004; 18:561–571.
26. Arriaga F, Paiva T. Clinical and EEG sleep changes in primary dysthymia and generalized anxiety disorder: a comparison with normal controls. Neuropsychobiology 1990–1991; 24:109–114.
27. Papdimitriou G, Kerkhofs M, Kempenaers C, et al. EEG sleep studies in patients with generalized anxiety disorder. Psychiatry Res 1988; 26:183–190.
28. Saletu-Zyhalrz G, Saletu B, Anderer P, et al. Nonorganic insomnia in generalized anxiety disorder. Controlled studies on sleep, awakening and daytime vigilance utilizing polysomnography and EEG mapping. Neuropsychobiology 1997; 36:117–129.
29. Spielberger C, Gorsuch R, Lushene R. Manual for the State-Trait Anxiety Inventory. Palo Alto, CA: Consulting Psychologists Press, 1970.
30. Meyer T, Miller M, Metzger R, et al. Development and validation of the Penn State Worry Questionnaire. Behav Res Ther 1990; 28:487–495.
31. Behar E, Alcaine O, Zuellig A, et al. Screening for generalized anxiety disorder using the Penn State Worry Questionnaire: a receiver operating characteristic analysis. J Behav Ther Exp Psychiatry 2003; 34:25–43.
32. Arriaga F, Paiva T, Matos-Pires A, et al. The sleep of non-depressed patients with panic disorder: a comparison with normal controls. Acta Psychiatr Scand 1996; 93:191–194.
33. Sloan E, Natarajan M, Baker B, et al. Nocturnal and daytime panic attacks-comparison of sleep architecture, heart rate variability, and response to sodium lactate challenge. Biol Psychiatry 1999; 45:1313–1320.
34. Mellman T, Uhde T. Patients with frequent sleep panic: clinical findings and response to medication treatment. J Clin Psychiatry 1990; 51:513–516.
35. Mellman T, Unde T. Electroencephalographic sleep in panic disorder. A focus on sleep-related panic attacks. J Clin Psychiatry 1989; 146:1204–1207.
36. Apeldorf W, Shear M, Leon A, et al. A brief screen for panic disorder. J Anxiety Disord 1994; 8:71–78.
37. Mellman T, Nolan B, Hebding J, et al. Sleep events among veterans with combat-related PTSD, depressed men, and non-ill controls. Sleep 1997; 20:46–51.
38. Ross R, Ball W, Dinges D, et al. Rapid eye movement sleep disturbance in posttraumatic stress disorder. Biol Psychiatry 1994; 35:195 202.
39. Ross R, Ball W, Dinges D, et al. Motor dysfunction during sleep in posttraumatic stress disorder. Sleep 1994; 17:723–732.
40. Lavie P. Current concepts: sleep disturbances in the wake of traumatic events. N Engl J Med 2001; 345:1825–1832.
41. Mellman T. Sleep and the pathogenesis of PTSD. In: Shalev A, Yehuda R, McFarlane A, eds. International Handbook of Human Response to Trauma. New York: Plenum Publishing, 2000.
42. Foa EB. Posttraumatic Stress Diagnostic Scale: Manual. Minneapolis, MN: National Computer System, 1995.
43. Sheeran T, Zimmerman M. Screening for posttraumatic stress disorder in a general psychiatric outpatient sample. J Consult Clin Psychol 2002; 70:961–966.
44. Ritsner M, Kurs R, Ponizovsky A, et al. Perceived quality of life in schizophrenia: relationships to sleep quality. Qual Life Res 2004; 13:783–791.
45. Haffmans P, Hoencamp E, Knegtering H, et al. Sleep disturbance in schizophrenia. Br J Psychiatry 1994; 165:697–698.
46. Chemerinski E, Ho B, Flaum M, et al. Insomnia as a predictor for symptom worsening following antipsychotic withdrawal in schizophrenia. Compr Psychiatry 2002; 43:393–396.
47. Benson K. Sleep in schizophrenia: impairments, correlates, and treatment. Psychiatr Clin North Am 2006; 29:1033–1045.

48. Chouinard S, Poulin J, Stip E, et al. Sleep in untreated patients with schizophrenia: a meta-analysis. Schizophr Bull 2004; 30:957–967.
49. Ferrarelli F, Huber R, Peterson M, et al. Reduced sleep spindle activity in schizophrenia patients. Am J Psychiatry 2007; 164:483–492.
50. Overall J, Gorham D. The Brief Psychiatric Rating Scale (BPRS): recent developments in ascertainment and scaling. Psychopharmacol Bull 1988; 24:97–99.
51. Kay S, Opler L, Fiszbein A. Positive and Negative Syndrome Scale Manual. North Tonawanda, NY: Multi-Health Systems, 1994.
52. Kohn L, Espie C. Sensitivity and specificity of measures of the insomnia experience: a comparative study of psychophysiologic insomnia, insomnia associated with mental disorder, and good sleepers. Sleep 2005; 28:104–112.
53. Lacks P, Rotert M. Knowledge and practice of sleep hygiene techniques in insomniacs and good sleepers. Behav Res Ther 1986; 24(3):365–368.
54. Morin C, Espie C. Insomnia: A Clinical Guide to Assessment and Treatment. New York: Kluwer, 2003.
55. Frank E. Treating Bipolar Disorder: A Clinician's Guide to Interpersonal and Social Rhythms Therapy. New York: Guilford Press, 2005.
56. Taylor D, Lichstein K, Weinstock J, et al. A pilot study of cognitive-behavioral therapy of insomnia in people with mild depression. Behav Ther 2007; 38:49–57.
57. DeMartinis N, Winokur A. Effects of psychiatric medications on sleep and sleep disorders. CNS Neurol Disord Drug Targets 2007; 6:17–29.
58. Argyropoulos S, Wilson S. Sleep disturbances in depression and the effects of antidepressants. Int Rev Psychiatry 2005; 17:237–245.
59. Lippmann S, Mazour I, Shahab H. Insomnia: therapeutic approach. South Med J 2001; 94:866–873.
60. Mayers AG, Baldwin, DS. Antidepressants and their effect on sleep. Hum Psychopharmacol 2005; 20:533–559.
61. Hofer A, Kemmler G, Eder U, et al. Attitudes toward antipsychotics among outpatient clinic attendees with schizophrenia. J Clin Psychiatry 2002; 63:49–53.
62. Armitage R, Cole D, Suppes T, et al. Effects of clozapine on sleep in bipolar and schizoaffective disorders. Prog Neuropsychopharmacol Biol Psychiatry 2004; 28:1065–1070.
63. Gimenez S, Clos S, Romero S, et al. Effects of olanzapine, risperidone and haloperidol on sleep after a single oral morning dose in healthy volunteers. Psychopharmacology 2007; 190:507–516.
64. Keshavan M, Prasad K, Montrose D, et al. Sleep quality and architecture in quetiapine, risperidone, or never-treated schizophrenia patients. J Clin Psychopharmcol 2007; 27:703–705.
65. Mendelson W, Caruso C. Pharmacology in sleep medicine. In: Pocete J, Mitler M, eds. Sleep Disorders: Diagnosis and Treatment. Totowa, NJ: Humana Press Inc, 1998:137–160.
66. Krakow B, Melendrez D, Ferreira E, et al. Prevalence of insomnia in patients with sleep-disordered breathing. Chest 2001; 120:1923–1929.
67. Ohayon M. The effects of breathing-related sleep disorders on mood disturbances in the general population. J Clin Psychiatry 2003; 64:1195–1200.
68. Winkelman J. Schizophrenia, obesity, and obstructive sleep apnea. J Clin Psychiatry 2001; 62:8–11.
69. Lesage S, Hening W. The restless legs syndrome and periodic limb movement disorder: a review of management. Semin Neurol 2004; 24:249–259.
70. Rottach K, Schaner B, Kirch M, et al. Restless legs syndrome as side effect of second generation antidepressants. J Psychiatr Res 2008; 43:70–75.
71. Yang C, White D, Winkleman J. Antidepressants and periodic leg movements of sleep. Biol Psychiatry 2005; 58:510–514.
72. Nofzinger E, Fasiczka A, Berman S, et al. Bupropion SR reduces periodic limb movements associated with arousals from sleep in depressed patients with periodic limb movement disorder. J Clin Psychiatry 2000; 61:858–862.
73. Taylor D, Jenni O, Acebo C, et al. Sleep tendency during extended wakefulness: insights into adolescent sleep regulation and behavior. J Sleep Res 2005; 22:571–584.
74. Mansour H, Wood J, Chowdari K, et al. Circadian phase variation in bipolar I disorder. Chronobiol Int 2005; 22:571–584.
75. Ahn Y, Change J, Joo Y, et al. Chronotype distribution in bipolar I disorder and schizophrenia in a Korean sample. Bioplar Disord 2008; 10:271–275.
76. Lack L, Wright H. Clinical management of delayed sleep phase disorder. Behav Sleep Med 2007; 5:57–76.
77. Bootzin, R. Stimulus control treatment for insomnia. In: Proceedings of the 80th Annual Convention of the American Psychological Association; 1972; 7:395–396.80

14 Insomnia in Chronic Pain

Emerson M. Wickwire
Center for Sleep Disorders, Pulmonary Disease and Critical Care Associates, Columbia, Maryland, U.S.A.

Michael T. Smith
Department of Psychiatry and Behavioral Sciences, Behavioral Sleep Medicine Program, Johns Hopkins University School of Medicine, Baltimore, Maryland, U.S.A.

INTRODUCTION: DEFINITION, PREVALENCE, AND COSTS OF CHRONIC PAIN

The International Association for the Study of Pain (IASP) defines *pain* as "an unpleasant sensory and emotional experience associated with actual or potential tissue damage, or described in terms of such damage" (1). Pain is the most common health-related complaint in the United States, accounting for over 80% of all doctor office visits (2). While acute pain serves a critical biologic survival mechanism, signaling injury, pain can develop from an acute, beneficial sensory phenomenon to a pathological, intractable condition. More than half of U.S. adults report experiencing some form of chronic pain during the past year and 50% of these individuals report pain lasting longer than one year (2). Chronic pain accounts for over $70 billion annually in health care costs and lost workplace productivity (2).

Chronic pain is often described as pain that persists beyond the expected time of healing, but the factors associated with the transition from acute to chronic pain are poorly understood and likely involve complex genetic, behavioral, societal, and peripheral and central nervous system interactions. Disorders associated with chronic pain are often classified by their presumed primary etiology, for example, inflammatory pain (e.g., rheumatory arthritis), nociceptive pain resulting from active stimulation of pain sensing neurons (i.e., nociceptors), and neuropathic pain, resulting from injury to nociceptors (e.g., postherpetic neuralgia). These categories, however, are not mutually exclusive, and chronic pain conditions often involve some combination of these classic categories of pain. Moreover, many chronic pain conditions such as fibromyalgia, irritable bowel syndrome, temporomandibular joint disorder, and others, are idiopathic, having no identifiable peripheral insult or pathology that explains the magnitude of pain and suffering.

Increasingly, data from neuroimaging and psychophysiologic studies implicate dysfunctional central pain processing mechanisms in the etiology and maintenance of many chronic pain disorders, particularly the idiopathic syndromes. A complex network of descending opioidergic and serotonergic systems have been shown to inhibit and facilitate afferent nociceptive input from second order neurons in the dorsal horn through key centers in the periaqueductal gray and the rostral ventral medulla (3). These systems are often dysregulated in chronic pain disorders, leading to a state of central sensitization, such that ascending pain signals are augmented at the level of the spinal cord (4). Specific higher order brain regions, often referred to as the pain neuromatrix, include the thalamus, anterior cingulate nucleus, insula, and prefrontal cortices, regions that are known to directly regulate brain stem pain modulatory centers (5). Individual differences in the functional integrity of these systems predict individuals at risk for the development of chronic pain (6). Many of the CNS systems involved in pain processing, particularly the limbic system, thalamus, and prefrontal cortices, are also critical to both affect and sleep regulation. It is therefore not surprising that both mood impairments and sleep disturbance are common to the experience of chronic pain. Moreover, both negative mood and sleep disturbance are increasingly identified as independent risk factors for the development of chronic pain syndromes (7–10), possibly contributing to a top–down pain amplification by impairing pain modulatory centers in the brain stem and spinal cord.

The vast majority of individuals with chronic pain report significant sleep problems, including delayed sleep onset, increased nocturnal awakenings, greater wake after sleep onset, and poorer quality sleep, relative to pain-free individuals (11). Evidence also suggests the possibility that rates of other intrinsic sleep disorders such as sleep disordered breathing may

(1) Traditional Linear View

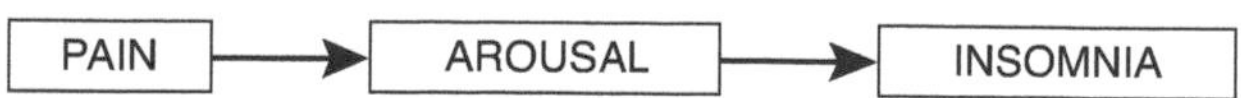

(2) Reciprocal View (Moldofsky, 1975)

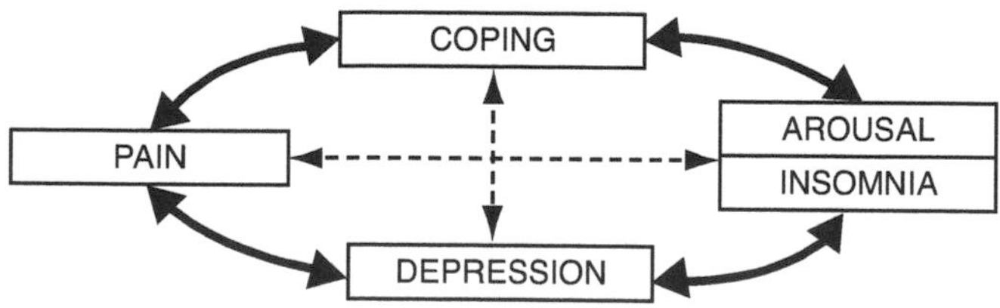

Figure 1 Reciprocal relations between sleep and pain.

be elevated in chronic pain patients (e.g., Ref. 12). Although it is commonly assumed that sleep disturbance associated with pain is primarily a consequence of pain, experimental and cross sectional evidence spanning over half a century, as well as emerging longitudinal data, support a bidirectional relationship between sleep and pain. Indeed, for patients with chronic pain a vicious cycle often develops, with pain disrupting sleep and poor sleep further exacerbating pain.

Importantly, mood disturbance and psychological distress are common among chronic pain patients (13). Evidence consistently supports elevated rates of both depression and anxiety in chronic pain populations, and as demonstrated in Figure 1, it is now known that the sleep–pain relationship is often mediated by cognitive and affective processes. This suggests that thorough assessment of emotional disturbance and sleep disorders is especially important in the evaluation and management of patients with chronic pain conditions. Further, despite high prevalence rates of insomnia complaints in patients suffering from chronic pain conditions, systematic empirical treatment approaches are not well developed and therefore clinical management can be especially challenging.

The purpose of this chapter is to review the relation between chronic insomnia and chronic pain. To this end, we will briefly summarize the literature evaluating the effect of experimental sleep disturbance on pain sensitivity, as well as the effects of the administration of pain during sleep to provide important background information. We will next consider evidence supporting prospective and reciprocal relations between sleep disturbance and pain. Sleep complaints in several common chronic pain conditions will be reviewed, and key findings from the extant clinical trials literature, including pharmacological and cognitive-behavioral approaches, will be discussed. The chapter concludes with clinical recommendations and suggestions for future research.

EXPERIMENTAL AND LONGITUDINAL RELATIONS BETWEEN SLEEP AND PAIN

Effects of Experimental Sleep Disruption on Pain

In the first third of the 20th century, researchers proposed a relation between sleep disruption and pain processing. Copperman (14) observed decreased skin sensitivity to touch and pain following 60 hours of sleep deprivation, with greater sleep loss being associated with lower pain thresholds. Nearly 40 years later, Moldofsky et al. evaluated the relation between sleep and pain by using auditory tones to disrupt slow wave sleep and REM sleep in uncontrolled studies of healthy subjects. They reported next day increases in musculoskeletal tenderness after SWS but not REM disruption, noting that the patterns of muscle tenderness resembled symptoms of fibrositis (fibromyalgia) (15,16). These authors were among the first to suggest a vicious cycle between sleep disturbance and chronic pain, with pain impairing sleep and poor sleep enhancing pain and disturbed mood. Since these reports in the mid-1970s, researchers have continued to evaluate the effects of sleep disruption on pain. Although results have been somewhat mixed (17), in aggregate these findings support a bidirectional, causal relationship between sleep and pain sensitivity (18). More recent studies have reported increased sensitivity to mechanical stimuli following 40 hours of total sleep deprivation (19), a 24% decrease in mechanical pain threshold, and an increase in inflammatory skin flare response following SWS disruption among women (20). Recent well-controlled experiments found that restriction to four hours of sleep and REM disruption (but not NREM disruption) caused thermal hyperalgesia (21). In a controlled study of 32 healthy females, sleep continuity disturbance induced via forced awakenings, but not simple sleep curtailment, impaired descending pain inhibitory functions and induced spontaneous reports of pain (22). While not enough systematic research is yet available to conclusively explain which types of sleep disruption or loss alter various dimensions of central pain processing, it is clear that insufficient sleep contributes to pain amplification and induces pain even in the absence of peripheral input.

Effects of Pain Administration During Sleep

A second line of experimental research has evaluated the effects of painful stimuli administered during sleep. All of these studies have found noxious stimuli to induce sleep microarousals (increases if high frequency EEG activity, often accompanied by autonomic changes) and concurrent decrease in slow wave activity (23–25). For example, Drewes et al. (24), administered painful stimuli to both muscles and joints and found decreased delta activity and increases in the alpha, beta, and sigma ranges. Other studies have found painful stimuli administered during sleep to produce transient tachycardia (26) as well as cortical arousal even in the absence of frank awakenings (25). These EEG findings are consistent with EEG profiles observed in chronic pain patients, which often show decreased slow wave sleep and increased alpha activity without frank awakenings. However, the stimuli administered in these studies were of brief duration (i.e., one millisecond) and therefore cannot be considered representative of clinical pain conditions, which are characterized by persistent pain of greater duration (23,24,27,28). In studies that have employed painful stimuli of greater duration, a dose–response relationship has been observed between stimuli duration and cortical arousal (24,26–28).

Despite the ability of noxious stimuli of sufficient intensity to fragment sleep, it should be noted that in healthy subjects the data also indicate that the nociceptive system is attenuated. The intensity of stimulation required to evoke arousal is much higher than the intensity of stimulation required to reach pain threshold during testing conducted when awake (27,28). It remains unknown whether chronic pain patients also have attenuated pain processing during sleep or whether this process itself becomes disrupted as part of neuroplastic changes associated with chronic pain. Although painful stimuli during sleep have not yet been administered in chronic pain populations, EEG arousal responses to painful stimuli suggest that sleep disturbances observed in chronic pain may in part be caused by pain itself and may not always reflect independent sleep or mood disturbance.

Longitudinal Relationship Between Sleep and Pain

Longitudinal clinical studies support a reciprocal relationship, such that pain interferes with sleep and disturbed sleep is associated with next day or longer-term increases in pain (29–34). Supporting the reciprocal nature of sleep–pain interactions, an increasing number of longitudinal studies suggest that poor sleep is an independent risk factor for increased pain severity (22,29,32,34,35). For example, in a sample of 333 hospitalized burn patients, insomnia complaints and pain severity were assessed at discharge and 6, 12, and 24-month follow-up (9). Individuals with sleep onset insomnia had significantly less improvement in pain symptoms and increased pain severity at follow-up, even after controlling for premorbid pain, pain severity at discharge, mental health, and total burn surface area. Similarly, burn pain during hospitalization predicted future insomnia complaints (9), although to a lesser extent. Hence the relationships between sleep and pain appear to be long term, prospective, and reciprocal. In a microlongitudinal study designed to assess these reciprocal relationships over multiple nights, Edwards et al. (36) recently reported results from a naturalistic telephone survey of representative sample of 971 U.S. adults in the general population. Over a one-week period, daily reports of sleep duration (<6 hours or >9 hours) were associated with greater next-day pain; in a reciprocal model daily pain reports were similarly although less strongly predictive of sleep duration that night (36). In addition to these self-report data, Drewes et al. (30) administered PSG to 35 patients with rheumatoid arthritis and found that time awake in bed predicted morning stiffness, joint tenderness, and subjective pain ratings six months later. Similarly, baseline ratings of pain and morning stiffness predicted nocturnal wake time as well as changes in sleep architecture at six months (30).

INSOMNIA IN CHRONIC PAIN CONDITIONS

Consistent with this experimental and longitudinal evidence, data obtained from clinical samples also support a strong relation between sleep disturbance and pain. High rates of sleep disturbance have been found in numerous chronic pain conditions, with insomnia being the most common presenting symptom. For example, large-scale studies consistently suggest that at least 50% or more of patients with osteoarthritis (OA) report significant difficulty initiating or maintaining sleep (37–42). Among cancer patients, high rates of insomnia complaints, depressive symptoms, and health anxiety have been reported (43). Because persistent pain, mood disturbance, and sleep complaints and nearly ubiquitous in these populations, a review of all chronic pain conditions is beyond the scope of this chapter. The following section, however, provides a brief overview of sleep in three broad categories of chronic pain conditions that are frequently seen in general clinical practice and highlight the complexities of sleep–pain interactions: (*i*) inflammatory and autoimmune conditions, (*ii*) idiopathic pain disorders (functional), and (*iii*) neuropathic pain syndromes.

Inflammatory and Autoimmune Conditions Associated with Chronic Pain

Patients with inflammatory and autoimmune conditions consistently report sleep disturbance. For example, adult rheumatoid arthritis (RA) patients frequently complain of sleep disruption, including decreased arousal threshold and increased time awake in the middle of the night. PSG findings have tended to corroborate these self-reports. For example, relative to healthy controls, RA patients have been found to have increased sleep fragmentation (44–50) and higher arousal indices as measured via PSG (45,48,49). Similarly, several studies have reported increased wake after sleep onset in RA (45,48). Importantly, evidence supports a relation between these sleep disturbances and pain severity in RA, with higher arousal indices and greater wake after sleep onset having been positively associated with self-reported pain and morning stiffness among adults (30,44,49). Not surprisingly, high frequency EEG activity (e.g., alpha intrusion) has also been consistently documented in the sleep of RA patients (44–50).

Data are more limited among other autoimmune conditions but also suggest disturbed sleep among patients with these diseases. For example, in a PSG study of 27 consecutive clinic patients with systemic sclerosis (scleroderma), results demonstrated decreased sleep efficiency, decreased REM sleep, increased SWS, and increased arousals, relative to normative data (51). This study also reported a high rate of periodic limb movement disorder and restless legs syndrome, indicating clinicians should actively assess and consider referral for these disorders in scleroderma. Likewise, persons with the autoimmune inflammatory disease sarcoidosis experience fatigue, insomnia, and daytime sleepiness, and PSG evidence supports both sleep apnea and periodic limb movements as common comorbid sleep disorders (52,53). Normalizing sleep in autoimmune diseases, inflammatory diseases, and other illnesses involving dysregulation of the immune system, such as cancer, may prove a critical and currently under appreciated component of disease management. Growing evidence from sleep deprivation studies suggests that insufficient sleep has detrimental consequences on immune system function, including causing elevation in proinflammatory cytokines, which sensitize nociceptors, thereby augmenting clinical pain and contributing to fatigue (54).

Idiopathic Pain Disorders

Idiopathic pain disorders are a group of highly comorbid syndromes with overlapping symptoms including chronic widespread pain, fatigue, psychological distress, and motor dysfunction. Neuroendocrine abnormalities and mild cognitive impairment can also be present. Common idiopathic pain conditions include fibromyalgia, irritable bowel syndrome, temporomandibular joint disorder, tension headache disorders, chronic pelvic pain, and interstitial cystitis (55,56). Although these disorders typically have no clear peripheral pathology, evidence suggests that they share a common central nervous system substrate characterized by heightened processing of noxious input. As a result, there is a great deal of overlap in symptoms between these conditions, which have been increasingly referred to as "central sensitivity syndromes" (57). Patients diagnosed with one of these disorders frequently meet diagnostic criteria for other syndromes in this cluster of conditions associated with intractable pain (58,59).

Subjective and objectively measured sleep disturbances are highly prevalent in these populations and may exacerbate symptoms through increased psychological distress or disturbed processing of noxious inputs (e.g., Ref. 22). In clinical settings, sleep disruption is among the most common of all symptoms reported in idiopathic pain disorders. For example, fibromyalgia (FM) has a consistent and well-replicated relation with disturbed sleep (11), with the majority of patients reporting difficulty maintaining sleep and characterizing their sleep quality as shallow and nonrestorative (60). Complaints of impaired sleep continuity in FM have been verified by PSG, including increased sleep onset latency (61), increased nocturnal arousals (62–64), more time awake during the night (62), greater sleep fragmentation (65), decreased sleep efficiency (64,66,67), and increased alpha intrusion during NREM sleep (64,68).

Patients with myofascial temporomandibular joint disorder (TMD) report similar sleep disturbances, and recent evidence suggests high rates of diagnosed sleep disorders in this population, including insomnia, obstructive sleep apnea, and sleep bruxism (69a,69b). Polysomnographically measured decrements in sleep efficiency have also been linked to psychophysical measures of impaired pain inhibitory processes in TMD (70). Sleep fragmentation has been shown to decrease endogenous pain inhibitory capacity, and dysfunction of these same descending pain inhibitory systems has been implicated in pathophysiologic models of idiopathic pain disorders (71).

Sleep disturbance and headache disorders, the most common category of episodic pain disorder, are also highly comorbid. Insomnia is the most common sleep complaint in this population (72) with over one half of all headache patients reporting difficulty initiating or maintaining sleep, early morning awakening, or nonrestorative sleep (73). Boardman et al. (74) surveyed 2662 adults living in the United Kingdom and found that after controlling for age and gender, sleep disturbance was monotonically related to headache complaints. Similarly, Ohayon (75) analyzed data from a large-scale telephone-based survey and found a significant association between morning headache and insomnia. Other studies have documented differences in sleep complaints between patients with migraine or tension-type headache, with tension-type headache generally being more strongly associated with complaints of insomnia (76,77). Among patients with tension-type headache, insomnia has also been associated with poorer prognosis (77). Patients with migraine have changes in the quality of sleep several days before the onset of a migraine attack, but have largely normal sleep patterns outside the attacks (78). Cluster headaches (attacks of severe unilateral orbital, supraorbital or temporal pain) frequently occur during sleep and are believed to be directly associated with chronobiologic mechanisms and sleep stage shifts. In addition to insomnia, sleep disordered breathing has often been linked to morning headaches, and current guidelines indicated that headache management should identify and treat sleep disorders, which may improve or prevent headaches (72). In general, the particularly strong association between sleep disturbance and central sensitivity syndromes suggests the possibility that sleep disturbances may play an integral role in the pathophysiology and clinical course of these syndromes. Research aimed at determining how treatment of sleep disturbances in these conditions alters pain and related symptoms is needed.

Neuropathic Pain Syndromes

Neuropathic pain syndromes are particularly treatment-refractory chronic pain conditions associated with damage to peripheral nerves. Like other intractable pain disorders, however, neuroplastic changes in pain processing systems play an integral role in their pathophysiology and maintenance. In addition to sensory loss associated with denervation, neuropathies also paradoxically involve positive symptoms, most commonly pain that is often qualitatively described as "burning" or "shooting." Spontaneous paresthesias/dysesthesias, hyperalgesia (exaggerated response to a noxious stimulus), and allodynia (in which previously non-noxious stimuli are perceived as painful) are common consequences of peripheral nerve damage. Allodynia can be particularly disruptive to sleep, and affected patients will often report that even light touch stimulation of the affected area by bed sheets can trigger exquisite pain. Common neuropathic pain conditions include diabetic neuropathies, complex regional pain syndrome, demyelinating diseases, virally mediated neuropathies (e.g., HIV and postherpetic neuralgia), spinal cord injuries, and iatrogenic nerve damage due to chemotherapies for cancer. Although there are many causes of neuropathic pain, treatment targeting neuropathic pain most commonly includes agents that stabilize cell membranes (e.g., Na+ and K+ channels) associated with aberrant nerve conduction. Anticonvulsant medications with sedating properties are commonly used and may improve sleep.

As is the case with other types of chronic pain, mood disturbance is common among patients experiencing neuropathic pain (79), and not surprisingly, many patients also complain of sleep disturbance. In one of the few systematic studies of sleep in neuropathic pain disorders, Zelman et al. (80) compared self-report sleep data from 255 patients with painful diabetic peripheral neuropathy (DPN). These authors found that relative to the general population ($P < 0.001$) and patients with chronic medical diseases ($P < 0.05$), patients with painful DPN reported significantly poorer sleep. The DPN group also reported greater sleep disturbance than subjects with postherpetic neuralgia. Average daily pain and anxiety and depression symptoms were all associated with poorer sleep in this cross sectional study. With increasing prevalence of obesity and diabetes worldwide and an estimated U.S. diabetes prevalence of 11.2% by the year 2030 (81), these data indicate that systematic research to assess and treat sleep and pain in this population is a health priority.

TREATMENT OF COMORBID INSOMNIA AND CHRONIC PAIN

The available experimental and longitudinal data strongly suggest the sleep–pain relationship is best described as bidirectional or reciprocal. Given this data, it is somewhat surprising that few clinical trials designed to determine analgesic efficacy and effectiveness have included sleep as a major outcome.

Pharmacologic Treatments for Sleep Disturbance in Chronic Pain

Several early studies have tested the short-term effects of benzodiazepine receptor agonists (BZRAs) on sleep and pain (44,82,83). These studies included patients with FM and RA, and results indicated that BZRAs improved sleep but had minimal impact on pain. Negative findings with respect to pain, however, are likely a function of very small sample sizes, insufficient treatment durations, and no follow-up investigation. Clinical trials designed to study the effects of these agents over longer periods of time (months rather than days) are needed.

Pharmacological Treatments for Pain and Effects on Sleep

Historically, sedating antidepressants have often been prescribed to treat comorbid chronic pain and insomnia. Older drugs, including tricyclic antidepressants, can be effective in improving sleep parameters when administered in doses lower than typically prescribed for treatment of depression (84). Nonetheless, given the ubiquitous overlap between sleep complaints and mood disturbance, it should be noted that it is not entirely clear whether these improvements are independent of changes in depressive symptoms (85). More recently, research has also evaluated the effectiveness of newer antidepressant compounds, particularly the selective serotonin and norepinephrine inhibitors. Fishbain et al. (86) pooled data from three double-blind, randomized, placebo-controlled clinical trials investigating the treatment of DPN with duloxetine. Results indicated that reductions in sleep interference were associated with less daily pain and less severe night pain. Clinicians should be cautioned that some patients may experience insomnia as a side effect of antidepressant medications.

In clinical practice, anticonvulsants have also often been prescribed for sleep disturbance within the context of chronic pain, and some evidence supports their effectiveness. Gordh et al. (87) conducted a randomized, double-blind, placebo-controlled trial of gabapentin among 120 traumatic nerve injury patients across nine treatment centers. Despite null findings for the primary outcome variable of pain intensity, gabapentin was associated with significant decreases in pain-related sleep interference. Similarly, Tolle et al. (88) found pregabalin to be associated with significant reductions in pain-related sleep interference in neuropathic pain. Arnold et al. (89) also reported significant improvements in self-reported sleep parameters in FM patients following 14 weeks of pregabalin administration.

Finally, some recent evidence also supports the use of weak opioid agonists for comorbid pain and sleep disturbance. In two large ($N > 1000$) posthoc studies of extended-release tramadol in adults with OA, significant improvement in self-reported sleep parameters were reported as early as one week and maintained throughout treatment (90). In another study of OA patients, Kivitz et al (91) reported that 40 and 50 mg, but not 10 mg, extended-release oxymorphone improved self-reported sleep.

Effects of Cognitive-Behavioral Therapy for Pain on Sleep

Like cognitive-behavioral treatments for insomnia, CBT interventions for pain typically include multiple components. These are likely to include training in relaxation, developing coping skills, and addressing maladaptive beliefs, and behavioral activation strategies including increasing physical activity, setting goals, and scheduling pleasurable activities. These protocols differ notably from typical CBT-I prescriptions, which are more likely to include sleep hygiene education, stimulus control, and sleep restriction. Relaxation is a shared component of the two approaches. Whereas treatment effects for CBT-I tend to be moderate to large, the impact of CBT-P on pain outcomes is more limited. Astin et al. (92) reported effect sizes of 0.20, and Morley et al. (93) found only slightly higher effect at 0.29. The effects of CBT-P on outcomes such as coping and self-efficacy are notably higher and in the moderate range and tend to increase over time (92,93).

Given the well-known relation among sleep complaints, pain severity, and mood disturbance, it is surprising that effects of CBT-P on sleep are generally not reported in treatment studies of chronic pain conditions (94). The studies that have considered these effects present a mixed picture. An early study (95) reported improvements in sleep complaints roughly equal to reductions in pain at posttreatment and six-month follow-up. Similarly, Singh et al. (96) reported improvements in sleep, pain, and depression following a treatment that included mindfulness meditation and movement therapy in FM patients. Thieme et al. (97,98) have reported similar results using operant behavioral and cognitive-behavioral approaches. Several clinical recommendations have been made in the literature. Based on a comprehensive literature review, Thieme et al. (99) recommended operant behavioral and cognitive-behavioral approaches to pain management, both of which have been associated with improvements in sleep. Dalton et al. (100) have described a tailored CBT-P for use in cancer pain patients and found that this approach was associated with a reduction in pain-related interference with sleep.

At the same time, a number of studies have detected no improvements in sleep following CBT-P. Among RA patients, two studies have failed to detect any improvement in sleep despite improvements in pain, self-efficacy, movement, and joint involvement (101,102). Whereas findings have been similar in adolescents with FM (103), Redondo et al. (104) employed a CBT-P and failed to find improvement in either pain or sleep in adults with FM. Others have also failed to detect improvement in sleep complaints following CBT-P among FM patients (105). Although CBT-P appears promising for improving sleep in patients with chronic pain, further research is needed before any clear conclusions can be drawn.

Effects of Cognitive-Behavioral Therapy for Insomnia in Chronic Pain Conditions

Although most CBT-I literature has excluded patients with comorbid conditions, a number of investigators have applied cognitive-behavioral models of insomnia to understanding insomnia in patients with chronic pain. Maladaptive coping strategies and compensatory sleep behaviors such as napping, spending excessive time awake in bed, and following an inconsistent sleep–wake schedule are common in patients with pain and may worsen insomnia. At the same time, pain patients are likely to catastrophize, or ruminate on the potential worst-case scenario outcomes of their condition. Similarly, Smith et al. (106) reported increased levels of presleep arousal and attention to bedroom stimuli such as temperature and noise among patients with chronic pain. These thought processes were more robust predictors than pain ratings of sleep complaints. Cognitive therapy techniques designed to manage these catastrophic cognitions may be particularly helpful in treating insomnia associated with chronic pain.

Early case reports of sleep restriction and stimulus control in chronic pain found large improvements in both subjective and objectively measured sleep onset latency and time awake in bed, and these changes were maintained at two- and six-month follow-up (107,108). Although mood improved concurrent with sleep, no changes were detected in subjective pain ratings. In a sample of cancer patients, Cannici et al. (109) found that PMR led to a significant, 90-minute reduction in diary-reported sleep onset latency, an improvement that was maintained at follow-up. Again, no improvements in pain were observed, although baseline pain ratings in this sample were low. A study of mixed diagnosis outpatients demonstrated that CBT-I could be effective even when the primary cause of sleep disturbance was believed to be medical or psychiatric (110). Moderate effect sizes were reportedly observed for improvements in wake time after sleep onset, sleep efficiency, and sleep quality ratings, and these changes were maintained at three-month follow-up (110). Others have reported similar results (111). Among older adults with mixed medical comorbidities including OA, CBT-I is associated with improvements in diary-reported but not actigraphically measured sleep onset latency, sleep efficiency, and sleep quality (112,113). In addition to these studies employing standard cognitive-behavioral treatment for insomnia, other studies have evaluated the impact of adding sleep education to routine medical care. For example, Calhoun and Ford (114) employed a randomized, placebo-controlled design and found that adding cognitive-behavioral instructions for improved sleep was associated with a significant reduction in headache complaints among 43 women with migraine. Further, improvement in headache symptoms was related to the number of changes in sleep behaviors reported. Although changes in sleep parameters were not reported, this study is nonetheless notable for the association of a sleep-focused intervention and reductions in report of chronic pain.

At least two randomized clinical trials have evaluated using CBT-I exclusively in chronic pain conditions. In the first of these, Currie et al. (115) reported improvements in the CBT-I condition relative to wait-list control in both diary and actigraphic measures of sleep latency, wake after sleep onset, sleep efficiency, and sleep quality. As is found in CBT-I for primary insomnia, effect sizes were large (in the range of 0.80), and treatment gains were maintained at three months. Although no significant group differences were observed in total sleep time, the CBT-I group tended to have larger gains that increased during the three-month follow-up period. More recently, Edinger et al. (116) employed an active control group to test the effectiveness of CBT-I in FM patients with chronic insomnia. Relative to the control condition, CBT-I was associated with improvements in diary-based measures of sleep onset latency, sleep efficiency, and total wake time. Actigraphy-measured sleep latency was also significantly improved in CBT-I relative to control. In addition, reductions in night-to-night sleep variability were also observed in the CBT-I group.

Preliminary evidence suggests effectiveness of standard CBT-I for improving sleep in patients with chronically painful conditions, although further research is needed. Several important limitations must also be noted. Only one of the aforementioned studies (116) employed a credible control condition. Thus, it cannot be concluded that observed changes were due to specific treatment elements rather than nonspecific factors such as therapist contact. It is particularly challenging to develop credible placebo control conditions for cognitive-behavioral interventions. Sleep hygiene, often employed as a control condition, has been associated with improvements in insomnia complaints (117), further highlighting the need for new approaches to experimental design in this area.

Relation Between Improved Sleep and Pain Complaints

Although they were not designed to address the issue, the Currie et al. (115) and Edinger et al. (116) studies provide some insight into the effect of improved sleep on pain complaints. For example, Currie et al. (115) reported a nonsignificant trend toward reduced pain complaints in the CBT-I group relative to wait-list at three-month follow-up. This study suggests that reductions in pain associated with improved sleep may be delayed. Although follow-up data were not reported in the Edinger et al. (116) study, it is common for studies evaluating cognitive-behavioral interventions for insomnia and pain, as well as other conditions, to find that treatment effects improve over time. Presumably, patients continue to learn and behavior change becomes more permanent with repeated practice. The issue of improvement over time is particularly important to CBT-I, as sleep restriction and stimulus control reduce total sleep time during the acute treatment phase before total sleep time is gradually extended. In the Currie et al. study, total sleep time had increased an additional duration of 24 minutes at three-month follow-up, concurrent with the nearly significant reduction in pain. This result raises the possibility that noticeable analgesic effects may require increases in consolidated sleep time. However, participants in the sleep hygiene condition of the Edinger et al. (116) study reported significantly reduced pain even by posttreatment, while those in the CBT-I condition did not. Posthoc analyses of this data revealed that a subset of patients in the sleep hygiene group actually restricted their sleep opportunity. These individuals reported reduced time in bed and total wake time, and also showed significant reductions in pain. In summary, although much remains to be learned, two studies suggest that improving sleep might reduce clinical pain, although these effects may require time for sleep consolidation to occur. Aggressively treating insomnia associated with chronic pain conditions clearly has the potential to improve sleep, pain, mood, and quality of life.

CLINICAL RECOMMENDATIONS

In clinical practice, a majority of patients suffering from chronic pain will report numerous overlapping symptoms including difficulty sleeping and psychological distress. Due to the numerous reciprocal relationships among these symptoms, their casual interactions are difficult to disentangle. Clinicians treating patients with chronic pain conditions will find themselves facing chicken-or-egg dilemmas in diagnosis: Are the patients having trouble sleeping because they are in pain, or do they are in pain because they are hardly sleeping? These relationships are likely to be dynamic and may change within the patients, requiring frequent re-evaluation for the treatment plan. It is strongly recommended that clinicians working with patients with chronic pain conditions adopt a biopsychosocial perspective for assessment and conceptualization. Treatment will frequently require flexibility on the part of the clinician, and providers will often be asked to employ a balanced treatment approach that addresses multiple complaints simultaneously. A multidisciplinary approach is highly desirable if not essential. Finally, because enhancing motivation is such an important component of many treatment approaches, an empathetic, patient-centered approach to maximize treatment outcomes is often most productive, as many chronic pain patients have experienced multiple frustrations in their search for pain relief.

When chronic pain patients seek care for their sleep disturbance, several areas must be addressed as part of a thorough biopsychosocial assessment (118,119). We review the primary categories below. In addition, medical records including current medications and previous sleep study results should be requested and reviewed.

- *Sleep disturbance.* In addition to thoroughly assessing insomnia complaints, the diagnostic priority should be to discern sleepiness from fatigue and whether referral for an overnight sleep study is warranted. Sleep disorders other than insomnia (e.g., sleep disordered breathing, restless legs) will require additional evaluation and treatment. Of note, actigraphy has recently been validated as a measure of sleep in patients with TMD and may be a useful adjunct in patients with chronic pain conditions (123).
- *Mood states and psychiatric distress.* Psychological distress is likely to impair patients' ability and motivation to care for themselves, undermining the self-efficacy that patients need to engage in routine self-care. Numerous validated screening instruments exist for the most common psychiatric disorders, including depression and anxiety, and clinicians should also inquire about suicidal ideation/behavior, which is not only elevated in chronic pain populations (120), but has also been linked to insomnia in chronic pain patients (121).
- *Cognitive processes and thought content.* Many patients with chronic pain report increased somatic focus and engage in catastrophic thinking, which predicts poorer functional outcomes. Clinicians should seek to understand these thought processes, which can be effectively addressed using cognitive restructuring, and patient attitudes that can similarly be explored and modified in treatment. For example, many pain patients perceive that exercise will exacerbate their pain experience. In reality, gradually building toward consistent moderate exercise is among the most reliable treatments associated with improvements in physical function and improved mood among chronic pain patients. Patient beliefs about the relations between their pain and sleep disturbance can also guide treatment planning. Treatment acceptability and readiness to change are other important areas for assessment.

- *Social function.* Understanding a patient's social support network is necessary to encourage their increased social interaction. Chronic pain patients are likely to experience depression and negative affect, and as a result many patients disengage from once-pleasurable activities. In addition to helping patients stay engaged, increasing social activity can be a good way to facilitate physical (e.g., exercise class) as well as intellectual activity among patients (e.g., playing bridge, book club).
- *Coping.* Because the strategies patients use to cope with pain can also have a detrimental impact on sleep (e.g., decreasing physical activity, staying in bed all day, etc.), it is important for clinicians to understand what patients do when they are in pain. This discussion often creates an excellent opportunity to discuss with the patient the relation between their sleep disturbance and pain, and to collaboratively decide on a treatment approach and objectives.

In terms of conceptualization and treatment, the blend of shared symptoms between sleep disturbance and chronic pain can make it difficult to determine which conditions to treat first. Providers should weigh and discuss with the patient the above factors as well as the patient's readiness to change and engage in potentially demanding cognitive-behavioral treatments. Clinical experience suggests that treatments that incorporate principles of motivational interviewing (122) are likely to be among the most effective at treating patients with chronic conditions. In addition, all treatments begin with comprehensive psychoeducation regarding the etiology and overlap between distinct but co-occurring disorders and symptoms.

CONCLUSIONS AND FUTURE DIRECTIONS

Sleep disturbances, particularly insomnia, are ubiquitous in patients suffering from most types of chronic pain. Although more research is needed, the available data indicate that the sleep–pain relationship is best described as reciprocal. Thus, aggressive evaluation and treatment of sleep disturbance in chronic pain is recommended. While some data suggest that interventions designed to treat pain may have some impact on pain-related sleep disturbance, the findings are mixed. Conversely, although additional data are needed, pharmacologic and behavioral interventions developed for primary insomnia improve sleep in chronic pain disorders. It is unclear whether improvements in sleep will translate into improvements in pain. Future research aimed at developing hybrid treatments that simultaneously maximize analgesia and improve sleep is needed, as are studies with sufficiently long follow-up periods and sample sizes necessary to determine how improving sleep in chronic pain might impact both pain and psychological symptoms.

REFERENCES

1. International Association for the Study of Pain. Pain terms: a list with definitions and notes on usage. Pain 1982; 14:205.
2. Gatchel RJ, Peng YB, Peters ML, et al. The biopsychosocial approach to chronic pain: scientific advances and future directions. Psychol Bull 2007; 133(4):581–624.
3. Basbaum AI, Fields HL. Endogenous pain control systems: brainstem spinal pathways and endorphin circuitry. Annu Rev Neurosci 1984; 7:309–338.
4. Edwards RR. Individual differences in endogenous pain modulation as a risk factor for chronic pain. Neurology 2005; 65(3):437–443.
5. Melzack R. Pain and the neuromatrix in the brain. J Dent Educ 2001; 65(12):1378–1382.
6. Diatchenko L, Slade GD, Nackley AG, et al. Genetic basis for individual variations in pain perception and the development of a chronic pain condition. Hum Mol Genet 2005; 14(1):135–143.
7. Gureje O, Von KM, Kola L, et al. The relation between multiple pains and mental disorders: results from the World Mental Health Surveys. Pain 2008; 135(1–2):82–91.
8. Smith MT, Huang MI, Manber R. Cognitive behavior therapy for chronic insomnia occurring within the context of medical and psychiatric disorders. Clin Psychol Rev 2005; 25(5):559–592.
9. Smith MT, Klick B, Kozachik S, et al. Sleep onset insomnia symptoms during hospitalization for major burn injury predict chronic pain. Pain 2008; 138(3):497–506.
10. von Korff M, Le Resche L, Dworkin SF. First onset of common pain symptoms: a prospective study of depression as a risk factor. Pain 1993; 55(2):251–258.
11. Smith MT, Haythornthwaite JA. How do sleep disturbance and chronic pain inter-relate? Insights from the longitudinal and cognitive-behavioral clinical trials literature. Sleep Med Rev 2004; 8(2):119–132.

12. Gold AR, Dipalo F, Gold MS, Broderick J. Inspiratory airflow dynamics during sleep in women with fibromyalgia. Sleep 2004; 27(3):459–466.
13. Bair MJ, Robinson RL, Katon W, et al. Depression and pain comorbidity: a literature review. Arch Intern Med 2003; 163(20):2433–2445.
14. Copperman NR, Mullin FJ, Kleitman N. Further observations on the effects of prolonged sleeplessness. Am J Physiol 1934; 107:589–594.
15. Moldofsky H, Scarisbrick P, England R, et al. Musculoskeletal symptoms and non-REM sleep disturbance in patients with "fibrositis syndrome" and healthy subjects. Psychosom Med 1975; 37:341–351.
16. Moldofsky H, Scarisbrick P. Induction of neurasthenic musculoskeletal pain syndrome by selective sleep stage deprivation. Psychosom Med 1976; 38(1):35–44.
17. Older SA, Battafarano DF, Danning CL, et al. The effects of delta wave sleep interruption on pain thresholds and fibromyalgia-like symptoms in healthy subjects; correlations with insulin-like growth factor I. J Rheumatol 1998; 25(6):1180–1186.
18. Lautenbacher S, Kundermann B, Krieg JC. Sleep deprivation and pain perception. Sleep Med Rev 2006; 10(5):357–369.
19. Onen SH, Alloui A, Gross A, et al. The effects of total sleep deprivation, selective sleep interruption and sleep recovery on pain tolerance thresholds in healthy subjects. J Sleep Res 2001; 10(1):35–42.
20. Lentz MJ, Landis CA, Rothermel J, et al. Effects of selective slow wave sleep disruption on musculoskeletal pain and fatigue in middle aged women. J Rheumatol 1999; 26(7):1586–1592.
21. Roehrs T, Hyde M, Blaisdell B, et al. Sleep loss and REM sleep loss are hyperalgesic. Sleep 2006; 29(2):145–151.
22. Smith MT, Edwards RR, McCann UD, et al. The effects of sleep deprivation on pain inhibition and spontaneous pain in women. Sleep 2007; 30(4):494–505.
23. Lavigne G, Zucconi M, Castronovo C,et al. Sleep arousal response to experimental thermal stimulation during sleep in human subjects free of pain and sleep problems. Pain 2000; 84(2–3):283–290.
24. Drewes AM, Nielsen KD, Arendt-Nielsen L, et al. The effect of cutaneous and deep pain on the electroencephalogram during sleep—an experimental study. Sleep 1997; 20(8):632–640.
25. Sandrini G, Milanov I, Rossi B, et al. Effects of sleep on spinal nociceptive reflexes in humans. Sleep 2001; 24(1):13–17.
26. Lavigne GJ, Zucconi M, Castronovo V, et al. Heart rate changes during sleep in response to experimental thermal (nociceptive) stimulations in healthy subjects. Clin Neurophysiol 2001; 112(3):532–535.
27. Bentley AJ, Newton S, Zio CD. Sensitivity of sleep stages to painful thermal stimuli. J Sleep Res 2003; 12(2):143–147.
28. Lavigne G, Brousseau M, Kato T, et al. Experimental pain perception remains equally active over all sleep stages. Pain 2004; 110(3):646–655.
29. Affleck G, Urrows S, Tennen H, et al. Sequential daily relations of sleep, pain intensity, and attention to pain among women with fibromyalgia. Pain 1996; 68:363–368.
30. Drewes AM, Nielsen KD, Hansen B, et al. A longitudinal study of clinical symptoms and sleep parameters in rheumatoid arthritis. Rheumatology (Oxford) 2000; 39(11):1287–1289.
31. Raymond I, Nielsen TA, Lavigne G, et al. Quality of sleep and its daily relationship to pain intensity in hospitalized adult burn patients. Pain 2001; 92(3):381–388.
32. Stone AA, Broderick JE, Porter LS, et al. The experience of rheumatoid arthritis pain and fatigue: examining momentary reports and correlates over one week. Arthritis Care Res 1997; 10(3):185–193.
33. Shaw IR, Lavigne G, Mayer P, et al. Acute intravenous administration of morphine perturbs sleep architecture in healthy pain-free young adults: a preliminary study. Sleep 2005; 28(6):677–682.
34. Raymond I, Ancoli-Israel S, Choiniere M. Sleep disturbances, pain and analgesia in adults hospitalized for burn injuries. Sleep Med 2004; 5(6):551–559.
35. Mikkelsson M, Sourander A, Salminen JJ, et al. Widespread pain and neck pain in schoolchildren. A prospective one-year follow-up study. Acta Paediatr 1999; 88(10):1119–1124.
36. Edwards RR, Almeida DM, Klick B, et al. Duration of sleep contributes to next-day pain report in the general population. Pain 2008; 137(1):202–206.
37. Leigh TJ, Bird HA, Hindmarch I, et al. A comparison of sleep in rheumatic and non-rheumatic patients. Clin Exp Rheumatol 1987; 5(4):363–365.
38. Wilcox S, Brenes GA, Levine D, et al. Factors related to sleep disturbance in older adults experiencing knee pain or knee pain with radiographic evidence of knee osteoarthritis. J Am Geriatr Soc 2000; 48(10):1241–1251.
39. Gallup Organization. Adult Public's Experiences with Nighttime Pain. Washington, DC: National Sleep Foundation, 1997.
40. Davis GC. Improved sleep may reduce arthritis pain. Holist Nurs Pract 2003; 17(3):128–135.
41. Gallup Organization. Sleep and Aging. Washington, DC: National Sleep Foundation, 1996.

42. Ohayon MM. Relationship between chronic painful physical condition and insomnia. J Psychiatr Res 2005; 39(2):151–159.
43. McMillan SC, Tofthagen C, Morgan MA. Relationships among pain, sleep disturbances, and depressive symptoms in outpatients from a comprehensive cancer center. Oncol Nurs Forum 2008; 35(4):603–611.
44. Drewes AM, Svendsen L, Taagholt SJ, et al. Sleep in rheumatoid arthritis: a comparison with healthy subjects and studies of sleep/wake interactions. Br J Rheumatol 1998; 37(1):71–81.
45. Hirsch M, Carlander B, Verge M, et al. Objective and subjective sleep disturbances in patients with rheumatoid arthritis. Arthritis Rheum 1994; 37(1):41–49.
46. Moldofsky H, Lue FA, Smythe HA. Alpha EEG sleep and morning symptoms in rheumatoid arthritis. J Rheumatol 1983; 10(3):373–379.
47. Lavie P, Epstein R, Tzischinsky O, et al. Actigraphic measurements of sleep in rheumatoid arthritis: comparison of patients with low back pain and healthy controls. J Rheumatol 1992; 19(3):362–365.
48. Mahowald MW, Mahowald ML, Bundlie SR, et al. Sleep fragmentation in rheumatoid arthritis. Arthritis Rheum 1989; 32(8):974–983.
49. Crosby LJ. Factors which contribute to fatigue associated with rheumatoid arthritis. J Adv Nurs 1991; 16(8):974–981.
50. Lavie P, Nahir M, Lorber M, et al. Nonsteroidal antiinflammatory drug therapy in rheumatoid arthritis patients. Lack of association between clinical improvement and effects on sleep. Arthritis Rheum 1991; 34(6):655–659.
51. Prado GF, Allen RP, Trevisani VM, et al. Sleep disruption in systemic sclerosis (scleroderma) patients: clinical and polysomnographic findings. Sleep Med 2002; 3(4):341–345.
52. Turner GA, Lower EE, Corser BC, et al. Sleep apnea in sarcoidosis. Sarcoidosis Vasc Diffuse Lung Dis 1997; 14(1):61–64.
53. Verbraecken J, Hoitsma E, van der Grinten CP, et al. Sleep disturbances associated with periodic leg movements in chronic sarcoidosis. Sarcoidosis Vasc Diffuse Lung Dis 2004; 21(2):137–146.
54. Haack M, Sanchez E, Mullington JM. Elevated inflammatory markers in response to prolonged sleep restriction are associated with increased pain experience in healthy volunteers. Sleep 2007; 30(9):1145–1152.
55. Management of temporomandibular joint disorders. National Institutes of Health Technology Assessment Conference Statement. J Am Dent Assoc 1996; 127(11):1595–1606.
56. Diatchenko L, Nackley AG, Slade GD, et al. Idiopathic pain disorders—pathways of vulnerability. Pain 2006; 123(3):226–230.
57. Yunus MB. Fibromyalgia and overlapping disorders: the unifying concept of central sensitivity syndromes. Semin Arthritis Rheum 2007; 36(6):339–356.
58. Aaron LA, Burke MM, Buchwald D. Overlapping conditions among patients with chronic fatigue syndrome, fibromyalgia, and temporomandibular disorder. Arch Intern Med 2000; 160(2):221–227.
59. Hudson JI, Goldenberg DL, Pope HG Jr.,et al. Comorbidity of fibromyalgia with medical and psychiatric disorders. Am J Med 1992; 92(4):363–367.
60. Moldofsky H. Sleep and fibrositis syndrome. Rheum Dis Clin North Am 1989; 15(1):91–103.
61. Horne J, Shackell B. Alpha-like EEG activity in non-REM sleep and the fibromyalgia (fibrositis) syndrome. Electroencephalogr Clin Neurophysiol 1991; 79:271–276.
62. Branco J, Atalaia A, Paiva T. Sleep cycles and alpha-delta sleep in fibromyalgia syndrome. J Rheumatol 1994; 21(6):1113–1117.
63. Jennum P, Drewes AM, Andreasen A, et al. Sleep and other symptoms in primary fibromyalgia and in healthy controls. J Rheumatol 1993; 20(10):1756–1759.
64. Drewes AM. Pain and sleep disturbances with special reference to fibromyalgia and rheumatoid arthritis. Rheumatology (Oxford) 1999; 38(11):1035–1038.
65. Shaver JL, Lentz M, Landis CA, et al. Sleep, psychological distress, and stress arousal in women with fibromyalgia. Res Nurs Health 1997; 20(3):247–257.
66. Delgado JA, Murali G, Goldberg R. Sleep disorders in fibromyalgia. Sleep 2004; 27:A339.
67. Khan SA, Goldberg R, Haber A. Sleep disorders in fibromyalgia. Sleep 2005; 28:A290.
68. Roizenblatt S, Moldofsky H, Benedito-Silva AA, et al. Alpha sleep characteristics in fibromyalgia. Arthritis Rheum 2001; 44(1):222–230.
69a. Wickwire EM, Kronfli T, Bellinger K, et al. The relations between objective sleep data, sleep disorders, and signs and symptoms of Temporomandibular Joint Disorder (TMD). Journal of Pain 2008; 9(Suppl 2):P14.
69b. Smith MT, Wickwire EM, Grace EG, et al. Sleep disorders and their association with laboratory pain sensitivity in temporomandibular joint disorder. Sleep 2009; 32(6):779–790.

70. Edwards RR, Grace E, Peterson S, et al. Sleep continuity and architecture associations with pain-inhibitory processes in patients with temporomandibular joint disorder. Eur J Pain 2009; 13(10):1043–1047.
71. Bradley LA, McKendree-Smith NL. Central nervous system mechanisms of pain in fibromyalgia and other musculoskeletal disorders: behavioral and psychologic treatment approaches. Curr Opin Rheumatol 2002; 14(1):45–51.
72. Rains JC, Poceta JS, Penzien DB. Sleep and headaches. Curr Neurol Neurosci Rep 2008; 8(2):167–175.
73. Rains JC, Poceta JS. Headache and sleep disorders: review and clinical implications for headache management. Headache 2006; 46(9):1344–1363.
74. Boardman HF, Thomas E, Millson DS, Croft PR. Psychological, sleep, lifestyle, and comorbid associations with headache. Headache 2005; 45(6):657–669.
75. Ohayon MM. Prevalence and risk factors of morning headaches in the general population. Arch Intern Med 2004; 164(1):97–102.
76. Rasmussen BK. Migraine and tension-type headache in a general population: precipitating factors, female hormones, sleep pattern and relation to lifestyle. Pain 1993; 53(1):65–72.
77. Lyngberg AC, Rasmussen BK, Jorgensen T, et al. Incidence of primary headache: a Danish epidemiologic follow-up study. Am J Epidemiol 2005; 161(11):1066–1073.
78. Jennum P, Jensen R. Sleep and headache. Sleep Med Rev 2002; 6(6):471–479.
79. Argoff CE. The coexistence of neuropathic pain, sleep, and psychiatric disorders: a novel treatment approach. Clin J Pain 2007; 23(1):15–22.
80. Zelman DC, Brandenburg NA, Gore M. Sleep impairment in patients with painful diabetic peripheral neuropathy. Clin J Pain 2006; 22(8):681–685.
81. Mainous AG III, Baker R, Koopman RJ, et al. Impact of the population at risk of diabetes on projections of diabetes burden in the United States: an epidemic on the way. Diabetologia 2007; 50(5): 934–940.
82. Drewes AM, Andreasen A, Jennum P, et al. Zopiclone in the treatment of sleep abnormalities in fibromyalgia. Scand J Rheumatol 1991; 20(4):288–293.
83. Moldofsky H, Lue FA, Mously C, et al. The effect of zolpidem in patients with fibromyalgia: a dose ranging, double blind, placebo controlled, modified crossover study. J Rheumatol 1996; 23(3): 529–533.
84. Arnold LM, Keck PE Jr, Welge JA. Antidepressant treatment of fibromyalgia. A meta-analysis and review. Psychosomatics 2000; 41(2):104–113.
85. O'Malley PG, Balden E, Tomkins G, et al. Treatment of fibromyalgia with antidepressants: a meta-analysis. J Gen Intern Med 2000; 15(9):659–666.
86. Fishbain DA, Hall J, Meyers AL, et al. Does pain mediate the pain interference with sleep problem in chronic pain? Findings from studies for management of diabetic peripheral neuropathic pain with duloxetine. J Pain Symptom Manage 2008; 36(6):639–647.
87. Gordh TE, Stubhaug A, Jensen TS, et al. Gabapentin in traumatic nerve injury pain: a randomized, double-blind, placebo-controlled, cross-over, multi-center study. Pain 2008; 138(2):255–266.
88. Tölle T, Freynhagen R, Versavel M, et al. Pregabalin for relief of neuropathic pain associated with diabetic neuropathy: a randomized, double-blind study. Eur J Pain 2008; 12(2):203–213.
89. Arnold LM, Russell IJ, Diri EW, et al. A 14-week, randomized, double-blinded, placebo-controlled monotherapy trial of pregabalin in patients with fibromyalgia. J Pain 2008; 9(9):792–805.
90. Florete OG, Xiang J, Vorsanger GJ. Effects of extended-release tramadol on pain-related sleep parameters in patients with osteoarthritis. Expert Opin Pharmacother 2008; 9(11):1817–1827.
91. Kivitz A, Ma C, Ahdieh H, et al. A 2-week, multicenter, randomized, double-blind, placebo-controlled, dose-ranging, phase III trial comparing the efficacy of oxymorphone extended release and placebo in adults with pain associated with osteoarthritis of the hip or knee. Clin Ther 2006; 28(3):352–364.
92. Astin JA, Beckner W, Soeken K, et al. Psychological interventions for rheumatoid arthritis: a meta-analysis of randomized controlled trials. Arthritis Rheum 2002; 47(3):291–302.
93. Morley S, Eccleston C, Williams A. Systematic review and meta-analysis of randomized controlled trials of cognitive behaviour therapy and behaviour therapy for chronic pain in adults, excluding headache. Pain 1999; 80(1–2):1–13.
94. Wilson KG, Eriksson MY, D'Eon JL, et al. Major depression and insomnia in chronic pain. Clin J Pain 2002; 18(2):77–83.
95. Basler HD, Rehfisch HP. Cognitive-behavioral therapy in patients with ankylosing spondylitis in a German self-help organization. J Psychosom Res 1991; 35(2–3):345–354.
96. Singh BB, Berman BM, Hadhazy VA, et al. A pilot study of cognitive behavioral therapy in fibromyalgia. Altern Ther Health Med 1998; 4(2):67–70.
97. Thieme K, Gromnica-Ihle E, Flor H. Operant behavioral treatment of fibromyalgia: a controlled study. Arthritis Rheum 2003; 49(3):314–320.

98. Thieme K, Flor H, Turk DC. Psychological pain treatment in fibromyalgia syndrome: efficacy of operant behavioural and cognitive behavioural treatments. Arthritis Res Ther 2006; 8(4):R121.
99. Thieme K, Hauser W, Batra A, et al. Psychotherapy in patients with fibromyalgia syndrome. Schmerz 2008; 22(3):295–302.
100. Dalton JA, Keefe FJ, Carlson J, et al. Tailoring cognitive-behavioral treatment for cancer pain. Pain Manag Nurs 2004; 5(1):3–18.
101. Appelbaum K, Blanchard E, Hickling E, et al. Cognitive behavioral treatment of a veteran population with moderate to severe rheumatoid arthritis. Behav Ther 1988; 19:489–502.
102. O'Leary JF, Mallory TH, Kraus TJ, et al. Mittelmeier ceramic total hip arthroplasty. A retrospective study. J Arthroplasty 1988; 3(1):87–96.
103. Kashikar-Zuck S, Swain NF, Jones BA, et al. Efficacy of cognitive-behavioral intervention for juvenile primary fibromyalgia syndrome. J Rheumatol 2005; 32(8):1594–1602.
104. Redondo JR, Justo CM, Moraleda FV, et al. Long-term efficacy of therapy in patients with fibromyalgia: a physical exercise-based program and a cognitive-behavioral approach. Arthritis Rheum 2004; 51(2):184–192.
105. Wigers SH, Stiles TC, Vogel PA. Effects of aerobic exercise versus stress management treatment in fibromyalgia. A 4.5 year prospective study. Scand J Rheumatol 1996; 25(2):77–86.
106. Smith MT, Perlis ML, Carmody TP, et al. Presleep cognitions in patients with insomnia secondary to chronic pain. J Behav Med 2001; 24(1):93–114.
107. Morin CM, Kowatch RA, Wade JB. Behavioral management of sleep disturbances secondary to chronic pain. J Behav Ther Exp Psychiatry 1989; 20(4):295–302.
108. Morin CM, Kowatch RA, O'Shanick G. Sleep restriction for the inpatient treatment of insomnia. Sleep 1990; 13(2):183–186.
109. Cannici J, Malcolm R, Peek LA. Treatment of insomnia in cancer patients using muscle relaxation training. J Behav Ther Exp Psychiatry 1983; 14(3):251–256.
110. Lichstein KL, Wilson NM, Johnson CT. Psychological treatment of secondary insomnia. Psychol Aging 2000; 15(2):232–240.
111. Perlis ML, Sharpe M, Smith MT, et al. Behavioral treatment of insomnia: treatment outcome and the relevance of medical and psychiatric morbidity. J Behav Med 2001; 24(3):281–296.
112. Rybarczyk B, Lopez M, Benson R, et al. Efficacy of two behavioral treatment programs for comorbid geriatric insomnia. Psychol Aging 2004; 17(2):288–298.
113. Rybarczyk B, Stepanski E, Fogg L, et al. A placebo-controlled test of cognitive-behavioral therapy for comorbid insomnia in older adults. J Consult Clin Psychol 2005; 73(6):1164–1174.
114. Calhoun AH, Ford S. Behavioral sleep modification may revert transformed migraine to episodic migraine. Headache 2007; 47(8):1178–1183.
115. Currie SR, Wilson KG, Pontefract AJ, et al. Cognitive-behavioral treatment of insomnia secondary to chronic pain. J Consult Clin Psychol 2000; 68(3):407–416.
116. Edinger JD, Wohlgemuth WK, Krystal AD, et al. Behavioral insomnia therapy for fibromyalgia patients: a randomized clinical trial. Arch Intern Med 2005; 165(21):2527–2535.
117. Edinger JD, Wohlgemuth WK, Radtke RA, et al. Cognitive behavioral therapy for treatment of chronic primary insomnia: a randomized controlled trial. JAMA 2001; 285(14):1856–1864.
118. Horowitz SH. The diagnostic workup of patients with neuropathic pain. Med Clin North Am 2007; 91(1):21–30.
119. Peat G, Croft P, Hay E. Clinical assessment of the osteoarthritis patient. Best Pract Res Clin Rheumatol 2001; 15(4):527–544.
120. Smith MT, Edwards RR, Robinson RC, et al. Suicidal ideation, plans, and attempts in chronic pain patients: factors associated with increased risk. Pain 2004; 111(1–2):201–208.
121. Smith MT, Perlis ML, Smith MS, et al. Sleep onset disturbance discriminates suicidal ideation in patients with chronic pain. Sleep 2000; 23(suppl #1).
122. Rollnick S, Miller WR, Butler CC, et al. Motivational Interviewing in Health Care: Helping Patients Change Behavior. COPD 2008; 5(3):203.
123. Wickwire EM, Saletin J, Hoehn J, et al. Performance of actigraphy in temporomandibular joint disorder. Sleep 2009; 32(Abstract Suppl):A340.

15 Insomnia Related to Medical and Neurologic Disorders

Brooke G. Judd and Glen P. Greenough

Dartmouth-Hitchcock Medical Center, Lebanon, New Hampshire, U.S.A.

Medical and neurological disorders frequently have a significant impact on sleep, affecting overall well-being and quality of life. Further, the lack of restful or sufficient sleep may exacerbate the underlying disease itself. Numerous investigators have demonstrated increased prevalence of insomnia in subjects with somatic diseases (1–7). Furthermore, a National Sleep Foundation survey found that participants' perception of their sleep quality was highly associated with their number of medical conditions (6). Although prevalence rates are variable, there is consensus that rates of chronic insomnia are higher in clinical populations than in the general population. While numerous disease processes may be associated with insomnia and poor sleep, some medical and neurological disorders have more consistent associations with sleep-related complaints. Chronic pain syndromes are also highly associated with insomnia and sleep disturbance, although this is not included in this chapter as it is discussed more fully in chapter 14.

MEDICAL DISORDERS

Chronic Obstructive Pulmonary Disease

Multiple studies have noted a high frequency of insomnia complaints in patients with chronic obstructive pulmonary disease (COPD) (8–13). In addition to higher frequency of subjective sleep complaints, patients with COPD have been found to have decreased total sleep time, increased arousals, and decreased rapid eye movement (REM) sleep, compared with matched controls without COPD (8,14). The etiology of the sleep architecture abnormalities and subjective complaints is likely multifactorial: Typical daytime symptoms of COPD such as cough, excessive mucus production, and breathlessness may also occur during sleep and cause sleep disruption. The alveolar gas exchange abnormalities associated with COPD are accentuated in sleep, during which time the normal ventilatory responses to hypercapnia and hypoxemia are blunted. During REM sleep, the ventilatory responses are blunted even further. Sleep-related hypoxemia has been postulated as a contributing factor to the poor sleep quality, as one study did correlate arterial oxygen desaturation with sleep fragmentation, particularly during REM sleep (8). It is not clear, however, that oxygen supplementation improves objective or subjective sleep abnormalities (8,15).

Medications used to treat COPD may also contribute to insomnia complaints and poor quality sleep. In particular, theophylline and the inhaled β-agonists have stimulant properties that could affect sleep quality. Alternatively, the inhaled anticholinergic agent, ipratropium bromide, has been shown to improve sleep quality in patients with COPD, perhaps related to improved respiratory status (16).

Patients with COPD may also have coexistent sleep apnea (also known as the overlap syndrome). Patients with overlap syndrome had more severe desaturations during sleep and worse sleep quality than patients with only one of these disorders (17). This too may contribute to sleep disruption in COPD, and treatment of sleep apnea may also help to improve sleep quality in these patients.

Treating insomnia in patients with COPD is similar to treating insomnia in the general population, although with a few additional considerations. First, as noted above, some of the medications used to treat COPD may contribute to sleep disruption and may present obstacles to treatment. It may be possible to alter the timing of the more stimulating medications so that they are less likely to interfere with sleep. Identifying and treating any concurrent sleep apnea is also an important consideration.

Medical treatment of insomnia in patients with COPD is also an option, although again with some special considerations. Benzodiazepines are commonly prescribed for insomnia, although they may pose additional risk in patients with COPD. A large number of studies (18) have reviewed the effects of the benzodiazepines on respiratory function in both normal individuals as well as those with COPD, with variable results. Most, though not all, studies demonstrated detrimental effects on a variety of respiratory parameters in patients with and without lung disease. Studies have been performed with the non-benzodiazepine benzodiazepine receptor agonist (BzRA) zolpidem (19–21), suggesting that there is not a significant impairment in respiratory parameters when administered to patients with COPD, although studies are limited in number and results must be interpreted cautiously. It remains reasonable to recommend that these medications may be used with caution in patients with underlying respiratory abnormalities, although the non-benzodiazepine BzRAs may be a better choice than standard benzodiazepines in this population. Recent studies have demonstrated the safety of ramelteon in patients with mild to moderate as well as severe COPD (22,23), although there is little information on the use of other designated sedative hypnotics in this specific group of patients.

Diabetes Mellitus

Sleep disturbances are common among individuals with diabetes due to a number of factors. There is a strong association between impaired glucose tolerance, insulin resistance, obesity, and sleep disordered breathing (24,25), increasing the likelihood of insomnia complaints related to nocturnal respiratory disturbances. Beyond this, however, are other factors that lead to increased insomnia complaints in diabetics and higher rates of hypnotic use (6,26,27).

Rapid changes in glucose levels during sleep have been postulated to cause awakenings in type 1 diabetics (28). Poor sleep in type 2 diabetics has been associated with poor glycemic control, with an inverse correlation between hemoglobin A1C and sleep efficiency (29). Thus, maintaining more constant levels of glucose control may help improve sleep quality in diabetic individuals.

Leg discomfort may also contribute to disrupted sleep in diabetics. Individuals with diabetes have not been found to have an increased risk for developing restless legs syndrome (26,30). Diabetic peripheral neuropathy with associated pain and paresthesias can lead to disturbed sleep (27,31) and treatments aimed at alleviating these symptoms may be helpful in improving sleep.

Chronic Kidney Disease

Chronic kidney disease (CKD) is associated with a high prevalence of disorders of sleep and wakefulness with estimates that range anywhere from 40% to 80%, depending on the assessment method and the type of population studied (32). There are numerous factors that can contribute to sleep–wake disturbances in this patient population, including biochemical and pathophysiological mechanisms, psychological problems, lifestyle, and treatment-related factors. Dialysis status and the role of uremia-related factors may play a role in poor sleep. A number of studies have attempted to correlate insomnia symptoms with numerous abnormal biochemical markers in CKD including altered melatonin levels, although there have been no consistent findings (33–35). One study (36) compared sleep disturbance complaints (including insomnia) with timing of dialysis (morning, afternoon or evening), finding no difference in sleep complaints with a dialysis shift. There has been evidence that insomnia complaints improve (though not resolve) after kidney transplantation (37,38), although it is not clear if this is due to improvements in biochemical markers or the other numerous factors that may contribute to insomnia in chronic illness.

Restless legs syndrome (RLS) is elevated in CKD and may contribute to insomnia complaints. A study that evaluated the association of RLS, insomnia, and quality of life in postrenal transplant patients (39) found that patients with RLS were three times more likely to have insomnia than those without RLS (29% vs. 9%). Patients with CKD also appear to be at an elevated risk for sleep apnea syndromes (40,41), and may be less likely to present with classic signs or symptoms such as elevated body mass index or snoring (42,43). The clinician therefore needs to be aware of the increased risk of comorbid sleep disorders, ask appropriate questions when obtaining a history, and consider polysomnography even if the patient does not report typical symptoms of sleep disordered breathing, as an occult respiratory or motor disorder may be contributing to insomnia symptoms.

Treatment of insomnia related to CKD is complex, given the multiple factors that may contribute to the symptoms. Further, extra care and caution has to be exercised when treating insomnia in this group of patients, given the potential altered metabolism of medications and potential interactions with the numerous medications often used in this population. Surprisingly little work has been done evaluating the use of sedative hypnotics in patients with CKD, despite their high prevalence of insomnia complaints. One analysis identified a 15% higher mortality rate in dialysis patients using benzodiazepines or zolpidem (44), although this did not further discern between the two medication classes or identify specific risks associated with these medications. The non-benzodiazepines, zaleplon, zolpidem, and zopiclone, are increasingly used to treat insomnia in the general population. As their primary mode of metabolism is hepatic and renal function does not contribute significantly to their excretion, these medications may be safer to use in patients with kidney disease. Both zolpidem (45) and zaleplon (46) have been evaluated in clinical studies involving patients with CKD and were found to be safe and effective; however, these were both small studies and sedative hypnotics should be used with caution given the numerous potential confounding factors in this population. Nonpharmacological interventions may also be appropriate and a recent study by Chen et al. (47) did demonstrate improvements in subjective sleep quality in a small group of peritoneal dialysis patients who underwent cognitive-behavioral therapy for insomnia.

Human Immunodeficiency Virus Infection

Sleep disturbances have been recognized as a prominent complaint in patients with human immunodeficiency virus (HIV) infection even in the earliest clinical reports of the disease (48). Multiple factors have been postulated to contribute to disturbed sleep and insomnia, although it remains unclear how much of the disturbance is due to the disease process itself and how much is due to other associated factors such as medications, concurrent illnesses, and the psychological effects of living with chronic illness. Of particular interest in patients with HIV infection as well as cancer patients is the observation that sleep deprivation results in alterations of immune system function (49–51), which may have implications in the recuperative process from infections and other illnesses.

Numerous studies have evaluated polysomnographic data in patients with HIV infection. These are described in detail in a review by Reid and Dwyer (52). While initial studies suggested an increase in slow wave sleep in HIV infection, this has not been confirmed in later studies. In fact, polysomnographic abnormalities have been inconsistent, with variable reports in regards to percentage of sleep stages, including slow wave sleep and REM, as well as spindle density. Thus, it does not appear that there is a definite change in sleep architecture that is associated with HIV infection.

The role of the multiple endogenous substances involved in sleep regulation, including neurotransmitters, hormones, and cytokines, has been evaluated in this population. For example, it is well documented that many changes occur in the hypothalamic-pituitary-adrenal axis in HIV infection (53–55). This subsequently leads to alterations in other substances such as growth hormone and other hormones, as well as multiple cytokines. These alterations may also contribute to sleep disturbance although there is no evidence at this point that targeting a particular chemical derangement will improve sleep.

Medications are another potential contributing factor in HIV-associated insomnia and antiretroviral therapy is often reported to include insomnia as an adverse effect. In general, however, multiple studies have not confirmed a class effect of the retroviral drugs (52). One notable exception is the nonnucleoside reverse transcriptase inhibitor efavirenz, a medication associated with a high number of neuropsychiatric complications. Studies with this medication have more clearly demonstrated an increased risk of sleep disturbance and insomnia complaints (56,57).

The factor most strongly associated with HIV infection and insomnia is underlying psychological morbidity. Given the strong relationship between psychiatric illnesses and insomnia in addition to the high prevalence of depression and anxiety in HIV infection, this association should not be surprising. Stage of illness has not necessarily correlated with insomnia symptoms. Asymptomatic seropositive patients with depression have been found to have a high likelihood for insomnia in clinical studies (52,58). Conversely, cognitive impairment due to Acquired Immune Deficiency Syndrome-related central nervous system involvement associated with more advanced disease is also highly predictive of insomnia (48).

Treatment of insomnia in this population may thus provide further challenges, given the multiple possible contributors to the sleep symptoms.

Malignancy

Sleep disturbance constitutes a significant source of suffering in patients with cancer, although prevalence rates vary depending on the type of cancer and method of assessing symptoms. Much of the work investigating insomnia and cancer has been with breast cancer patients. In this group, using standardized criteria as defined by Savard and Morin (59) insomnia rates were found to be double that of the general population. As with the general population, sleep disturbances can significantly impact quality of life in cancer patients. Women with metastatic breast cancer rated sleep in the highest quartile of quality of life items (59) and patients undergoing radiation therapy ranked sleep disturbance as one of the 10 most troubling difficulties of their illness (60). However, despite the distress associated with insomnia, many patients do not report the problem to their health care providers, perhaps assuming it is an inevitable aspect of their illness or that nothing can be done for the symptoms. In fact, one study found that almost 85% of cancer patients with sleep disturbance did not discuss the problem with their provider (61). The same study also noted that approximately half of the patients experienced their symptoms on a nightly basis.

Although the nature of the sleep disturbance may be as heterogeneous as the underlying illness, frequent awakenings appear to be the most commonly reported disturbance, described in multiple studies (62–66). In Davidson's survey (66), 52% of patients attributed their insomnia to "intrusive thoughts" and 45% attributed their sleep disturbance to physical discomfort. Although there is limited objective evaluation of sleep in cancer patients, the studies available would generally concur with subjective reports demonstrating decreased sleep efficiency and increased awakenings on polysomnography (67) as well as actigraphy (68,69).

As with many of the other illnesses discussed in this chapter, the etiology of insomnia related to cancer is likely multifactorial. Physical symptoms, psychological distress, and medications may all play a role in the sleep disturbance and may be targets for treatment. Cancer-related fatigue is also a highly prevalent and persistent problem in patients with cancer, as well as cancer survivors. Roscoe et al. (70) provides a detailed description of the interrelationship between fatigue and sleep disturbance in cancer patients. The relationship between the two may be bidirectional. The fatigue may be due at least in part to the poor sleep, although other factors such as cytokines associated with tumors have also been reported as possible contributors to cancer-related fatigue. However, the fatigue may cause patients to extend their sleep opportunity, spending excessive time in bed with subsequent reductions in sleep efficiency and worsening feelings of poor sleep. Thus, measures aimed at improving daytime fatigue may also help with the nocturnal disturbance.

Treatment of insomnia in cancer has typically focused on pharmacologic agents, although there have been a number of studies demonstrating the effectiveness of cognitive-behavioral therapy for insomnia (CBT-I). This is particularly important, given that insomnia symptoms can persist for several years after the end of treatment. More recent studies (71,72) in particular have modified CBT-I to meet the special needs of cancer patients, more specifically using strategies to help cope with fatigue (such as encouraging physical activity) and employing education and cognitive restructuring to address the fatigue.

NEUROLOGICAL DISORDERS

Neurodegenerative Diseases

As the pathophysiology of neurodegenerative diseases becomes better understood there has been a shift in classification. Traditional classification systems were based on clinical symptom complexes. More recently many neurodegenerative diseases can be classified as tauopathies or synucleinopathies based on which protein is dysfunctional. Interestingly this breakdown seems to correlate with sleep symptoms as well. Patients with tauopathies and synucleinopathies may be afflicted with different sleep disorders or complaints. In general, the characteristic sleep disturbance in the tauopathies appears to be insomnia and circadian dysfunction as opposed to REM sleep behavior disorder (RBD) and hypersomnias in the synucleinopathies (73). That being said, insomnia is still a significant problem in Parkinson's disease (PD), the most common synucleinopathy.

Tauopathies

The prototypic tauopathy is Alzheimer's disease (AD). AD is the most common form of dementia. Short-term memory loss, the hallmark of the disease, tends to be progressive. Other areas of impairment include executive dysfunction, language, abstraction, and mood. The classic pathologic findings in this disorder include extracellular plaques of the peptide β-amyloid and intracellular neurofibrillary tangles composed of the protein tau. The most prominent biochemical change is the loss of choline acetyltransferase activity. This enzyme is responsible for the production of acetylcholine in cholinergic neurons.

Patients with AD exhibit abnormal sleep architecture on polysomnography. These changes generally reflect lower quality sleep with a reduction in sleep efficiency and total sleep time and an elevation in stage one sleep along with an increased number of arousals and awakenings (73). The formed elements of sleep, K-complexes, and sleep spindles may also be reduced. Late in the disease, a decrease in REM sleep percentage and a prolongation of the latency to REM sleep develop (73). Cholinesterase inhibitors used to treat dementia have been shown to increase REM sleep in nondemented patients and may have the same effect in AD patients. Reports of vivid dreaming in AD patients on cholinesterase inhibitor support this notion (74). The cholinesterase inhibitor, donepezil, may lead to insomnia whereas this does not appear to be the case with rivastagmine and galantamine (74).

Degeneration of neurons in the suprachiasmatic nucleus and decreased melatonin secretion may lead to circadian rhythm disruption in AD (75). Circadian rhythm abnormalities characteristic of this disorder include daytime sleepiness and nocturnal wakefulness (75). Patients with dementia may develop the irregular sleep–wake type circadian sleep disorder (76). This disorder is characterized by a lack of clearly defined sleep and wake periods with at least three sleep episodes in a 24-hour period. The severity of dementia has been correlated with the severity of the circadian rhythm disturbance (77). Other factors such as medications that lead to confusion, lack of environmental cues (e.g., limited light exposure), other medical conditions (e.g., pain), psychiatric conditions (e.g., depression), and inadequate sleep hygiene (e.g., time spent in bed watching television) may exacerbate or mimic the circadian rhythm disruption. Use of sleep logs and actigraphy can help provide diagnostic clues. This disruption of the circadian pattern of sleep and wake is particularly important, as the majority of caregivers point to nocturnal problems as a factor in their decision to institutionalize elderly relatives (78).

Sleep disordered breathing may lead to an insomnia complaint. An association between AD and obstructive sleep apnea (OSA) has been demonstrated. The APOE4 allele commonly associated with AD has also been associated with OSA (79).

When considering therapies for insomnia in AD patients one must first consider the etiology. Addressing the underlying problem driving the insomnia may then lead to improvement in the symptom of insomnia. For example, a delirium secondary to a medical condition or medication could be the driving force behind the insomnia in an AD patient (74). A primary sleep disorder such as RLS or OSA should be addressed directly if possible before addressing the symptom of insomnia. Assuming these conditions have been met, symptom management of insomnia can be undertaken. Information on the use of sedative hypnotics in AD patients is sparse. There are limited data to suggest that the short acting benzodiazepine, triazolam, and the BzRA, zolpidem, may help with insomnia in AD patients (74). Concerns, however, about adverse events such as unsteadiness, falls, and worsening of cognitive impairment have limited their usage. A meta-analysis of hypnotic use in people aged 60 or over concluded there were small improvements in the sleep quality but an increased risk of adverse events (80). Antipsychotic medications have been used off-label as hypnotics, especially if nocturnal agitation is also present. The safety of these medications for this purpose, however, remains largely unexplored with some evidence to suggest increased cerebrovascular adverse events (81,82), cognitive decline (83), and mortality (84) in patients with dementia. Because of the reduction in melatonin secretion that is greater than expected for age in AD, melatonin supplementation has been attempted as a therapy (85). Studies evaluating melatonin replacement's effect on sleep in elderly and AD patients have been mixed (85). In 2003, a multicenter, randomized, double-blind, placebo-controlled clinical trial suggested no benefit of melatonin up to 10 mg on actigraphically derived measure of sleep in an AD population (86). This may be explained by the observation that the number of melatonin-1 receptor containing neurons in the suprachiasmatic nucleus in patients with AD is reduced (85). The data on the use of ramelteon, a melatonin-1 and 2 receptor agonist, is limited (85). Phototherapy may be helpful in the management of the circadian disruption in patients with AD but the specifics on the timing, duration, and intensity have yet to be determined (75). Some success has been achieved through a combination of environmental and behavioral changes in nursing home residents. Such changes have included increased daytime bright light exposure, avoidance of daytime time in bed, structured bedtime routines, and increased physical activity as well as sleep hygiene education for the caregiver (87,88).

Progressive supranuclear palsy (PSP), another tauopathy, is a disorder characterized by parkinsonism, dystonia, gait disturbance, and a supranuclear gaze palsy (impaired voluntary vertical eye movements initially). Insomnia is common in this disorder and tends to be more severe than the insomnia in AD or PD (89,90). Insomnia in PSP disorder correlates most closely with motor impairment and to a lesser degree with cognitive or eye movement impairment (90,91). Polysomnographic findings demonstrate a reduced sleep efficiency of 58% in one study (90). The etiology of the insomnia complaint may be a direct result of brain stem pathology, immobility, depression, dysphagia, and/or nocturia (90,92). Sleep-related breathing disorders and REM sleep behavior disorder are probably not common in PSP but data are limited (89,90). Besides the reduced sleep efficiency, other polysomnographic findings in PSP include reduced or absent eye movements, poorly formed or absent sleep spindles and K-complexes, and increased alpha activity in stage 1 and 2 sleep (90). Corticobasal degeneration, another tauopathy, has been associated with periodic limb movements and REM sleep behavior disorder in case reports only (89). Little is known about sleep in this rare disorder.

Synucleinopathies

Parkinson's disease is characterized by a resting tremor, bradykinesia, masked fascies, loss of postural reflexes, and an increased incidence of depression. The hallmark pathologic finding is loss of dopaminergic neurons in the substantia nigra in the brainstem. Sleep complaints and problems are multiple in this disorder and are more common with more severe disease (93). The frequency of reported sleep problems in PD varies among studies from 25% to 98% (93). RBD is seen in one-third of newly diagnosed patients with PD (76). Hypersomnia, whether it is from the disease process itself, the dopaminergic agents used to treat PD or coexistent sleep disorders known to cause excessive sleepiness, is common in PD (94–96). The frequency of the RLS and OSA appears to be elevated in PD as well and may lead to insomnia and/or daytime sleepiness (94).

While the sleep complaints are multiple in patients with PD the two most problematic appear to be sleep maintenance insomnia and nocturia (93). Almost two-thirds of PD patients complain of sleep onset difficulties but almost 90% may complain about sleep maintenance issues (97). Akathisia, dystonia, freezing, tremor, nocturia, muscle cramps, and off period-related urinary incontinence and pain can all play a role in insomnia in PD (94). Some of the medications used to treat PD, such as selegiline or the dopamine agonists, can be alerting and contribute to insomnia. The depression associated with PD may also be associated with insomnia complaints (96).

Polysomnographic findings in patients with PD include decreased sleep efficiency, increased wake after sleep onset, sleep fragmentation, decreased SWS, decreased REM sleep, decreased sleep spindles, and increased EMG activity. Findings consistent with RBD such as REM sleep without atonia may also be present (97). Periodic limb movements consistent with RLS as well as obstructive respiratory events consistent with OSA may also play a role in sleep disruption in PD and have been demonstrated at an increased frequency on polysomnography in this population (94,98).

Treatment of specific sleep disorders, such as OSA, RLS with or without periodic limb movements or RBD, can be undertaken directly and may lead to improved symptom control. Treating the parkinsonian symptoms at night can also be helpful in improving nocturnal mobility among other symptoms. That being said one must be aware that dopaminergic agents, particularly at higher doses, may be arousing (75). Improving sleep quality theoretically may also lead to improvement in mobility and motor function especially in the morning. This is based on the observation that some patients with PD experience improved mobility upon awakening from a night of sleep (99).

Dementia with Lewy Body Disease is a degenerative disorder characterized by parkinsonism, dementia, and hallucinations. The sleep problem most closely associated with this disorder is RBD (76). Multisystem atrophy (MSA) is a disorder characterized by parkinsonism, autonomic dysfunction, and cerebellar signs. MSA is also strongly associated with RBD in that 90% of patients with MSA have RBD (76). MSA patients may also have fragmented sleep on the basis of sleep disordered breathing that may manifest in various forms with nocturnal stridor being the most characteristic (89).

Fatal Familial Insomnia

Fatal familial insomnia (FFI) is a fatal progressive prion disease characterized by sleep onset and maintenance insomnia with lapses from quiet wakefulness into a sleep-like state with dream enactment (76). It is inherited in an autosomal dominant fashion although sporadic cases have been reported. Thalamic hypometabolism is characteristic on PET scans (100). Pathologic findings include reactive gliosis of the anterior and dorsomedial thalamic nuclei and neuronal loss and reactive astrogliosis in the inferior olives (76). Patients homozygous for the defect have a rapid course with a mean 9 to 10 month survival whereas patients heterozygous for the defect have a mean disease duration of 30 months (100). Age of onset is typically in the fifth and sixth decades of life. Early symptoms include apathy and drowsiness. Other characteristic symptoms include dream enactment, dysautonomia (pyrexia, salivation, tachycardia, tachypnea, hyperhydrosis, and dyspnea), and motor symptoms (dysarthria, dysphagia, tremor, myoclonus, and dystonia) (76). Polysomnographic features include reductions in SWS and sleep spindles. Stage one sleep and REM sleep predominate (76). There is no directly effective medical therapy. Treatment is limited to supportive measures.

Cerebrovascular Disease

Strokes have been associated with a number of disorders of sleep and wake. Insomnia complaints, specifically, are common in the poststroke period. Approximately 2/3 of ischemic stroke patients had insomnia early on and that insomnia persisted for at least 18 months in almost half of the patients in one study (101). Damage to specific regions of the brain may lead to an insomnia complaint. Inversion of the sleep–wake cycle with nocturnal agitation and daytime hypersomnolence may occur in association with subcortical, thalamic, thalamomesencephalic, and large tegmental pontine strokes (102). Two patients with locked-in syndromes had prolonged periods of polysomnographically confirmed insomnia lasting over one month. One had a pontomesencephalic stroke and the other had a bilateral basal pontine stroke with extension to the pontine tegmentum (102). Insomnia in the poststroke period may be related to depression. Depression is a well-documented consequence of stroke (103). Just as in nonstroke patients, sleep disordered breathing may lead to an insomnia complaint (102). Inadequate sleep hygiene (i.e., extended periods in bed) secondary to a lack of mobility or independence may lead to insomnia. Other causes of insomnia in the poststroke period include other medical disorders, other sleep disorders, medications, inactivity, and environmental disturbances (104). Directly treating any underlying disorder such as depression or pain that could be leading to insomnia may also lead to improvement in the insomnia. No large-scale trials of therapy for insomnia in stroke populations have been undertaken. If pharmacotherapy is used one must take into account the respiratory suppressant effects as sleep-related breathing disorders are common in poststroke populations (102).

Multiple Sclerosis

Multiple sclerosis (MS) is a disorder characterized by central nervous system demyelination. Difficulty initiating or maintaining sleep is a complaint in approximately 40% of MS patients (105). This insomnia in MS may have multiple possible causes such as pain, nocturia, medications, depression, or classic sleep disorders such as RLS and periodic limb movement disorder (106). Depression may be present in up to 50% of patients with MS and a symptom of that depression may be insomnia (107). Pain is also very common in MS and may take different forms such as neuropathic pain or pain related to muscle spasm. Nocturia or urinary incontinence related to a spastic bladder is also very common in MS and may also disrupt sleep (106). Immunomodulating medications such as interferon and steroids that are commonly used in MS have been associated with insomnia (106). Addressing the underlying etiology of the insomnia is the principal means of treatment in MS.

Traumatic Brain Injury

Traumatic brain injury (TBI) has been associated with a wide spectrum of sleep disorders and complaints both soon after the trauma and chronically. Patients hospitalized after TBI are likely to have insomnia complaints (108). While hypersomnias may be a more common complaint in chronic TBI populations, insomnia still is a frequent complaint (109). Ouellet et al. (110) found that 50% of TBI patients, 7.8 years on average after their trauma, had an insomnia complaint while almost 30% met diagnostic criteria for an insomnia syndrome. There are multiple potential causes for insomnia in chronic TBI including posttraumatic mood disorder, sleep disordered breathing, periodic limb movements, narcolepsy and parasomnias (109) as well as pain from other injuries. Evidence for a posttraumatic circadian rhythm disorder has been mixed (111). Recently, Ayalon et al. (112) have provided evidence of either a delayed sleep phase syndrome or irregular sleep–wake pattern in 36% of mild TBI patients with an insomnia complaint. From a therapeutic standpoint, cognitive-behavioral therapy has been shown efficacious in treating insomnia in TBI. Concerns have been raised about side effects in TBI populations with benzodiazepines. Non-benzodiazepine receptor agonists have fewer complications in non-TBI populations so it has been theorized that this would also be the case in TBI populations (113). There is little data on the subject of pharmacotherapy for insomnia in patients with TBI. Lorazepam and zopiclone had similar effects on insomnia and daytime cognition in a population with stroke or brain injury (114).

CONCLUSION

A wide range of medical and neurologic diseases have been associated with insomnia complaints. The etiology of the insomnia in these conditions varies with the condition and is also often multifactorial. The pathologic process of the disease itself may directly lead to the insomnia complaint as may be the case in AD. Other symptoms or problems attributable to the condition such as pain, impaired respiration or immobility may also lead to insomnia. In chronic diseases in particular, the insomnia may be associated with a coexistent mood disorder, rather than directly with the neurologic or medical disorder. Some of the medications used to treat medical and neurological disorders can also lead to insomnia, such as β-agonist inhalers in COPD. Primary sleep disorders, such as OSA or the RLS, among others, may occur more frequently in patients with certain conditions. These primary sleep disorders may manifest as an insomnia complaint. Therapy for insomnia in medical or neurologic disease is often highly dependent on the etiology of the insomnia.

REFERENCES

1. Mellinger G, Balter M, Uhlenhuth E. Insomnia and its treatment: prevalence and correlates. Arch Gen Psychiatry 1985; 42(3):225–232.
2. Gislason T, Almqvist M. Somatic diseases and sleep complaints. Acta Med Scand 1987; 221(5):475–481.
3. Klink M, Quan S, Kaltenborn W, et al. Risk factors associated with complaints of insomnia in a general adult population. Arch Intern Med 1992; 152(8):1634–1637.
4. Kuppermann M, Lubeck D, Mazonson, P, et al. Sleep problems and their correlates in a working population. J Gen Intern Med 1995; 10(1):25–32.

5. Katz D, McHorney C. Clinical correlates of insomnia in patients with chronic illness. Arch Intern Med 1998; 158(10):1099–1106.
6. Foley D, Ancoli-Israel S, Britz P, et al. Sleep disturbances and chronic disease in older adults: results of the 2003 National Sleep Foundation Sleep in America Survey. J Psychosom Res 2004; 56(5):497–502.
7. Taylor DJ, Mallory LJ, Lichstein KL, et al. Comorbidity of chronic insomnia with medical problems. Sleep 2007; 30(2):213–218.
8. Fleetham J, West P, Mezon B, et al. Sleep, arousals and oxygen desaturation in chronic obstructive pulmonary disease. Am Rev Respir Dis 1982; 126(3):429–433.
9. Klink M, Quan S. Prevalence of reported sleep disturbances in a general adult population and their relationship to obstructive airway diseases. Chest 1987; 91(4):540–546.
10. Saaresranta T, Irjala K, Aittokallio T, et al. Sleep quality, daytime sleepiness and fasting insulin levels in women with chronic obstructive pulmonary disease. Respir Med 2005; 99(7):856–863.
11. George CF, Bayliff CD. Management of insomnia in patients with chronic obstructive pulmonary disease. Drugs 2003; 63(4):379–387.
12. van Manen JG, Bindels PJ, IJzermans CJ, et al. Prevalence of comorbidity in patients with a chronic airway obstruction and controls over the age of 40. J Clin Epidemiol 2001; 54(3):287–293.
13. George CF. Perspectives on the management of insomnia in patients with chronic respiratory disorders. Sleep 2000; 23(suppl 1):S31–S35.
14. Cormick W, Olsen LG, Hensley MJ, et al. Nocturnal hypoxemia and quality of sleep in patients with chronic obstructive lung disease. Thorax 1986; 41(11):846–851.
15. Calverley PM, Brezinova V, Douglas NJ, et al. The effect of oxygenation on sleep quality on chronic bronchitis and emphysema. Am Rev Respir Dis 1982; 126(2):206–210.
16. Martin RJ, Bartelson BLB, Smith P, et al. Effect of ipratropium bromide on oxygen saturation and sleep quality in COPD. Chest 1999; 115(5):1338–1345.
17. Sanders MH, Newman AB, Haggerty CL, et al. Sleep and sleep-disordered breathing in adults with predominantly mild obstructive airway disease. Am J Respir Crit Care Med 2003; 167(1):7–14.
18. Stege G, Vos PJE, van den Elshout FJJ,et al. Sleep, hypnotics and chronic obstructive pulmonary disease. Respir Med 2008; 102(6):801–814.
19. Girault C, Muir JF, Mihaltan F, et al. Effect of repeated administration of zolpidem on sleep, diurnal and nocturnal respiratory function, vigilance, and physical performance in patients with COPD. Chest 1996; 110(5):1203–1211.
20. Steens RD, Pouliot Z, Millar TW, et al. Effect of zolpidem and triazolam on sleep and respiration in mild to moderate chronic obstructive pulmonary disease. Sleep 1993; 16(4):318–326.
21. Murciano D, Armengaud MH, Cramer PH, et al. Acute effects of zolpidem (Z), triazolam (T), and flunitrazepam (F) on arterial blood gasses and control of breathing in severe COPD. Eur Respir J 1993; 6(5):625–629.
22. Kryger M, Roth T, Wang-Weigand S, et al. The effects of ramelteon on respiration during sleep in subjects with moderate to severe chronic obstructive pulmonary disease. Sleep Breath 2009; 13(1): 79–84.
23. Kryger M, Wang-Weigand S, Zhang J, et al. Effect of ramelteon, a selective MT(1)/MT(2) -receptor agonist on respiration during sleep in mild to moderate COPD. Sleep Breath 2008; 12(3): 243–250.
24. Punjabi NM, Shahar E, Redline S, et al. Sleep disordered breathing, glucose intolerance, and insulin resistance: the Sleep Heart Health Study. Am J Epidemiol 2004; 160(6):521–530.
25. Seicean S, Kirchner HL, Gottlieb DJ, et al. Sleep-disordered breathing and impaired glucose metabolism in normal-weight and overweight/obese individuals: the Sleep Heart Health Study. Diabetes Care 2008; 31(5):1001–1006.
26. Skomro RP, Ludwig S, Salamon E, et al. Sleep complaints and restless leg syndrome in adult type 2 diabetics. Sleep Med 2001; 2(5):417–422.
27. Sridhar GR, Madhu K. Prevalence of sleep disturbances in diabetes mellitus. Diabetes Res Clin Pract 1994; 23(3):183–186.
28. Pillar G, Schuscheim G, Weiss R, et al. Interactions between hypoglycemia and sleep architecture in children with type 1 diabetes mellitus. J Pediatr 2003; 142(2):163–168.
29. Trento M, Broglio F, Riganti F, et al. Sleep abnormalities in type 2 diabetes may be associated with glycemic control. Acta Diabetol 2008; 45(4):225–229.
30. Garcia-Borreguero D, Egatz R, Winkelmann J, et al. Epidemiology of restless legs syndrome: the current status. Sleep Med Rev 2006; 10(3):153–167.
31. Schmader KE. Epidemiology and impact of quality of life of postherpetic neuralgia and painful diabetic neuropathy. Clin J Pain 2002; 18(6):350–354.
32. Gusbeth-Tatomir P, Boisteanu D, Seica A, et al. Sleep disorders: a systematic review of an emerging major clinical issue in renal patients. Int Urol Nephrol 2007; 39:1217–1226.

33. Iliescu EA, Yeates KE, Holland DC. Quality of sleep in patients with chronic kidney disease. Nephrol Dial Transplant 2004; 19(1):95–99.
34. De Santo RM, Bartiromo M, Cesare CM, et al. Sleep disorders occur very early in chronic kidney disease. J Nephrol 2008; 21(suppl 13):S59–S65.
35. Merlino G, Gigli GL, Valente M. Sleep disturbances in dialysis patients. J Nephrol 2008; 21(suppl 13):S66–S70.
36. Bastos JPC, de Sousa RB, Nepumuceno LA, et al. Sleep disturbances in patients on maintenance hemodialysis: role of dialysis shift. Rev Assoc Med Bras 2007; 53(6):492–496.
37. Novak M, Molnar MZ, Ambrus C, et al. Chronic insomnia in kidney transplant recipients. Am J Kidney Dis 2006; 47(4):655–665.
38. Sabbatini M, Pisani A, Crispo A, et al. Renal transplantation and sleep: a new life is not enough. J Nephrol 2008; 21(suppl 13):S97–S101.
39. Molnar MZ, Novak M, Szeifert L, et al. Restless legs syndrome, insomnia and quality of life after renal transplantation. J Psychosom Res 2007; 63(6):591–597.
40. Kraus MA, Hamburger RJ. Sleep apnea in renal failure. Adv Perit Dial 1997; 13:88–92.
41. Zoccali C, Mallamaci F, Tripepi G, et al. Autonomic neuropathy is linked to nocturnal hypoxaemia and to concentric hypertrophy and remodeling in dialysis patients. Nephrol Dial Transplant 2001; 16(1):70–77.
42. Jean G, Piperno D, Francois B, et al. Sleep apnea incidence in maintenance hemodialysis patients: influence of dialysate buffer. Nephron 1995; 71(2):138–142.
43. Parker KP, Bliwise DL. Clinical comparison of hemodialysis and sleep apnea patients with excessive daytime sleepiness. ANNA J 1997; 24(6):663–665.
44. Winkelmayer WC, Mehta J, Wang PS. Benzodiazepine use and mortality of incident dialysis patients in the United States. Kidney Int 2007; 72(11):1388–1393.
45. Fillastre JP, Geffroy-Josse S, Etienne I, et al. Pharmacokinetics and pharmacodynamics of zolpidem following repeated doses in hemodialyzed uraemic patients. Fundam Clin Pharmacol 1993; 7(1):1–9.
46. Sabbatini M, Crispo A, Pisani A, et al. Zaleplon improves sleep quality in maintenance hemodialysis patients. Nephron Clin Pract 2003; 94(4):c99–c103.
47. Chen H, Chiang C, Wang H, et al. Cognitive behavioral therapy for sleep disturbance in patients undergoing peritoneal dialysis: a pilot randomized control trial. Am J Kidney Dis 2008; 52(2): 314–323.
48. Rubinstein ML, Selwyn PA. High prevalence of insomnia in an outpatient population with HIV infection. J Acquir Immune Defic Syndr Hum Retrovirol 1998; 19(3):260–265.
49. Bryant PA, Trinder J, Curtis N. Does sleep have a vital role in the immune system? Nat Rev Immunol 2004; 4(6):457–467.
50. Irwin M. Effects of sleep and sleep loss on immunity and cytokines. Brain Behav Immun 2002; 16(5):503–512.
51. Majde JA, Krueger JM. Links between the innate immune system and sleep. J Allergy Clin Immunol 2005; 116(6):1188–1198.
52. Reid S, Dwyer J. Insomnia in HIV infection: a systematic review of prevalence, correlates and management. Psychosom Med 2005; 67(2):260–269.
53. Freda PU, Bilezikian JP. The hypothalamus-pituitary-adrenal axis in HIV disease. AIDS Read 1999; 9(1):46–47.
54. Silverman MN, Pearce BD, Biron CA, et al. Immune modulation of the hypothalamic-pituitary-adrenal (HPA) axis during viral infection. Viral Immunol 2005; 18(1):41–78.
55. Zapanti E, Terzidis K, Chrousos G. Dysfunction of the hypothalamic-pituitary-adrenal axis in HIV infection and disease. Hormones 2008; 7(3):205–216.
56. Nuñez M, de Requena DG, Gallego L, et al. Higher efavirenz plasma levels correlate with development of insomnia. J Acquir Immune Defic Syndr Hum Retrovirol 2001; 28(4):399–400.
57. Fumaz CR, Tuldra A, Ferrer MJ, et al. Quality of life, emotional status, and adherence of HIV-1 infected patients treated with efavirenz versus protease inhibitor-containing regimens. J Acquir Immune Defic Syndr Hum Retrovirol 2002; 29(3):244–253.
58. Perkins DO, Leserman J, Stern RA, et al. Somatic symptoms and HIV infection: relationship to depressive symptoms and indicators of HIV disease. Am J Psychiatry 1995; 152(12):1776–1781.
59. Savard J, Morin CM. Insomnia in the context of cancer: a review of a neglected problem. J Clin Oncol 2001; 19(3):895–908.
60. Sutherland HJ, Lockwood GA, Boyd NF. Ratings of the importance of quality of life variables: therapeutic implications for patients with metastatic breast cancer. J Clin Epidemiol 1990; 43(7):661–666.
61. Munro AJ, Biruls R, Griffin AV, et al. Distress associated with radiotherapy for malignant disease: a quantitative analysis based on patient perceptions. Br J Cancer 1989; 60(3):370–374.

62. Engstrom CA, Strohl RA, Rose L, et al. Sleep alterations in cancer patients. Cancer Nurs 1999; 22(2):143–148.
63. Kaye J, Kaye K, Madow L. Sleep patterns in patients with cancer and patients with cardiac disease. J Psychol 1983; 114(1st half):107–113.
64. Koopman C, Nouriani B, Erickson V, et al. Sleep disturbances in women with metastatic breast cancer. Breast J 2002; 8(6):362–370.
65. Savard J, Simard S, Blanchet J, et al. Prevalence, clinical characteristics and risk factors for insomnia in the context of breast cancer. Sleep 2001; 24(5):583–590.
66. Davidson JR, MacLean AW, Brundage MD, et al. Sleep disturbance in cancer patients. Soc Sci Med 2002; 54(9):1309–1321.
67. Silberfarb PM, Hauri PJ, Oxman TE, et al. Assessment of sleep in patients with lung cancer and breast cancer. J Clin Oncol 1993; 11(5):997–1004.
68. Ancoli-Israel S. The impact and prevalence of chronic insomnia and other sleep disorders associated with chronic illness. Am J Manag Care 2006; 12(suppl 8):S221–S219.
69. Fernandes R, Stone P, Andrews P, et al. Comparison between fatigue, sleep disturbance and circadian rhythm in cancer patients and healthy volunteers: evaluation of diagnostic criteria for cancer-related fatigue. J Pain Symptom Manage 2006; 32(3):245–254.
70. Roscoe JA, Kaufman ME, Matteson-Rusby SE, et al. Cancer-related fatigue and sleep disorders. Oncologist 2007; 12(suppl 1):35–42.
71. Quesnel C, Savard J, Simard S, et al. Efficacy of cognitive-behavioral therapy for insomnia in women treated for non-metastatic breast cancer. J Consult Clin Psychol 2003; 71(1):189–200.
72. Savard J, Simard S, Ivers H, et al. Randomized study on the efficacy of cognitive-behavioral therapy for insomnia secondary to breast cancer, part I: sleep and psychological effects. J Clin Oncol 2005; 23(25):6083–6096.
73. Avidan AY. Clinical neurology of insomnia in neurodegenerative and other disorders of neurological function. Rev Neurol Dis 2007; 4(1):21–34.
74. Bliwise DL. Sleep disorders in Alzheimer's disease and other dementias. Clin Cornerstone 2004; 6(suppl 1A):S16–S28.
75. Avidan AY. Sleep and neurologic problems in the elderly. Sleep Med Clin 2006; 1:273–292.
76. Sateia MJ, ed. The International Classification of Sleep Disorders. 2nd ed. Westchester, IL: American Academy of Sleep Medicine, 2005.
77. Ancoli-Israel S, Klauber MR, Jones DW, et al. Variations in circadian rhythms of activity, sleep and light exposure related to dementia in nursing-home patients. Sleep 1997; 20(1):18–23.
78. Pollak CP, Perlick D. Sleep problems and institutionalization of the elderly. J Geriatr Psychiatry Neurol 1991; 4 (4):204–210.
79. Gottlieb DJ, Destefano AL, Foley DJ, et al. APOE E4 is associated with obstructive sleep apnea/hypopnea, The Sleep Heart Health Study. Neurology 2004; 63:664–668.
80. Glass J, Lanctot KL, Herrmann N, et al. Sedative hypnotics in older people with insomnia: meta-analysis of risks and benefits. BMJ 2005; 331(7526):1169.
81. Wooltorton E. Risperidone (Risperdal): increased rate of cerebrovascular events in dementia trials. CMAJ 2002; 167:1269–1270.
82. Wooltorton E. Olanzapine (Zyprexa): increased incidence of cerebrovascular events in dementia trials. CMAJ 2004; 170:1395.
83. McShane R, Keene J, Gedline K, et al. Do neuroleptic drugs hasten cognitive decline in dementia? Prospective study with necropsy follow up. BMJ 1997; 314:266–270.
84. Singh S, Wooltorton E. Increased mortality among elderly patients with dementia using atypical antipsychotics. CMAJ 2005; 173:252.
85. Wu YH, Swaab DF. Disturbance and strategies for reactivation of the circadian rhythm system in aging and Alzheimer's disease. Sleep Med 2007; 8:623–636.
86. Singer C, Tractenber RE, Kaye J, et al. A multicenter, placebo-controlled trial of melatonin for sleep disturbance in Alzheimer's disease. Sleep 2003; 26:893–901.
87. Alessi CA, Martin JL, Webber AP, et al. Randomized, controlled trial of a nonpharmacological intervention to improve abnormal sleep/wake patterns in nursing home residents. J Am Geriatr Soc 2005; 53(5):803–810.
88. Martin JL, Marler MR, Harker JO, et al. A multicomponent nonpharmacological intervention improves activity rhythms among nursing home resident with disrupted sleep/wake patterns. J Gerontol A Biol Sci Med Sci 2007; 62(1):67–72.
89. Bhatt MH, Podder N, Chokroverty S. Sleep and neurodegenerative diseases. Semin Neurol 2005; 25(1):39–51.
90. Aldrich MS, Foster NL, White RF, et al. Sleep abnormalities in progressive supranuclear palsy. Ann Neurol 1989; 25:577–581.

91. Perrett JL, Jouvet M. Sleep study of progressive supranuclear paralysis. Electroencephalogr Clin Neurophysiol 1980; 49:323–329.
92. DeBruin VS, Machado C, Howard RS, et al. Nocturnal and respiratory disturbances in Steele-Richardson-Olszewski syndrome (progressive supranuclear palsy). Postgrad Med J 1996; 72:293–296.
93. Porter B, Macfarlane R, Walker R. The frequency and nature of sleep disorders in a community-based population of patients with Parkinson's disease. Eur J Neurol 2008; 15:50–54.
94. Dhawan V, Healy DG, Pal S, et al. Sleep-related problems of Parkinson's disease. Age Ageing 2006; 35:220–228.
95. Chaudhuri KR, Martinez-Martin P, Schapira AH, et al. International multicenter pilot study of the first comprehensive self-completed nonmotor symptoms questionnaire for Parkinson's disease: the NMSQuest study. Mov Disord 2006; 21(7):916–923.
96. Chaudhuri KR. Nocturnal symptom complex in PD and its management. Neurology 2003; 61(suppl 3):S17–S23.
97. Chokroverty S. Sleep and degenerative neurological disorders. Neurol Clin 1996; 14(4):807–826.
98. Dhawan V, Dhoat S, Williams AJ. The range and nature of sleep dysfunction in untreated Parkinson's disease (PD). A comparative controlled clinical study using the Parkinson's disease sleep scale and selective polysomnography. J Neurol Sci 2006; 248:158–162.
99. Hogl BE, Gomez-Arevalo G, Garcia S. A clinical, pharmacologic, and polysomnographic study of sleep benefit in Parkinson's disease. Neurology 1998; 50:1332–1339.
100. Provini F, Lombardi C, Lugaresi E. Insomnia in neurological disease. Semin Neurol 2005; 25(1):81–89.
101. Palomaki H, Berg A, Meririnne E. Complaints of poststroke insomnia and its treatment with mianserin. Cerebrovasc Dis 2003; 15:56–62.
102. Bassetti CL. Sleep and Stroke. Semin Neurol 2005; 25(1):19–32.
103. Kotila M, Numminen H, Waltimo O, et al. Depression after stroke. Results for the FINNSTROKE study. Stroke 1998; 29:368–372.
104. Bassetti CL. Sleep and stroke. In: Kryger MH, Roth MH, Dement WC, eds. Principles and Practice of Sleep Medicine. 4th ed. Philadelphia: Elsevier Saunders, 2005:811–830.
105. Tachibana N, Howard RS, Hirsch NP, et al. Sleep problems in multiple sclerosis. Eur Neurol 1994; 34:320–323.
106. Fleming WE, Pollak CP. Sleep disorders in multiple sclerosis. Semin Neurol 2005; 25(1):64–68.
107. Sadovnick AD, Remick RA, Allen J, et al. Depression and multiple sclerosis. Neurology 1996; 46:628–632.
108. Cohen M, Oksenberg A, Snir D, et al. Temporally related changes of sleep complaints in traumatic brain injured patients. J Neurol Neurosurg Psychiatry 1992; 55:313–315.
109. Verma A, Anand V, Verma NP. Sleep disorders in chronic traumatic brain injury. J Clin Sleep Med 2007; 3(4):357–362.
110. Ouellet MC, Beaulieu-Bonneau S, Morin CM. Insomnia in patients with traumatic brain injury. J Head Trauma Rehabil 2006; 21(3):199–212.
111. Baumann CR, Werth E, Stocker R, et al. Sleep-wake disturbances 6 months after traumatic brain injury: a prospective study. Brain 2007; 130:1873–1883.
112. Ayalon L, Borodkin MA, Dishon L, et al. Circadian rhythm sleep disorders following mild traumatic brain injury. Neurology 2007; 68:1136–1140.
113. Flanagan SR, Greenwald B, Weber S, et al. Pharmacological treatment of insomnia for individuals with brain injury. J Head Trauma Rehabil 2007; 22 (1):67–70.
114. Li Pi Shan RS, Ashworth NL. Comparison of lorazepam and zopiclone for insomnia in patients with stroke and brain injury: a randomized, crossover, double-blinded trial. Am J Phys Med Rehabil 2004; 83:421–427.

16 Substance-Induced Insomnia

Deirdre A. Conroy
Department of Psychiatry, University of Michigan, Ann Arbor, Michigan, U.S.A.

J. Todd Arnedt
Department of Psychiatry and Neurology, University of Michigan, Ann Arbor, Michigan, U.S.A.

Kirk J. Brower
Department of Psychiatry, University of Michigan, Ann Arbor, Michigan, U.S.A.

EPIDEMIOLOGY OF SUBSTANCE-INDUCED INSOMNIA

Substance-induced insomnia (SII) is characterized by disruption of sleep and adverse daytime consequences during periods of use or withdrawal from illicit drugs, prescription medications, or licit substances (i.e. alcohol, caffeine, toxins or food items). SII does not result exclusively from substance abuse, but can also develop over time through repeated exposure to a prescribed dosage of a medication. SII is found in approximately 0.2% of the general population, but can comprise up to 3.5% of the sleep disorders clinic population (1). Not unexpectedly, rates are considerably higher in patients presenting for substance abuse treatment. Up to 91% of alcohol-dependent patients, for example, have symptoms of insomnia (2).

Nearly all substances can disrupt sleep and a number of toxins and food allergies can lead to insomnia. A complete description of all potential sleep-disruptive substances is outside the scope of this chapter. Here, we focus on the illicit and licit substances most commonly associated with substance-induced insomnia.

Individuals with insomnia may use substances to either self-medicate (e.g. with alcohol or hypnotics) or to treat the side effects of a poor night's sleep. According to the National Sleep Foundation's (NSF) 2008 Sleep in America poll, 8% percent of the respondents reported current use of alcohol to help them fall asleep (3). It has also been found that a much higher percentage of patients diagnosed with insomnia use alcohol as a sleep aid, with 15% to 28% reporting the use of alcohol to fall asleep (4). In addition, 58% of respondents to the NSF survey reported that they were at least somewhat likely to use caffeinated beverages such as coffee, soda, or tea to cope with sleepiness during the day (3).

The evolution of SII can be difficult to establish. This chapter focuses on how substance use directly affects sleep, but the reverse should also be considered. One can have insomnia before developing substance abuse or dependence. In a longitudinal epidemiological study, Breslau et al. (5) found that young adults that had insomnia at baseline were twice as likely to develop an alcohol use disorder, seven times more likely to develop an illicit drug use disorder, and twice as likely to develop nicotine dependence 3.5 years later (5). These findings raise important questions about the cyclical nature of insomnia and SII.

SII is a relatively understudied area. As will be evident in the evaluation and treatment sections of this chapter, the majority of research has focused on alcohol-induced insomnia to the exclusion of other substances. Much more research is needed on these other substances that can lead to chronic sleep difficulties.

Alcohol

Intoxication

Acute administration of alcohol to normal healthy volunteers decreases sleep onset latency (SOL) (6–8), prolongs rapid eye movement onset latency (ROL) (9) and increases slow wave sleep (SWS) in the first half of the night (6,7,10). In the second half of the night, stage 1 (N1) sleep, wakefulness, and the percentage of REM sleep increase (6), while SWS decreases (6,7,10) (Table 1).

Table 1 Effect of Substances of Abuse on Sleep and Wakefulness

	Sleep continuity			Sleep architecture				Sleep disorders		Sleepiness[a]	
Substance of Abuse	**SOL**	**TST**	**SE**	**ROL**	**REM**	**SWS**	**S1**	**SDB**	**PLMS**	**MSLT**	**MWT**
ALCOHOL											
Intoxication[b]	⇓6–8	⇓8,13[c]	⇑8	⇑9	⇓7,9,14,15	⇑6–8,15,16	⇓8	⇑15,17[d]	⇑18	⇑11 ⇓19	
Withdrawal	⇑20 ⇓16	⇓16 ⇑21[e]	⇑21	⇓22,23 ⇔16	⇑16	⇓10,22		⇑24	⇑25	⇓14[f]	
NICOTINE											
Intoxication	⇑26–28	⇓26	⇓26	⇑29	⇓26	⇔26	⇔26	⇔26	⇓30	—	
Withdrawal	⇑31 ⇓27[g]	31–33 ⇑ ⇓ ⇓	27,31[g]	⇓31	⇑27,31	⇑32[h]⇓ 31⇓ 33⇔	⇓31 ⇔ 32,33[i]		⇑33[j]	⇓33	
CAFFEINE											
Intoxication	⇑34,35 ⇔	⇓34,36	⇓34,35	⇓34[k]	⇔34[k]	⇓35,36[l] ⇔	⇑36			⇑34,37	
Withdrawal	34	⇔34	⇔34	⇔34	⇔34	34	⇔34			⇔34	
MARIJUANA											
Intoxication	⇑38	⇑38[m] ⇓	⇑38 ⇓	⇑38 ⇓39	⇓40	⇑40,41	⇑38[m] ⇓	⇓38			
Withdrawal	⇑42				⇑43	⇓42,43	⇓41				
OPIOIDS											
Intoxication	⇑44	⇔45,46 ⇓44	⇔45,46 ⇓47	⇑46	⇓46–49	⇓45–47	⇑48 49 ⇓46	⇑46,47,50 ⇔51 ⇓45			
Withdrawal			⇑52		⇑49,52,53	⇔52 ⇓					
MDMA “ECSTASY”											
Intoxication	⇔54	⇓55	⇓54 ⇑		⇓54	⇑56	⇑57				
Withdrawal	⇑57	⇓57	⇓57[j]	⇓57	⇑57[j]	⇔57		⇑57			

COCAINE												
Intoxication	⇑58	⇓58	⇓58	⇑58	⇓58	⇑59 ⇔60	⇔58					
Withdrawal	⇓58,59[g] ⇔61 ⇑59[e]	⇓ 59,62– 64[e] ⇑ 58,59[g]	⇓62,63 ⇔ 61 ⇑59[g]	⇓62,65 ⇔63	⇑62,64 ⇔63[n]	⇓59,61	⇑61				⇓65	
AMPHETAMINES												
Intoxication											⇑66–68	
Withdrawal	⇑64	⇓64	⇓64[g]	⇓64	⇓64[g]	⇓64	⇑64					
GHB												
Intoxication	⇑69	⇓69	⇑69	⇓69	⇓69 ⇑	⇑69	⇓69	⇑70				⇑69
Withdrawal												

[a]Decrease in sleep onset on the MSLT indicates more sleepiness.
[b]Alcohol's effects on sleep stages change from the 1st half to the 2nd half of the night.
[c]Increased number of wake periods in sleep.
[d]Only in men.
[e]Late withdrawal (>3 weeks).
[f]Increased SOL during first 75 min after consumption.
[g]Early withdrawal (<3 weeks).
[h]Wetter et al (2000) shows SWS decreases at day 3 but then increases from day 3–10.
[i]Initially increased, but decreased over time.
[j]Not significant.
[k]Decreased shortly after caffeine intake but increase with late caffeine (see Table 1, pg. 530 of Bonnet and Arand 34).
[l]During the first 1/3rd of the sleep period.
[m]Depending on dose of THC and CBD variables; include dose and time into withdrawal.
[n]Pace –Schott et al (63) is a binge abstinence protocol.
⇑= Increase, ⇓= Decrease, ⇔= No change, = No data. *Abbreviations*: MSLT, Multiple Sleep Latency Test; MWT, Maintenance of Wakefulness Test. PLMS, Periodic Limb Movements in Sleep; REM%, Rapid Eye Movement percentage; ROL, Rapid Eye Movement Sleep Latency; S1, Stage 1 sleep; SDB, Sleep Disordered Breathing; SE, Sleep efficiency; SOL, Sleep onset latency; SWS, Slow Wave Sleep; TST, Total sleep time.

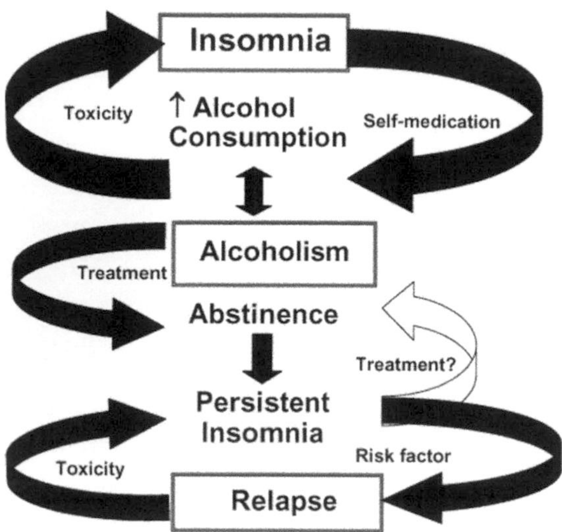

Figure 1 The reciprocal relationship between insomnia and alcoholism. Insomnia may lead to increased alcohol consumption by self-medication. Increased alcohol consumption can have neurotoxic effects on the same neurotransmitters that are involved in sleep regulation. Both insomnia and high alcohol intake may lead to alcoholism. Insomnia can persist despite treatment and can lead to relapse. Treatment of insomnia may facilitate abstinence. Studies are ongoing.

Tolerance to alcohol's acute effects can develop quickly, within one week in healthy volunteers (11), resulting in increased alcohol intake to derive the same sleep-promoting effects. Insomnia may persist even after alcohol use has stopped and treatment has been initiated. In fact, an estimated 36% to 91% of patients in early recovery from alcohol dependence complain of insomnia (2,12) Figure 1 provides a schematic describing the bidirectional relationship of alcohol use and sleep disturbance.

Withdrawal

Polysomnographic (PSG) irregularities during alcohol withdrawal have been well characterized. There is typically an increase in SOL (14,22), a decrease in SWS percentage (%) (16,22) and an increase in REM sleep (16). Returning to drinking was found to temporarily increase SWS or decrease REM sleep; however, upon repeat withdrawal, these changes reverted to baseline or below baseline levels (71).

Sleep architecture (SWS and REM) and sleep continuity (sleep latency, total sleep time, sleep efficiency) during withdrawal have been studied extensively as predictors of relapse (22). Reduced SWS percentage was implicated in some early studies, (10,72) but these findings were only partially replicated in a larger sample (22). REM variables have been consistently linked to relapse in alcoholic patients (23). Increased REM pressure and reduced ROL, have been shown to differentiate relapsers from abstainers after follow-up as long as six months (22,73). A recent study using spectral EEG analysis found evidence for increased hyperarousal in the REM sleep of alcoholic patients who relapsed within three months compared to abstinent alcoholics and controls (74). In addition to the consistent REM findings, most clinical studies have also identified sleep continuity measures, (increased SOL and reduced TST) as being strongly predictive of relapse (21,22). Sleep disturbances during withdrawal can persist for up to two years (16).

Comparisons between subjective and objective data may highlight important perceptual distinctions in SII. Alcohol dependent patients with insomnia who overestimated SOL and underestimated wake time after sleep onset (WASO) were more likely to relapse (75).

Several mechanisms have been proposed to explain the sleep disruptive properties of alcohol. Sleep-generating systems in the brain, including the GABAergic system, adapt to chronic alcohol administration by downregulation, whereas arousal-generating systems involving glutamate and other neurotransmitters are upregulated. During alcohol withdrawal, dysregulated neurotransmitter systems such as these are postulated to disrupt sleep (71). One study found that alcoholics' homeostatic response (measured via SWS and delta power) to partial sleep deprivation was impaired compared to controls (76). Circadian rhythm mechanisms are also disturbed by alcohol (77–79). Insomnia may also be related to alcohol-related sleep disordered breathing (SDB) (18) or periodic limb movements in sleep (PLMS) (25,80), both of which are elevated in alcoholic patients.

Nicotine

Nicotine increases catecholamines, vasopressin, growth hormone, ACTH, and endorphins in the brain, which can disturb sleep. The average cigarette contains 8 to 9 mg of nicotine, but the amount delivered varies because smokers can adjust dose by puffing volume, depth, rate or intensity. Many studies, therefore, have employed the nicotine patch to better regulate dose-dependent effects.

Intoxication

Smokers (particularly females (81)) report more difficulty sleeping compared to nonsmokers independent of health, demographics, behavioral, and psychological variables (81). Laboratory studies show that nonsmokers with a nicotine patch took longer to fall asleep, had shorter TST, lower sleep efficiency (SE), and lower REM sleep % compared to participants with a placebo patch (26).

Depression history is associated with differences in REM sleep during nicotine exposure and withdrawal. A randomized controlled trial found that depressed nonsmokers wearing nicotine patches showed increased REM sleep and short-term mood improvements compared to nondepressed nonsmokers (29). The increased REM sleep persisted during withdrawal in depressed patients, while REM sleep in nondepressed patients decreased (32).

Withdrawal

Sleep and mood disturbances have been documented for up to one year following smoking cessation. Heavy smokers (mean smoking history of 24 years) were studied across a smoking week and a withdrawal week. During the withdrawal week, smokers had more arousals, awakenings, and stage changes compared to the smoking week (33). In the first long-term study across one year of abstinence, seven former smokers underwent PSG at months 1, 2, 4, 6, 9, and 12. There was a reduction of REM latency, N1 sleep, and SWS coupled with an increase in REM sleep and N2 sleep (31). Interestingly, depression measures were increased and correlated with REM, ROL from sleep onset and N2, and stage shifts (31). The authors posit that the increases in REM sleep and levels of depression may be due in part to an increased sensitivity of serotonergic neurons during withdrawal.

Caffeine

Caffeine, a phosphodiesterase inhibitor with a half-life ranging from three to seven hours, promotes wakefulness by blocking adenosine receptors (82) and is the most widely used substance for counteracting the daytime effects of sleep loss.

Intoxication

Caffeine attenuates the progressive increase in sleepiness across the day and reduces the quality of recovery sleep (83), but effects vary depending on an individual's history of caffeine consumption (84). Administration of caffeine at bedtime has been shown to prolong SOL, shorten TST, and reduce total SWS and S4 sleep in a dose-dependent manner (34,35,85) During sleep deprivation, low to moderate caffeine doses (100–200 mg) have been found to increase stage 1 sleep and reduce the slow component of EEG power (0.75–2.0 Hz) relative to placebo; during recovery sleep, fast EEG components (11.25–20.0 Hz) were enhanced (35). Higher caffeine doses during sleep deprivation (300 mg) reduce TST, increase S1 sleep, and reduce SWS in the first third of the night (36).

Low-dose caffeine improves daytime performance more than placebo (86). Concomitant subjective sleepiness data has been more variable. For example, a recent double-blind parallel-group design using a forced desynchrony protocol found that low doses of repeated caffeine (0.3 mg per hour) across an extended 28.57 hour "day" reduced objective sleepiness compared to placebo, but increased subjective sleepiness (86).

Chronic caffeine use can lead to a physiological state of hyperarousal, a common characteristic in patients with insomnia. One study used caffeine to model insomnia by giving repeated doses of 400 mg of caffeine to healthy volunteers across one week. The study reported prolonged SOL, reduced S4, and shortened TST (34). Metabolic rate measured via VO_2 also increased, consistent with the hyperarousal theory of insomnia. A later study by the same group examined electrocardiograms (ECGs) during sleep in 15 healthy volunteers who took 400 mg of caffeine a half-hour before bedtime. Heart rate variability, defined as the integration of the low frequency (LF)/high frequency (HF) ratio band was significantly higher during REM sleep in the caffeine group than in the placebo group. The investigators interpreted this finding as suggestive of a predominance of sympathetic nervous system activity and an increased risk for adverse cardiac events (87).

Withdrawal

Withdrawal from chronic caffeine use is associated with distinct physiological and subjective withdrawal symptoms, due in large part to the hypersensitivity of adenosine receptors during abstinence (82). Within 12 to 16 hours into caffeine withdrawal, sleepiness, lethargy, headaches, decreased alertness, depressed mood, irritability, and mental fogginess may occur (83,84). Withdrawal symptoms usually dissipate within 3 to 5 days, but can last as long as one week (88). In summary, the ability of caffeine to attenuate decrements in performance across prolonged wakefulness makes it a highly desired substance. However, caffeine can contribute to impairments in sleep if consumed in close proximity to bedtime and withdrawal can be associated with impairment in cognitive functioning.

Marijuana

The psychoactive ingredient in marijuana, delta-9-tetrahydrocannabinol (THC), binds to type 1 cannabinoid (CB_1) G protein-coupled receptors located in the nociceptive areas of the brain, spinal cord, and peripheral nervous system (89).

Intoxication

Overall, THC effects on sleep have been found to be variable, owing to variability in methodology and samples studied (see also Table 1 –substance table).

Marijuana can induce sleep (38) and decrease REM sleep (40). Administration of THC at doses of 10, 20, and 30 mg prior to sleep onset decreased SOL after subjects reported achieving a "high" (90). When large doses (15 mg) of cannabidiol (a major component in marijuana thought to have minimal psychoactive effects) were added to THC and administered to participants before sleep, the amount of wakefulness in the night increased (38). Conflicting evidence exists with respect to the acute effect of THC on SWS [for review see Schierenbeck et al. 2008 (91)]. Some studies have reported an increase in stage 4 (S4) (40) sleep, while others have reported a decrease in overall SWS (38).

Withdrawal

Sleep disturbance is one of the most common symptoms associated with marijuana withdrawal. Other common symptoms may include strange dreams, depression, chills, and irritability. Among 1735 frequent users of marijuana (>21 occasions in a single year), 235 (13.5%) reported difficulty sleeping during withdrawal (92). Laboratory studies show prolonged SOL (42) and decreased SWS% (42,43) during withdrawal. REM sleep rebound has been documented, but only in withdrawal from higher doses of THC (70–210 mg) (43). One study tracking common cannabis withdrawal symptoms, including sleep problems, in 36 cannabis-dependent subjects reported that these symptoms were not predictive of relapse after an approximately 26-month period (93).

Opioids

Intoxication

Opioids, (e.g. methadone, morphine, heroin) are perceived as sedating, but can disrupt sleep quality. In healthy adults, morphine sulfate and methadone have been found to reduce SWS (45,47) and REM sleep (48,49) When compared to naltrexone in a group of recovering addicts, methadone patients had increased SOL (44) and WASO and reduced TST (44), SWS (47), and

REM sleep (44). Heroin-dependent patients detoxified with methadone reported even greater sleep problems than those maintained on methadone during the first months of heroin abstinence (94). Sleep disturbance, increased dreams, and nightmares were also associated with opioids in palliative care patients (95).

Withdrawal

Abstinent morphine-dependent patients showed a dose-related effect of morphine on sleep with decreases in TST, SWS, and REM sleep (96). Methadone-maintained patients had more awakenings (44) lower sleep efficiency (SE), and lower SWS (47) than controls. One early study of six male heroin-dependent prisoners compared sleep for three months prior to methadone induction, during titration and stabilization of 100 mg daily of methadone, and finally up to 22 weeks after withdrawal. During methadone administration, awake time during the night decreased and delta bursts increased significantly (53). Across 22 weeks of abstinence, wake-up time decreased further while REM sleep and delta sleep increased significantly (53).

Animal data suggest that opioids may disrupt sleep by decreasing GABA neurotransmission in the pontine reticular nucleus (97). Symptoms of insomnia may also result from opioid-induced central sleep apnea (46,47,98), occurring in about 30% of chronic users (99).

"Ecstacy" (±) 3, 4- Methylenedioxymethamphetamine (MDMA)

MDMA (3, 4 –methylenedioxymethamphetamine), or "ecstasy" is a stimulant with hallucinogenic properties and commonly called a "club drug". It stimulates the release and inhibits the reuptake of serotonin (5HT), among other effects on various neurotransmitter systems, which can generate feelings of elation and pleasure (56,100). This abrupt surge in neurotransmitters can acutely affect sleep as well as regulation of mood, aggression, sexual activity, and sensitivity to pain. The repeated surge in serotonin levels can have neurotoxic effects with possible implications for sleep, circadian rhythms, anxiety, impulsivity, cognitive deficits, and mood disorders (57).

Intoxication

Persistent use of ecstasy shortens TST and impairs NREM sleep, particularly S2 sleep (100,101). An early study examined the effects of MDMA on the sleep of 23 MDMA abstinent users compared to age- and sex-matched controls with no history of use (55). The MDMA users had a 19-minute reduction of TST and a slightly shorter ROL than controls (60 minutes versus 75 minutes). In a more recent study, alpha-methyl-para-tyrosine (AMPT), which decreases brain catecholamines, was administered to abstinent MDMA users to determine whether AMPT would differentially affect sleep and cognitive performance in abstinent users. Results showed that exposure to AMPT at 4 PM and 10 PM before a 12 AM bedtime resulted in a trend towards decreased TST, ROL and significantly lower S2 sleep (102).

MDMA exposure has lasting effects on circadian rhythms in animal experiments. Rats exposed to MDMA had alterations in sleep and circadian pattern of activity (wheel running) for up to five days after dosage. In addition, SWS was still altered after one month (103). In vitro administration of MDMA to rat brain slices impaired the resetting ability of cells in the SCN to a serotoinin receptor agonist 20 weeks after initial exposure (60).

Cocaine

Cocaine is a stimulant that blocks reuptake of DA, NE, and 5HT and can cause increased energy and euphoria.

Intoxication

Acute administration of cocaine in a laboratory setting causes sleep impairment, including increased SOL by several hours, decreased SE, and decreased REM sleep (58). In chronic cocaine users, administration of cocaine actually increased SWS during cocaine administration (59). Spectral analyses of the sleep EEG showed that during binge periods, slower EEG bandwidths, e.g., delta and theta, were higher than the faster bands, e.g., sigma and beta (59).

Withdrawal

Sleep disturbance is one of the most common symptoms of cocaine withdrawal, reported in 71% of a sample of recovering cocaine addicts (20). Sleep quality appears to change from early abstinence (≤3 weeks) to late abstinence (>3 weeks). Early abstinence in cocaine withdrawal is associated with decreased SOL (59), increased TST (58,59,62), shortened ROL (61,62), and increased REM% (62). Late abstinence is associated with prolonged SOL (59,62), decreased TST (63) and decreased SE (63).

Finally, there appears to be a discrepancy between objective sleep and subjective perception of sleep during early withdrawal from cocaine. Subjective ratings, including overall sleep quality, feeling well rested, depth of sleep, and mental alertness all increased over protracted abstinence in one study, but objectively measured sleep did not (59). Other studies have found that despite deterioration of sleep quality across cocaine abstinence, estimates of sleep quality improved (104) or remained unchanged (63). The authors posit that this finding may reflect a dysregulation of homeostatic sleep drive in chronic cocaine users. Similar discrepancies between objective and subjective measures have been documented in early abstinence from alcohol (74).

While cocaine is a known stimulant of monoamine neurotransmitter systems via reuptake blockade, animal studies suggest that circadian mechanisms may also be involved in its rewarding effects, if not sleep impairment *per se* (105,106).

Amphetamines

The exact mechanisms of how amphetamines, a major class of stimulants, increase EEG arousal are uncertain, but are thought to involve adrenergic or dopaminergic transmission (107). Increased alertness is also highly dependent on the dose and the type of amphetamine.

Intoxication

D-amphetamine is three times more potent than L-amphetamine and 12 times more potent than L-methamphetamine in increasing wakefulness and reducing SWS (108). Three studies have examined the effect of amphetamines on daytime sleepiness using the Multiple Sleep Latency Test (MSLT). All three showed prolonged SOL on nap opportunities across the day (66–68). Sleep deprivation appears to increase the drug-seeking behaviors associated with amphetamines. Another similarly acting stimulant, methylphenidate, was chosen more often (88% of days) after a four-hour time in bed time than it was after an 8-hour time in bed (29%) (68).

Withdrawal

Early amphetamine withdrawal is associated with initial long bouts of sleep and reports of poor quality sleep. Sleep records obtained by nurses' observations in abstinent amphetamine-dependent subjects showed an initial increase in TST followed by reduced TST across 20 nights following cessation of use (109). Sleep questionnaires given to 21 patients in the first three weeks of methamphetamine withdrawal showed that TST (day and night) peaked on the fifth day of abstinence (110). One study evaluated objective sleep parameters across acute (days 3–10) and subacute withdrawal (days 11–14) in stimulant abusers. From acute to subacute withdrawal, stimulant abusers had less TST and REM sleep. However, subjective reports of sleep improved across abstinence. Another study found that self-reported SOL, number of awakenings in the night, quality of sleep, clear-headedness on awakening, satisfaction with sleep, and depth of sleep all improved significantly across the three weeks of continued abstinence (110).

EVALUATION

Preliminary Assessment

SII may have varying clinical presentations depending on the patient's age, gender, weight, genetics, psychological traits and states, and health status. For example, stimulant-induced insomnia may be diagnosed more in younger patients (typically adolescents) whereas SII due to alcohol or hypnotics may be found more in older patients. Substances may also have indirect effects by exacerbating preexisting medical conditions (e.g. caffeine may worsen gastroesophageal reflux disease, which can disrupt sleep).

When assessing substance-using patients for insomnia, several principles should be borne in mind. First, substances may not be the only cause of the insomnia. Other medical or psychiatric disorders, sleep-impairing medications, inadequate sleep hygiene, and dysfunctional beliefs about sleep may play a role. This issue is particularly relevant to patients with substance use disorders, who have high rates of co-occurring psychiatric and medical disorders. It should be assumed that substances are part of the problem, even if not necessarily the only cause of insomnia. Second, PSG should be considered if there is high suspicion of other sleep disorders, particularly sleep apnea and periodic limb movement (PLM) disorder. Third, assessment of sleep complaints is aided by asking patients to keep a sleep log for two weeks during early recovery after acute substance withdrawal symptoms have subsided. Sleep logs have several advantages, including an assessment of sleep patterns over time, documenting improvement with abstinence, and engaging the patient in the treatment process.

Differential Diagnoses

In addition to other medical or psychiatric disorders, differential diagnoses of SII include inadequate sleep hygiene and psychophysiological insomnia. To distinguish SII from these two disorders, specific inquiry about substance tolerance, dosage escalation, rebound insomnia in the absence of the substance, fear of not sleeping (or staying awake) without the substance, and sporadic use of hypnotics, will help distinguish SII from other sleep disorders. Use of the Diagnostic and Statistical Manual or the ICSD can be used to diagnose SII, but certain diagnostic criteria may vary (see Table 2).

Inadequate sleep hygiene is characterized by daily activities that are not compatible with maintenance of quality sleep. This diagnosis is appropriate when the timing of substance use is incompatible with the preferred sleep time. For example, a patient's use of alcohol or nicotine in the hours before bedtime is clearly associated with the sleep disturbance. However, SII should be considered if the sleep problem began or got worse after initiation of the substance use or the sleep difficulties improve markedly during periods of abstinence, or the individual feels unable to sleep without the substance. Some of the distinguishing characteristics of psychophysiological insomnia are the perpetuating factors that serve to maintain the insomnia, i.e., heightened arousal in bed. Substance use may have contributed to poor sleep in the acute and early stages of the insomnia, but when the maladaptive thoughts and behaviors persist even after the patient stops using the substance, the diagnosis is more consistent with psychophysiological insomnia

Table 2 Diagnostic Criteria for Substance-Induced Sleep Disorders

A. SUBSTANCE-INDUCED SLEEP DISORDERS	DSM-IV[a]	ICSD-2[b]
Must identify sleep disturbance as:		
Insomnia due to drug or substance	✓	✓
Hypersomnia due to drug or substance	✓	✓
Parasomnia due to drug or substance	✓	✓
Mixed due to drug or substance	✓	
Circadian rhythm sleep disorder due to drug or substance		✓
Central sleep apnea due to drug or substance		✓
B. SUBSTANCE-INDUCED INSOMNIA		
Meets the criteria for insomnia		✓
Insomnia developed within one month of substance exposure, use or abuse, or acute withdrawal	✓	✓
There is current ongoing dependence on or abuse of a substance known to disrupt sleep either during use or withdrawal or there is exposure to a toxin known to disrupt sleep.	✓	✓
Insomnia is temporally associated with the substance use, exposure or withdrawal	✓	✓
Insomnia is not better accounted for by a sleep disorder that is not substance induced, medical, neurological, or mental disorder	✓	✓

[a]DSM-IV, Diagnostic and Statistical Manual of Mental Disorders, 4th ed. American Psychiatric Association, DSM-IV-TR: Diagnostic and Statistical Manual of Mental Disorders, 4th ed, Text Revision, American Psychiatric Association, Washington DC, 2000.
[b]ICSD-2, International Classification of Sleep Disorders, 2nd edition (1).

than SII. Therefore, a timeline with respect to the use of the substance(s) and the onset of the insomnia is important to obtain.

Finally, insomnia may predate the substance use/dependence; however, there must be convincing evidence based on the sleep history that the sleep disturbance and substance use/abuse are intricately related.

TREATMENT

Pharmacological Treatments

Special considerations are required when considering hypnotic therapy with patients recovering from substance dependence. First, physicians who treat patients with a history of substance abuse or dependence are reticent to prescribe medications for sleep. This is especially true for the Schedule IV hypnotics (including benzodiazepine receptor agonists), which are first-line agents for insomnia in nonabusing patients with insomnia, but their reluctance to prescribe may also generalize to other available hypnotics. A recent postal survey of addiction medicine physicians found that less than one-third of alcoholic patients with sleep disturbances during the first three months of recovery were offered a sleep medication (111). Second, although the most widely used hypnotic agents have low addiction potential for most patients with insomnia (112), the benzodiazepine receptor agonist medications have moderate to high abuse liability in patients with a history of substance abuse and dependence (113).

We outline the most commonly available hypnotic medications and their efficacy for substance-induced insomnia below. These studies have been conducted almost exclusively with alcohol-dependent patients. Pharmacological treatment options for patients with other types of substance use disorders are needed.

Benzodiazepines and Benzodiazepine Receptor Agonists (BzRAs)

Benzodiazepines and other benzodiazepine receptor agonists (e.g., zolpidem) are safe, efficacious, sedative-hypnotics and often the medications of choice for treating transient insomnia in non-SII patients (114). They also may have beneficial effects on sleep during subacute alcohol withdrawal (115), but confer increased risk for sedative-hypnotic abuse in patients with a history of substance abuse or dependence (116–118). Accordingly, most addiction treatment specialists recommend against the use of sedative-hypnotics in alcoholic patients (except for benzodiazepines during acute alcohol withdrawal), because of their abuse potential, withdrawal effects, rebound insomnia, and potential for overdose when mixed with alcohol (119–122).

Anticonvulsants

Anticonvulsant agents do not lower seizure threshold, which makes them appealing for treating insomnia in the substance-abusing population. At least two anticonvulsants—carbamazepine and gabapentin—have been studied specifically for their effects on sleep in alcoholics. Carbamazepine was superior to lorazepam for treating sleep disturbance associated with acute alcohol withdrawal (123). Gabapentin has the advantages of sleep promotion, non-liver metabolism, noninterference with metabolism or excretion of other medications, and it does not require blood monitoring for therapeutic concentrations, hepatotoxicity, and hematological toxicity. Furthermore, it has a favorable side effects profile, low abuse potential, and is not protein-bound. It exerts its CNS effects by binding to alpha-2-delta receptors, resulting in voltage-sensitive calcium channel inhibition (124).

Gabapentin may improve the sleep of recovering alcoholic patients (125–127). Karam-Hage and Brower (125) found that self-reported sleep quality improved after four to six weeks of treatment with gabapentin (mean dose 953 mg/day) in 15 of 17 consecutively evaluated alcoholic patients with persistent insomnia. A recent placebo-controlled study, however, found that, while six weeks of gabapentin 1500 mg nightly delayed the onset to heavy drinking, no subjective or objective sleep differences were found between the gabapentin and placebo groups (128). Although gabapentin and pregabalin, a newer anticonvulsant agent, increase SWS in healthy control subjects, similar evidence is lacking in patients with alcohol dependence.

Antidepressants

Trazodone is the most frequently prescribed medication for sleep by addiction medicine physicians (111). It is effective acutely in the treatment of depressed patients with insomnia (129–132) and has been used safely in several samples of alcoholics (126,133). In a placebo-controlled study of trazodone in 16 abstinent alcoholic patients, trazodone significantly reduced wake time after sleep onset (WASO) and improved SE compared to placebo, but only improvements in WASO were sustained at night 28. Depression scores were also more improved in the trazodone group (134). A recently completed study also found superior sleep outcomes of trazodone vs. placebo more than 12 weeks of treatment in alcohol-dependent patients, but heavy drinking was *higher* in the trazodone-treated group compared to the placebo group (135).

Antipsychotics

Quetiapine is an atypical antipsychotic with sedative effects (136) that has been used as a treatment for insomnia in alcohol-dependent patients. In one of the only studies in substance users, Monnelly et al (137) found that alcohol-dependent veterans who reported difficulty sleeping and were treated with 25 to 200 mg of quetiapine had an increased number of days of abstinence and fewer hospitalizations, but no subjective or objective sleep measure was included. Moreover, any benefit of quetiapine for use in this population must be weighed against its potential for akathisia (138) and increased PLMs when used to promote sleep (136).

Other Hypnotics

Melatonin is a sleep-promoting agent that may be particularly useful to treat circadian rhythm disorders (139). Because the manufacturing and quality of melatonin is not currently regulated in the U.S., the melatonin receptor agonist, ramelteon, may be a better candidate for study. Over-the-counter remedies such as antihistamines, valerian root extract (from the herbal plant, *Valeriana officinalis*), and melatonin have not been widely evaluated in substance-abusing patients, although they are commonly used.

Nonpharmacological Treatments for Substance-Induced Insomnia

Few studies have evaluated the efficacy of nonpharmacological sleep treatments for substance-induced insomnia. An initial study compared progressive muscle relaxation to no treatment in 22 alcoholic inpatients with insomnia (140). At the end of treatment, the relaxation group reported better sleep quality on a nonvalidated 10-point rating scale.

The benefits of cognitive behavioral therapy for insomnia (CBT-I) for reducing relapse in alcoholic patients have been studied. Currie and colleagues (141) randomized sixty alcoholic outpatients to individual CBT therapy (5 sessions more than 7 weeks), self-help manual with telephone support calls, or wait-list control. Patients in both active treatment groups reported greater improvements than controls on diary measures of sleep quality and sleep continuity at posttreatment and follow-up, but no differences in relapse rates were found (141). An uncontrolled trial of an individual eight-session cognitive behavioral therapy for insomnia found posttreatment improvements in both sleep quality and daytime functioning and no one relapsed to drinking (142).

The use of CBT-based interventions has also been explored in adolescent users of alcohol, marijuana, hallucinogens, cocaine, opioids, and stimulants. A six-session multicomponent behavioral sleep intervention (stimulus control, bright light therapy, sleep hygiene, cognitive therapy, mindfulness-based stress reduction) improved sleep, reduced aggression, and decreased drug use after one year in adolescents who had received treatment for substance abuse (143,144). These findings indicate that CBT-I may be efficacious for improving sleep and daytime functioning in adolescents and adults with SII. More controlled trials of nonpharmacological sleep interventions are needed and the relationship between improved sleep and future substance use remains to be more clearly elucidated.

CONCLUSIONS

There are a number of licit and illicit substances that can lead to SII. Although substance-induced sleep problems improve with continued abstinence, persistent sleep problems may occur for at least two reasons. First, long-lasting alterations to the sleep centers of the brain may occur due to chronic drug exposure. Second, chronic sleep disturbance is typically associated with multiple perpetuating causes and substance use may be just one of many reasons for sleep complaints. Assessment should consider the many causes of sleep disturbance. Pharmacological and nonpharmacological treatments to target insomnia associated with substance use disorders do exist, but many are either inappropriate or have been inadequately tested in this patient population. More well-controlled studies are needed to characterize the phenomenology of sleep during recovery, to determine the efficacy of monotherapy and combined approaches to sleep treatment in patients with addiction, and to evaluate the impact of such treatments on relapse and recovery.

REFERENCES

1. The International Classification of Sleep Disorders, Diagnostic and Coding Manual, 2nd ed. American Academy of Sleep Medicine. Westchester, IL; 2005.
2. Cohn T, Foster J, Peters T. Sequential studies of sleep disturbance and quality of life in abstaining alcoholics. Addict Biol 2003; 8:455–462.
3. National Sleep Foundation. 2008. Sleep in America poll: summary of findings. http://www.sleepfoundation.org/sites/default/files/2008%20POLL%20SOF.PDF (Accessed February 17, 2010).
4. Roehrs T, Papineau K, Rosenthal L, et al. Ethanol as a hypnotic in insomniacs: Self administration and effects on sleep and mood. Neuropsychopharmacology 1999; 20:279–286.
5. Breslau N, Roth T, Rosenthal L, et al. Sleep disturbance and psychiatric disorders: A longitudinal epidemiological study of young adults. Biol Psychiatry 1996; 39:411–418.
6. MacLean A, Cairns J. Dose response effects on ethanol on the sleep of young men. J Stud Alcohol 1982; 43:434–444.
7. Williams D, MacLean A, Cairns J. Dose-response effects of ethanol on the sleep of young women. J Stud Alcohol 1983; 44:515–523.
8. Feige B, Gann H, Brueck R, et al. Effects of alcohol on polysomnographically recorded sleep in healthy subjects. Alcohol Clin Exp Res 2006; 30:1527–1537.
9. Miyata S, Noda A, Atarashi M, et al. REM sleep is impaired by a small amount of alcohol in young women sensitive to alcohol. Intern Med 2004; 43:679–684.
10. Allen R, Wagman A, Funderburk F. Slow wave sleep changes: Alcohol tolerance and treatment implications Adv Exp Med Biol 1977; 85A:629–640.
11. Roehrs T, Zwyghuizen-Doorenbos A, Knox M, et al. Sedating effects of ethanol and time of drinking. Alcohol Clin Exp Res 1992; 16:553–557.
12. Brower KJ, Aldrich M, Robinson EAR,et al. Insomnia, self-medication, and relapse to alcoholism. Am J Psychiatry 2001; 158:399–404.
13. Van Reen E, Jenni O, Carskadon M. Effects of alcohol on sleep and the sleep electroencephalogram in healthy young women. Alcohol Clin Exp Res 2006; 30:974–981.
14. Papineau K, Roehrs T, Petrucelli N, et al. Electrophysiological assessment (The Multiple Sleep Latency Test) of the biphasic effects of ethanol in humans. Alcohol Clin Exp Res 1998; 22:231–235.
15. Prinz P, Roehrs T, Vitaliano P, et al. Effect of alcohol on sleep and nighttime plasma growth hormone and cortisol concentrations. J Clin Endocrinol Metab 1980; 51:759–764.
16. Drummond S, Gillin J, Smith T, et al. The sleep of abstinent pure primary alcoholic patients: Natural course and relationship to relapse. Alcohol Clin Exp Res 1998; 22:1796–1802.
17. Peppard P, Austin D, Brown R. Association of alcohol consumption and sleep disordered breathing in men and women. J Clin Sleep Med 2007; 3:265–270.
18. Aldrich MS, Brower KJ, Hall JM. Sleep-disordered breathing in alcoholics. Alcohol Clin Exp Res 1999; 23:134–140.
19. Roehrs T, Claiborue D, Knox M, et al. Residual sedating effects of alcohol. Alcohol Clin Exp Res 1994; 18:831–834.
20. Brower K, Maddahian E, Blow F, et al. A comparison of self reported symptoms and DSM-III-R criteria for cocaine withdrawal. Am J Drug Alcohol Abuse 1988; 14:347–356.
21. Clark CP, Gillin JC, Golshan S, et al. Increased REM sleep density at admission predicts relapse by three months in primary alcoholics with a lifetime diagnosis of secondary depression. Biol Psychiatry 1998; 43:601–607.
22. Brower KJ, Aldrich MS, Hall JM. Polysomnographic and subjective sleep predictors of alcoholic relapse. Alcohol Clin Exp Res 1998; 22:1864–1871.
23. Gillin JC, Smith TL, Irwin M, et al. Increased pressure for rapid eye movement sleep at time of hospital admission predicts relapse in nondepressed patients with primary alcoholism at 3-month follow-up. Arch Gen psychiatry 1994; 51:189–197.

24. Aldrich M, Shipley J, Tandon R, et al. Sleep-disordered breathing in alcoholics: Association with age. Alcohol Clin Exp Res 1993; 17:1179–1183.
25. Gann H, Feige B, van Calker D, et al. Periodic limb movements during sleep in alcohol dependent patients. Eur Arch Psychiatry Neurosci 2002; 252:124–129.
26. Davila D, Hurt R, Offord K, et al. Acute effects of transdermal nicotine on sleep architecture, snoring, and sleep disordered breathing in nonsmokers. Am J Respir Crit Care Med 1994; 150:469–474.
27. Soldatos C, Kales J, Scharf M, et al. Cigarette smoking associated with sleep difficulties. Science 1980; 207:551–552.
28. Gothe B, Strohl K, Levin S, et al. Nicotine: A different approach to treatment of obstructive sleep apnea. Chest 1985; 87:11–17.
29. Salin-Pascual R, de la Fuente J, Galicia-Polo L, et al. Effects of transdermal nicotine on mood and sleep in nonsmoking major depressed patients. Psychopharmacology (Berl) 1995; 121:476–479.
30. Wetter DW, Young TB. The relation between cigarette smoking and sleep disturbance. Prev Med 1994a; 23:328–334.
31. Moreno-Coutino A, Calderon -Ezquerro C, Drucker-Colin R. Long-term changes in sleep and depressive symptoms of smokers in abstinence. Nicotine Tob Res 2007; 9:389–396.
32. Wetter DW, Carmack C, Anderson C, et al. Tobacco withdrawal signs and symptoms among women with and without a history of depression. Exp Clin Psychopharmacol 2000; 8:88–96.
33. Prosise G, Bonnet M, Berry R, et al. Effects of abstinence from smoking on sleep and daytime sleepiness. Chest 1994; 105:1136–1141.
34. Bonnet M, Arand D. Caffeine use as a model of acute and chronic insomnia. Sleep 1992; 15:526–536.
35. Landolt H, Retey J, Tonz K, et al. Caffeine attenuates waking and sleep electroencephalographic markers of sleep homeostasis in humans. Neuropsychopharmacology 2004; 29:1933–1399.
36. LaJambe C, Kamimori G, Belenky G, et al. Caffeine effects on recovery sleep following 27 hours of total sleep deprviation. Aviat Space Environ Med 2005; 76:108–113.
37. Zwyghuizen-Doorenbos A, Roehrs T, Lipschutz L, et al. Effects of caffeine on alertness. Psychopharmacology (Berl) 1990; 100:36–39.
38. Nicholson A, Turner C, Stone B, et al. Effect of delta-9- tetrahydrocannabinol and cannabidiol on nocturnal sleep and early morning behavior in young adults. J Clin Psychopharmacol 2004; 24:305–313.
39. Freemon F. The effect of delta-9-tetrahydrocannabinol on sleep. Psychopharmacology 1974; 35:39–44.
40. Feinberg I, Jones R, Walker J, et al. Effects of marijuana extract and tetrahydrocannabinol on electroencephalographic sleep patterns. Clin Pharmacol Ther 1976; 19:782–794.
41. Pivik R, Zarcone V, Dement W, et al. Delta-9-tetrahydrocannabinol and synhexyl; effects on human sleep patterns. Clin Pharmacol Ther 1972; 13:426–435.
42. Freemon F. The effect of chronically administered delta-9-tetrahydrocannabinol upon the polygraphically monitored sleep of normal volunteers. Drug Alcohol Depend 1982; 10:345–353.
43. Feinberg I, Jones R, Walker J, et al. Effects of high dosage delta -9-tetrahydrocannabinol on sleep patterns in man. Clin Pharmacol Ther 1975; 17:458–466.
44. Staedt J, Wassmuth F, Stoppe G. Effects of chronic treatment with methadone and naltrexone on sleep in addicts. Eur Arch Psychiatry Clin Neurosci 1996; 246:305–309.
45. Dimsdale J, Norman D, DeJardin D, et al. The effect of opioids on sleep architecture. J Clin Sleep Med 2007; 3:33–36.
46. Wang D, Teichtahl H, Drummer O, et al. Central sleep apnea in stable methadone maintenance treatment patients. Chest 2005; 128:1348–1356.
47. Teichtahl H, Prodromidis A, Miller B, et al. Sleep-disordered breathing in stable methadone programme patients: A pilot study. Addiction 2001; 96:395–403.
48. Kay D, Pickworth W, Neider G. Morphine-like insomnia from heroin in nondependent human addicts. Br J Clin Pharmacol 1981; 11:159–169.
49. Lewis S, Oswald I, Evans J, et al, Tompsett S. Heroin and human sleep. Electroencephalogr Clin Neurophysiol 1970; 28:374–381.
50. Farney R, Walker J, Cloward T, et al. Sleep-disordered breathing associated with long-term opioid therapy. Chest 2003; 123:623–639.
51. Shaw I, Lavigne G, Mayer P, et al. Acute intravenous administration of morphine perturbs sleep architecture in healthy pain -free young adults: A preliminary study. Sleep 2005; 28:677–682.
52. Wang D, Teichtahl H. Opioids, sleep architecture, and sleep-disordered breathing. Sleep Med Rev 2007; 11:35–46.
53. Kay D. Human sleep and EEG through a cycle of methadone dependence. Electroencephalogr Clin Neurophysiol 1975; 38:35–43.
54. Gouzoulis E, Steiger A, Ensslin M, et al. Sleep EEG effects of 3, 4-⇔⇓methylenedioxyethamphetamine (MDE;"eve") in healthy volunteers. Biol Psychiatry 1992; 32:1108–1117.

55. Allen R, McCann U, Ricaurte G. Persistent effects of 3, 4-Methylenedioxymethamphetamine (MDMA, "Ecstasy") on human sleep. Sleep 1993; 16:560–564.
56. Ricaurte G, McCann U. Experimental studies on 3, 4-methylenedioxymethamphetamine (MDMA, "Ecstasy") and its potential to damage brain serotonin neurons. Neurotox Res 2001; 3:85–99.
57. McCann U, Ricaurte G. Effects of (±) 3, 4- methylenedioxymethamphetamine (MDMA) on sleep and circadian rhythms. Scientific WorldJournal 2007; 7:231–238.
58. Watson R, Bakos L, Compton P, et al. Cocaine use and withdrawal: Effect on sleep and mood. Am J Drug Alcohol Abuse 1992; 18:21–28.
59. Morgan P, Pace-Schott E, Sahul Z, et al. Sleep, sleep-dependent procedural learning and vigilance in chronic cocaine users: Evidence for occult insomnia. Drug Alcohol Depend 2006; 82:283–349.
60. Biello S, Dafters R. MDMA and fenfluramine alter the response of the circadian clock to a serotonin agonist in vitro. Brain Res 2001; 920:202–209.
61. Valladares E, Eljammal S, Lee J, et al. Sleep dysregulation in cocaine dependence during acute abstinence. Sleep 2006; 29 (suppl) A334.
62. Kowatch R, Schnoll S, Knisely J, et al. Electroencephalographic sleep and mood during cocaine withdrawal. JAddict Dis 1992; 11:21–45.
63. Pace-Schott E, Stickgold R, Mazur A, et al. Sleep quality deteriorates over a binge-abstinence cycle in chronic smoked cocaine users. Psychopharmacology 2005; 179:873–883.
64. Thompson P, Gillin J, Golshan S, et al. Polygraphic sleep measures differentiate alcoholics and stimulant abusers during short term abstinence. Biol Psychiatry 1995; 38:831–836.
65. Johanson C, Roehrs T, Schuh K, et al. The effects of cocaine on mood and sleep in cocaine-dependent males. Exp Clin Psychopharmacol 1999; 7:338–346.
66. Bishop C, Roehrs T, Rosenthal L, et al. Alerting effects of methylphenidate under basal and sleep deprived conditions. Exp Clin Psychopharmacol 1997; 5:344–352.
67. Mitler M, Hajdukovic R, Erman M. Treatment of narcolepsy with methamphetamine. Sleep 1993; 16:306–317.
68. Roehrs T, Papineau K, Rosenthal L, et al. Sleepiness and the reinforcing and subjective effects of methylphenidate. Exp Clin Psychopharmacol 1999; 7:145–150.
69. Mamelak M, Black J, Montplaisir J, et al. A pilot study on the effects of sodium oxybate on sleep architecture and daytime alertness in narcolepsy. Sleep 2004; 27:1327–1334.
70. U.S. Food and Drug Administration. Xyrem (sodium oxybate) oral solution prescribing information. http://www.fda.gov/ohrms/dockets/dockets/05n0479/05N-0479-EC9-Attach-2.pdf (Accessed February 17, 2010).
71. Brower KJ. Alcohol's effects on sleep in alcoholics. Alcohol Res Health 2001; 25:110–125.
72. Aldrich MS, Hall JM, Eiser AS, et al. Slow wave sleep decrement and relapse tendency in alcoholics in treatment. Sleep Res 1994; 23:185.
73. Gann H, Feige B, Hohagen F, et al. Sleep and the cholinergic Rapid Eye Movement sleep induction test in patients with primary alcohol dependence. Biol Psychiatry 2001; 50:383–390.
74. Feige B, Scaal S, Hornyak M, et al. Sleep Electroencephalographic Spectral Power After Withdrawal from Alcohol in Alcohol-Dependent Patients. Alcohol Clin Exp Res 2007; 31:19–27.
75. Conroy D, Arnedt J, Brower K, et al. Perception of sleep in recovering alcohol dependent patients with insomnia: Relationship with future drinking. Alcohol Clin Exp Res 2006; 30:1986–1999.
76. Irwin M, Gillin J, Dang J, et al. Sleep deprivation as a probe of homeostatic sleep regulation in primary alcoholics. Biol Psychiatry 2002; 51:632–641.
77. Farnell Y, West J, Chen W, et al. Developmental alcohol exposure alters light-induced phase shifts of the circadian activity rhythm in rats. Alcohol Clin Exp Res 2004; 28:1020–1027.
78. Chen C, Kuhn P, Advis J, et al. Chronic ethanol consumption impairs the circadian rhythm of pro-opiomelanocortin and period genes mRNA expression in the hypothalamus of the male rat. J Neurochem 2004; 88:1547–1554.
79. Prosser R, Mangrum C, Glass J. Acute ethanol modulates glutamatergic and serotonergic phase shifts of the mouse circadian clock in vitro. Neuroscience 2007; 152:837–848.
80. Aldrich M, Shipley J. Alcohol use and periodic limb movements of sleep. Alcohol Clin Exp Res 1993; 17:192–196.
81. Riedel B, Durrence H, Lichstein K, et al. The relation between smoking and sleep: The influence of smoking level, health, and psychological variables. Behav Sleep Med 2004; 2:63–78.
82. Biaggioni I, Paul S, Puckett A, et al. Caffeine and theophylline as adenosine receptor antagonists in humans. J Pharmacol Exp Ther 1991; 258:588–593.
83. Roehrs T, Roth T. Caffeine: Sleep and daytime sleepiness. Sleep Med Rev 2008; 12:153–162.
84. James J, Keane M. Caffeine, sleep, and wakefulness: Implications of new understanding about withdrawal reversal. Hum Psychopharmacol 2007; 22:549–558.
85. Nicholson A, Stone B. Heterocyclic amphetamine derivative and caffeine on sleep in man. Br J Clin Pharmacol 1980; 9:195–203.

86. Wyatt J, Cajochen C, Ritz-De Cecco A, et al. Low-dose repeated caffeine administration for circadian-phase dependent performance degredation during extended wakefulness. Sleep 2004; 27: 374–381.
87. Bonnet M, Tancer M, Uhde T, et al. Effects of caffeine on heart rate and QT variability during sleep. Depress Anxiety 2005; 22:150–155.
88. Hughes J, Oliveto A, Bickel W, et al. Caffeine self-administration and withdrawal: Incidence, individual differences and interrelationships. Drug Alcohol Depend 1993; 32:239–246.
89. Pertwee R. Cannabinoid receptors and pain. Prog Neurobiol 2001; 63:569–611.
90. Cousens K, Dimascio A. Delta-9- THC as an hypnotic. An experimental study of 3 dose levels. Psychopharmacologia 1973; 33:355–364.
91. Schierenbeck T, Riemann D, Berger M, et al. Effect of illicit recreational drugs upon sleep: Cocaine, ecstasy, and marijuana. Sleep Med Rev 2008; 12:381–389.
92. Wiesbeck G, Schuckit M, Kalmijn J, et al. An evaluation of the history of marijuana withdrawal syndrome in a large population. Addiction 1996; 91:1469–1478.
93. Arendt M, Rosenberg R, Foldager L, et al. Withdrawal symptoms do not predict relapse among subjects treated for cannabis dependence. Am J Addict 2007; 16:461–467.
94. Shi J, Zhao L, Epstein D, et al. Long-term methadone maintenance reduces protracted symptoms of heroin abstinence and cue-induced craving in Chinese heroin abusers. Pharmacol Biochem Behav 2007; 87:141–145.
95. Vella-Brincat J, Macleod A. Adverse effects of opioids on the central nervous systems of palliative care patients. J Pain Palliat Care Pharmacother 2007; 21:15–25.
96. Kay D, Einstein R, Jasinski D. Morphine effects on human REM state, waking state and NREM sleep. Psychopharmacologia 1969; 14:404–416.
97. Watson C, Lydic R, Baghdoyan H. Sleep and GABA levels in the oral part of rat pontine reticular formation are decreased by local and systemic administration of morphine. Neuroscience 2007; 144:375–386.
98. Walker J, Farney R, Rhondeau S, et al. Chronic opioid use is a risk factor for the development of central sleep apnea and ataxic breathing. J Clin Sleep Med 2007; 3:455–461.
99. Teicher M, Wang D. Sleep disordered breathing with chronic opioid use. Expert Opin Drug Saf 2007; 6:641–649.
100. Parrott A. Human psychopharmacology of Ecstasy (MDMA): A review of 15 years of empirical research. Hum Psychopharmacol 2001; 16:557–577.
101. Jansen K. Ecstasy (MDMA) dependence. Drug Alcohol Depend 1999; 53:121–124.
102. McCann U, Peterson S, Ricaurte G. The effect of catecholamine depletion by alpha-methyl-para-tyrosine on measures of cognitive performance and sleep in abstinent MDMA users. Neuropsychopharmacology 2007; 32:1695–1706.
103. Balogh B, Molnar E, Jakus R, et al. Effects of a single dose of 3,4 methylenedioxymethamphetamine on circadian patterns, motor activity and sleep in drug naive rats and rats previously exposed to MDMA. Psychopharmacology (Berl) 2004; 173:296–309.
104. Morgan P, Mailison R. Cocaine and sleep:early abstinence. Scientific WorldJournal 2007; 7:223–230.
105. Lynch W, Girgenti M, Breslin F, et al. Gene profiling the response to repeat cocaine self-administration in dorsal striatum: A focus on circadian genes. Brain Res 2008; 1213:166–177.
106. Roybal K, Theobold D, Graham A, et al. Mania-like behavior induced by disruption of CLOCK. Proc Natl Acad Sci U S A 2007; 104:6406–6411.
107. Nishino S, Mignot E. Wake-promoting medications: Basic mechanisms and pharmacology. In: Kryger M, Roth T, Dement W, eds. Principles and Practice of Sleep Medicine, 4th ed. Philadelphia, PA: Elsevier Saunders, 2005:468–483.
108. Kanbayashi T, Honda K, Kodama T, et al. Implication of dopaminergic mechanisms in the wake-promoting effects of amphetamine: a study of D- and L-derivatives in canine narcolepsy. Neuroscience 2000; 99:651–659.
109. Gossop M, Bradley B, Brewis R. Amphetamine withdrawal and sleep disturbance. Drug Alcohol Depend 1982; 10:177–183.
110. McGregor C, Srisurapanont M, Jittiwutikarn J, et al. The nature, time course and severity of methamphetamine withdrawal. Addiction 2005; 100:1320–1329.
111. Friedmann PD, Herman DS, Freedman S, et al. Treatment of sleep disturbance in alcohol recovery: A national survey of addiction medicine physicians. J Addict Dis 2003; 22:91–103.
112. Mendelson WB, Roth T, Cassella J, et al. The treatment of chronic insomnia: Drug indications, chronic use and abuse liability. Summary of a 2001 New Clinical Drug Evaluation Unit Meeting Symposium. Sleep Med Rev 2004; 8:7–17.
113. Griffiths RR, Johnson MW. Relative abuse liability of hypnotic drugs: A conceptual framework and algorithm for differentiating among compounds. J Clin Psychiatry 2005; 66:31–41.
114. Roehrs T, Roth T. Hypnotics: An update. Curr Neurol Neurosci Rep 2003; 3:181–184.

115. Aubin H-J, Goldenberg F, Benoit O, et al. Effects of tetrabamate and of diazepam on sleep polygraphy during subacute withdrawal in alcohol-dependent patients. Hum Psychopharmacol 1994; 9:191–195.
116. Graham AW. Sleep disorders. In: Graham AW, Schultz T, eds. Principles of Addiction Medicine. Chevy Chase, MD: American Society of Addiction Medicine, 1998:793–808.
117. Ciraulo DA, Nace EP. Benzodiazepine treatment of anxiety or insomnia in substance abuse patients. Am J Addict 2000; 9:276–284.
118. Hajak G, Müller WE, Wittchen HU, et al. Abuse and dependence potential for the non-benzodiazepine hypnotics zolpidem and zopiclone: A review of case reports and epidemiological data. Addiction 2003; 98:1371–1378.
119. Johnson B, Longo LP. Considerations in the physician's decision to prescribe benzodiazepines to patients with addiction. Psychiatr Ann 1998; 28:160–165.
120. Kranzler HR. Evaluation and treatment of anxiety symptoms and disorders in alcoholics. J Clin Psychiatry 1996; 57:15–21.
121. Schuckit MA. Recent developments in the pharmacotherapy of alcohol dependence. J Consult Clin Psychol 1996; 64:669–676.
122. Swift RM. Pharmacologic treatment for drug and alcohol dependence: Experimental and standard therapies. Psychiatr Ann 1998; 28:697–702.
123. Malcolm R Jr., Myrick H, Roberts J, et al. The differential effects of medication on mood, sleep disturbance, and work ability in outpatient alcohol detoxification. Am J Addict 2002; 11:141–150.
124. LaRoche S, Helmers S. The new antiepileptic drug. JAMA 2004; 291:605–614.
125. Karam-Hage M, Brower KJ. Gabapentin treatment for insomnia associated with alcohol dependence. Am J psychiatry 2000; 157:151.
126. Karam-Hage M, Brower KJ. Open pilot study of gabapentin versus trazodone to treat insomnia in alcoholic patients. Psychiatry Clin Neurosci 2003; 57:542–544.
127. Rosenberg KP. Gabapentin for chronic insomnia. Am J Addict 2003; 12:273–274.
128. Brower KJ, Kim HB, Strobbe S, et al. A randomized double-blind pilot trial of gabapentin vs. placebo to treat alcohol dependence and comorbid insomnia. Alcohol Clin Exp Res. 2008; 32:1429–1438.
129. Armitage R. The effects of antidepressants on sleep in patients with depression. Can J Psychiatry 2000; 45:803–809.
130. Mendelson WB. A review of the evidence for the efficacy and safety of trazodone for insomnia. J Clin Psychiatry 2005; 66:469–476.
131. Kaynak H, Kaynak D, Gozukirmizi E, et al. The effects of trazodone on sleep in patients treated with stimulant antidepressants. Sleep Med 2004; 5:15–20.
132. Nierenberg AA, Adler LA, Peselow E, et al. Trazadone for antidepressant-associated insomnia. Am J Psychiatry 1994; 151:1069–1072.
133. Janiri L, Hadjichristos A, Buonanno A, et al. Adjuvant trazodone in the treatment of alcoholism: An open study. Alcohol Alcohol 1998; 33:362–365.
134. Le Bon O, Murphy J, Staner L, et al. Double-blind, placebo controlled study of the efficacy of trazodone in alcohol post-withdrawal sydrome: Polysomnography and clinical evaluations. J Clin Psychopharmacol 2003; 23:377–383.
135. Friedmann PD, Rose JS, Swift RM, et al. Trazodone for sleep disturbance after detoxification from alcohol dependence: A double-blind, placebo-controlled trial. In: American Academy of Addiction Psychiatry 18th Annual Meeting & Symposium. 2007; Coronado, CA.
136. Cohrs S, Rodenbeck A, Guan Z, et al. Sleep-promoting properties of quetiapine in healthy subjects. Psychopharmacology 2004; 174:421–429.
137. Monnelly EP, Ciraulo DA, Knapp C, et al. Quetiapine for treatment of alcohol dependence. J Clin Psychopharmacol 2004; 24:532–535.
138. Catalano G, Grace JW, Catalano MC, et al. Acute akathisia associated with quetiapine use. Psychosomatics 2005; 46:291–301.
139. Cajochen C, Krauchi K, Wirz-Justice A. Role of melatonin in the regulation of human circadian rhythms and sleep. J Neuroendocrinol 2003; 15:432–437.
140. Greeff AP, Conradie WS. Use of progressive relaxation training for chronic alcoholics with insomnia. Psychol Rep 1998; 82:407–412.
141. Currie SR, Clark S, Hodgins DC, et al. Randomized controlled trial of brief cognitive-behavioural interventions for insomnia in recovering alcohlics. Addiction 2004; 99:1121–1132.
142. Arnedt J, Conroy D, Rutt J, et al. An open trial of cognitive-behavioral treatment for insomnia comorbid with alcohol dependence. Sleep Med 2007; 8:176–180.
143. Bootzin RR, Stevens S. Adolescents, substance abuse, and the treatment of insomnia and daytime sleepiness. Clin Psychol Rev 2005; 25:629–644.
144. Haynes PL, Bootzin RR, Smith L, et al. Sleep and aggression in substance-abusing adolescents: Results from an integrative behavioral sleep-treatment pilot program. Sleep 2006; 29:512–520.

17 Insomnia in Circadian Rhythm Sleep Disorders: Shift Work/Jet Lag/DSP/ASP/Free-Running—Blindness

Robert L. Sack
Oregon Health and Science University, Portland, Oregon, U.S.A.

INTRODUCTION

Circadian rhythm sleep disorders (CRSDs) arise from either an alteration in the function of the circadian timing system or a misalignment between the circadian rhythm of sleep propensity and the requirements of the environmental or socially structured sleep schedule. There are six recognized CRSDs: (*i*) delayed sleep phase disorder (DSPD), (*ii*) advanced sleep phase disorder (ASPD), (*iii*) irregular sleep–wake disorder (ISWD), (*iv*) free-running disorder (FRD), also called nonentrained or non–24-hour sleep–wake disorder, (*v*) jet lag disorder (JLD), and (*vi*) shift work disorder (SWD). Insomnia (difficulty falling asleep or staying asleep) is a major symptom of all the CRSDs, as well as sleepiness and dysphoria while awake. To meet the full diagnostic criteria for a sleep disorder, the symptoms must be persistent and involve a significant impairment in social, occupational, or other areas of function.

DIAGNOSTIC CONSIDERATIONS

Although the formal diagnostic criteria developed by the American Academy of Sleep Medicine (AASM) (1) are intended to distinguish clinical disorders from normal variability, the dividing line is not always sharp. Symptoms are likely to occur in otherwise unaffected people if the circadian system is significantly challenged, as in long distance jet travel or shift work. There is ambiguity about the relevance of the formal diagnostic criteria to a clinical population since the criteria have rarely been used in research studies (2,3). In any case, the principles of treatment are similar whether the symptoms are mild (subclinical) or more severe. The clinician needs to judge whether a patient meets criteria for a formal diagnosis and decide how aggressive treatment should be.

EPIDEMIOLOGY AND CONSEQUENCES

Data on the epidemiology of CRSDs are quite limited, but considering that millions of people work unconventional schedules and travel across time zones, the prevalence of SWD and JLD must be high. In addition, many young people have a tendency for DSPD, and older people, for ASPD, whether or not they meet full criteria.

Although CRSDs are common, patients with these disorders do not seek medical attention as frequently as patients with other sleep disorders. There could be a number of reasons. Patients with SWD and JLD often accept their symptoms as an inevitable burden of their circumstance, which will ultimately remit when their situation changes. Patients with DSPD or ASPD may consider their sleep pattern as so ingrained in their makeup that it would be very difficult to change. Perhaps a more important reason that these patients do not present to the sleep clinic is a lack of public awareness regarding the safe and effective treatments that are available. It is unfortunate that severely affected patients may suffer recurrent educational or occupational failure, or endure lifelong impairment, when simple treatments are available. The theme of this chapter is that the therapy of CRSDs can be based on well-developed principles derived from circadian science.

CIRCADIAN MISALIGNMENT: THE UNDERLYING PATHOPHYSIOLOGY OF CIRCADIAN RHYTHM SLEEP DISORDERS

Although the CRSDs have different etiologies, they share a common pathophysiology; namely, a misalignment between the endogenous circadian rhythms and the desired (or required) time for sleep. This misalignment in timing can arise from either exogenous or endogenous factors (or both). For example, in JLD and SWD, rhythms are misaligned because of an externally imposed shift in the timing of sleep. In the other CRSDs, misalignment is hypothesized to involve abnormalities of the circadian system itself; for example, in DSPD the intrinsic circadian period may be unusually long, and in ASPD, unusually short; or there may be subsensitivity to the usual circadian time cues. In ISWD associated with dementia, the amplitude of the circadian signal may be diminished. However, the distinction between exogenous and endogenous factors is not always sharp; for example, an "owl" (a person with a tendency for DSPS) may have no problem with insomnia until the requirements of a new job involve going to bed earlier and getting up earlier.

The opponent process model of sleep regulation, as formulated by Edgar et al. (4), readily explains the consequences of circadian misalignment. The model postulates that, during the day, homeostatic sleep drive accumulates in proportion to the duration of prior wakefulness (Fig. 1). However, the accumulation of sleep drive is not manifest as sleepiness during the day because it is counteracted (opposed) by a circadian alerting process. As bedtime approaches, this circadian alerting process wanes, the accumulated sleep drive is unopposed, and normally a person becomes sleepy and ready for bed. Whether the circadian system actively promotes sleep at night, or simply does not oppose it, is debated by circadian scientists. During sleep, the accumulated sleep drive is discharged, and in the morning the cycle begins again. These homeostatic and circadian processes are normally synchronized with each other and with the 24-hour solar and social day–night cycle.

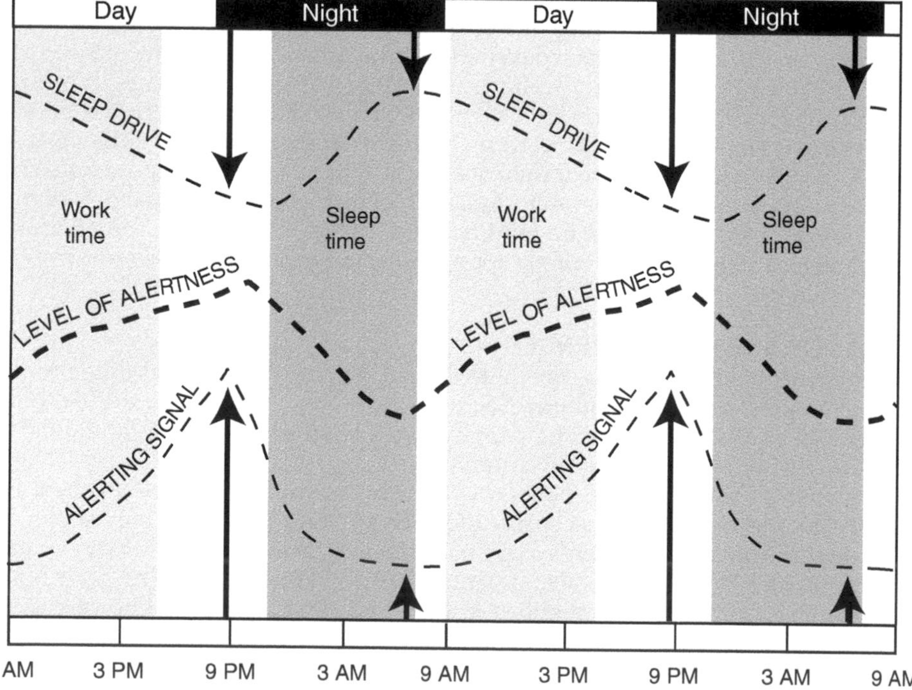

Figure 1 The opponent process model of sleep regulation on a conventional sleep schedule. The opponent process model proposed by Edgar et al. (4) is illustrated in a double-plotted hypothetical diagram. According to the model, the level of alertness (sleepiness) is a vector sum derived from the opposing forces of sleep drive, which accumulates in proportion to the duration of prior wakefulness (shown as a downward force), and an alerting signal, generated by the circadian pacemaker in the SCN (shown as an upward force). During the day, sleep drive accumulates, but is counteracted by the opposing alerting signal. In the early evening, the alerting signal peaks and, even though sleep drive is strong, initiating sleep is difficult. Prior to bedtime, the alerting signal recedes, sleepiness emerges, sleep commences, and sleep drive dissipates. At the time of final awakening, sleep drive is at a minimum. After sleep inertia has receded, the daytime level of alertness is restored to a normal zone.

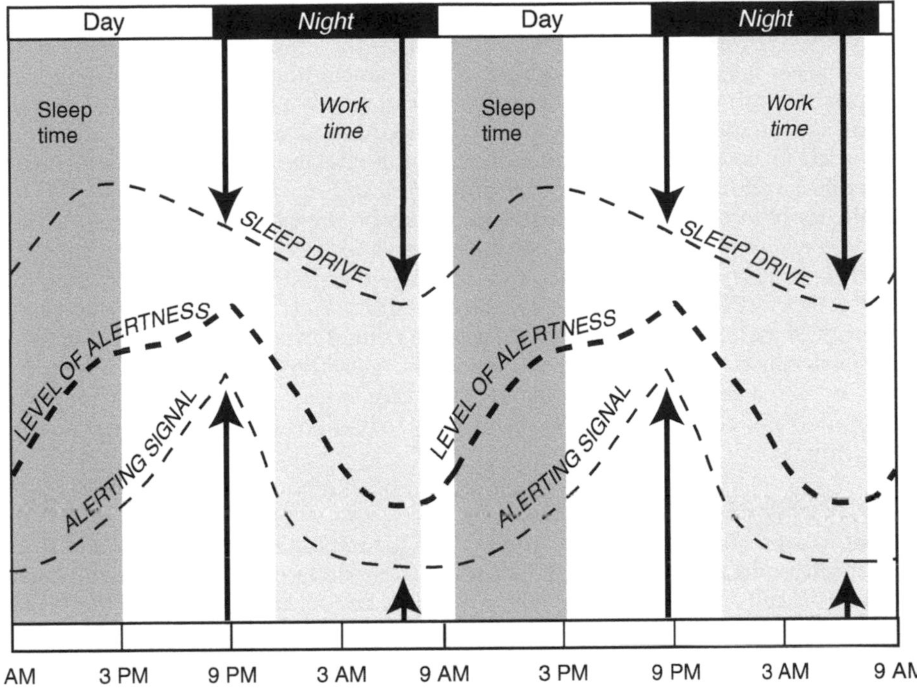

Figure 2 The opponent process model of sleep regulation in a night shift worker. This diagram illustrates the role of the opponent process on alertness in a night shift worker that has made no circadian adaptation. Daytime sleep is undermined and shortened by the circadian alerting process: consequently, overall sleep drive is increased due to insufficient, nonrestorative sleep. Furthermore, the timing of work is coincident with a recession of the alerting signal; consequently, the accumulated sleep drive is unopposed by the SCN alerting. With the combination of a high burden of sleep drive and a lack of circadian alerting, sleep may be very difficult to resist toward the end of the night or on the drive home.

When homeostatic and circadian processes are out of alignment, the inappropriately timed circadian alerting process interferes with sleep. Depending on the relationship of the circadian alerting signal to the timing of attempted sleep, there can be difficulties getting to sleep, staying asleep, as well as waking up too early. Moreover, during the intervening periods of wake, the circadian alerting signal is weak or absent, and does not sufficiently counteract the accumulated sleep drive (or may actively promote sleep) resulting in unwelcome sleepiness and dysphoria.

A multitude of physiological processes are driven by the circadian pacemaker, including cyclic variations in core body temperature, melatonin, and cortisol secretion, as well as glucose and lipid metabolism. These abnormalities in circadian synchrony may increase the risk for cardiovascular and metabolic disorders.

In addition to these endogenous mechanisms, sleep at nonstandard times can be interrupted by ambient noise and light, as well as pressing social obligations. Furthermore, there is an unavoidable degree of sleep deprivation associated with sudden transitions in the sleep schedule as occur in SWD and JLD. The various consequences of circadian misalignment as exemplified in SWD are illustrated in Figure 2 and discussed in the accompanying legend.

DIAGNOSTIC ASSESSMENT

The treatment of CRSDs needs to be preceded by a careful history to rule out other primary sleep disorders and to characterize behavior patterns (e.g., ill-timed recreational or social activities) or other factors (e.g., chronic illness, medication side effects, caffeine intake) that may be exacerbating the problem. Difficulty falling asleep or waking up too early may suggest a CRSD, but other causes of sleep onset or maintenance insomnia need to be considered, especially psychophysiological insomnia as well as anxiety and depressive disorders.

A sleep diary is always a useful assessment instrument when a CRSD is suspected. Data should be collected for at least two weeks and include the times of "light's off" and "light's on," estimated sleep latency, final awakening, and the recording of medications, alcohol use, or other factors that influence sleep. Actigraphy, if available, is extremely useful to corroborate diary data and to provide objective assessment of sleep timing and quality. The Morningness–Eveningness scale (5) can corroborate the preference for a delayed or advanced sleep schedule, but cannot replace a clinical interview and evaluation.

An indicator of internal circadian timing ("hands on the clock") would provide the most objective way to evaluate the alignment between sleep and circadian phase. However, the two methods most frequently used in the research setting—the timing of melatonin secretion and the core body temperature rhythm under constant conditions—have not been applied clinically. Measuring onset of melatonin secretion in the evening either in serial plasma or saliva samples (dim light melatonin onset or *DLMO*) (6) would be feasible in a sleep laboratory, but the melatonin assay is not readily available as yet. The constant routine protocol (7) required for valid measurements of core temperature rhythms is very labor intensive and not suitable for the clinical setting.

GENERAL PRINCIPLES OF TREATMENT

It is important to set realistic goals for treatment that the patient is clearly motivated to accomplish. For example, some patients with DSPD have a strong preference for their atypical schedule and may have difficulty understanding why others do not accommodate it. If the problem is impacting the family, they should be involved in the treatment as well.

There are three general treatment strategies that have been used to treat CRSDs: (1) prescribed sleep scheduling, designed to either improve the alignment between sleep and the underlying rhythms, or to minimize the consequences of misalignment. (2) Pharmacotherapy (using hypnotic or alerting medication) aimed at counteracting the symptoms of insomnia and/or sleepiness that are generated by circadian misalignment. (3) Circadian phase shifting ("resetting the body clock"); that is, realigning circadian rhythms with the desired sleep schedule by administering appropriately timed bright light exposure or melatonin. Combining two or more of these intervention strategies may be warranted. Circadian phase shifting is a treatment that is quite specific for CRSDs and therefore its basis, derived from circadian science, will be explained in more detail.

Phase Shifting with Appropriately Timed Light Exposure

In all mammals, the fundamental intrinsic circadian rhythm is generated by the activity of *clock genes* that regulate a translational–transcription feedback cycle within individual neurons of the suprachiasmatic nucleus (SCN) in the hypothalamus. The output of the SCN (the circadian signal) represents the summation of rhythms generated by a population of SCN neurons, and is usually slightly longer or shorter than 24 hours. Therefore normal synchronization (entrainment) of the circadian pacemaker to the 24-hour day requires recurrent timing adjustments (phase resetting) that, in turn, depend on exposure to relevant environmental time cues (zeitgebers)—most importantly, the solar light/dark cycle. Signals from specialized photoreceptors in the retina carry information about the level of illumination directly to the SCN via a retinal-hypothalamic tract that is separate from the visual pathway. If a person is isolated from environmental times cues (or is totally blind, with no light perception), circadian rhythms will typically "free-run" on a non–24-hour cycle reflecting the intrinsic period of the nonentrained circadian pacemaker.

In nature, the solar light–dark cycle is the most potent environmental time cue for synchronizing the circadian pacemaker, for humans, as well as most other species. If circadian rhythms drift out of alignment, exposure to the solar light–dark cycle will normally provide a corrective advance or delay, thereby maintaining a stable relationship of the circadian system to the 24-hour day. Specifically, light exposure in the morning will reset the body clock to an earlier time (cause a phase advance), while light exposure in the evening will reset the body clock to a later time (cause a phase delay) (Fig. 2). These timing (phase)-dependent effects of light exposure can be plotted as a light phase response curve (PRC). The magnitude of the phase shifts is greatest around the inflection point of the PRC (around 5 AM in normally entrained individuals) and is least (but not absent) with light exposure in mid-day [reviewed by Duffy and Wright (8)].

Appropriately timed bright light exposure (3000–10,000 lux) has been shown to produce robust phase shifts, but even modest intensities (100–550 lux) can produce substantial phase shifts if subjects have been living in a constant dim light environment. Also, intermittent bright light exposure can produce almost as much phase shifting as continuous exposure (9). Recently, specialized nonrod, noncone photoreceptors, associated with the ganglion cells of the retina, that are maximally sensitive to blue-green light, have been shown to be important for the circadian phase resetting (10). Clinical trials are underway to determine if exposure to blue-green light has advantages. Reports of phase shifting with light exposure to the skin (11) have not been replicated (12,13).

People usually sleep at night, in a dark room, with eyelids closed; thus, the timing of sleep structures (or "gates") an individual's exposure to the light/dark cycle and in this way sleep can indirectly (but importantly) influence circadian timing. Because sleep and reduced light exposure occur together, it has been difficult to determine if sleep itself, apart from its gating effect on light exposure, influences rhythms. Other possible nonphotic time cues, for example, timed physical activity, may have some influence on circadian rhythms, but are not as potent as light exposure.

Timed light exposure as a treatment modality usually involves a bright artificial light source (3000 to 10,000 lux). There have been some safety concerns with light of this intensity, especially the possibility of phototoxic effects on the lens and/or the retina, but it can be argued that the intensities are no greater than sunlight on a clear, sunny day. Nevertheless, bright light sources should be used with caution in patients with ocular pathology (e.g., lenticular cataracts or retinal degeneration). In early experiments with light therapy "full spectrum" sources that included UV radiation were employed for light therapy, but UV wavelengths are unnecessary and should be avoided (14). A diffuser panel placed over the light sources effectively filters UV radiation.

In summary, the phase-resetting effects of light are dependent on intensity, timing, wavelength, pattern (intermittent or continuous), duration, exposure history, and the level of contrast with background light exposure. In clinical practice, it is customary to employ light exposure from a commercially available light source that generates diffuse illumination with an intensity of 3000 to 10,000 lux for 30 to 60 minutes, at a time of day that will promote the desired phase-shifting effect. If light exposure is to be carried out on a regular basis, compliance will be poor if it is not integrated into some other daily activity (e.g., eating, watching television, reading, etc.). The light can be indirect; that is, patients do not need to fix their gaze at a light source. Used in this way, timed bright light exposure appears to be safe within the parameters that have been tested. Appropriately timed exposure to ordinary daylight, when feasible, can be just as effective, and is less expensive than an artificial light source.

If the goal is to synchronize the circadian system to the desired (or required) sleep schedule, appropriately timed light exposure should, in principle, be a helpful intervention for almost all of the CRSDs, although it may be impractical or even impossible to implement in some circumstances. Likewise, eliminating (or reducing) the unwanted effects of light on the circadian system (by staying indoors or wearing goggles) has been shown to inhibit unwanted phase shifting (15).

Phase Shifting with Timed Melatonin Administration

Melatonin is a hormone produced by the pineal gland at night, in the dark. Its effects on the circadian system are opposite to light exposure, so it is useful to think of it as a "darkness signal." Hence, melatonin administration in the morning shifts rhythms later, while melatonin administration in the evening shifts rhythms earlier (16) (Fig. 3). In other words, the melatonin PRC is about 180 degrees out of phase with the light PRC. Melatonin administration to both animals and humans has been shown to be sufficiently potent to entrain free-running rhythms.

The use of melatonin and melatonin agonists to directly promote sleep (a soporific effect as distinct from a phase-shifting effect) is discussed in a later chapter. In general, the soporific activity of melatonin appears to be more prominent with higher doses, and when it is administered at

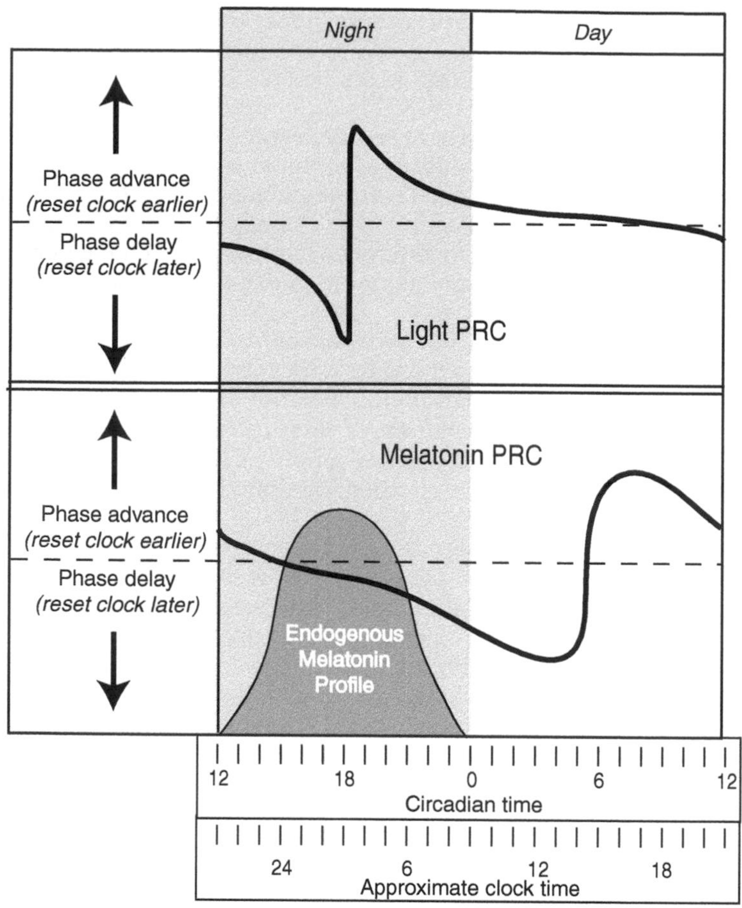

Figure 3 Schematic phase response curves (PRCs) for light and melatonin administration. The effects of light and melatonin are dependent on the timing (phase) of administration, a relationship that can be plotted as a phase response curve (PRC). Light exposure late in the day or melatonin administration in the morning will cause the circadian clock to shift later (a phase delay); on the other hand, light exposure in the morning or melatonin administration late in the day will cause the circadian clock to shift earlier (a phase advance). Both light and melatonin PRCs have an inflection point, the crossover time between advances and delays. According to convention, circadian time 0 is the beginning of the light phase (daytime) and circadian time 12 is the beginning of the dark phase (nighttime).

those times of the day when endogenous melatonin is not being secreted. Sleep promoting and phase-shifting effects may occur concurrently, depending on the timing and dose, and in some instances, one or the other may be considered undesirable; for example, an early morning dose of melatonin may promote an intended phase delay but an associated hypnotic effect would be unwelcome. Likewise, melatonin taken at bedtime for sleep maintenance insomnia related to an advanced circadian phase might exacerbate the problem by promoting a further phase advance.

Appropriately timed melatonin and light exposure may have synergistic phase-shifting effects (17), and melatonin can counteract, to some extent, the effect of light exposure on the circadian system if light and melatonin are promoting shifts in opposite directions.

A variety of doses of melatonin have been used for phase shifting, and it appears that the shape of a dose response curve for this effect is rather flat; that is, there is not a great deal of difference between lower and higher doses. Timing of administration appears to be more important than dose. Paradoxically, it is possible for a high dose to be less effective than a low dose. In one report, a low dose (0.5 mg per day) was able to normally entrain a blind person with free-running rhythms after a high dose (up to 20 mg) had failed (18). The authors suggested that the higher dose overlapped both the advance and delay portions of the melatonin PRC, canceling out a phase-resetting effect, while the lower dose targeted just the phase advance region.

Melatonin is widely available in the United States as a "nutritional supplement" but has not been approved by the FDA as a drug. Concerns have been raised about the purity of the available preparations, as well as the reliability of stated doses. Labels that feature a GMP seal, which stands for *Good Manufacturing Practice*, provide some assurance of the purity and accuracy of stated doses.

Commonly available melatonin formulations of 3 mg produce blood levels that are at least 10-fold higher than physiological concentrations; however, no serious adverse reactions have been attributed to these supra-physiological doses. Recently, a melatonin agonist, ramelteon has been licensed as a hypnotic in the United States and other melatonin agonists are in development. Animal studies suggest that ramelteon has phase-shifting effects that are analogous to melatonin (19) but, at this time, no studies have been reported in humans.

Other Phase-Shifting Treatments

Timed vigorous exercise has been tested for its phase-shifting effects, but does not appear to be as potent as appropriately timed light or melatonin administration. In some experiments, animals have been entrained to the time of feeding, but this has not been demonstrated to be effective in humans.

Prescribed Sleep Scheduling

It is sometimes possible to devise a sleep schedule, based on an understanding of circadian physiology that will minimize or remediate CRSD symptoms for example. Some examples will be provided under the sections regarding the treatment of DSPS and SWD.

Symptomatic Treatment

Counteracting Insomnia

As discussed above, the circadian pacemaker generates an alerting signal during the day (in diurnal species) that counteracts the expression of accumulated homeostatic sleep drive (4). During the normal time for sleep at night, this alerting signal is withdrawn. In CRSDs, there is a mismatch so that the circadian alerting signal occurs during the desired (or required) time for sleep, potentially generating insomnia, usually manifested as foreshortened sleep. Hypnotic drugs or other treatments for insomnia can be used to counteract the unwelcome clock-dependent alerting in patients with CRSDs.

Counteracting Excessive Sleepiness

Circadian misalignment can produce excessive sleepiness in at least two ways: (*i*) insomnia (see above) shortens time asleep resulting in an accumulation of homeostatic sleep drive, (*ii*) the activity of the circadian alerting process is reduced when the person desires to be awake.

Caffeine is the most widely used alerting agent in our culture and is effective in counteracting sleepiness from almost any cause, but if over-used, can worsen insomnia. Amphetamine-related drugs are more potent than caffeine and may be indicated in some patients with CRSDs. Modafanil is the only drug that has been specially approved by the FDA for a CRSD; namely, SWD.

Having discussed the general principles of circadian biology and modalities of treatment, the remainder of this chapter will focus on specific CRSDs.

DELAYED SLEEP PHASE SYNDROME

DSPD is characterized by a recurrent or chronic complaint of not being able to fall asleep at a desired or conventional time, as well as an extreme inability to awaken when desired or required [for a recent review, see Wyatt (20)]. When there are no constraints on the timing of sleep, patients with DSPD may sleep quite normally, albeit at a delayed time frame. They typically seek help when unable to conform to conventional work schedules or other social demands. A tendency for a delayed sleep schedule is very common in adolescence and young adulthood, but this could reflect life style issues as well as a biological tendency.

DSPD is the most common CRSD diagnosis among patients presenting to a sleep disorders center; nevertheless, these individuals represent but a small percentage of the patients who would qualify for the diagnosis that is estimated to be between 360,000 to several million people in the United States alone (20). The disorder is more common in men than women. Weitzman, who first described the syndrome (21), originally proposed that a significant number of patients with a diagnosis of sleep onset insomnia may, in fact, have underlying subsyndromal DSPD. If true, it would imply that an appreciable subgroup of insomnia patients should respond to circadian-based interventions.

It is often suggested that patients with DSPS have an intrinsic circadian period that is longer than average and that is why they have such difficulty resetting their circadian pacemaker (and sleep schedule) to an earlier time frame; however, other mechanisms; such as a subsensitivity to the phase-advancing effects of light could explain the disorder. Okawa and Uchiyama have recently published a detailed review of possible mechanisms (22).

Timed Light Exposure

Bright light exposure in the morning, on the advance portion of the light PRC, would be expected to shift circadian rhythms to an earlier time, thereby correcting a pathological phase delay. Although the evidence is limited, this hypothesis has been supported in a few clinical trials. For example, Rosenthal et al. (23) in a cross-over design, compared bright light (2500 lux) to dim light (300 lux) exposure, two hours per day (6 AM to 9 AM), for two weeks in 20 patients with DSPD. The bright light treatment produced a greater benefit, as judged by self-report. In addition, bright light produced a larger advance in the core body temperature rhythm and increased morning alertness as measured with an MSLT.

The optimal intensity and duration of morning bright light exposure for DSPD remains undefined, and practical, realistic arrangements need to be negotiated with the patient. In our clinic, we aim for at least 3000 lux for at least 30 minutes, beginning shortly after awakening, and integrated with other morning activities such as eating breakfast or applying makeup. We provide a schedule on a spreadsheet that starts with the patient's current sleep schedule, and advances the timing of sleep and light exposure gradually (15 to 30 minutes, every few days). Since advancing the circadian system in these patients is challenging, attempting to normalize the schedule too quickly can lead to failure and frustration. Limiting light exposure in the evening (when it has a delaying effect) may augment the response.

In clinical practice, an artificial light source may be unnecessary if the wake-up time occurs after sunrise; simply going outside into sunlight for 20 to 30 minutes upon awakening may provide the required exposure. Compliance with light therapy is a major challenge as patients with DSPD because their notorious sleep inertia is reflected in their extraordinary difficulty waking up in the morning when the light exposure is needed.

Timed Melatonin Administration

Melatonin administration in the afternoon or evening would be expected to shift rhythms earlier, thereby correcting a pathological phase delay. In an early double-blind crossover study, Dahlitz et al. (24) gave eight patients with DSPD melatonin (5 mg), or placebo at 22:00, five hours before the average sleep onset time for four weeks. Melatonin treatment shifted sleep onset times 82 minutes earlier (on average) and wake-up times 117 minutes earlier. In a large ($N = 61$), open-label study, those receiving 5 mg of melatonin given at 22:00 for six weeks reported significant benefit, but also a high rate of relapse when treatment was discontinued (level 4) (25).

In a double-blind trial, Kayumov et al. (26) administered melatonin (5 mg between 19:00 and 21:00) for four weeks. Treatment normalized the melatonin rhythm, and significantly reduced sleep onset latency as determined by PSG. However, total sleep time as measured by PSG, was not improved, nor were self-reported measures of daytime alertness.

In a recent double-blind study, two doses of melatonin (0.3 and 3 mg) were administered between 1.5 and 6.5 hours prior to the pretreatment DLMO for four weeks. Both doses advanced the DLMO and CBT rhythm. On further analysis, the earlier the melatonin was administered relative to DLMO, the larger was the phase advance.

The optimal time for melatonin administration would be at the peak of the phase advance portion of the melatonin PRC, but until circadian marker such as the DLMO becomes clinically available, appropriate timing has to be estimated. In our clinic, we provide the patient with a schedule (like the one for light therapy) that initiates treatment (0.5 to 3 mg) at about three to four hours prior to habitual bedtime, and then gradually shifts the timing of both melatonin administration and bedtime earlier (15 to 30 minutes every few days).

Prescribed Sleep Schedule

The term *chronotherapy* was originally coined to describe a prescribed sleep schedule treatment for DSPD in which patients are instructed to intentionally, and systematically, delay their sleep several hours per day until it is aligned to a targeted bedtime (27). After the patient achieves this goal, they are instructed to scrupulously maintain their new sleep schedule lest they relapse and the procedure has to be repeated. Chronotherapy is based on the hypothesis that the human circadian period is usually longer than 24 hours and might be exceptionally long in patients with DSPD. This would account for the great difficulty DSPD patients have in shifting their sleep schedule to an earlier time, and why delaying sleep would be easier.

Pharmacologic Symptom Control

Hypnotic medications have not been systematically tested for DSPS, and are not recommended as monotherapy, but can be a reasonable adjunctive measure for those nights when the patient's sleep latency extends 30 minutes beyond the prescribed bedtime.

Combination Treatment

In our clinic, evening melatonin and morning bright light are often prescribed in tandem, utilizing a schedule (provided by a computer-generated worksheet) that gradually advances the timing of attempted sleep and the timing of both treatments by 15 to 30 minutes every few days. These gradual shifts in schedule are based on an understanding that large circadian "phase jumps" are difficult to achieve, especially phase advances, and therefore attempting to shift sleep times too quickly may lead to failure and the abandonment of treatment. Once the desired schedule is accomplished, maintenance treatment with light and melatonin can be continued on a stable, fixed schedule.

Many patients with DSPS have a strong personal preference for being awake late at night (e.g., they may enjoy the solitude at this time of day) and unless there is a serious consequence such as failing in school or losing a job, they may not want to change their sleep schedule. Consequently, cultivating patient motivation is important for the success of any treatment for DSPD. With adolescents, a great deal of tension has often developed with their parents regarding sleep schedules. In order to reduce unproductive blaming, an effort may be needed to educate patients and their parents about the factors that regulate circadian rhythms and sleep, attempting to frame the problem in a more dispassionate way.

ADVANCED SLEEP PHASE DISORDER

Advanced sleep phase syndrome (ASPD) is characterized by a sleep schedule that is persistently several hours earlier than the conventional or desired time. ASPD is thought to be much less common than DSPD, but may be underestimated because an early sleep pattern is less likely to generate social conflicts. A familial form of ASPD has been described (28), associated with a specific clock gene mutation that would be expected to shorten circadian period (29). In fact, a member of the originally described family was studied in a temporal isolation facility and found to have a circadian period less than 24 hours (28).

As normal people age, bedtimes, wake times and circadian markers often shift earlier (30,31). Experimental treatment with timed bright light exposure has been tested in this population on the assumption that these patients have a variant of ASPD although the etiology might be different from younger people; for example, older people may awaken early because of a decrease in homeostatic sleep drive that results in a secondary phase advance due to early morning light exposure.

Timed Light Exposure

According to circadian principles, light exposure in the evening should counteract the tendency for phase-advanced rhythms. A number of clinical trials have been conducted, and subjective reports have been encouraging; however, PSG outcome data have been mixed. For example, one group reported that bright light treatment (4000 lux for two hours in the late evening for 12 days) produced a delay in the core body temperature rhythm of more than two hours and substantial improvements in PSG-documented sleep efficiency and sleep architecture (32). However, in a subsequent report the same group, using an identical protocol, reported comparable circadian phase delays but no improvement in PSG monitored sleep (33). Another group reported that two nights of late evening light therapy (2500 lux for four hours) produced both an acute delay in circadian phase and continued benefits for sleep. In follow-up at one week and at four weeks, improvement in wake after sleep onset (WASO) persisted (34).

In summary, late evening light exposure is likely to delay circadian phase, and can be used in patients with ASPD. It may also be tried as an adjunctive treatment in patients with sleep maintenance insomnia who may have a secondarily phase-advanced circadian rhythms due to early awakening.

Timed Melatonin Administration

Although there are no systematic reports of melatonin administration for ASPD, it would be expected to promote phase delays if administered in the latter half of the night or early morning. The dose should be kept low (0.5 mg) in order to minimize unwanted soporific effects and patients should be cautioned about the possibility of drowsiness that could carry over into the daytime hours.

Prescribed Sleep Schedule

Chronotherapy (systematic sleep scheduling), shifting sleep around the clock in an advance direction, was found to be effective in one case of ASPS (35).

Pharmacologic Symptom Control

If a patient with ASPS is unable to stay up to enjoy social or cultural activities in the evening, the intermittent use of a low-dose, short-acting stimulant (e.g., methylphenidate 5 mg) to counteract evening sleepiness may be justified. A short-acting hypnotic such as zaleplon could be used as a middle-of-the-night sleeping aid for premature awakening. Neither of these treatments has been systematically studied in clinical trials.

Combination Treatment

As with DSPD, a combination of the treatments can be employed as there are no known adverse interactions.

SHIFT WORK DISORDER

Shift work is a term that applies to a broad range of nonstandard work schedules including permanent night shifts, rotating shifts, intermittent night duty, and jobs that require an early awakening from nocturnal sleep. Daytime sleep in night workers is shorter (4 to 6 hours in one study) and less efficient (36). Day sleep insomnia is due, in large part, to circadian misalignment although ambient light, noise, childcare duties, and social conflicts also play a role.

Rapidly rotating shifts clearly do not allow sufficient time for circadian adaptation, but even permanent night workers typically undermine circadian adaptation by adopting a conventional day active schedule on their days off. Shift workers appear to be at greater risk for certain medical problems, including peptic ulcer disease, coronary artery disease, and obesity. In addition, sleepiness on the job can lead to accidents that affect both the worker and other people.

SWD is a clinical diagnosis that presumably applies to a subgroup of night workers who fail to adapt to their atypical schedule (37); however, the difference between a normal response to an unnatural sleep schedule and a diagnosable disorder is not easy to determine. Most of the descriptive research studies on shift work have been done without regard to clinical diagnosis. Furthermore, many of the interventional studies have been carried out in a laboratory setting with recruited volunteers as subjects. Therefore, the precise nature and boundaries of this disorder remain rather undefined.

The degree to which night workers reset their circadian rhythms to match their daytime sleep schedule appears to be quite variable and may depend on a number of factors, especially baseline circadian phase and the pattern of light exposure. In general, realignment of rhythms so they are congruent with a day sleep schedule improves the quantity and quality of sleep (36), although one study of actual shift workers found an unexpectedly weak correlation between sleep quality and work satisfaction (38). Even if phase congruence could be accomplished, some night workers would find it undesirable because they would be out of phase on their days off.

Timed Light Exposure

Most night workers go to bed in the morning after their shift, so circadian adaptation requires a phase delay. In a series of elegant experiments employing subjects on a simulated night shift schedule, Eastman and colleagues have shown that individuals, who have an early circadian phase while on a conventional schedule, will have greater difficulty re-entraining to a night work schedule. They also showed that strategically timed bright light exposure during the night can substantially facilitate adaptive phase days (39). Furthermore, wearing dark goggles on the commute home, to block the phase-advancing effect of morning light exposure, also facilitates phase delays. In recent studies, they demonstrated that 20 minutes pulses of bright light, if presented in a gradually delaying pattern (one hour later per day), combined with dark goggles worn on the morning commute, was a highly effective treatment regimen that was practical and could be adapted by actual shift workers.

While complete resynchronization of the circadian clock to a nocturnally active schedule is probably unrealistic, the Eastman group showed that phase delays that were sufficient to move the temperature minimum into the first half of the sleep cycle could produce as much benefit for sleep and alertness as more robust delays (40). In order to optimize the congruence of circadian phase and sleep, night workers should go to bed as quickly as possible after they get home.

There are only a few field studies of light treatment tested in actual shift workers, but they have generally supported the findings derived from simulation studies. For example, Boivin and James (41) treated 10 night duty nurses for the first six hours of their shift with intermittent bright light exposure administered when the subjects were working at their nurse's station. The bright light treatment, combined with strategic light avoidance (by wearing goggles on the commute home and sleeping in absolute darkness), produced robust phase shifts in the melatonin and body temperature rhythms.

Despite these kinds of encouraging results, light treatment (or avoidance) has not been widely adopted by night workers. For many occupations, bright lights are considered too difficult and expensive to incorporate into the work environment, and may be unpleasant for the worker. Wearing goggles on the morning commute may not be safe for people who are driving home. These are not insurmountable obstacles, and with modification to the realities of a particular setting, strategically patterning light exposure offers a potent nonpharmacological treatment for SWD that is based on sound circadian science.

Timed Melatonin Administration

In one shift work simulation study, melatonin (0.5 or 3.0 mg) administered to subjects who went to bed in the afternoon (7.5 hours earlier than their usual bedtime) potentiated a desired phase advance (42). However, in another study in which melatonin (1.8 mg) was administered prior to a morning (0830) bedtime, their was no augmentation of a desired phase delay (43).

A study from our program illustrates not only the efficacy, but also the complexity of melatonin treatment for shift work sleep problems (44). Melatonin (0.5 mg) or placebo was administered at bedtime for seven consecutive days at a time to permanent night nurses ($N = 24$) who worked seven night shifts alternating with seven days off (*7/70 schedule*). In other words, each subject received both a melatonin trial and a placebo trial for both a work-week and a week-off (a four-week protocol). At the end of each week, DLMOs were assessed to determine circadian phase. Nine of the subjects had similar phase shifts on melatonin compared to placebo, and eight failed to shift with either treatment. Seven were specific melatonin responders; that is, they shifted with melatonin treatment but not with placebo. In summary, it appears that some night workers do not need treatment, others fail melatonin treatment, and some respond specifically to melatonin treatment.

Melatonin given just prior to daytime sleep may have both a direct hypnotic effect (perhaps by counteracting the unwelcome daytime circadian alerting signal) as well as a circadian phase-resetting effect. To date, there have been no studies comparing melatonin to a standard hypnotic medication for daytime sleep.

Pharmacologic Symptom Control

Counteracting Insomnia

Hypnotic medications have been shown to promote daytime sleep in several simulated shift work studies (45,46). However, it was somewhat surprising that the increase in total sleep time did not necessarily counteract the circadian-mediated dip in nighttime alertness, as measured with MSLT. In another study, treatment did not improve nighttime alertness as assessed by MSLT, but did improve scores on the Maintenance of Wakefulness Test (MWT), suggesting a differential effect on these two dimensions of sleepiness (47).

There is little question that hypnotic medications can lengthen daytime sleep in night workers, but there is not yet a consensus as to when such treatment would be appropriate (or inappropriate). For short runs or occasional night shifts, a short course of hypnotic medication would seem consistent with the generally accepted guidelines for their use. The use of hypnotics for permanent night workers is more controversial.

Counteracting Excessive Sleepiness

In the largest ($N = 209$) double-blind, placebo-controlled study of shift workers to date, Czeisler et al. (48) tested modafinil (300 mg) as a treatment to counteract excessive sleepiness during night work. At baseline, and then on three occasions, one month apart, MSLTs, clinical symptom ratings, and simple reaction time performance testing were performed. Modafinil produced a modest, but statistically significant, lengthening of nighttime sleep latency (1.7 ± 0.4 vs. 0.3 ± 0.3 minutes; $P = 0.002$). Self-rated symptom improvement occurred in 74% of those treated versus 36% on placebo. There were concomitant improvements in performance measures. Although modafinil counteracted nighttime sleepiness, it did not restore alertness to a daytime level. It is unknown whether a higher dose would have produced a more robust effect.

In several studies, caffeine has been shown to be an effective countermeasure for sleepiness during night work or experimentally induced sleep deprivation (49,50).

Treating SWD with Prescribed Sleep Scheduling

Designing a shift work schedule, based on sleep and circadian science, can be considered a form of prescribed sleep scheduling. However, there remains a lack of consensus as to the optimal schedule for night work – all have advantages and disadvantages. For example, if a rapidly rotating schedule minimizes time in a desynchronized state, then a schedule with more consecutive days of shift work would provide an opportunity to achieve a degree of circadian synchrony.

Because the human circadian period is longer than 24 hours, it is easier for most people to phase shift in a delay direction than in an advance direction. This understanding of human circadian physiology is consistent with the finding that a clockwise (delaying) shift work rotation was better tolerated than a counterclockwise (advancing) rotation (51). In another example of basing a work schedule on circadian physiology (15), Eastman et al. showed that gradual, rather than abrupt, shifts in a night work schedule allowed the circadian system to adapt. This schedule was designed with the understanding that the circadian pacemaker can be reset only an hour or two per day however. Although consistent with circadian physiology, a gradually shifting work/sleep schedule would be difficult to implement in most settings. In the "real world," circadian physiology is often secondary to other considerations in shift work scheduling; for example, worker seniority status, labor-management relations, time-off preferences.

Prescribed napping, either before (*prophylactic napping*) or during a night shift (*recuperative napping*), has been shown to improve alertness on the job, and has been used more extensively in Europe than in the United States. In order to minimize sleep inertia, naps should be kept relatively brief.

Combination Treatment

Given the wide variety shift work schedules and the various desires of patients, treatment will need to be tailored to meet the needs of the individual worker. For an occasional overnight duty (e.g., 24-hour duty in the Emergency Room), phase resetting would not be possible or desirable. A stimulant medication to maintain alertness during the shift and perhaps a hypnotic for daytime sleep might be indicated. For workers on a steady night shift (who maintain a relative nocturnal orientation on the their days off), promoting phase resetting with light exposure or melatonin would be more logical. For a worker who is at risk for costly mistakes (e.g., a nuclear power plant supervisor) more aggressive treatment may be required. Recently, Eastman et al. have shown that using light treatment to reset rhythms to a compromise phase, along with prescribed sleep scheduling, in between a night work and conventional schedule, may be the best way to maximize sleep and alertness for both work days and days off. Some people are very intolerant of shift work and may need a medical authorization to be excused.

JET LAG DISORDER

JLD results from crossing time zones too rapidly for the circadian system to keep pace. It can take days or even weeks for the circadian system to resynchronize, depending on a number of factors: (*i*) the number of time zones crossed, (*ii*) the direction of travel, (*iii*) the availability and intensity of local circadian time cues upon arrival, and (*iv*) individual differences in circadian adaptability or tolerance to circadian misalignment. Attempting to sleep in upright position in an uncomfortable airplane seat adds the burden of sleep deprivation to the mix, and excessive alcohol or caffeine intake while in transit can make it worse. Although JLD is naturally self-limited, preventative measures and treatment can diminish its intensity and duration.

Timed Light Exposure

Numerous laboratory-based studies (which can be considered as jet travel simulations) have shown that appropriately timed bright light exposure can accelerate circadian phase shifting. So it makes sense, in most instances, to get as much sunlight after arrival at the destination as possible, but there are possible exceptions (52). When traveling across eight time zones or more, it would be prudent to avoid light in the early morning for the first few days, as it would be illuminating the "wrong" portion of the light PRC; that is, delaying rhythms when an advance is needed. Likewise, after a very long westward flight, it would make sense to avoid and advance when a delay is needed. After a few days, there will be enough circadian adaptation (shift in the light PRC) that light avoidance should be unnecessary. While light avoidance is rational, it is difficult for travelers to do. Wearing dark sunglasses and staying in dimly lit hotel room might help, but no studies have been done. After eastward flight of more than eight time zones, an eight-hour advance would be needed for resynchronization to local time and some experts suggest that it would be easier to promote a delay, even though this would involve up to a 16-hour phase shift (53).

Another approach is to use timed bright light exposure to reset the body clock in anticipation of jet travel. Aiming to develop a practical light treatment for use prior to eastward flight, Eastman et al. (54) showed that shifting the sleep schedule earlier by one or two hours per day, combined with bright morning light (5000 lux), advanced rhythms up to 1.8 hours in three days. If a formal light treatment program is too difficult, getting up progressively earlier than usual for a few days into a brightly lit environment should begin to advance rhythms before eastward travel; staying up progressively later with exposure to bright light should begin to delay rhythms for westward travel.

Melatonin Administration

The benefits of melatonin for jet lag have been demonstrated in a number of double-blind, placebo-controlled studies (55). Improvement in sleep, accelerated phase shifting, and a decrease in jet lag symptoms have been reported in various studies. Doses ranging from 0.5 to 10 mg for up to three days prior to departure and up to five days upon arrival at the destination have been employed. Most of these studies have tested melatonin for eastward flight, when a bedtime dose would promote a desired phase advance and might have a hypnotic effect as well. With westward flight melatonin should be taken (according to the melatonin PRC) upon early morning awakening in order to facilitate phase delays; if taken at bedtime, it could stimulate the advance portion of the melatonin PRC and thereby inhibit clock resetting in the desired delay direction. In order to minimize a sleep-promoting effect, a morning dose should be low; for example, 0.5 mg.

Prescribed Sleep Scheduling

For brief trips, maintaining the home base schedule (if feasible) and avoiding phase shifts is logical. Many travelers feel that immediately adopting local time upon arrival (not thinking about what time it is back home) reduces jet lag symptoms, but this has never been systematically studied.

Pharmacologic Symptom Control

Counteracting Insomnia

JLD-related insomnia is the result, not only of circadian misalignment, but also of attempting to sleep in an upright, sometimes noisy, airplane seat, and later, in an unfamiliar hotel bed. Because JLD-insomnia is self-limited, a short course of hypnotic medication can be readily justified. A few studies that have tested hypnotics for this indication and they were shown to be generally safe and effective (56). Occasional adverse events have been reported; for example, global amnesia following the use of triazolam (and some alcohol) during flight (57). Also, hypnotic use during a flight could increase immobility and raise the risk for deep vein thrombosis.

Counteracting Excessive Sleepiness

Many travelers increase their caffeine consumption as a countermeasure for JLD daytime sleepiness, but this could exacerbate jet lag-induced insomnia. In a clinical trial of slow-release caffeine (300 mg), daytime alertness was improved but the treated group also had longer sleep latencies and more awakenings at night (58). In phase-shifting experiments that simulate jet lag (as well as shift work), modafinil has been shown to improve daytime alertness, but there have been no field trials to date. There appears to be relatively few contraindications to its use.

Combination Treatment

Melatonin, for its phase-resetting effect, and a hypnotic medication, for insomnia, could be taken together as there are no known adverse pharmacological interactions. The hypnotic effects might be additive.

FREE-RUNNING DISORDER (NON–24-HOUR SLEEP DISORDER) – SIGHTED

In patients with FRD, the timing of sleep persistently delays by about 30 to 90 minutes per day, expressing a *free-running* circadian cycle that is greater than 24 hours. FRD is uncommon in sighted people, and the available literature consists mostly of single case reports. Most of the cases have been young males. Some of these patients had a history of severe DSPD prior to developing a free-running pattern, and the two disorders might well have similar etiologies (22).

Timed Light Exposure

Bright light exposure was found to successfully entrain circadian rhythms in several case reports; however, no placebo-controlled trials have been conducted (2).

Timed Melatonin Administration

There are reports of successful treatment with daily melatonin administration at the desired bedtime (when it would be predicted to promote a corrective phase advance). The most common dose was 3 mg and the duration of treatment ranged from one month to six years (2).

Prescribed Sleep Scheduling

An early study of four children with FRD related to neurological disorders suggested that increasing the regularity of sleep and potency of environmental time cues could improve the sleep–wake rhythms (2).

Combination Treatment

Non–24-hour CRSD may be an extreme form of DSPS and similar treatment strategies can be tried; for example, morning light exposure, evening melatonin administration, and intermittent hypnotics (as described above).

FREE-RUNNING DISORDER (NON–24-HOUR SLEEP DISORDER) – BLIND

Although Non–24-hour CRSD is very rare in normally sighted people, about half of the totally blind, those with no light perception, have free-running circadian rhythms (59). The recurrent symptoms of daytime sleepiness and nighttime insomnia, when their rhythms are out of phase, can be very burdensome.

Timed Melatonin Administration

Daily melatonin administration has been shown to entrain free-running rhythms in totally blind subjects (60–63) and is the current treatment of choice. A physiological dose (0.5 mg) appears to be as effective as a pharmacological dose (5 to 10 mg), and in some cases, more effective (18).

IRREGULAR SLEEP–WAKE DISORDER

Irregular sleep–wake disorder (ISWD) is characterized by a relative absence of a circadian pattern, with sleep and wake randomly distributed over the night and day, mimicking the pattern seen in animals with SCN lesions. The diagnosis is uncommon in healthy adults and is usually associated with dementia [particularly Alzheimer's disease (AD)], mental retardation, or brain injury. In these cases, damage to the SCN is thought to underlie a circadian amplitude (rather than phase) disturbance. Demented patients with ISWD cause their caretakers to lose sleep, and consequently, and this is the most common reason these cases are brought to medical attention. More rarely, the pattern is seen in otherwise normal individuals with either very poor sleep hygiene or without apparent etiology. The goal of therapy is to consolidate sleep, as much as possible, into a major nighttime bout.

Timed Light Exposure

Older adults living in an institutional setting are exposed to less daylight than elderly people living in the community. In addition, the retina and optic nerve may be compromised. These considerations have provided the rationale for using daytime bright light treatment (sometimes combined with more intense social activity) for Alzheimer's patients in nursing home settings. Most studies of this treatment have found a modest beneficial effect (2), but the increased attention associated with light therapy may explain some of results.

Timed Melatonin Administration

The nocturnal secretion of melatonin is reduced with normal aging; even greater reductions are seen with AD, providing the rationale for melatonin treatment in this population. Several large trials have been disappointing. For example, Singer et al. (64) randomized 157 AD patients to 2.5 mg sustained release melatonin, 10 mg of immediate release, or placebo. The primary outcome variable was actigraphically monitored sleep. The protocol involved two to three weeks of baseline measurement, eight weeks of treatment, and two weeks of placebo washout. Neither formulation of melatonin was better than placebo.

More favorable results have been reported using melatonin (2 to 20 mg) for brain-injured, mentally retarded children with ISWD (65). However, a trial of melatonin to improve the timing and quality of sleep in young girls with Rett syndrome was negative (66).

Prescribed Sleep Scheduling

McCurry et al. (67) conducted a study in which family caregivers of AD patients were instructed in the standard principles of good sleep hygiene, including regularized sleep schedules, and were provided training in behavior management skills. A control group received education about dementia and caregiver support. Sleep was monitored actigraphically. The active treatment group had fewer nighttime awakenings and a reduction in total wake time during the night. These benefits persisted to six-month follow-up.

Pharmacologic Symptom Control

A number of studies have concluded that sedative–hypnotic drugs are inappropriately prescribed or overprescribed to demented patients. On the other hand, no controlled studies of benzodiazepine receptor agonists have been conducted to assess efficacy and safety in AD. A clinical trial with one of the usual sedative/hypnotic drugs might be justified in difficult cases, but may exacerbate confusion and disorientation. Stimulant medications during the day have not been tested but might be justified in some individuals.

SUMMARY AND CONCLUSIONS

The symptom of insomnia in CRSDs is usually related to a misalignment of the circadian alerting process and the sleep schedule. Understanding the basic principles of circadian physiology can provide the basis for intervention. The delineation of the PRCs for light exposure and melatonin administration has provided a scientific basis for resetting of the body clock so that it is more congruent with the desired or required time for sleep. If clock resetting is impractical, unsuccessful, or undesirable, insomnia (however unconventional the sleep–wake schedule) can be counteracted with judicious use of hypnotic medications.

REFERENCES

1. Evans R. Letter to the editor: practicing under the influence of fatigue [comment]. Adv Neonatal Care 2006; 6(2):61–62.
2. Sack RL, Auckley D, Auger RR, et al. Circadian rhythm sleep disorders: part II, advanced sleep phase disorder, delayed sleep phase disorder, free-running disorder, and irregular sleep-wake rhythm. An American Academy of Sleep Medicine review. Sleep 2007; 30(11):1484–1501.
3. Sack RL, Auckley D, Auger RR, et al. Circadian rhythm sleep disorders: part I, basic principles, shift work and jet lag disorders. An American Academy of Sleep Medicine review. Sleep 2007; 30(11):1460–1483.
4. Edgar DM, Dement WC, Fuller CA. Effect of SCN lesions on sleep in squirrel monkeys: evidence for opponent processes in sleep-wake regulation. J Neurosci 1993; 13(3):1065–1079.
5. Horne JA, Ostberg O. A self-assessment questionnaire to determine morningness-eveningness in human circadian rhythms. Int J Chronobiol 1976; 4(2):97–110.
6. Lewy AJ, Sack RL. The dim light melatonin onset as a marker for circadian phase position. Chronobiol Int 1989; 6(1):93–102.
7. Czeisler CA, Duffy JF, Shanahan TL, et al. Stability, precision, and near-24-hour period of the human circadian pacemaker. Science 1999; 284(5423):2177–2181.
8. Duffy JF, Wright KP Jr. Entrainment of the human circadian system by light. J Biol Rhythms 2005; 20(4):326–338.
9. Gronfier C, Wright KP Jr, Kronauer RE, et al. Efficacy of a single sequence of intermittent bright light pulses for delaying circadian phase in humans. Am J Physiol Endocrinol Metab 2004; 287(1):E174–E181.
10. Hankins MW, Peirson SN, Foster RG. Melanopsin: an exciting photopigment. Trends Neurosci 2008; 31(1):27–36.
11. Campbell SS, Murphy PJ. Extraocular circadian phototransduction in humans. Science 1998; 279(5349):396–399.
12. Eastman CI, Martin SK, Hebert M. Failure of extraocular light to facilitate circadian rhythm reentrainment in humans. Chronobiol Int 2000; 17(6):807.
13. Wright KP Jr, Czeisler CA. Absence of circadian phase resetting in response to bright light behind the knees. Science 2002; 297(5581):571.
14. Reme CE, Rol P, Grothmann K, et al. Bright light therapy in focus: lamp emission spectra and ocular safety. Technol Health Care 1996; 4(4):403–413.
15. Revell VL, Eastman CI. How to trick mother nature into letting you fly around or stay up all night. J Biol Rhythms 2005; 20(4):353–365.
16. Lewy AJ, Ahmed S, Jackson JM, et al. Melatonin shifts human circadian rhythms according to a phase-response curve. Chronobiol Int 1992; 9(5):380–392.

17. Revell VL, Burgess HJ, Gazda CJ, et al. Advancing human circadian rhythms with afternoon melatonin and morning intermittent bright light. J Clin Endocrinol Metab 2006; 91(1):54–59.
18. Lewy AJ, Emens JS, Sack RL, et al. Low, but not high, doses of melatonin entrained a free-running blind person with a long circadian period. Chronobiol Int 2002; 19(3):649.
19. Hirai K, Kita M, Ohta H, et al. Ramelteon (TAK-375) accelerates reentrainment of circadian rhythm after a phase advance of the light-dark cycle in rats. J Biol Rhythms 2005; 20(1):27–37.
20. Wyatt JK. Delayed sleep phase syndrome: pathophysiology and treatment options. Sleep 2004; 27(6):1195.
21. Weitzman ED, Czeisler CA, Coleman RM, et al. Delayed sleep phase syndrome. A chronobiological disorder with sleep-onset insomnia. Arch Gen Psychiatry 1981; 38(7):737.
22. Okawa M, Uchiyama M. Circadian rhythm sleep disorders: characteristics and entrainment pathology in delayed sleep phase and non-24-h sleep-wake syndrome. Sleep Med Rev 2007; 11(6):485–496.
23. Rosenthal NE, Joseph-Vanderpool JR, Levendosky AA, et al. Phase-shifting effects of bright morning light as treatment for delayed sleep phase syndrome. Sleep 1990; 13(4):354.
24. Dahlitz M, Alvarez B, Vignau J, et al. Delayed sleep phase syndrome response to melatonin. Lancet 1991; 337(8750):1121.
25. Dagan Y, Yovel I, Hallis D, et al. Evaluating the role of melatonin in the long-term treatment of delayed sleep phase syndrome (DSPS). Chronobiol Int 1998; 15(2):181.
26. Kayumov L, Brown G, Jindal R, et al. A randomized, double-blind, placebo-controlled crossover study of the effect of exogenous melatonin on delayed sleep phase syndrome. Psychosom Med 2001; 63(1):40.
27. Czeisler CA, Richardson GS, Coleman RM, et al. Chronotherapy: resetting the circadian clocks of patients with delayed sleep phase insomnia. Sleep 1981; 4(1):1–21.
28. Jones CR, Campbell SS, Zone SE, et al. Familial advanced sleep-phase syndrome: a short-period circadian rhythm variant in humans [see comment]. Nat Med 1999; 5(9):1062.
29. Toh KL, Jones CR, He Y, et al. An hPer2 phosphorylation site mutation in familial advanced sleep phase syndrome. Science 2001; 291(5506):1040.
30. Dijk DJ, Duffy JF. Circadian regulation of human sleep and age-related changes in its timing, consolidation and EEG characteristics. Ann Med 1999; 31(2):130–140.
31. Carrier J, Paquet J, Morettini J, et al. Phase advance of sleep and temperature circadian rhythms in the middle years of life in humans. Neurosci Lett 2002; 320(1–2):1–4.
32. Campbell SS, Dawson D, Anderson MW. Alleviation of sleep maintenance insomnia with timed exposure to bright light. J Am Geriatr Soc 1993; 41(8):829–836.
33. Suhner AG, Murphy PJ, Campbell SS. Failure of timed bright light exposure to alleviate age-related sleep maintenance insomnia. J Am Geriatr Soc 2002; 50(4):617–623.
34. Lack L, Wright H, Kemp K, et al. The treatment of early-morning awakening insomnia with 2 evenings of bright light [see comment]. Sleep 2005; 28(5):616–623.
35. Moldofsky H, Musisi S, Phillipson EA. Treatment of a case of advanced sleep phase syndrome by phase advance chronotherapy. Sleep 1986; 9(1):61.
36. Boivin DB, Tremblay GM, James FO. Working on atypical schedules. Sleep Med 2007; 8(6): 578–589.
37. Ohayon MM, Lemoine P, Arnaud-Briant V, et al. Prevalence and consequences of sleep disorders in a shift worker population. J Psychosom Res 2002; 53(1):577.
38. Roden M, Koller M, Pirich K, et al. The circadian melatonin and cortisol secretion pattern in permanent night shift workers. Am J Physiol 1993; 265(1, pt 2):R261–R267.
39. Burgess HJ, Sharkey KM, Eastman CI. Bright light, dark and melatonin can promote circadian adaptation in night shift workers. Sleep Med Rev 2002; 6(5):407–420.
40. Crowley SJ, Lee C, Tseng CY, et al. Complete or partial circadian re-entrainment improves performance, alertness, and mood during night-shift work. Sleep 2004; 27(6):1077–1087.
41. Boivin DB, James FO. Circadian adaptation to night-shift work by judicious light and darkness exposure. J Biol Rhythms 2002; 17(6):556.
42. Sharkey KM, Eastman CI. Melatonin phase shifts human circadian rhythms in a placebo-controlled simulated night-work study. Am J Physiol Regul Integr Comp Physiol 2002; 282(2):R454.
43. Smith L, Tanigawa T, Takahashi M, et al. Shiftwork locus of control, situational and behavioural effects on sleepiness and fatigue in shiftworkers. Ind Health 2005; 43(1):151–170.
44. Sack RL, Lewy AJ. Melatonin as a chronobiotic: treatment of circadian desynchrony in night workers and the blind. J Biol Rhythms 1997; 12(6):595–603.
45. Hart CL, Ward AS, Haney M, et al. Zolpidem-related effects on performance and mood during simulated night-shift work. Exp Clin Psychopharmacol 2003; 11(4):259.
46. Monchesky TC, Billings BJ, Phillips R, et al. Zopiclone in insomniac shiftworkers. Evaluation of its hypnotic properties and its effects on mood and work performance. Int Arch Occup Environ Health 1989; 61(4):255.

47. Porcu S, Bellatreccia A, Ferrara M, et al. Performance, ability to stay awake, and tendency to fall asleep during the night after a diurnal sleep with temazepam or placebo. Sleep 1997; 20(7):535.
48. Czeisler CA, Walsh JK, Roth T, et al. Modafinil for excessive sleepiness associated with shift-work sleep disorder [see comment]. N Engl J Med 2005; 353(5):476–486.
49. McLellan TM, Bell DG, Kamimori GH. Caffeine improves physical performance during 24 h of active wakefulness. Aviat Space Environ Med 2004; 75(8):666–672.
50. Wyatt JK, Cajochen C, Ritz-De Cecco A, et al. Low-dose repeated caffeine administration for circadian-phase-dependent performance degradation during extended wakefulness. Sleep 2004; 27(3):374.
51. Czeisler CA, Moore-Ede MC, Coleman RH. Rotating shift work schedules that disrupt sleep are improved by applying circadian principles. Science 1982; 217(4558):460–463.
52. Daan S, Lewy AJ. Scheduled exposure to daylight: a potential strategy to reduce "jet lag" following transmeridian flight. Psychopharmacol Bull 1984; 20(3):566–568.
53. Waterhouse J, Reilly T, Atkinson G, et al. Jet lag: trends and coping strategies. Lancet 2007; 369(9567):1117–1129.
54. Eastman CI, Gazda CJ, Burgess HJ, et al. Advancing circadian rhythms before eastward flight: a strategy to prevent or reduce jet lag. Sleep 2005; 28(1):33–44.
55. Herxheimer A. Jet lag. Clin Evid 2005; 13:2178–2183 [update of Clin Evid 2004; 12:2394–2400; PMID: 15865798].
56. Jamieson AO, Zammit GK, Rosenberg RS, et al. Zolpidem reduces the sleep disturbance of jet lag. Sleep Med 2001; 2(5):423–430.
57. Morris HH III, Estes ML. Traveler's amnesia. Transient global amnesia secondary to triazolam. JAMA 1987; 258(7):945–946.
58. Pierard C, Beaumont M, Enslen M, et al. Resynchronization of hormonal rhythms after an eastbound flight in humans: effects of slow-release caffeine and melatonin. Eur J Appl Physiol 2001; 85(1–2):144.
59. Sack RL, Lewy AJ, Blood ML, et al. Circadian rhythm abnormalities in totally blind people: incidence and clinical significance. J Clin Endocrinol Metab 1992; 75(1):127–134.
60. Lockley SW, Skene DJ, James K, et al. Melatonin administration can entrain the free-running circadian system of blind subjects. J Endocrinol 2000; 164(1):R1–R6.
61. Sack RL, Brandes RW, Kendall AR, et al. Entrainment of free-running circadian rhythms by melatonin in blind people. N Engl J Med 2000; 343(15):1070–1077.
62. Lewy AJ, Bauer VK, Hasler BP, et al. Capturing the circadian rhythms of free-running blind people with 0.5 mg melatonin. Brain Res 2001; 918(1–2):96.
63. Hack LM, Lockley SW, Arendt J, et al. The effects of low-dose 0.5-mg melatonin on the free-running circadian rhythms of blind subjects. J Biol Rhythms 2003; 18(5):420–429.
64. Singer C, Tractenberg RE, Kaye J, et al. A multicenter, placebo-controlled trial of melatonin for sleep disturbance in Alzheimer's disease. Sleep 2003; 26(7):893.
65. Jan JE, Freeman RD. Melatonin therapy for circadian rhythm sleep disorders in children with multiple disabilities: what have we learned in the last decade? [see comment]. Dev Med Child Neurol 2004; 46(11):776–782.
66. McArthur AJ, Budden SS. Sleep dysfunction in Rett syndrome: a trial of exogenous melatonin treatment. Dev Med Child Neurol 1998; 40(3):186.
67. McCurry SM, Gibbons LE, Logsdon RG, et al. Nighttime insomnia treatment and education for Alzheimer's disease: a randomized, controlled trial. J Am Geriatr Soc 2005; 53(5):793–802.

18 Insomnia in Other Sleep Disorders: Movement Disorders

Michael H. Silber

Center for Sleep Medicine and Department of Neurology, Mayo Clinic College of Medicine, Rochester, Minnesota, U.S.A.

RESTLESS LEGS SYNDROME

Definition

Restless legs syndrome (RLS) is a major cause of comorbid insomnia. It is characterized by four basic symptoms: an urge to move the legs, usually accompanied by unpleasant sensations; worsening of symptoms by rest; relief of symptoms by activity; and worsening of symptoms in the evening or night (1,2). The unpleasant sensations are typically described as creepy-crawly or worm-like, but patients use varied descriptors and not uncommonly find it hard to label the quality of the discomfort. A minority will describe the sensations as painful and some will experience only the need to move without associated sensations. Usually the symptoms are experienced bilaterally, but one limb may predominate, with discomfort sometimes alternating between different sides. In some patients the symptoms may also be experienced in other areas of the body, especially the arms (3). The urge to move is precipitated by physical rest such as sitting or lying down and may be especially severe in prolonged situations of enforced quiescence, such as traveling in a car or plane or sitting in a theater. Reduced alertness may enhance the severity of RLS and, conversely, stimulating mental activities may help alleviate the discomfort. Activities such as walking, stretching or bicycling result in relief but symptoms recommence after the activity is discontinued. Soaking or massaging the affected limb may also provide temporary relief. The characteristic circadian rhythmicity of RLS results in symptoms frequently being most severe in bed, either before sleep onset or on waking during the night.

Additional Clinical Features

Three other features of the disorder may provide added confirmation of the diagnosis (1). First, the probability of a correct diagnosis of RLS may be increased by the identification of a family history of the disorder in a first degree relative. Second, a sustained therapeutic response to a dopaminergic drug may provide indirect evidence that the diagnosis is correct. Third, RLS is frequently accompanied by periodic limb movements of sleep (PLMS) with polysomnographic studies showing their occurrence in 80% to 88% of patients (4). PLMS are repetitive contractions of the legs during sleep with dorsiflexion of the ankle and flexion of the knee and hip. Each movement typically lasts 0.5 to 10 seconds with an intermovement interval of 5 to 90 seconds (2). PLMS are not confined to patients with RLS and may accompany a wide range of other sleep and neurological disorders, including obstructive sleep apnea (5), narcolepsy (6), REM sleep behavior disorder (7), and Parkinson's disease (8). They may also occur in isolation, either as an asymptomatic phenomenon especially in older people (9–11), or rarely as a primary disorder causing sleep disruption.

Diagnostic Assessment

The diagnosis of RLS can be made in most patients by obtaining a careful history and diagnostic testing is not generally needed. Polysomnography to detect PLMS has low sensitivity and specificity and immobilization tests (12) to detect periodic limb movements of wakefulness are rarely used clinically. Other potentially confusing conditions have different clinical features, usually allowing easy differentiation. Nocturnal leg cramps abruptly awaken the patient with severe pain in a palpably contracted muscle. Arthritis pain is localized to joints and the discomfort of a sensory peripheral neuropathy is predominantly felt in the feet. While neurogenic pain may be worse at night or at rest, it is not generally associated with an urge to move. Fibromyalgia is accompanied by tender muscle trigger points in a characteristic distribution. Discomfort from transient compression neuropathies is associated with numbness and tingling and is confined to specific peripheral nerve distributions. Jiggling of the legs during wakefulness is not associated with an urge to move and can be voluntarily discontinued without discomfort. Akathisia, most commonly associated with neuroleptic use, is neither worse at rest nor relieved by movement. Painful legs and moving toes syndrome is a rare disorder characterized by typical wandering toe movements.

Epidemiology

The prevalence of RLS has been identified as 5% to 10% in a variety of population based epidemiological studies (13–17). In one study based on a primary care practice, 6.6% of patients described RLS occurring more than three times a week (18). The incidence of RLS increases with age but symptoms may develop as early as childhood. RLS is twice as frequent in women as in men and is especially frequent during pregnancy. At least 50% of patients have a family history of a relative with the disorder, especially if symptoms started early in life (4,19). The genetics of RLS are complex and much further work will be needed to fully understand the hereditary underpinnings of the disorder. Studies have shown linkage to sites on five different chromosomes (12q, 14q, 9p, 20p and 2q) with four reports suggesting an autosomal dominant inheritance pattern and one an autosomal recessive pattern (20–24). Genome wide studies have suggested an association of RLS or PLMS with a number of genes on chromosomes 2p, 6p and 15q, some of which affect spinal motor neuron connectivity or the development of spinal cord sensory pathways (25,26).

Associated Conditions and Pathogenesis

A number of acquired factors are associated with RLS. The best studied is that of iron deficiency, with studies showing a relationship between RLS severity and low or low- normal serum ferritin concentration (27,28). Even in RLS patients with ostensibly normal systemic iron stores, CSF ferritin levels are lower than in normal controls (29). MRI (30) and pathological (31) studies have also revealed lower concentration of iron in the basal ganglia in RLS. Current hypotheses link low cerebral iron stores to dopamine deficiency. The exact nature of the relationship is uncertain, but iron is a cofactor for tyrosine hydroxylase, the rate-limiting step of dopamine synthesis, and is also necessary for the functioning of the dopamine D2 receptor. RLS is also associated with chronic renal failure, but the exact pathophysiology has not been determined. In one study, 23% of 138 dialysis patients had definite RLS (32). RLS has been linked to peripheral neuropathy, especially in patients with older onset disease and no family history of the disorder (33). Evidence of small fiber neuropathy has been detected in some RLS patients by measurement of intraepidermal nerve fiber density on skin biopsy (34). It has been suggested that Parkinson's disease may also predispose to the development of RLS (35).

Insomnia in Restless Legs Syndrome

RLS is classified as a sleep disorder (2) because patients frequently report difficult initiating and maintaining sleep. This observation gives rise to the question of how frequently RLS actually causes insomnia and what form the sleep disturbance takes. Controlled and uncontrolled questionnaire and polysomnographic studies have addressed these issues.

Uncontrolled, questionnaire studies of the consequences of RLS on sleep have been reported in sleep clinic, primary care practice and population settings. In a large, clinic-based study of 133 consecutive RLS patients, 84.7% reported difficulty falling asleep and 86% difficulty staying asleep (4). Of 55 patients in a sleep clinic practice, insomnia was reported in 67% of those with onset at ≤20 years of age and 55% of those with onset >20 years of age (36). RLS patients with symptoms at least twice a week and at least some negative impact on quality of life were studied in primary care centers in the USA and four European countries (37). Of 551 patients, 88% reported at least one sleep-related symptom (including inability to fall asleep, inability to stay asleep and disturbed sleep). A sleep latency of 30 minutes or longer on symptomatic nights was reported by 68.6%, while 60.1% reported waking three or more times a night. Sleep disturbances were rated the most troublesome symptom in 43.4% of patients. A population based study of 15,391 subjects in the USA and five European countries revealed 416 (2.7%) respondents with moderate or severe RLS causing at least moderate distress and occurring a minimum of twice weekly (17). Sleep-related symptoms were noted by 75.5% of patients, with 48.1% describing difficulty falling asleep, 39.2% difficulty staying asleep, 60.6% experiencing disturbed or interrupted sleep and 40.1% insufficient sleep. The most troublesome symptom was listed as sleep disturbance by 37.8% of patients.

Several controlled, population-based studies of RLS symptoms have been reported. A study of 1000 randomly selected adults from Norway and 1005 from Denmark revealed a prevalence of RLS of 11.5% (38). Of those subjects indicating that insomnia was usually or always present, 23% had RLS compared to 9.3% of those indicating insomnia to be sometimes or never present. Multivariate analysis demonstrated that RLS was significantly associated with insomnia that was always present (odds ratio 2.75), usually present (odds ratio 3.16) and sometimes present (odds ratio 1.71). Depressive mood did not correlate significantly with the presence of RLS. Of 1000 randomly selected Swedish adults, 5% were diagnosed with RLS (39). Symptoms of insomnia were described by 51% of the RLS patients compared to 24.3% of the controls ($p = 0.0001$), whereas depressed mood was present in 18% of the RLS patients compared to 6.7% of the controls ($p = 0.01$). As part of the 2005 National Sleep Foundation Poll, 1506 randomly selected United States adults were interviewed. RLS was identified in 9.7% of the sample (40). Compared to controls, RLS subjects were more likely to sleep <6 hours a night, to endorse symptoms of insomnia, to stay up longer than they planned more than a few nights a week and to take >30 minutes to fall asleep.

A few polysomnographic (PSG) studies of RLS patients have addressed the question of sleep disruption. In an uncontrolled study of 133 consecutive patients with RLS (4), the mean PSG sleep latency was 20.5 minutes and the mean sleep efficiency was 75%. A mean of 7.4 awakenings per night greater than two minutes was reported. The PSG findings correlated with the patients' subjective reports. The mean sleep latency for those complaining of difficulty falling asleep was 22.9 minutes compared to 10.6 minutes for those reporting no initial insomnia. The mean sleep efficiency was 73.2% for those complaining of difficulty maintaining sleep compared to 86.4% for those reporting no sleep maintenance problems. The periodic limb movement index did not, however, correlate with patients' complaints of sleep onset or maintenance insomnia, the number of objective awakenings or sleep efficiency, suggesting that periodic limb movements are not the primary cause of the sleep disturbances in RLS patients. In a study of the effects of ropinirole on moderate to severe RLS, baseline PSG data was reported for 59 patients (41). Mean preintervention sleep efficiency was 81.2% for the drug group and 81.9% for the placebo group. However, preintervention mean sleep latency was relatively short: only 16.7 minutes for the drug group and 8.9 minutes for the placebo group.

A small controlled PSG study of 12 RLS patients compared to 12 controls showed increased wake time after sleep onset (mean 92.4 minutes compared to 36.2 minutes), reduced sleep efficiency (73.2% compared to 86.6%), shorter total sleep time (326.3 minutes compared to 383.3 minutes) and more awakenings (12.2 compared to 7.4) (42). A larger controlled PSG study of 45 RLS patients and controls showed that the patients had significantly reduced sleep efficiency (80% compared to 87.6%), higher arousal index (23.4 compared to 12.4), more awakenings (26.8 compared to 20.8) and more wake after sleep onset (15.6% compared to 7.9%) (43). Percentage stages 2 and REM sleep were significantly reduced in the RLS group and REM latency was prolonged. Sleep onset latency did not differ between the groups, but latency to 10 minutes persistent sleep was significantly longer in the RLS subjects (41.6 minutes compared to 25.4 minutes).

In summary, questionnaire and PSG studies show conclusively that untreated RLS causes serious disruption of sleep. In population based studies, approximately one half to three quarters of RLS patients describe sleep-related symptoms, with higher percentages reported in studies based on primary care or specialist practices. Both sleep onset and sleep maintenance difficulties are described. In objective PSG studies, sleep maintenance difficulties are confirmed, with reduced sleep efficiency together with increased arousals and awakenings. Conventionally calculated sleep latency is less consistently prolonged but latency to sustained sleep lengthens, suggesting that many patients fall asleep rapidly but wake shortly thereafter with recurrence of symptoms. While there is limited data on the role of periodic limb movements, one study suggests that they do not significantly contribute to the sleep disturbances of RLS (4).

Management of Restless Legs Syndrome

Insomnia due to RLS is generally managed by treating the underlying disorder. Nonpharmacological approaches (44) include iron replacement when systemic iron deficiency is detected, usually indicated by a low or low-normal serum ferritin concentration. Ferrous sulphate, ferrous fumarate or ferrous gluconate may be used in combination with Vitamin C to enhance absorption. Mental alerting activities and physical exercise may alleviate symptoms adequately in mild cases of RLS. Dopaminergic agents have been shown in controlled trials to be very effective in relieving RLS and are the first line of therapy in patients with severe enough disease to require daily therapy (45). Levodopa, the first drug shown to be effective, is rarely used currently except on an intermittent basis because of the high risk of inducing daytime augmentation, defined as the worsening of symptoms earlier in the day after an evening dose of medication. The nonergot dopamine agonists pramipexole and ropinirole, both approved by the U.S. Food and Drug Administration for RLS treatment, are most widely prescribed. Potential side-effects include daytime sleepiness and the development of impulse control disorders, such as compulsive gambling or excessive shopping (15). Other agents shown to be effective include gabapentin and opioids, such as oxycodone (44). Benzodiazepines may also help to relieve symptoms.

Do the therapeutic agents, which reduce restless legs, also help the associated insomnia? Most information comes from studies of dopaminergic drugs. In four large multicenter, controlled studies of 202 to 380 patients with moderate to severe RLS (46–49), the effects of ropinirole after 12 weeks administration were compared to those of placebo using the Medical Outcomes Study (MOS) sleep scale domains. In all studies there was a significant improvement in sleep disturbance, sleep adequacy and sleep quantity with the drug. The mean degree of improvement in sleep time ranged between 0.3 and 1.3 hours. A similar study of 345 patients treated with pramipexole or placebo showed significant decrease in the severity of sleep disturbance and increased satisfaction with sleep after six weeks use of the drug compared to placebo (50). The effects of levodopa were assessed in a crossover trial of 32 patients with RLS (51). Quality of sleep, refreshment after sleep, sleep latency, and sleep duration assessed by questionnaire were all improved with the drug compared to placebo. Sleep latency was shortened by a mean of 25.2 minutes and total sleep time lengthened by a mean of 0.9 hours. A combination of regular release and slow release levodopa before bed resulted in significantly better quality of sleep, longer time asleep and fewer awakenings compared to regular release levodopa alone (52). In a PSG study of 29 patients taking ropinirole for RLS and 30 taking placebo, adjusted mean total sleep time increased by 20.5 minutes and sleep efficiency by 4.3% but these changes did not reach statistical significance. In contrast, mean sleep latency fell significantly by a mean of 6.1 minutes (41). In summary, RLS patients report definite benefit in sleep from dopaminergic agents. Little additional objective PSG data is available.

In a controlled PSG study of the effect of gabapentin on 22 RLS patients compared to 22 on placebo, significantly increased total sleep time (0.5 hour) and sleep efficiency (9.8%) were noted in the drug group but sleep latency was not significantly different (53). Interpretation of studies of the effects of other agents on sleep is limited by small numbers of patients and inconsistent diagnostic criteria, especially lack of distinction between RLS and PLMS. A crossover study of 11 RLS patients showed that oxycodone resulted in significantly higher sleep efficiency than placebo (mean difference 24.7%) (54). A crossover study of clonazepam (6 patients) showed significantly better quality sleep by questionnaire with the drug compared to placebo (55).

The Medical Advisory Board of the Restless Legs Syndrome Foundation has developed an algorithm for the management of RLS, based on classifying the disorder into intermittent, daily and refractory forms (56). Intermittent RLS can be managed by nonpharamacological therapies or intermittent use of levodopa, low-potency opoids or benzodiazepines. Daily RLS is usually treated with dopamine agonists, but gabapentin or low-potency opioids can be used. Refractory RLS is defined as RLS in which the use of a dopamine agonist has failed due to inadequate response, intolerable side effects, or development of tolerance or uncontrollable augmentation. Options include substituting another dopamine agonist, changing to gabapentin, adding a second drug, or using a high potency opioid. There are several practical considerations regarding the management of insomnia associated with RLS. It is important that dopamine agonists be administered one to two hours before the usual onset of symptoms to allow for adequate absorption. In particular, the drugs should not be given at bedtime to patients whose symptoms are maximal in bed before sleep onset. If the initial dose is given in the afternoon or early in the evening, a second dose before bed may be needed. In patients who have both RLS and primary insomnia, a benzodiazepine agonist may be helpful, either as a first-line or supplementary drug. Similarly, gabapentin is generally sedating and may be helpful in these circumstances.

PERIODIC LIMB MOVEMENT DISORDER

Periodic Limb Movements of Sleep

PLMS are motor phenomena recordable during polysomnography and frequently visible to bed partners and other observers. The original definition by Coleman has been recently modified (57,58), based on new quantitative approaches (59). A PLM lasts 0.5 to 10 seconds with minimum amplitude of 8 μv increase in anterior tibial surface electromyographic voltage above the resting EMG. A minimum of four leg movements, separated by 5 to 90 seconds between onsets of successive movements, must occur in succession to be considered PLMS.

PLMS may accompany a wide range of other disorders. As discussed above, more than five PLMS/hr are found in 80 to 88% of RLS patients (4). PLMS are found in 80% of patients with narcolepsy and 71% of patients with REM sleep behavior disorder (6). They appear to be common in association with obstructive sleep apnea (5,60). They occur more frequently in Parkinson's disease than in controls (61). In addition, PLMS are frequently seen in asymptomatic older subjects. A study of 100 normal subjects using a cut-off of 30 movements over the course of a night found that no subjects younger than 30 years, 5.2% of subjects 30 to 49 years old and 29% of subjects older than 49 years, had PLMS (10). In a study of 100 community dwelling subjects aged 60 years or older, 58% showed PLMS ≥5/hr (11). A similar community-based study of 420 volunteers found that 45% had five or more PLMS/hr (9).

Periodic Limb Movement Disorder and Insomnia

In view of the association of PLMS with multiple other disorders and the high frequency of PLMS in normal older subjects, the clinical significance of PLMS alone has been a matter of confusion and controversy (6,62–64). The term periodic limb movement disorder (PLMD) has been used in widely different ways but was standardized in the second edition of the International Classification of Sleep Disorders (ICSD) (2). In order for a diagnosis of PLMD to be made, PLMS must be present on PSG at a frequency of >5/hr in children and >15/hr in most adult cases. In addition, there must be a clinical sleep disturbance or complaint of daytime fatigue not better explained by any other current sleep, medical, neurologic, mental or substance use disorder or the use of medications. Thus PLMS in the setting of RLS should not be diagnosed as PLMD and considerable caution should be exercised in diagnosing PLMD in the setting of sleep apnea or narcolepsy. But how common is true PLMD and, in particular, how frequently do PLMS alone cause insomnia?

In an early study of 441 successive patients seen at an academic sleep center, 53 had 40 or more PLMS during a night of PSG monitoring. There was no significant difference between the frequency of insomnia diagnosed in the patients with PLMS (18%) compared to the frequency in patients with diagnoses of narcolepsy, sleep apnea or other hypersomnias. Similarly, the frequency of insomnia as the chief complaint (17%) was no higher than that of excessive daytime sleepiness or other disorders (65). Of 1692 patients seen in an academic sleep center, 67 had PLMS in the absence of RLS. There was no association between the PLM arousal index and sleep efficiency on the PSG but wake time after sleep onset was increased in the PLMS patients. However, no association was found between the presence of PLMS and complaints of insomnia, sleepiness, or unrefreshing sleep (66). In a study of 22 older subjects with insomnia or depression, no significant associations were found between the PLM index and total sleep time or wake time after sleep onset on PSG, or subjective measures of insomnia (67). The PLMS index was similar in 20 middle-aged patients complaining of insomnia compared to 20 age and gender matched controls (6). A group of 61 patients referred for insomnia or hypersomnia with PLM index of five or greater and RLS, sleep apnea and narcolepsy excluded was compared to 61 control patients, mainly with sleep apnea. Symptoms of insomnia or sleepiness predicted neither the presence nor severity of PLMS (68). No association was found between sleep quality assessed on a standardized questionnaire and the PLMS index in 78 patients with PLMS (narcolepsy and sleep apnea patients excluded). There was also no association detected in a subgroup of 22 patients diagnosed with primary insomnia (69). A study of 34 patients with daytime sleepiness and PLMS showed no correlation between the PLMS index and mean latencies on a multiple sleep latency test (70).

Similar results have been found in studies of normal subjects. In a study of 100 community dwelling older subjects, the presence of PLMS was not significantly associated with complaints of insomnia or sleepiness, nor with any abnormal sleep log measurements (11). However, in a similar study of 420 subjects, PLMS were associated with complaints of reduced sleep satisfaction (9). Seventy healthy middle-aged subjects were assessed by PSG and sleep questionnaires. There was no association between PLMS severity and any PSG measure, including sleep latency and sleep efficiency. Sleep quality assessed with the Pittsburgh Sleep Quality Index was significantly lower in men with higher numbers of PLMS but not for women (71).

Another approach to understanding the significance of PLMS comes from analysis of arousals. In a detailed study of 10 patients complaining of insomnia or sleepiness, including six with RLS, the relationship between PLMS and arousal phenomena was assessed. Of 3916 EEG arousals occurring 10 seconds before or after the onset of a PLMS, 49.2% occurred before leg movements, 30.6% simultaneous with leg movements and 23.2% after leg movements. Alpha activity was significantly higher during the 10 seconds before movements compared to the 10 seconds after movements. These data suggest that PLMS may be manifestations of an underlying arousal disorder rather than the primary cause (72). Six patients with RLS were treated with levodopa or placebo and the effect on PLMS and arousals assessed. Levodopa resulted in a significant reduction in the PLMS index compared to placebo but the frequency of K-alpha complexes remained unchanged, suggesting that the leg movements were not responsible for the arousals (73). Transient increases in heart rate (74,75) and changes in EEG theta and delta activity (74) have been reported following PLMS, even when unassociated with EEG arousals. However, the clinical relevance, if any, of these physiologic changes has not been established.

Thus, in summary, there is little data to suggest that PLMS alone play an important role in causing insomnia or sleepiness in the absence of other sleep disorders. PLMD appears to be a rare condition and should be diagnosed with care. A sustained response of the primary complaint of insomnia or hypersomnia with the use of dopaminergic agonists can result in increased confidence in the correctness of the initial diagnosis (62). However, while it may seem intuitive to treat PLMD with drugs known to improve RLS and the associated PLMS, no controlled clinical trials of any agents for pure PLMD have been reported (76), apart from studies using clonazepam (77) and ropinirole (78) for a single night compared to a night with placebo.

SLEEP-RELATED BRUXISM

Sleep-related bruxism (tooth grinding or clenching) is associated with either tonic contraction of the masseter muscle or rhythmic masticatory muscle activity (RMMA), a series of repetitive contractions at approximately 1 Hz each lasting 0.25 to 2 seconds (57). Bruxism can occur in any stage of sleep, but occurs most frequently in light NREM sleep. Bruxism is common, but in order to qualify as a disorder, not only must the patient report or be aware of tooth grinding sounds or tooth clenching in the night, but one or more clinical consequence must occur. According to the second edition of the ICSD, these are abnormal wear of the teeth; jaw muscle discomfort, fatigue or pain and jaw lock on awakening; and masseter muscle hypertrophy. In adults the prevalence of sleep related tooth grinding has been estimated at 8% in a Canadian sample of 2,019 subjects, with prevalence dropping from 13% at ages 18 to 29 years to 3% at ages 60 years and older (13). In a European sample of 13,057 subjects, the prevalence of sleep-related bruxism was 8.8% in women and 7.5% in men (79). Prevalence was 5.5% in the 15 to 18 year age group, 8.8% to 10.5% in adults aged 19 to 64 years and 3% in subjects older than 64 years. It should be understood that these figures (13,79) reflect the motor phenomenon alone and not its consequences. In the European study, the prevalence of bruxism as a disorder using the ICSD (second edition) criteria was also assessed (79). Overall prevalence was 4.6% in women and 4.1% in men with the lowest prevalence (1.1%) in subjects older than 64 years and maximal prevalence in those age 19 to 44 years (5.8%).

It should be noted that the ICSD criteria for bruxism do not include any resultant changes in sleep or wakefulness. In an age and gender matched PSG study of 18 patients with bruxism and 18 controls, there was no significant difference in total sleep time, sleep efficiency, sleep latency or arousals between the two groups (80). In a similar study of six patients and six controls, again no significant differences in total sleep time, wake time after sleep onset or sleep latency were noted (81). A further PSG study of 10 patients and 10 controls also failed to detect any differences between sleep duration, sleep efficiency and arousals (82). In a European study of 13,057 subjects, the disorder of sleep bruxism was not associated with insomnia disorder diagnoses but tooth grinding was associated with perception of disrupted sleep in a multivariate model (79). In a study of 917 subjects, mostly shift workers, frequent occurrence of bruxism was associated with symptoms of difficulty initiating sleep and disrupted sleep (83) Thus, there is no evidence that bruxism, either as a motor phenomenon or an arbitrarily defined disorder, causes significant insomnia. It is possible that there may be an association with perceived disrupted sleep, but other data suggests that bruxism may actually be the result of sleep fragmentation rather than its cause.

In a study of 10 patients with bruxism, a significant increase in EEG alpha band activity was seen in a four second window preceding the onset of RRMA (82). Similarly, during the 10 heart beats preceding onset of RRMA, the mean heart rate significantly increased. These findings suggest that a microarousal occurred before the start of an episode of bruxism and thus may have been instrumental in its causation. Similarly, in a study of six patients with bruxism, EMG activity commenced during phase A of the cyclic alternating pattern and especially during subtype A3 (81). Phase A indicates a state of arousal and subtype A3 specifically suggests the presence of microarousals. The results of these studies match with the clinical observation that episodes of bruxism sometimes occur with arousals from episodes of obstructive sleep apnea. Because the major consequences of bruxism are related to dental damage and not to sleep disruption, management usually involve the use of oral appliances rather than medications.

RHYTHMIC MOVEMENT DISORDER

Rhythmic movement disorder (RMD) consists of stereotyped, rhythmic and repetitive movements of large muscles during drowsiness or sleep. The movements take the form of rocking the head or body from side to side or from front to back, resulting in alternative names of head banging, body rocking or jactatio capitis nocturna. The movements are common in infancy and early childhood and in some people persist into later childhood or adulthood. The movements occur at a frequency of 0.5 to 2 Hz and are easily recognizable on a PSG and video recording (57). The ICSD (second edition) definition of RMD requires the movements to be predominantly sleep related, occurring near bedtime or when the person appears drowsy or asleep. In addition, the movements must interfere with normal sleep, significantly impair daytime function or result in self-inflicted injury that would require medical treatment (2). However, whether RMD actually disturbs sleep is controversial.

Rhythmic movements occur during light NREM sleep, especially stage N2, as well as during REM sleep (84), but also frequently occur during drowsiness before sleep onset and following arousals from sleep. Many patients will explain that they have used the soothing and rhythmic nature of the movements to induce sleep, usually from early childhood onwards. In a questionnaire study of 1413 children aged 6.2 to 10.9 years, RMD was significantly associated with a complaint of sleep onset insomnia (odds ratio 2.4), but causation could not be determined (85). Further studies of the clinical consequences of the phenomenon are needed, but at present there is little evidence that rhythmic movements cause insomnia. Unless there is a risk of body injury or the sleep of a bed partner is disrupted, RMD generally does not need treatment although associated primary insomnia may need to be independently addressed. No trials of therapy for RMD have been reported, although the use of benzodiazepines such as clonazepam has been suggested (86).

SLEEP RELATED LEG CRAMPS

Leg cramps are painful contractions of muscles of the leg or foot with resultant tightness or hardness. The pain is relieved by stretching the muscle, often induced by standing on the affected leg (2). Sleep-related leg cramps wake patients abruptly from sleep. While cramps can occur in some neuromuscular disorders, idiopathic cramps are common, especially in older persons (87). Their pathophysiology is uncertain. Leg cramps, when frequent, can cause clinically relevant arousals and may precipitate periods of sleep maintenance insomnia. However, no systematic studies of these potential consequences have been reported.

Treatment of leg cramps can be challenging. While quinine has been recommended, controlled trials have shown at most modest benefits. A meta-analysis showed a relative risk reduction of only 21% with frequent side effects reported, especially tinnitus (88). The potential for more serious complications of therapy, such as thrombocytopenia and cardiac arrhythmias, should also be noted. Gabapentin and verapamil have been suggested as alternative possible therapies, but adequate trials have not been performed (89).

SUMMARY

Restless legs syndrome is a common disorder and is one of the most important causes of comorbid insomnia. It can usually be diagnosed clinically with a careful history. The pathogenesis is not fully understood, but involves genetic factors, low brain iron stores and dopamine deficiency. Population studies show that 50% to 75% of RLS patients complain of insomnia, confirmed by PSG studies showing reduced sleep efficiency, increased arousals and prolonged latency to sustained sleep. Appropriate treatment of RLS can be a vital component in managing insomnia.

Periodic limb movements of sleep accompany RLS but probably play little role in the sleep disturbances. True periodic limb movement disorder is uncommon and, in the absence of other disorders, rarely results in insomnia. Bruxism, while common, has not been shown to cause sleep disruption, but may sometimes occur as a motor phenomenon accompanying arousals from other causes. Rhythmic movement disorder consists of rhythmic movements of large muscle groups but there is little evidence that the movements cause sleep disruption. On the contrary, they may be seen as a sleep induction technique by patients with other causes of insomnia. Sleep related leg cramps are little understood and their severe pain can disrupt sleep. Treatment can be challenging.

REFERENCES

1. Allen RP, Picchietti D, Hening WA, et al. Restless legs syndrome: Diagnostic criteria, special considerations, and epidemiology. A report from the restless legs syndrome diagnosis and epidemiology workshop at the National Institutes of health. Sleep Med 2003; 4:101–119.
2. American Academy of Sleep Medicine. Sleep Related Movement Disorders. International Classification of Sleep disorders, 2nd ed. Diagnostic and Coding Manual. Westchester, IL: American Academy of Sleep Medicine, 2005.
3. Michaud M, Chabli A, Lavigne G, et al. Arm restlessness in patients with restless legs syndrome. Mov Disord 2000; 15:289–293.
4. Montplaisir J, Boucher S, Poirier G, et al. Clinical, polysomnographic, and genetic characteristics of restless legs syndrome: A study of 133 patients diagnosed with new standard criteria. Mov Disord 1997; 12:61–65.
5. Fry JM, DiPhillipo MA, Pressman MR. Periodic leg movements in sleep following treatment of obstructive sleep apnea with nasal continuous positive airway pressure. Chest 1989; 96:89–91.
6. Montplaisir J, Michaud M, Denesle R, et al. Periodic leg movements are not more prevalent in insomnia or hypersomnia but are specifically associated with sleep disorders involving a dopaminergic mechanism. Sleep Med 2000; 1:163–167.
7. Fantini ML, Michaud M, Gosselin N, et al. Periodic leg movements in REM sleep behavior disorder and related autonomic and EEG activation. Neurology 2002; 59:1889–1894.
8. Wetter TC, Collado-Seidel V, Pollmacher T, et al. Sleep and periodic leg movement patterns in drug-free patients with Parkinson's disease and multiple system atrophy. Sleep 2000; 23:361–367.
9. Ancoli-Israel S, Kripke DF, Klauber MR, et al. Periodic limb movements in sleep in community-dwelling elderly. Sleep 1991; 14(6):496–500.
10. Bixler EO. Nocturnal myoclonus and nocturnal myoclonic activity in a normal population. Res Commun Chem Path Pharmacol 1982; 36:129–140.
11. Dickel MJ, Mosko SS. Morbidity cut-offs for sleep apnea and periodic leg movements in predicting subjective complaints in seniors. Sleep 1990; 13:155–166.
12. Montplaisir J, Boucher S, Nicolas A, et al. Immobilization tests and periodic leg movements in sleep for the diagnosis of restless leg syndrome. Mov Disord 1998; 13:324–329.

13. Lavigne GJ, Montplaisir JY. Restless legs syndrome and sleep bruxism: Prevalence and association among Canadians. Sleep 1994; 17:739–743.
14. Phillips B, Young T, Finn L, et al. Epidemiology of restless legs symptoms in adults. Arch Int Med 2000; 160:2137–2141.
15. Tippmann-Peikert M, Silber MH, Park JP, et al. Pathologic gambling in patients with restless leg syndrome treated with dopaminergic agnostics. Neurology 2007; 68: 301–303.
16. Hogl B, Kiechl S, Willeit J, et al. Restless legs syndrome: A community-based study of prevalence, severity and risk factors. Neurology 2005; 64:1920–1924.
17. Allen RP, Walters AS, Montplaisir J, et al. Restless legs syndrome prevalence and impact. REST general population study. Arch Intern Med 2005; 165:1286–1292.
18. Nichols DA, Allen RP, Grauke JH, et al. Restless legs syndrome symptoms in primary care. A prevalence study. Arch Intern Med 2003; 163:2323–2329.
19. Walters AS, Hickey K, Maltzman J, et al. A questionnaire study of 138 patients with restless legs syndrome: The 'Night-Walkers' survey. Neurology 1996; 46:92–95.
20. Desautels A, Turecki G, Montplaisir J, et al. Identification of a major susceptibility locus for restless legs syndrome on chromosome 12q. Am J Hum Genet 2001; 69:1266–1270.
21. Bonati MT, Ferini-Strambi L, Aridon P, et al. Autosomal dominant restless legs syndrome maps on chromosome 14q. Brain 2003; 126:1485–1492.
22. Chen S, Ondo WG, Rao S, et al. Genome wide linkage scan identifies a novel susceptibility locus for Rls on chromosome 9p. Am J Hum Genet 2004; 74:876–885.
23. Levchenko A, Provost S, Montplaisir JY, et al. A novel autosomal dominant restless legs syndrome locus maps to chromosome 20p13. Neurology 2006; 67:900–901.
24. Pichler I, Marroni F, Volpato CB, et al. Linkage analysis identifies a novel locus for restless legs syndromeon chromosome 2q in a South Tyrolean population isolate. Am J Hum Genet 2006; 79: 716–723.
25. Winkelmann J, Schormair B, Lichtner P, et al. Genome-wide association study of restless legs syndrome identifies common variants in three genomic regions. Nat Genet 2007; 39:1000–1006.
26. Stefansson H, Rye DB, Hicks A, et al. A genetic risk factor for periodic limb movements in sleep. N Eng J Med 2007; 357:639–647.
27. O'Keeffe ST, Gavin K, Lavan JN. Iron status and restless legs syndrome in the elderly. Age Ageing. 1994; 23:200–203.
28. Sun ER, Chen CA, Ho G, et al. Iron and the restless legs syndrome. Sleep 1998; 21:371–377.
29. Earley CJ, Connor JR, Beard JL, et al. Abnormalities in CSF concentrations of ferritin and transferrin in restless legs syndrome. Neurology 2000; 54:1698–1700.
30. Allen RP, Barker PB, Wehrl F, et al. MRI measurement of brain iron in patients with restless legs syndrome. Neurology 2001; 56(2):263–265.
31. Connor JR, Boyer PJ, Menzies SL, et al. Neuropathological examination suggests impaired brain iron acquisition in restless legs syndrome. Neurology 2003; 61:304–309.
32. Collado-Seidel V, Kohnen R, Samtleben W, et al. Clinical and biochemical findings in uremic patients with and without restless legs syndrome. Am J Kidney Dis 1998; 31:324–328.
33. Ondo W, Jankovic J. Restless legs syndrome: Clinicoetiologic correlates. Neurology 1996; 47: 1435–1441.
34. Polydefkis M, Allen RP, Hauer P, et al. Subclinical sensory neuropathy in late-onset restless legs syndrome. Neurology 2000; 55:1115–1121.
35. Ondo WG, Vuong KD, Jankovic J. Exploring the relationship between Parkinson's disease and restless legs syndrome. Arch Neurol 2002; 59:421–424.
36. Bassetti CL, Mauerhofer D, Gugger M, et al. Restless legs syndrome: A clinical study of 55 patients. Eur Neurol 2001; 45:67–74.
37. Hening W, Walters AS, Allen RP, et al. Impact, diagnosis and treatment of restless legs syndrome (RLS) in a primary care population: The REST (RLS epidemiology, symptoms, and treatment) primary care study. Sleep Med 2004; 5:237–246.
38. Bjorvatn B, Leissner L, Ulfberg J, et al. Prevalence, severity and risk factors of restless legs syndrome in the general adult population in two Scandinavian countries. Sleep Med 2005; 6:307–312.
39. Ulfberg J, Bjorvatn B, Leissner L, et al. Comorbidity in restless legs syndrome among a sample of Swedish adults. Sleep Med 2007; 8:768–772.
40. Phillips B, Hening W, Britz P, et al. Prevalence and correlates of restless legs syndrome. Results from the 2005 National Sleep Foundation poll. Chest 2006; 129:76–80.
41. Allen R, Becker PM, Bogan R, et al. Ropinirole decreases periodic leg movements and improves sleep parameters in patients with restless legs syndrome. Sleep 2004; 27:907–914.
42. Saletu B, Anderer P, Saletu M, et al. EEG mapping, psychometric, and polysomnographic studies in restless legs syndrome (RLS) and periodic limb movement disorder (PLMD) patients as compared with normal controls. Sleep Med 2002; 3:S35–S42.

43. Hornyak M, Feige B, Voderholzer U, et al. Polysomnography findings in patients with restless legs syndrome and in healthy controls: A comparative observational study. Sleep 2007; 30:861–865.
44. Hening W, Allen R, Earley C, et al. The treatment of restless legs syndrome and periodic limb movement disorder. An American Academy of Sleep Medicine Review. Sleep 1999; 22:970–999.
45. Hening W, Allen R, Earley C, et al. An update on the dopaminergic treatment of restless legs syndrome and periodic limb movement disorder. An American Academy of Sleep Medicine review. Sleep 2004; 27:560–583.
46. Bogan RK, Fry JM, Schmidt MH, et al; TREAT RLS US Study Group. Ropinirole in the treatment of patients with restless legs syndrome: A US-based randomized, double-blind, placebo-controlled clinical trial. Mayo Clin Proc 2006; 81:17–27.
47. Montplaisir J, Karrasch J, Haan J, et al. Ropinirole is effective in the long-term management of restless legs syndrome: A randomized controlled trial. Mov Disord 2006; 21:1627–1635.
48. Trenkwalder C, Garcia-Borreguero D, Montagna P, et al. Ropinirole in the treatment of restless legs syndrome: Results from the TREAT RLS 1 study, a 12 week, randomised, placebo controlled study in 10 European countries. J Neurol Neurosurg Psychiatry 2004; 75:92–97.
49. Walters AS, Ondo W, Dreykluft T, et al. Ropinirole is effective in the treatment of restless legs syndrome. TREAT RLS 2: A 12-week, double blind, randomized parallel-group, placebo-controlled study. Mov Disord 2004; 19:1414–1423.
50. Oertel WH, Stiasny-Kolster K, Bergtholdt B, et al. Efficacy of pramipexole in restless legs syndrome: A six-week, multicenter, randomized, double-blind study (effect-RLS study). Mov Disord 2007; 22: 213–219.
51. Benes H, Kurella B, Kummer J, et al. Rapid onset of action of levodopa in restless legs syndrome: A double-blind, randomized, multicenter, crossover trial. Sleep 1999; 22:1073–1081.
52. Collado-Seidel V, Kazenwadel J, Wetter TC, et al. A controlled study of additional sr-L-dopa in L-dopa-responsive restless legs syndrome with late-night symptoms. Neurology 1999; 52: 285–290.
53. Garcia-Borreguero D, Larrosa E, De la Llave Y, et al. Treatment of restless legs syndrome with gabapentin. A double-blind, cross-over study. Neurology 2002; 59:1573–1579.
54. Walters AS, Wagner M, Hening W, et al. Successful treatment of the idiopathic restless legs syndrome in a randomized double-blind trial of oxycodone versus placebo. Sleep 1993; 16:327–332.
55. Montagna P, Sassoli de Bianchi L, Zucconi M, et al. Clonazepam and vibration in restless legs syndrome. Acta Neurol Scand 1984; 69:428–430.
56. Silber MH, Ehrenberg BL, Allen RP. An algorithm for the management of restless legs syndrome. Mayo Clin Proc 2004; 79:916–922.
57. Iber C, Ancoli-Israel S, Chesson A, et al; for the American Academy of Sleep Medicine. The AASM Manual for the Scoring of Sleep and Associated Events: Rules, Terminology and Technical Specifications. Westchester, Illinois: American Academy of Sleep Medicine, 2007.
58. Zucconi M, Ferri R, Allen R, et al. The official World Association of Sleep Medicine (WASM) standards for recording and scoring periodic leg movements in sleep (PLMS) and wakefulness (PLMW) developed in collaboration with a task force from the International Restless Legs Syndrome Study Group (IRLSSG). Sleep Med 2006; 7:175–183.
59. Ferri R, Zucconi M, Manconi M, et al. New approaches to the study of periodic leg movements during sleep in restless legs syndrome. Sleep 2006; 29:759–769.
60. Al-Awali A, Mulgrew A, Tench E, et al. Prevalence, risk factors and impact on daytime sleepiness and hypertension of periodic leg movements with arousals in patients with obstructive sleep apnea. J Clin Sleep Med 2006; 2:281–287.
61. Wetter TC, Collado-Seidel V, Pollmacher T, et al. Sleep and periodic leg movement patterns in drug-free patients with Parkinson's disease and multiple system atrophy. Sleep 2000; 23:361–367.
62. Silber MH. Controversies in Sleep Medicine: Periodic limb movements. Sleep Med 2001; 2:367–369.
63. Mahowald MW. Assessment of periodic leg movements is not an essential component of an overnight sleep study. Am J Respir Crit Care Med 2001; 164:1340–1341.
64. Walters AS. Assessment of periodic leg movements is an essential component of an overnight sleep study. Am J Respir Crit Care Med 2001; 164:1339–1340.
65. Coleman RM, Pollack CP, Weitzman ED. Periodic movements in sleep (nocturnal myoclonus): Relation to sleep disorders. Ann Neurol 1980; 8:416–421.
66. Mendelson W. Are periodic limb movements associated with clinical sleep disturbances? Sleep 1996; 19:219–223.
67. Youngstedt SD, Kripke DF, Klauber MR, et al. Periodic leg movements during sleep and sleep disturbances in elders. J Gerontol A Biol Sci Med Sci 1998; 53:M391–M394.
68. Hilbert J, Mohsenin V. Can periodic limb movement disorder be diagnosed without polysomnography? A case-control study. Sleep Med 2003; 4:35–41.

69. Hornyak M, Riemann D, Voderholzer U. Do periodic leg movements influence patients' perception of sleep quality? Sleep Med 2004; 5:597–600.
70. Nicolas A, Lesperance P, Montplaisir J. Is excessive daytime sleepiness with periodic leg movements during sleep a specific diagnostic category? Eur Neurol 1998; 40:22–26.
71. Carrier J, Frenette S, Montplaisir J, et al. Effects of periodic leg movements during sleep in middle-aged subjects without sleep complaints. Mov Disord 2005; 20:1127–1132.
72. Karadeniz D, Ondze B, Besset A, et al. EEG arousals and awakenings in relation with periodic leg movements during sleep. J Sleep Res 2000; 9:273–277.
73. Montplaisir J, Boucher S, Gosselin A, et al. Persistence of repetitive EEG arousals (K-alpha complexes) in RLS patients treated with L-DOPA. Sleep 1996; 19:196–199.
74. Sforza E, Nicolas A, Lavigne G, et al. EEG and cardiac activation during periodic leg movements in sleep: Support for a hierarchy of arousal responses. Neurology 1999; 52:786–791.
75. Winkelman JW. The evoked heart rate response to periodic leg movements of sleep. Sleep 1999; 22:575–580.
76. Hornyak M, Feige B, Riemann D, et al. Periodic leg movements in sleep and periodic limb movement disorder: Prevalence, clinical significance and treatment. Sleep Med Rev 2006; 10:169–177.
77. Saletu M, Anderer P, Saletu-Zyhlarz G, et al. Restless legs syndrome (RLS) and periodic limb movement disorder (PLMD): Acute placebo-controlled sleep laboratory studies with clonazepam. Eur Neuropsychopharmacol 2001; 11(2):153–161.
78. Saletu M, Anderer P, Saletu B, et al. Sleep laboratory studies in periodic limb movement disorder (PLMD) patients as compared with normals and acute effects of ropinirole. Hum Psychopharmacol 2001; 16:177–187.
79. Ohayon MM, Li KK, Guilleminault C. Risk factors for sleep bruxism in the general population. Chest 2001; 119:53–61.
80. Lavigne GJ, Rompre PH, Montplaisir JY. Sleep bruxism: Validity of clinicial research diagnostic criteria in a controlled polysomnographic study. J Dent Res 1996; 75:546–552.
81. Macaluso GM, Guerra P, Di Giovanni G, et al. Sleep bruxism is a disorder related to periodic arousals during sleep. J Dent Res 1998; 77:565–573.
82. Kato T, Rompre P, Montplaisir JY, et al. Sleep bruxism: An oromotor activity secondary to micro-arousal. J Dent Res 2001; 80:1940–1944.
83. Ahlberg K, Jahkola A, Savolainen A, et al. Associations of reported bruxism with insomnia and insufficient sleep symptoms among media personnel with or without irregular shift work. Head Face Med 2008; 4:4
84. Dyken ME, Lin-Dyken DC, Yamada T. Diagnosing rhythmic movement disorder with video-polysomnography. Pediatr Neurol 1997; 16:37–41.
85. Neveus T, Cnattingius S, Olsson U, et al. Sleep habits and sleep problems among a community sample of schoolchildren. Acta Paediatr 2001; 90:1450–1455.
86. Jankovic SM, Sokic DV, Vojvodic NM, et al. Multiple rhythmic movement disorders in a teenage boy with excellent response to clonazepam. Mov Disord 2008; 23:767–775.
87. Butler JV, Mulkerrin EC, O'Keeffe ST. Nocturnal leg cramps in older people. Postgrad Med 2002; 78:596–598.
88. Man-Son-Hing M, Wells G, Lau A. Qunine for nocturnal leg cramps. A meta-analysis including unpublished data. J Gen Intern Med 1998; 13:600–606.
89. Guay DR. Are there alternatives to the use of quinine to treat nocturnal leg cramps? Consult Pharm 2008; 23:141–156.

19 Insomnia in Other Sleep Disorders: Breathing Disorders

Emerson M. Wickwire
Center for Sleep Disorders, Pulmonary Disease and Critical Care Associates, Columbia, Maryland, U.S.A.

Michael T. Smith
Department of Psychiatry and Behavioral Sciences, Behavioral Sleep Medicine Program, Johns Hopkins University School of Medicine, Baltimore, Maryland, U.S.A.

Nancy A. Collop
Division of Pulmonary and Critical Care, Johns Hopkins University School of Medicine, Baltimore, Maryland, U.S.A.

INTRODUCTION

Recent years have seen a rapidly growing interest in the frequent co-occurrence of insomnia disorder and sleep related breathing disorders (SRBD) (1). The two conditions were once considered orthogonal, or insomnia was considered a symptom of SRBD. However, evidence from clinical, research, and population samples, as well as clinical experience, consistently suggest that insomnia disorder and SRBD co-exist as distinct disease entities and warrant independent treatment in many patients. The purpose of this chapter is to review the association between insomnia and SRBD, the two most common sleep disorders among adults. The chapter begins with a review of the causes and consequences of SRBD, followed by a discussion of the literature regarding the cooccurrence of chronic insomnia and SRBD. Treatment of these disorders when they are comorbid is considered, along with the potential interactions among treatments, including pharmacological approaches. Clinical recommendations and suggestions for future research are offered.

DEFINITION OF SLEEP-RELATED BREATHING DISORDER

Upper airway obstructive SRBD exists on a continuum from narrowing of the upper airway to snoring to complete obstruction. Snoring, the least severe form, occurs when air is forced through the restricted space of a narrowed airway, causing the surrounding tissues to vibrate. As the airway becomes increasingly more restricted, increased work of breathing, even in the absence of actual flow decrement or oxyhemoglobin desaturation, may result in repetitive arousals. Such events are classified as respiratory effort-related arousals or RERAs. Hypopneas are partial restrictions of airflow due to obstruction. A hypopnea is defined as $\geq$ 30% reduction in airflow followed by $\geq$ 4% reduction in oxyhemoglobin saturation and/or an EEG arousal. At the most severe end of the SRBD continuum, frank obstructive apnea occurs when the upper airway completely collapses during sleep. As presented in Figure 1, several consequences result from these obstructive events. First, significant hypoxemia may develop. Second, increased respiratory effort results in frequent EEG arousals, causing sleep fragmentation, a nonrestorative pattern of sleep, and daytime symptoms (See below). Each of these outcomes has been associated with negative health effects. Further, even without distinct hypopneas and apneas, increased airway resistance and flow limitation during sleep [Upper Airway Resistance Syndrome (UARS)] has been identified as a distinct sleep-related breathing disorder (2) and is associated with negative health consequences.

Although Obstructive sleep apnea (OSA) accounts for more than 95% of apnea cases, central sleep apnea, characterized by the absence of both effort and airflow, is not uncommonly observed in certain populations such as congestive heart failure patients or opioid users. For the purposes of this Chapter, we will focus most of our discussion on OSA.

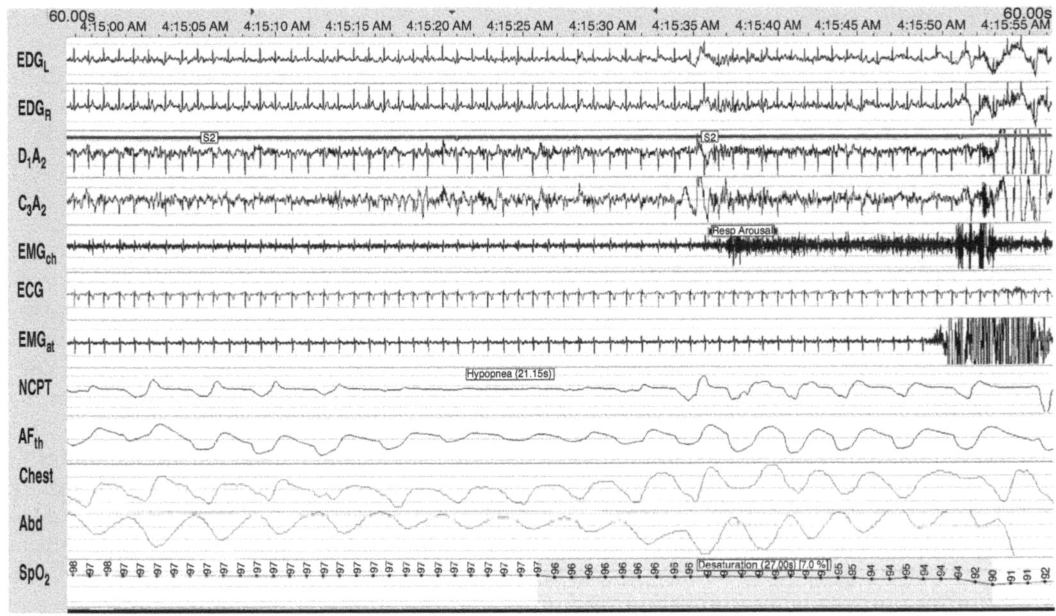

Figure 1 Hypopnea This figure shows a polysomnographic recording of an obstructive hypopnea lasting 21 seconds. Airflow (NCPT and AF_{th}) is decreased but effort (Chest and Abd) increases as the event proceeds. The event is terminated with an arousal from sleep and oxygen saturation falls by 7%. *Abbreviations:* EOG_L, EOG_R, electrooculogram; O_1A_2, Occipital electroencephalogram; C_3A_2, Central electroencephalogram; EMG_{ch}, Chin electromyogram; ECG, Electrocardiogram; EMG_{at}, Anterior tibialis (leg) electromyogram; NCPT, Airflow as measured by a nasal cannula pressure transducer; AF_{th}, Airflow as measured by a thermocouple; Chest Abd, Respiratory effort of chest and abdomen; SpO_2, Pulse oxygen saturation.

Sequelae of SRBD

The short and long-term health consequences of OSA can be severe. Common short-term symptoms of OSA include excessive daytime sleepiness, irritability, depressed mood, poor executive function including cognitive and memory impairment, and other performance deficits. For example, a recent review reported that 23 of 27 studies found a significant relation between OSA and risk for motor vehicle accident (3). Equally striking are the long-term disease correlates of OSA. Well-documented relationships exist between OSA and hypertension, stroke, cardiovascular death, and overall mortality (4).

Of particular relevance to health care professionals working with insomnia patients is the complex and often subtle presentation of SRBD. Symptoms of OSA can include restless or nonrestorative sleep, rapid weight gain, lethargy, excessive daytime sleepiness, reduced libido, irritability, difficulty concentrating, and hyperactivity in children. Such complaints can easily be mistaken for numerous psychological or medical disorders, including depression, anxiety, attention deficit hyperactivity disorder and cognitive impairment (5). At the very least, to maximize diagnostic accuracy, routine assessments across medical and psychological disciplines should include the question, "Do you snore?"

Epidemiology of SRBD

Obstructive sleep apnea (OSA) is the second most common sleep disorder, with overall population prevalence estimates ranging from 3% to 7% (6). Men suffer OSA at roughly two to three times the rate of women (7), although clinic referrals display a greater gender discrepancy, with five or more times as many men being referred for evaluation than women. Perhaps due to decreasing patency in the upper airway and changes in the pharyngeal structure (8,9), the prevalence of OSA increases steadily with age until the sixth decade of life, when a plateau appears to be reached (7). Although obstructive apnea increases with age for both genders, in women, menopause is associated with significant increases in incidence. In addition to age and gender, members of certain ethnic and socioeconomic groups are also at increased risk relative to the general population. Although additional data is needed, African-Americans younger than 25 years or older than 65 years in age have been found to have higher rates of OSA than middle-aged African-Americans or members of other racial or ethnic groups (10,11). Similarly, after controlling for age, body mass, and other factors, Asians are at increased risk for the development of OSA (12,13), perhaps due to differences in craniofacial structures (14). High rates of snoring have been reported among both Hispanic men and women (15).

Causes of SRBD

The exact cause of OSA is unknown. However, certain anatomical and behavioral factors have been consistently associated with this condition (16). There also appears to be a genetic predisposition for obstructive sleep apnea (17). Craniofacial structures differ across racial groups, and these differences have also been associated with higher prevalence of OSA. In terms of behavior, weight gain has consistently been associated with increased prevalence of the disorder. In one community-based longitudinal study, individuals whose weight increased by 10% were found to have a 32% increase in AHI and were at six times the risk for development of moderate or severe obstructive sleep apnea, relative to individuals whose weight remained constant (18). Other factors may also contribute to development or exacerbation of OSA. Alcohol consumption decreases muscle tone in the upper airway and can precipitate apneic episodes in otherwise normal breathing individuals, or worsen the severity of apneic events and oxyhemoglobin desaturation in patients with established OSA (19). Smoking and exposure to second-hand smoke have been associated with snoring and obstructive sleep apnea (20). (Readers are referred to reference #7, Punjabi 2008, for a detailed review of the epidemiology of OSA.)

Clinical Presentation of SRBD

Most patients referred for evaluation of SRBD do not recall their repeated airway obstructions and arousals during the night. Although some patients do awaken choking or gasping for air, a majority of referred individuals present based on complaints of fatigue and daytime sleepiness or concerns expressed by a bed partner about their snoring and breathing pauses during sleep. Not surprisingly, daytime sleepiness impacts many areas of a patient's life, and complaints of difficulty concentrating and staying awake at work are common. Sleep-deprived individuals report poor cognitive functioning and mood disturbance. Relationship difficulties are also common complaints, due to both nighttime disturbance (i.e., sharing a bed with someone who snores loudly) as well as conflict caused by increased irritability during the day. SRBD has also been associated with decreased libido and impotence.

Assessment of SRBD

An overnight sleep study, or polysomnogram (PSG), is usually performed to confirm the diagnosis. The PSG is a test that records a number of parameters during sleep: brain activity (via electroencephalogram); electrical activity of muscles (via surface electromyography); eye movements (via electrooculogram); leg movement; heart rate and rhythm; airflow, snoring; blood oxygen saturation; and chest and abdominal movement. Most sleep centers also use video recording, which allows treatment providers to observe sleeping position, body movements, or other unusual behaviors during sleep.

A diagnosis of sleep apnea is made based on the number of breathing "events" (i.e., apneas and hypopneas) observed during the night, which are calculated into an apnea-hypopnea index (AHI—the number of events/hr of sleep time). Unfortunately, there is a lack of consensus in interpreting the significance of the AHI, and this is reflected in inconsistent diagnostic cutoffs among various sleep centers. Centers for Medicare and Medicaid Services (CMS) define mild sleep apnea as having an AHI between 5 and 15 events/hr, with an associated daytime complaint; an AHI of 15 to 30 is labeled moderate disease severity, and individuals with an AHI greater than 30 are described as having severe sleep apnea (21). In terms of prevalence estimates and determining the relationship between SRBD and insomnia, the sensitivity of these cutoffs is important and can lead to notably divergent results, as will be discussed below.

Treatment of SRBD

Depending on disease severity and individual patient characteristics, most SRBD patients are currently treated using one of four approaches. For mild cases of OSA, conservative treatment includes weight loss, careful monitoring of symptom progression, and mechanical interventions, such as sleeping with additional pillows or sewing a tennis ball into the back of a t-shirt, to prevent the patient from sleeping on his or her back. The next least invasive approach involves the use of a customized oral appliance designed to keep the airway open by pulling the lower jaw forward. In a recent metaanalysis, Lim and colleagues (22) reported significant reduction in disease severity when use of an oral appliance was compared to a control condition. Surgical alternatives such as uvulopalatopharyngoplasty (UPPP) represent the most invasive treatments. Although surgery may be effective in certain carefully selected patients, a recent review (23) found insufficient evidence to support the use of surgical treatment approaches in SRBD.

Continuous positive airway pressure (CPAP) is the currently the most commonly employed and "gold standard" treatment for SRBD and an overwhelming majority of SRBD patients are treated using positive airway pressure therapy. CPAP consists of small machine that generates a prescribed level of air pressure, delivered to the upper airway via a hose and mask that covers the nose or nose and mouth. The air pressure functions as a pneumatic splint, pushing the airway open and allowing the patient to breathe normally. CPAP is the most effective first-treatment available. The major challenge to successful long-term therapy is patient adherence. Careful follow-up and resolution of complicating factors is required to achieve compliance. Readers are referred to Reference (24) for review of minimally invasive treatments of SRBD as well as modifiable psychological factors related to CPAP adherence.

RELATION BETWEEN INSOMNIA AND SRBD

Guilleminault (25) first documented comorbid insomnia and sleep related breathing disorder 35 years ago. With few exceptions, studies of the phenomenon since then have employed one of two designs. Nine reports have retrospectively reviewed charts of patients referred to sleep disorder centers for evaluation of suspected sleep apnea, and several other studies have considered the relations between insomnia and SRBD among older adults. Here the issue of diagnostic criteria is particularly important. Although both SRBD and insomnia complaints increase over the lifespan, there is a lack of consensus regarding the relation between various SRBD cutoffs and functional impairment among older adults. Studies by Krakow and Gold have considered the co-occurrence of insomnia disorder and SRBD in specific patient populations including trauma survivors and women with fibromyalgia. Not surprisingly these studies have varied in patient demographics, criteria for insomnia complaints, and criteria for OSA diagnosis.

Prevalence of Insomnia Complaints Among Patients Referred for Evaluation of SRBD

A majority of studies reporting on the cooccurrence of insomnia and SRBD have retrospectively analyzed charts of patients referred to a sleep disorder center for suspected SRBD. All studies evaluating these patient populations have utilized some form of screening questionnaire to identify insomnia complaints, and none has included a diagnostic interview. Table 1 presents a summary of these studies.

Of the clinic studies, Smith et al. (28) conducted the most thorough assessment of insomnia complaints. In a retrospective review of 105 consecutive patients referred for suspected SRBD, these authors required four criteria for a diagnosis of insomnia: a score of 15 or greater on the Insomnia Severity Index (34), complaint duration of at least six months, objective sleep onset latency or wake after sleep onset of at least 30 minutes (as documented by PSG), and a daytime complaint. Thirty-nine percent of SRBD patients met criteria for moderately severe insomnia. Unfortunately, the AHI threshold used to define OSA was not included in this report.

In a representative study, Krell and Kapur (31) assessed subjective sleep latency, nocturnal awakenings, and early morning awakenings via three individual items, scored on a four-point scale. Just more than half of patients diagnosed with OSA (AHI > 10) reported at least one insomnia-related complaint. In this study, among the patients with SRBD the most common complaint was difficulty maintaining sleep (36.4%), followed by difficulty initiating sleep (29.4%) and early morning awakening (28.9%). Interestingly, a significantly greater percentage (81.5%) of patients without SRBD (i.e., AHI < 10) reported at least one insomnia complaint,

Table 1 Retrospective Chart Review Studies of Insomnia Complaints in Patients Referred for Evaluation of SRBD

References	*N*	Insomnia criteria	OSA criteria	Prevalence of insomnia	Major findings
26	358	Questionnaire items	RDI > 5	OI in women: 27.9%; OI in men: 21.9%	Profile of SRBD-related sleep disturbances may differ b/t men and women, (e.g., women more SOL complaints than men but not snoring or EDS; Women also complain ↑ EDS and ↑ SOL together, more often than men.
27	157	4 questionnaire items	AHI > 5, AHI > 15	42% ≥1 complaint: OI (6%), MI (26%), EMA (19%)	OI: ↓ AHI; MI: ↑ EDS; results similar w/AHI > 5 and AHI > 15
28	105	ISI > 15, duration > 6 mo, SOL or WASO > 30 m on PSG	self-report, chart review (AHI not reported)	39%	Suspected OSA: 2x likely INS; INS + SRBD vs. SRBD alone: ↑ depression, ↑ anxiety, ↑ stress
29	357	3 questionnaire items	AHI > 10	OI: 15.6% if AHI > 60, 18.2% if AHI > 30, 20.9% if AHI > 10; MI: 73.9% if AHI > 60, 62.9% if AHI > 30, 58.2% if AHI > 10	OI: ↓ SRBD; lie awake w/intense thoughts: ↓ SRBD; MI: ↑ SRBD
30	231	3 questionnaire items	AHI > 5	50%	INS + SRBD vs SRBD alone: ↑ SOL (65 vs 17 m), ↓ TST (5.6 vs 7.2 h), ↑ psych probs
31	255	3 questionnaire items	AHI > 5, AHI > 15	54.9% ≥1 complaint: OI (33.4%), MI (38.8%), EMA (31.4%)	INS: ↓ SRBD; INS: ↑ pain, psych probs, RLS, PLMS; AHI > 10 vs AHIÃ10: ↓ INS (51.8% vs 81.5%)
32	119	4 questionnaire items	AHI > 5	33% NOA, 21% EMA, 16% WASO, 9% SOL	OI: ↓ AHI vs MI or no insomnia; MI is most common complaint in SRBD; many SRBD pts have OI
33	232	3 questionnaire items	AHI > 5	37% > 1 complaint: OI (16.6%), MI (23.7%), EMA (20.6%)	Patients reporting maintenance insomnia were less adherent to CPAP prescription at clinical follow-up. Insomnia complaints were unrelated to AHI.

Abbreviations: INS, insomnia; SRBD, sleep related breathing disorder; OI, onset insomnia; MI, maintenance insomnia; EMA, early morning awakenings; SOL, sleep onset latency; WASO, wake after sleep onset; NOA, number of nocturnal awakenings; PSG, polysomnogram; AHI, apnea-hypopnea index; ISI, insomnia severity index; RLS, restless legs syndrome; PLMS, periodic limb movements.

Table 2 Sleep Related Breathing Disorder in Insomnia Patients

References	Study design	*N*	Insomnia criteria	Prevalence of SRBD
35	RCT	45 older adults	TST < 6.5 h, SOL or WASO > 30 m, 6 m duration	40% had RDI > 10, 35.6% had RDI < 5, 24.4% had RDI between 5–9
36	RCT	80 older adults	SOL or WASO > 30 m w/daytime complaint for 6 m duration	29% had AHI > 15, 43% had AHI > 5
38	chart review	394 older women insomniacs	30 m SOL; >20 m WASO, 3x/wk, >1 m duration, + daytime complaint; >30 m SOL at least 1x/wk as measured by actigraphy	67% had AHI > 5; 15.7% had UARS

including significantly more difficulty initiating sleep (66.7%), maintaining sleep (59.2%), and early morning awakenings (51.8%).

Other investigators have reported an inverse relationship between insomnia complaints and severity of SRBD. Gold et al. (29) analyzed data collected from 357 consecutive patients, including 220 OSA (AHI > 10) patients and 137 patients diagnosed with UARS. Insomnia complaints were quantified using three Likert items from an intake questionnaire. Consistent with previous findings (31), greater sleep onset latency was associated with less severe SRBD. Similarly, Chung (27) also found that complaints of onset insomnia were associated with lower respiratory disturbance. In this study, an insomnia complaint was reported by 42% of 157 patients diagnosed with OSA (AHI > 5). Individuals with more severe SRBD likely experience greater daytime sleepiness, which may explain the inverse relationship between SRBD and onset insomnia. We will return to this issue in a later section.

SRBD Among Older Adults with Complaints of Insomnia

As indicated previously, a PSG is not necessary for a diagnosis of insomnia and is in fact often denied for insurance reimbursement. Therefore, PSG data is not typically available for clinic patients whose primary presenting complaint is insomnia. Further, because of the cost involved in administering PSG, insomnia researchers typically screen potential participants for the most common signs of OSA: excessive daytime sleepiness, snoring, choking during sleep or waking gasping for air. As a result most research evaluating SRBD among insomnia patients has been conducted within the context of controlled insomnia research.

In one of the earliest studies to administer PSG to insomniacs, 40% of 45 recruited older adults were found to have OSA (AHI>10) while 35.6% had no OSA (AHI > 5; (35) (Table 2). Similarly, even after screening out obvious cases of OSA, 29% to 43% (based on AHI cutoffs of 5 and 15, respectfully) of older adults recruited for an insomnia study were diagnosed with previously undetected OSA (36). Guilleminault, et al (37) found 67% of 394 postmenopausal women complaining of insomnia had OSA (AHI>5), and an additional 15.7% were diagnosed with UARS. In aggregate, these data suggest high rates of SRBD in older adults complaining of insomnia.

Among the general population the picture is less clear. In a large-scale study of more than 1700 participants, Bixler (39) found no differences in AHI based on insomnia status. Similarly, Gooneratne et al. (40) matched 99 older adults with insomnia with 100 controls. Based on two PSG nights, fewer insomniacs (29.3%) than controls (38.0%) were diagnosed with OSA (AHI>15). Although the later finding may be related to sleepiness associated with SRBD, these discrepant findings warrant more detailed consideration.

Consequences of Comorbid SRBD and Insomnia

Beyond determining the prevalence of comorbid insomnia and SRBD, it is important to evaluate how the two disorders may interact. In terms of sleep disruption, there appear to be additive effects of insomnia and SRBD. Individuals with both insomnia and SRBD report worse habitual sleep than patients with only SRBD (28), and several studies have documented worse sleep during the PSG evaluation. In the Smith et al. (28) study, individuals with both insomnia and SRBD experienced lower sleep efficiency and total sleep time, as well as more time awake in bed. This finding is consistent with Krakow et al. (30), who observed that patients with both insomnia and OSA (AHI>5) reported significantly longer SOL (17 m vs. 65 m), shorter TST (5.6 h vs. 7.2 h), and lower SE (75% vs. 92%) as measured during PSG.

A similar pattern emerges in daytime performance. Patients with both insomnia and SRBD report significantly more depression, anxiety, and stress than did patients with only SRBD (28). Gooneratne et al. (40) found that individuals with both insomnia and SRBD had slower psychomotor reaction times and greater functional impairment, including daytime sleepiness as measured by MSLT, than did patients with SRBD alone. At least one study has found no significant differences between individuals with insomnia and SRBD versus individuals with insomnia alone (35); however, small samples size in this study limited power to identify differences between groups.

Central Sensitization: A Potential Shared Mechanism Between Insomnia and OSA

Although traditionally conceptualized as distinct disorders, insomnia and SRBD have recently been proposed to share a common pathogenesis. For example, Gold et al. (29) suggest that mild SRBD can result in inspiratory flow limitation and increased alpha intrusion into the sleeping EEG. The result is a chronic hyperarousal similar to that experienced by insomniacs. This hyperarousal is believed to account for the increased SOL among patients with mild SRBD.

Additional data support this hypothesis. Chung (27) found that individuals who experienced extended sleep latencies reported less daytime sleepiness, while patients who reported nocturnal awakenings and more time awake in the middle of the night were more likely to be sleepy both by subjective and objective measures. In this study ($n = 157$), only 6% of participants reported extended SOL, while WASO and NOA were reported by 26% and 19% of participants, respectively.

In a sample of trauma survivors presenting for complaints of insomnia and PTSD-related nightmares, 40 of 44 had AHI>15 (41). Similarly, 95% of patients who underwent PSG had an AHI>15 (42). In this study, SRBD, psychophysiological insomnia, and nightmares accounted for 37% of variance in PTSD symptoms, suggesting that sleep complaints are more complex than simply a symptom or complaint related to psychological distress.

TREATMENT OF COMORBID INSOMNIA AND OSA

SRBD in Insomnia and/or Insomnia in SRBD

Although the true prevalence of SRBD cooccurring with chronic insomnia is not known, the above literature review and clinical experience indicates that the two disorders coexist in a substantial number of patients. Yet very little research has been conducted to develop appropriate treatment approaches when both disorders are present. The lack of systematic research is likely due in part to the fact that the two disorders have traditionally been conceptualized as orthogonal. Researchers developing insomnia therapies routinely exclude patients with the diagnosis of sleep apnea to avoid confound and visa versa.

This mutual exclusion is unfortunate, as clinical experience suggests that insomnia and SRBD often interact in complex ways that may compromise outcomes for the treatment of either condition. For example, patients with chronic insomnia who present with subclinical anxiety and more focused on sleep and the consequences of poor sleep, may be less likely to adhere to CPAP interventions and experience the PAP device as sleep interfering. Conversely, patients sometimes perceive insomnia as a stigmatization associated with mental health problems. They therefore may be more inclined to over-attribute all their sleep problems to SRBD, and neglect needed insomnia interventions. A recent study by Machado and colleagues highlights the fact that chronic insomnia, left unaddressed, may be associated with poor outcome in patients with sleep related breathing disorder (43). These authors conducted telephone interviews of 188 clinic patients previously treated for OSA with a mandibular device. Although a majority reported subjective improvement, 20 individuals were identified as treatment nonresponders who perceived a lack of improvement. These patients were matched on age, gender, and OSA severity with 20 "improved" patients from the same sample. In a multivariate logistic regression model, insomnia symptoms were the only predictors of nonimprovement. Similarly, in a sample of 232 patients referred for evaluation of SRBD and seen in clinical follow-up, complaints of sleep maintenance insomnia at baseline independently predicted poorer rates of CPAP acceptance at follow-up (33). This study was the first to provide empirical support for the very common clinical phenomenon of patients ascribing difficulty acclimating to CPAP to difficulty initiating or maintaining sleep.

Only a few pioneering studies (summarized in Table 3) have explored the use of behavioral interventions for insomnia in patients with SRBD, or interventions for SRBD in patients with insomnia. In perhaps the first related study, Guilleminault and colleagues (47) subdivided a sample of older adult females with chronic insomnia into those with upper airway resistance syndrome versus those with no sleep related breathing disorder. None of the sample met criteria for obstructive sleep apnea, however. Half of the subjects with UARS received either CPAP or turbinectomy and the other half received a six-week CBT-I intervention. The group without UARS received either CBT-I or a sleep hygiene education control condition. Interestingly none of the groups showed improvement in Epworth sleepiness scores, and all groups showed improvement in sleep quality, PSG sleep latency, and PSG wake after sleep onset time. This suggests that CBT-I alone may have some long-term benefit for patients with UARS. Only the group receiving CPAP or turbinectomy demonstrated significant reduction in fatigue and actigraphic measure of arousal at six months. This indicates that in select cases intervening on upper airway resistance may be a critical intervention to add to traditional interventions for insomnia. Another major finding from the study was that subjects who underwent CBT-I outperformed the sleep hygiene control groups as well as the SRBD treatment only groups on PSG measures of sleep latency and total sleep time. While this study did not contrast a treatment package that combined CPAP or turbinectomy with CBT-I, the differential gains with both interventions suggest that a combination approach may prove superior.

The only other studies exploring treatment approaches to patients with chronic insomnia and signs/symptoms of sleep related breathing disorder were conducted by Krakow and colleagues (45). In the only study of patients meeting criteria for obstructive sleep apnea, Krakow and colleagues (45) conducted a chart review of patients who had initially presented with symptoms of insomnia but who had achieved only partial remission of insomnia symptoms from standard CBT-I. Nineteen patients subsequently underwent PSG and an adequate CPAP titration trial. Comparing the titration night PSG against the diagnostic baseline, these authors found that CPAP was associated with decreased sleep latency, decreased sleep wake transitions and increased percentage of REM sleep.

In a prospective open label study of trauma survivors with OSA and insomnia, Krakow and colleagues (45) studied outcomes at the end of CBT-I. Patients without complete cure from CBT-I were then enrolled in a CPAP or mandibular positioning device (MPD) arm with outcomes assessed three months posttreatment. Only subjects showing good adherence to CPAP or the MPD (one subject had turbinectomy) were included in the analyses. At the end of CBT-I, all groups demonstrated subjective improvement in insomnia. Improvement increased further at three months on all measures. Of particular interest is that the vast majority of insomniacs (88%) treated for sleep related breathing disorder demonstrated subclinical levels of insomnia symptoms at three months posttreatment. This suggests that insomniacs refractory to insomnia therapies may benefit from further evaluation and treatment of sleep related breathing disorder.

More recently, Krakow and colleagues (46) studied the effects of an external nasal dilator strip in normal weight, sleep maintenance insomniacs reporting some symptoms of sleep disordered breathing. Subjects were randomly assigned to four weeks of nasal dilator strips versus a contact educational control condition. At one month, the nasal dilator group showed large differential effects on self-reported insomnia severity and improvements in sleep quality. Moderate but significant improvements were observed on measures of quality of life, sleepiness impact, and diary symptoms of sleep related breathing disorder. While this study is suggestive, conclusions must be tempered as no diagnostic PSGs were conducted and there was no placebo condition. Since only subjective measurements were conducted with no blinded placebo control, it remains possible that these data might be a function of expectancies for improvement or lack of improvement. This said, the effect sizes were large and future placebo controlled studies using objective measurement and diagnosis is warranted.

Table 3 Studies Treating Sleep Related Breathing Disorder in Patients with Chronic Insomnia

References	Sample	Design	Endpoints	OSA criteria	Major findings	Comments
44	Two groups of Post menopausal females with chronic insomnia: 1. With UARS ($n = 62$) 2. Without UARS ($n = 68$); Mean Age = 62	Clinical Trial, 4 conditions: a. UARS + CPAP ($n = 15$) or Radiofrequncy / turbinectomy ($n = 15$) b. UARS + CBT-I (6 weeks, $n = 32$) c. No UARS + CBT-I ($n = 34$) d. No UARS + Sleep hygiene Waitlist	Baseline & 6 mo - VAS Sleep Quality & Fatigue - Actigraphy (7 days) - PSG	No OSA, AHI < 5 Note: mean baseline ESS ≈7.9 all groups, i.e., normal baseline level of sleepiness.	No group showed improved sleepiness (ESS) All groups ↑SQ & TST (ACT &PSG) All groups ↓PSG SL & PSG WASO Therapy for UARS (Group A) ↓VAS fatigue and actigraphy arousal index with only turbinate sig. ↓ relative to B,C, & D CBT-I > PSG SL reductions CBT-I in non UARS had > ↑PSG TST	combined RX of CBT-I +UARS RX, although not tested may hold particular promise Unclear whether 4 groups randomly allocated
45	<u>Study 1:</u> Chronic Insomnia, failed CBT-I with sleep apnea (N = 19) <u>Study 2:</u> Trauma survivors with insomnia, refractory to CBT-I, and compliant with SRBD RX (N = 17)	<u>Study 1</u>: Uncontrolled, chart review comparing CPAP titration night versus DX night <u>Study 2:</u> Open label trial CBT-I followed sequentially by SRBD RX (CPAP, 3 mo, oral appliance, turbinectomy)	<u>Study 1</u>: PSG sleep continuity & architecture <u>Study 2</u>: Self-report sleep quality, insomnia severity, & sleepiness impairment @ baseline, post CBT-I and @ 3 mo: ISI, PSQI, FOSQ	AHI ≥ 5 plus daytime SX	<u>Study 1</u>: Compared to DX night, CPAP Night : ↓ Sleep-wake transition; ↓ AHI; ↓ SL↑ REM% <u>Study 2:</u> Both CBT-I and SRBD Rx phase demonstrated improvement on all measures. ↓ Insomnia severity post SRBD RX @ 3 mo FU 88% achieved nonclinical ISI score after SRBD RX	Highly selected groups of treatment compliant subjects and lack of control limit conclusions & generalizability
46	Nonobese, Sleep maintenance insomnia with self-reported mild-moderate sleep related breathing disorder symptoms (N = 80)	Randomized controlled clinical trial of nasal dilators strips (4 wk ($n = 42$) vs. contact, SRBD education control ($n = 38$)	Baseline and 4 wk. <u>Primary outcomes</u>: Self-report sleep quality, insomnia severity, & sleepiness impairment (ISI, PSQI, FOSQ, and quality of life QLSEQ) <u>Secondary Outcomes</u>: prospective diaries of sleep-related SX	Self-reported SX consistent with mild to moderate, uncomplicated SRBD. No PSG assessment.	Nasal dilator strips associated with large (effect sizes >1) reductions in insomnia severity ISI, and improvements in sleep quality. Moderate improvements in sleepiness impact and quality of life FOSQ. Diary data revealed self-reported improvement in sleep quality and sleep related breathing symptoms	Lack of PSG diagnosis of SRBD, a placebo condition, and objective measurement limits conclusions.

Abbreviations: FOSQ, Functional outcomes of sleep questionnaire; ISI, Insomnia severity index; PSQI, Pittsburgh Sleep Quality Index; QLSEQ, Quality of Life Enjoyment and Satisfaction Questionnaire.

Drug Effects on OSA

Many drugs can have an adverse effect on SRBD patients. Drugs that depress the central nervous system often result in worsening SRBD. The literature on this subject comes predominantly from the study of anesthesia in OSA patients. The worsening of OSA when CNS depressants are used is due to respiratory depression with resultant changes in neuromuscular tone and loss of protective reflexes. Caution should be utilized when considering the use of any sedative, narcotic or hypnotic drug in OSA patients.

Sedatives

Benzodiazepines including diazepam and midazolam, have been shown to preferentially reduce upper airway muscle tone more than diaphragmatic muscle tone (48–50) This is thought to worsen OSA due to the imbalance of muscle tone. Benzodiazepines also reduce the arousal threshold so patients may have longer events prior to arousing from sleep. Finally, these medications likely also reduce hypoxic and hypercapneic ventilatory responses.

Alcohol

Many patients with insomnia use alcohol to induce sleep. Alcohol has numerous effects on sleep, both in terms of breathing and architecture. Alcohol induces deep (slow wave) sleep but as the alcohol wears off, REM sleep rebound occurs, although this rebound is typically fragmented by arousal and awakenings (51). In addition to its effects on sleep, alcohol is a respiratory depressant and has been shown in several studies to induce sleep apnea in susceptible persons, and worsen the degree of apnea in patients known to have the disorder (19,52,53). Specifically, alcohol has been shown to cause selective reduction in genioglossus and hypoglossal motor nerve activity increased edema of the nasal mucosa, and reduction of the arousal response (54–57). These depressant effects have been shown to occur even with levels of alcohol below the "legal blood alcohol concentration" (58).

Narcotics

There are a number of case reports describing adverse events in OSA patients following surgery in which narcotics were used for pain control (59–62). In general, most textbooks and guidelines suggest caution in prescribing opioids to OSA patients due to their respiratory depressive effects. In fact, however, there are relatively few studies that have actually examined the use of these drugs in OSA (63).

Hypnotics

Medications specifically formulated as sleep aids have been studied in relation to their effects on SRBD. Trials are usually short (1–5 nights) and placebo-controlled. Table 4 lists many of the trials that have evaluated hypnotic use in patients with OSA. Some of the trials evaluated using hypnotics while patients were on CPAP, to determine if the CPAP requirements changed when under the influence of those drugs.

In general, the newer hypnotic agents (zolpidem, eszopiclone/zopiclone, zaleplon, ramelteon) appear to have minimal effects on OSA. Typically, apnea-hypopnea indices do not change significantly and changes in oxygen saturation are minimal and likely not clinically significant. Some of the older agents, which were in the benzodiazepine class, did show some more significant changes in AHI and oxygen saturation, but these were not dramatic. Of particular interest, use of a hypnotic in one study did not show any improvement in CPAP usage, although patients were unselected and insomnia complaints not utilized as a screen for enrollment. (Ref 61, Table 4)

In summary, it appears that some medications (benzodiazepines, opioids) should be used with caution in OSA patients unless they are undergoing concomitant treatment with CPAP. Further studies should be performed to determine their effects under that condition however. Alcohol should also be avoided in OSA patients around the sleep hours, as it clearly worsens SRBD. Using CPAP following alcohol ingestion does not appear to change CPAP efficacy—but again, more study is needed (76). Finally, the newer hypnotic agents appear to be relatively safe to use in OSA patients although, again, caution should be exercised in patients with severe OSA or with other respiratory disorders.

Table 4 Studies Investigating Effects of Medication on Respiration

References	Intervention	Trial type	*N*	Length	Findings
64	Triazolam (0.25 mg)	R/DB/PC/CO	12	1 nt	↑ NREM AHI, ↓ SpO_2 nadir
65	Flurazepam (30 mg)	R/DB/PC	20	1 nt	↑ # apnea and apnea duration, ↑degree of SpO_2 desaturation
66	Nitrazepam (5, 10 mg)	R/DB/PC/CO	11	1 nt each dose	No difference between doses in AI or SpO_2 nadir
67	Temazepam (15–30 mg)	R/PC	15	8 wks	No difference in AHI
68	Eszopiclone (3 mg)	R/DB/PC/CO	21	2 nts	No difference in AHI or SpO_2
69	Zolpidem/CPAP (10 mg)	R/PC vs standard care	16	1 nt each	No improvement in CPAP usage with zolpidem
70	Zolpidem/CPAP (10 mg)	R/DB/PC/CO	72	4 wks	No difference in AHI, ODI, or SpO_2 nadir
71	Zolpidem (10 mg)	DB/PC/CO	10	1 nt	↑ AHI (3 vs 1.5), no difference in SpO2 parameters
72	Zolpidem (20 mg)/ Flurazepam (30 mg)	R/DB/PC/CO	12	1 nt each drug	↓ SpO_2 nadir and mean low SpO_2 with zolpidem
73	Zopiclone (7.5 mg)	R/DB/PC	8	7 nts	No difference in AHI or SpO_2
74	Zaleplon/CPAP (10 mg)	R/ PC/CO	15	5 nts	No difference in AHI, ↓ SpO_2 nadir
75	Ramelteon	R/DB/PC/CO	26	1 nt	No difference in AHI or mean SpO_2

Abbreviations: R, randomized; DB, double blind; PC, placebo-controlled; CO, crossover.

CLINICAL RECOMMENDATIONS

Patients experiencing both sleep related breathing disorder and insomnia are likely to be seen in a variety of health care environments. In each setting, health care providers should inquire, at minimum, about difficulty initiating and maintaining sleep, as well as snoring and witnessed apnea. The diagnostic priority should be to distinguish sleepiness from fatigue, while keeping in mind that patients with comorbid insomnia disorder and SRBD will be likely to report complex symptoms that may involve sleepiness *and* fatigue. Further, patient self-reports will be affected by their knowledge of sleep and sleep disorders. Due to the nature of insomnia as a subjective and highly distressing condition, patients may self-diagnose with insomnia when in reality, SRBD or other factors play an equal or larger role in the overall sleep pathology. In addition, the influence of social desirability factors must not be overlooked. For some patients, both male and female, insomnia may be a more socially acceptable condition than snoring and sleep apnea, or the opposite may be equally true. Practitioners are encouraged to consider their patients' symptom and disease awareness and to elicit as much corroborating information as necessary to reliably discern sleepiness from fatigue.

In terms of treatment, the overlap between insomnia and SRBD presents the equally challenging dilemma of selecting the first targets for treatment. Not surprisingly, there are a number of factors for providers to consider: severity of sleep complaints, comorbid medical or psychiatric conditions, and patient preference or readiness for demanding treatments such as CBT-I or CPAP, to name just a few although clinical judgment should guide the decision-making process, there are a few rules of thumb. Regardless of the severity of insomnia complaints, patients who report sleepiness while driving, who have fallen asleep unexpectedly during daytime hours, or who exhibit other overt signs of sleepiness should be referred for a sleep study, especially if they snore or have witnessed apneas during sleep. Similarly, if patients describe chronic problems falling asleep or staying asleep, referral to behavioral sleep medicine specialist should be considered. A recent report (77) of combined insomnia and poor CPAP adherence documented the psychoeducation, motivational approach (78), and give and take often necessary when treating patients with complicated presentations.

CONCLUSIONS AND FUTURE DIRECTIONS

Insomnia is the second most common medical complaint after pain, and sleep related breathing disorder is the second most common sleep disorder. Health care providers in all areas, including physicians, psychologists, nurses, social workers, and especially sleep medicine professionals, will see patients with combined insomnia and sleep related breathing disorder. In terms of practice, accurate assessment is essential to ensure patients receive state of the art, appropriate treatment. Students and health care providers should be trained in the basics of assessing fatigue and sleepiness and realize that symptoms of both insomnia and SRBD can appear as other medical or psychological disorders. Future research will help illuminate any potential shared mechanisms underlying comorbid insomnia and SRBD and guide the further development and refinement of effective treatments.

REFERENCES

1. Smith MT, Huang MI, Manber R. Cognitive behavior therapy for chronic insomnia occurring within the context of medical and psychiatric disorders. Clin Psychol Rev 2005; 25(5):559–592.
2. Exar EN, Collop NA. The upper airway resistance syndrome. Chest 1999; 115(4):1127–1139.
3. Ellen RL, Marshall SC, Palayew M, et al. Systematic review of motor vehicle crash risk in persons with sleep apnea. J Clin Sleep Med 2006; 2(2):193–200.
4. Collop N. The effect of obstructive sleep apnea on chronic medical disorders. Cleve Clin J Med 2007; 74(1):72–78.
5. Haynes PL. The role of behavioral sleep medicine in the assessment and treatment of sleep disordered breathing. Clin Psychol Rev 2005; 25(5):673–705.
6. Punjabi NM. The epidemiology of adult obstructive sleep apnea. Proc Am Thorac Soc 2008; 5(2): 136–143.
7. Young T, Palta M, Dempsey J, et al. The occurrence of sleep-disordered breathing among middle-aged adults. N Engl J Med 1993; 328(17):1230–1235.
8. Malhotra A, Huang Y, Fogel R, et al. Aging influences on pharyngeal anatomy and physiology: The predisposition to pharyngeal collapse. Am J Med 2006; 119(1):72–14.
9. Eikermann M, Jordan AS, Chamberlin NL, et al. The influence of aging on pharyngeal collapsibility during sleep. Chest 2007; 131(6):1702–1709.
10. Redline S, Kirchner HL, Quan SF, et al. The effects of age, sex, ethnicity, and sleep-disordered breathing on sleep architecture. Arch Intern Med 2004; 164(4):406–418.
11. Ancoli-Israel S, Klauber MR, Stepnowsky C, et al. Sleep-disordered breathing in African-American elderly. Am J Respir Crit Care Med 1995; 152(6Pt 1):1946–1949.
12. Li KK, Powell NB, Kushida C, et al. A comparison of Asian and white patients with obstructive sleep apnea syndrome. Laryngoscope 1999; 109(12):1937–1940.
13. Ong KC, Clerk AA. Comparison of the severity of sleep-disordered breathing in Asian and Caucasian patients seen at a sleep disorders center. Respir Med 1998; 92(6):843–848.
14. Lam B, Ip MS, Tench E, et al. Craniofacial profile in Asian and white subjects with obstructive sleep apnoea. Thorax 2005; 60(6):504–510.
15. O'Connor GT, Lind BK, Lee ET, et al. Variation in symptoms of sleep-disordered breathing with race and ethnicity: The Sleep Heart Health Study. Sleep 2003; 26(1):74–79.
16. Peppard PE, Young T, Palta M, et al. Longitudinal study of moderate weight change and sleep-disordered breathing. JAMA 2000; 284(23):3015–3021.
17. Redline S, Tosteson T, Tishler PV, et al. Studies in the genetics of obstructive sleep apnea. Am Rev Respir Dis 1992; 145:440–444.
18. Newman AB, Foster G, Givelber R, et al. Progression and regression of sleep-disordered breathing with changes in weight: The Sleep Heart Health Study. Arch Intern Med 2005; 165(20): 2408–2413.
19. Taasan VC, Block AJ, Boysen PG. Alcohol increase in sleep apnea and alcohol desaturation in asymptomatic men. Am J Med 1981; 71:240–245.
20. Wetter DW, Young TB, Bidwell TR, et al. Smoking as a risk factor for sleep-disordered breathing. Arch Intern Med 1994; 154(19):2219–2224.
21. Kushida CA, Littner MR, Hirshkowitz M, et al. Practice parameters for the use of continuous and bilevel positive airway pressure devices to treat adult patients with sleep-related breathing disorders. Sleep 2006; 29(3):375–380.

22. Lim J, Lasserson TJ, Fleetham J, et al. Oral appliances for obstructive sleep apnoea. Cochrane Database Syst Rev 2006; (1):CD004435.
23. Sundaram S, Bridgman SA, Lim J, et al. Surgery for obstructive sleep apnoea. Cochrane Database Syst Rev 2005; (4):CD001004.
24. Wickwire EM. Behavioral management of sleep-disordered breathing. Prim Psychiatry 2009; 16(2):34–41.
25. Guilleminault C, Eldridge FL, Dement WC. Insomnia with sleep apnea: A new syndrome. Science 1973; 181(102):856–858.
26. Lavie P. Insomnia and sleep-disordered breathing. Sleep Med 2007; 8(suppl 4):S21–S25.
27. Chung KF. Insomnia subtypes and their relationships to daytime sleepiness in patients with obstructive sleep apnea. Respiration 2005; 72(5):460–465.
28. Smith S, Sullivan K, Hopkins W, et al. Frequency of insomnia report in patients with obstructive sleep apnoea hypopnea syndrome (OSAHS). Sleep Med 2004; 5(5):449–456.
29. Gold AR, Gold MS, Harris KW, et al. Hypersomnolence, insomnia and the pathophysiology of upper airway resistance syndrome. Sleep Med 2007; 9(6):675–683.
30. Krakow B, Melendrez D, Ferreira E, et al. Prevalence of insomnia symptoms in patients with sleep-disordered breathing. Chest 2001; 120(6):1923–1929.
31. Krell SB, Kapur VK. Insomnia complaints in patients evaluated for obstructive sleep apnea. Sleep Breath 2005; 9(3):104–110.
32. Chung KF. Relationships between insomnia and sleep-disordered breathing. Chest 2003; 123(1):310–311.
33. Wickwire EM, Smith MT, Birnbaum S, et al. The relation between insomnia complaints and CPAP use in a patient sample. Sleep. 2009; 31(Abstract suppl):A227.
34. Morin CM. Insomnia: Psychological Assessment and Management. New York, NY: Guilford Press, 1993.
35. Stone J, Morin CM, Hart RP, et al. Neuropsychological functioning in older insomniacs with or without obstructive sleep apnea. Psychol Aging 1994; 9(2):231–236.
36. Lichstein KL, Riedel BW, Lester KW, et al. Occult sleep apnea in a recruited sample of older adults with insomnia. J Consult Clin Psychol 1999; 67(3):405–410.
37. Guilleminault C, Palombini L, Poyares D, et al. Chronic insomnia, postmenopausal women, and sleep disordered breathing: Part 1. Frequency of sleep disordered breathing in a cohort. J Psychosom Res 2002; 53(1):611–615.
38. Guilleminault C, Palombini L, Poyares D, et al. Chronic insomnia, postmenopausal women, and sleep disordered breathing: Part 1. Frequency of sleep disordered breathing in a cohort. J Psychosom Res 2002; 53(1):611–615.
39. Bixler EO, Vgontzas AN, Lin HM, et al. Insomnia in central Pennsylvania. J Psychosom Res 2002; 53(1):589–592.
40. Gooneratne NS, Gehrman PR, Nkwuo JE, et al. Consequences of comorbid insomnia symptoms and sleep-related breathing disorder in elderly subjects. Arch Intern Med 2006; 166(16):1732–1738.
41. Krakow B, Melendrez D, Pedersen B, et al. Complex insomnia: Insomnia and sleep-disordered breathing in a consecutive series of crime victims with nightmares and PTSD. Biol Psychiatry 2001; 49(11):948–953.
42. Krakow B, Haynes PL, Warner TD, et al. Nightmares, insomnia, and sleep-disordered breathing in fire evacuees seeking treatment for posttraumatic sleep disturbance. J Trauma Stress 2004; 17(3): 257–268.
43. Machado MA, de Carvalho LB, Juliano ML, et al. Clinical co-morbidities in obstructive sleep apnea syndrome treated with mandibular repositioning appliance. Respir Med 2006; 100(6):988–995.
44. Guilleminault C, Palombini L, Poyares D, et al. Chronic insomnia, premenopausal women and sleep disordered breathing: Part 2. Comparison of nondrug treatment trials in normal breathing and UARS post menopausal women complaining of chronic insomnia. J Psychosom Res 2002; 53(1):617–623.
45. Krakow B, Melendrez D, Lee SA, et al. Refractory insomnia and sleep-disordered breathing: A pilot study. Sleep Breath 2004; 8(1):15–29.
46. Krakow B, Melendrez D, Sisley B, et al. Nasal dilator strip therapy for chronic sleep-maintenance insomnia and symptoms of sleep-disordered breathing: A randomized controlled trial. Sleep Breath 2006; 10(1):16–28.
47. Guilleminault C, Palombini L, Poyares D, et al. Chronic insomnia, premenopausal women and sleep disordered breathing: Part 2. Comparison of nondrug treatment trials in normal breathing and UARS post menopausal women complaining of chronic insomnia. J Psychosom Res 2002; 53(1):617–623.
48. Nishino T, Shirahata M, Yonezawa T, et al. Comparison of changes in the hypoglossal and the phrenic nerve activity in response to increasing depth of anesthesia in cats. Anesthesiology 1984; 60(1):19–24.
49. Drummond GB. Comparison of sedation with midazolam and ketamine: Effects on airway muscle activity. Br J Anaesth 1996; 76(5):663–667.

50. Nozaki-Taguchi N, Isono S, Nishino T, et al. Upper airway obstruction during midazolam sedation: Modification by nasal CPAP. Can J Anaesth 1995; 42(8):685–690.
51. Guilleminault C. Benzodiazepines, breathing, and sleep. Am J Med 1990; 88(3A):25S–28S.
52. Landolt HP, Roth C, Dijk DJ, et al. Late-afternoon ethanol intake affects nocturnal sleep and the sleep EEG in middle-aged men. J Clin Psychopharmacol 1996; 16(6):428–436.
53. Berry RB, Bonnet MH, Light RW. Effect of ethanol on the arousal response to airway occlusion during sleep in normal subjects. Am Rev Respir Dis 1992; 145(2 Pt 1):445–452.
54. Collop NA. Medroxyprogesterone acetate and ethanol-induced exacerbation of obstructive sleep apnea. Chest 1994; 106(3):792–799.
55. Krol RC, Knuth SL, Bartlett D. Selective reduction of genioglossal muscle activity by alcohol in normal human subjects. Am Rev Respir Dis 1984; 129(2):247–250.
56. Robinson RW, White DP, Zwillich CW. Moderate alcohol ingestion increases upper airway resistance in normal subjects. Am Rev Respir Dis 1985; 132(6):1238–1241.
57. Bonora M, Shields GI, Knuth SL, et al. Selective depression by ethanol of upper airway respiratory motor activity in cats. Am Rev Respir Dis 1984; 130(2):156–161.
58. St John WM, Bartlett D Jr., Knuth KV, et al. Differential depression of hypoglossal nerve activity by alcohol. Protection by pretreatment with medroxyprogesterone acetate. Am Rev Respir Dis 1986; 133(1):46–48.
59. Scanlan MF, Roebuck T, Little PJ, et al. Effect of moderate alcohol upon obstructive sleep apnoea. Eur Respir J 2000; 16(5):909–913.
60. Samuels SI, Rabinov W. Difficulty reversing drug-induced coma in a patient with sleep apnea. Anesth Analg 1986; 65(11):1222–1224.
61. Keamy MF III, Cadieux RJ, Kofke WA, et al. The occurrence of obstructive sleep apnea in a recovery room patient. Anesthesiology 1987; 66(2):232–234.
62. Etches RC. Respiratory depression associated with patient-controlled analgesia: A review of eight cases. Can J Anaesth 1994; 41(2):125–132.
63. Ostermeier AM, Roizen MF, Hautkappe M, et al. Three sudden postoperative respiratory arrests associated with epidural opioids in patients with sleep apnea. Anesth Analg 1997; 85(2):452–460.
64. Berry RB, Kouchi K, Bower J, et al. Triazolam in patients with obstructive sleep apnea. Am J Respir Crit Care Med 1995; 151(2 Pt 1):450–454.
65. Dolly FR, Block AJ. Effect of flurazepam on sleep-disordered breathing and nocturnal oxygen desaturation in asymptomatic subjects. Am J Med 1982; 73(2):239–243.
66. Hoijer U, Hedner J, Ejnell H, et al. Nitrazepam in patients with sleep apnoea: A double-blind placebo-controlled study. Eur Respir J 1994; 7(11):2011–2015.
67. Camacho ME, Morin CM. The effect of temazepam on respiration in elderly insomniacs with mild sleep apnea. Sleep 1995; 18(8):644–645.
68. Rosenberg R, Roach JM, Scharf M, et al. A pilot study evaluating acute use of eszopiclone in patients with mild to moderate obstructive sleep apnea syndrome. Sleep Med 2007; 8(5):464–470.
69. Bradshaw DA, Ruff GA, Murphy DP. An oral hypnotic medication does not improve continuous positive airway pressure compliance in men with obstructive sleep apnea. Chest 2006; 130(5): 1369–1376.
70. Berry RB, Patel PB. Effect of zolpidem on the efficacy of continuous positive airway pressure as treatment for obstructive sleep apnea. Sleep 2006; 29(8):1052–1056.
71. Quera-Salva MA, McCann C, Boudet J, et al. Effects of zolpidem on sleep architecture, night time ventilation, daytime vigilance and performance in heavy snorers. Br J Clin Pharmacol 1994; 37(6): 539–543.
72. Cirignotta F, Mondini S, Zucconi M, et al. Zolpidem-polysomnographic study of the effect of a new hypnotic drug in sleep apnea syndrome. Pharmacol Biochem Behav 1988; 29(4):807–809.
73. Lofaso F, Goldenberg F, Thebault C, et al. Effect of zopiclone on sleep, night-time ventilation, and daytime vigilance in upper airway resistance syndrome. Eur Respir J 1997; 10(11):2573–2577.
74. Coyle MA, Mendelson WB, Derchak PA, et al. Ventilatory safety of zaleplon during sleep in patients with obstructive sleep apnea on continuous positive airway pressure. J Clin Sleep Med 2005; 1(1):97.
75. Kryger M, Wang-Weigand S, Roth T. Safety of ramelteon in individuals with mild to moderate obstructive sleep apnea. Sleep Breath 2007; 11(3):159–164.
76. Berry RB, Desa MM, Light RW. Effect of ethanol on the efficacy of nasal continuous positive airway pressure as a treatment for obstructive sleep apnea. Chest 1991; 99(2):339–343.
77. Wickwire E, Schumacher J, Richert A, et al. Combined insomnia and poor CPAP compliance: A case study and discussion. Clinical Case Studies 2008; 4(7):267–286.
78. Aloia MS, Arnedt JT, Riggs RL, et al. Clinical management of poor adherence to CPAP: Motivational enhancement. Behav Sleep Med 2004; 2(4):205–222.

20 Insomnia in the Elderly

Philip Gehrman

Department of Psychiatry, University of Pennsylvania, Philadelphia, Pennsylvania, U.S.A.

Sonia Ancoli-Israel

Department of Psychiatry, University of California, San Diego, La Jolla, California, U.S.A.

INTRODUCTION

Insomnia is the most common sleep-related complaint in the elderly and its prevalence increases with age. In one study of more than 9000 older adults, 42% reported difficulty falling or staying asleep (1). The high frequency of insomnia has led to a popular myth that disturbed sleep is a part of the normal aging process. In fact, it is the factors associated with aging, but not aging per se, that contribute to poor sleep. Therefore, it is not surprising that insomnia is so prevalent in the elderly given the multiplicity of both internal and external factors that can have a negative impact on sleep.

Aside from the increased prevalence, insomnia is of particular concern in the elderly because of its related consequences. In addition to the sequelae seen in younger adults, such as problems with concentration and poor quality of life, insomnia in older adults is associated with greater risk of falls, difficulty with ambulation and balance, and visual impairment, over and above the effects of medications (2,3). The increased fall risk is particularly concerning since this is a strong predictor of nursing home placement (4). Compared to older adults without sleep complaints, those with insomnia demonstrate slower reaction times and greater cognitive dysfunction in domains such as memory (5). Thus age-related cognitive decline can be exacerbated by insomnia. Perhaps most significantly, disturbed sleep increases the risk of all-cause mortality, even after controlling for important covariates (6).

It is important to keep in mind the definition of insomnia. For an individual to receive a diagnosis of insomnia (7,8) there must be both disturbed sleep and a subjective complaint that the disturbance is associated with daytime distress or impairment. Not all individuals with disturbed sleep meet criteria for insomnia. Although this phenomenon occurs at all ages it may be particularly salient for older adults who might not express distress over poor sleep because of the belief that it is just a natural consequence of aging. Fichten and colleagues separated subjects in a study of older adults into three groups defined as good sleepers, poor sleepers with a sleep-related distress, and poor sleepers without distress (9). The largest groups consisted of clear good and poor sleepers (i.e., reported sleep quantity and rating of sleep-related distress were in agreement). However, there was also a sizeable group who had disturbed sleep based on quantitative criteria but who did not complain of poor sleep. The field of sleep research contains a number of studies of 'insomnia' that did not assess for distress or impairment and hence can only be considered studies of 'disturbed sleep' or 'insomnia symptoms' which represents a more heterogeneous phenotype. As such an effort will be made in this chapter to use the term insomnia only for studies that utilized this criterion.

AGE-RELATED CHANGES IN SLEEP/WAKE PROCESSES

Sleep Architecture

There are both quantitative and qualitative changes in sleep changes with age. Polysomnographic studies of older adults that did not focus exclusively on those with insomnia complaints found longer sleep onset latency, decreased total sleep time, and greater number of awakenings during the night, despite greater time spent in bed (10). There is an associated change in the distribution of sleep stages with more time spent in lighter stages N1 and N2 and less time spent in REM sleep. There is also a gradual decline in slow wave sleep (SWS), beginning earlier in life during young and middle adulthood, resulting in reduction of delta wave amplitude (11). The fact that these sleep changes occur with age irrespective of complaints of poor sleep has led to a popular myth that sleep need declines with age. However, evidence suggests that it is not sleep need but rather sleep *ability* that changes (12).

There are also changes in sleep/wake patterns during the day. The frequency and duration of napping increase with age (13). This trend is maintained even within the elderly population such that "old old" individuals reported more napping than the "young old" (14). Napping is often a coping strategy used to compensate for poor sleep as suggested by data demonstrating a relationship between nighttime sleep fragmentation and increased daytime napping (15). There are some data to indicate that napping can improve daytime functioning. For example, Monk and colleagues found that an afternoon nap decreased objective sleepiness as measured on the Multiple Sleep Latency Test (16). However, this same study found that napping was associated with reduced total sleep time and earlier wake times the following night. It has been argued that daytime napping reduces homeostatic sleep drive that has accumulated prior to the nap, so at bedtime there is less drive available to initiate and maintain sleep, although data examining this relationship are mixed (13).

Homeostatic Processes

Age-related changes in sleep architecture are likely a reflection of changes in underlying brain processes for sleep and wakefulness. According to current models of sleep/wake regulation, arousal state is determined by *homeostatic* (process S) and *circadian* (process C) mechanisms (17). The homeostatic process is a drive for sleep that accumulates during wakefulness and is discharged during sleep. Insomnia, in particular sleep onset complaints, could be produced by an insufficient build-up of sleep drive such that at bedtime sleep-promoting processes are weaker than those promoting wakefulness. Sleep maintenance complaints, on the other hand, could be the result of a decline in process S during sleep that is too rapid. This would create a situation in which there is not sufficient sleep drive to keep the individual asleep in the latter part of the night, particularly after the minimum of core body temperature when the drive for wakefulness increases. There is evidence that homeostatic processes change with age. Delta activity during sleep is a marker of sleep drive, so the age-related decline in SWS can be interpreted as indicating reduced drive (18). Theta EEG activity, which acts similarly as a marker of homeostatic drive during wakefulness (19), has been found to decline with age although this may reflect an overall decline in EEG power across frequency bands and not a decline in homeostatic drive (20). Sleep deprivation experiments also provide evidence of reduced homeostatic drive in the elderly. Following a period of sleep deprivation, and therefore enhanced accumulation of sleep drive, good sleepers exhibit subsequent recovery sleep that is of longer duration and is characterized by greater delta EEG activity compared to baseline sleep. In contrast, studies of individuals with insomnia have found reduced rebound in delta activity following sleep deprivation compared to good sleepers, although the effects on total sleep time were mixed (18). In contrast to research on the accumulation of sleep drive in insomnia, no studies have examined the rate of decline of slow wave activity during the night. Given the high prevalence of sleep maintenance complaints in the elderly this possible etiological mechanism need to be explored.

Circadian Rhythms

The second sleep/wake regulatory process is circadian rhythmicity. Most physiological processes follow predictable rhythmic patterns with a periodicity of approximately 24 hours. These circadian rhythms are generated endogenously by the suprachiasmatic nucleus (SCN) of the hypothalamus and are influenced by environmental factors that act as *zeitgebers* or 'time cues,' both of which can change with age. There is a substantial body of research documenting age-related changes in circadian rhythms in humans and various animal species. Some have even speculated that deterioration of circadian rhythms may be a central component of the aging process (21). Early free-running studies in animals (22) and humans (23) suggested that there is a decrease in the intrinsic period of circadian rhythms. The human data have been criticized, however, because of more recent findings that demonstrate that self-selected light exposure during free-running protocols affects estimates of period derived from these studies (24). In a more recent constant routine study comparing core body temperature rhythms in younger and older subjects, Czeisler and colleagues found almost identical periods in the two groups (25). This and similar studies suggest that, at least in humans, there is no decrease in period associated with aging.

A second age-related change is a decrease in the amplitude of the circadian rhythms, including in the rhythm of body temperature, melatonin, urinary electrolytes, and prolactin (10). In one study younger subjects had an average core body temperature amplitude that was 40% greater than in older subjects (26). Data on the amplitude of rest-activity rhythms, which are less of a 'pure' measure of circadian rhythmicity, are mixed (e.g., 27).

A phase advance of circadian rhythms has been consistently found in older compared to younger adults. During constant routine studies, a phase advance of approximately 90 minutes was found in older adults (10). These results are in accordance with those found for circadian rhythms of melatonin (28) and cortisol (29) in older adults. This phase advance manifests as difficulties with sleepiness in the evening prior to the desired bedtime and early morning awakenings with difficulty returning to sleep (see below).

Lastly, there is some evidence that there is a desynchronization of circadian rhythms with age. Wever found that 70% of subjects between the ages of 40 and 70 years became internally desynchronized during free running compared to only 22% of younger subjects (30). In another study, it was found that 18% of younger subjects met criteria for desynchronization of rhythms compared to 50% of older adults (31).

There are several etiological pathways for the age-related decline in circadian rhythmicity including reductions in endogenous circadian drive, environmental cues, and entrainment. Swaab et al. found that the volume of the SCN decreased by 41% with age in subjects more than 80 years of age (32). In animals, lesions that destroy a large portion of the SCN are sufficient to cause disruptions in circadian rhythms that produced nocturnal wakefulness and daytime napping, similar to sleep changes seen in aging (33). Recently Malatesta and colleagues found evidence for changes in CLOCK protein activity in older compared to younger animals (34), suggesting that there may be age-related declines in the fundamental molecular pathways that generate circadian rhythms.

According to the "environmental hypothesis," deficient zeitgebers, which entrain endogenous rhythms to the external environment, are the cause of disrupted circadian rhythms in aging (35). Bright light plays an important role as a zeitgeber and studies have found that many older adults receive very little exposure to bright light. One study reported that older adults were exposed to bright light (>1000 lux) for only 35 minutes/day compared to 102 minutes in younger adults (36). In a study of community-dwelling elderly, investigators reported that the median duration of exposure to light more than 1000 lux was only 4% (37). Exposure to bright light is the strongest, but not the only environmental cue that can entrain circadian rhythms. Older adults have also been shown to have less exposure to other zeitgebers such as physical activity (36).

Whereas light acts as the primary zeitgeber during the day, melatonin plays an important role in sleep/wake regulation at night. A number of investigators have reported age-related decreases in melatonin production. Kennaway and colleagues conducted a meta-analysis of these studies and found a decrease of peak plasma melatonin levels of 36% and 43% in adults age 50 to 65 and 65 to 80, respectively, compared to adults between the ages of 20 and 35 (38). Several theories have been proposed to explain the decline in melatonin with age including decreased beta-adrenergic receptors in the pineal, increased clearance of melatonin in the brain, and reduced exposure to bright light (39). Recent data also suggest that there is an age-related decline in responsiveness of the SCN to melatonin (40). However, data on the relationship between melatonin production and insomnia complaints in the elderly are very mixed. Lushington and colleagues found no differences in urinary melatonin metabolites between elderly with sleep maintenance insomnia and good sleepers (41). The therapeutic effects of exogenous melatonin on insomnia have been equally variable, with several large controlled studies failing to find any significant benefit (42). The relationship between melatonin and sleep in older adults is clearly complex and further research will be necessary to untangle the intricacies.

Aging may be associated with a failure of the entrainment process itself. Light exposure affects activity of the SCN via the retinohypothalamic tract, which is the primary neural pathway by which bright light entrains circadian rhythms. Once photic (light-related) information reaches the SCN it induces the expression of immediate early genes, such as c-*fos* and *jun*-B, at times of day that correspond to the phase response curve to light (43). Sutin et al. found that there was an age-related decrease in the response of immediate early genes to photic stimuli (44) suggesting a possible site of molecular changes with age that impact the entrainment of circadian rhythms.

The results of these and other studies suggest that there are definite changes in circadian rhythms with age that reflect a variety of etiological pathways. Coupled with the changes in homeostatic processes, it is clear that increasing age is associated with a greater vulnerability to insomnia due to alterations in basic sleep/wake regulation. This is consistent with the concept of *predisposing* factors in Spielman's 3-P's model of insomnia (45). Increased vulnerability to insomnia in older adults can interact with *precipitating* events that trigger an episode of disturbed sleep.

CORRELATES OF INSOMNIA IN THE ELDERLY

Several prior chapters have addressed the most common correlates of insomnia that act as precipitating factors including medical illness, psychiatric illness, and the effects of medications and substances. The mechanisms by which these factors contribute to insomnia are not thought to change with age except to the extent that older adults may be more vulnerable to their effects due to the previously reviewed changes in sleep/wake regulatory processes. The difference in the elderly is the higher prevalence of these factors compared to younger adults.

Medical Factors

Advancing age is associated with, on average, a greater number of physical health problems. In the 2003, National Sleep Foundation poll of sleep in older adults it was found that the likelihood of disturbed sleep increased in parallel with increases in the number of medical conditions reported (46). This relationship exists across a wide range of medical conditions including cardiac and pulmonary disease, but the strongest relationships are found in conditions associated with pain. Sleep maintenance is particularly affected with 81% of arthritis patients and 85% of chronic pain patients reported difficulty staying asleep (47). Aside from pain, chronic medical conditions more prevalent in the older adult such as nocturia secondary to an enlarge prostate, shortness of breath in congestive heart failure or chronic obstructive pulmonary disease, and neurological damage related to cerebrovascular accidents or dementia can negatively impact sleep in other ways (48–50). As the number of medical conditions increases these factors can have a cumulative effect on sleep.

Psychiatric Disorders

Psychiatric illness is a frequent comorbidity with insomnia. Insomnia is a diagnostic criterion for major depression and generalized anxiety disorder, and sleep disturbance is a common correlate of psychopathology in general (51). The relationship between insomnia and depression/anxiety is bi-directional. The onset of psychiatric illness is often associated with a worsening of sleep. However, several longitudinal studies have now found that insomnia in psychiatrically healthy individuals is a risk factor for later development of psychopathology, particularly depression and anxiety (52). The prevalence of psychiatric illness is lower in the elderly compared to younger and middle-aged adults (53) so the higher rate of insomnia in the aged population is not a consequence of greater psychopathology. Although insomnia often occurs in the context of psychiatric illness (so called 'secondary insomnia') data are emerging that resolution of the illness is often not associated with an improvement in sleep (54). It appears that over time the insomnia develops into an independent condition requiring sleep-specific interventions. It is likely that a portion of the elderly insomnia population first experienced disturbed sleep in the context of psychopathology earlier in life, with perpetuation of the insomnia over time despite the absence of ongoing comorbid psychopathology.

Dementia

Although the prevalence of psychopathology in general declines with age, there is an increase in dementia (53), which is often associated with insomnia. In one study of community dwelling adults with dementia, between 19% and 44% complained of disturbed sleep (55). Polysomnographic studies have documented lower sleep efficiency, greater nocturnal awakenings, and more time spent in lighter stages of sleep compared to nondemented older adults (10). Fragmentation of sleep at night is accompanied by disruption of wakefulness during the day. Patients with dementia often sleep during the day, with one study of institutionalized patients with Alzheimer's dementia finding that patients were rarely asleep for a full hour at night or awake for a full hour during the day (56). Insomnia can exacerbate the difficulties of providing care for an individual with dementia because they may be awake and wandering around during the night. Pollak and Perlick found that disturbed sleep was one of the primary reasons caregivers cited for decisions regarding institutionalization (57). During the day, cognitive functioning may be further impaired as a result of poor sleep.

It is not clear if the sleep disturbance is the result of neurological damage associated with the dementia or if it is related to the other factors such as pain or depression (58). Many of the age-related changes in sleep/wake processes are magnified in dementia including deterioration of the SCN (32) and reduced circadian rhythmicity of melatonin (59) and activity (60). There is often also a paucity of exposure to zeitgebers, particularly bright light. Campbell et al found that community-dwelling elderly with mild Alzheimer's dementia received, on average, less than 30 minutes of bright light exposure per day (61). The situation is even worse for those in nursing institutions that are often dimly lit (62). Increased prevalence of sleep disordered breathing (SDB) and periodic limb movements in sleep (PLMS) in patients with dementia further complicates the situation (63).

Sleep Disorders

In the older adult, primary sleep disorders also contribute to the decreased ability to get sufficient sleep, and may present with a primary complaint of insomnia. SDB is characterized by recurrent apneic events throughout the night due to obstruction of airflow or reduced respiratory effort. Reduced blood oxygen triggers an arousal that stimulates a resumption of normal airflow. These arousals are often very brief and are typically not remembered the next day; however they often can lead to full awakenings. Even if each awakening is brief, their cumulative impact can be experienced as a sleep maintenance problem. This may be further compounded by increasing difficulty returning to sleep in some individuals. The apnea/insomnia comorbidity is particularly relevant in older adults, as both conditions occur with higher prevalence than in younger adults. In a randomly selected community sample of older adults Ancoli-Israel and colleagues found that 81% had an apnea hypopnea index (AHI) of at least five events/hr (64). Even at a more stringent cutoff of 20 events/hr, 44% of the samples were categorized as having SDB. These rates are considerably higher than in young and middle aged adults. In one case-control study of older adults with insomnia complaints there was an additive impact of daytime functioning such that impairment was greatest in subjects with both conditions compared to those with only one or zero conditions (65). Rates of SDB are even higher in the portion of the elderly population with dementia (see below). The gold standard treatment for SDB is continuous positive airway pressure (CPAP), with oral appliances and upper airway surgery as alternatives. There is currently little known regarding the impact of CPAP treatment on insomnia for individuals with both conditions, although it is unlikely that CPAP alone will eliminate difficulties falling or staying asleep (see Collop chapter for further discussion of this issue).

Similarly, the prevalence of PLMS, the core feature of periodic limb movement disorder (PLMD), and restless legs syndrome (RLS) increases with age. Rates of the disorders in the elderly have been found to be as high as 45% for PLMS (66) and between 9% and 20% for RLS (67). PLMS are characterized by repetitive limb movements throughout the night, usually in the legs. As in sleep disordered breathing, PLMS can cause repetitive awakenings from sleep and lead to a complaint of sleep maintenance insomnia. RLS, on the other hand, is associated with uncomfortable, tingling sensations in the legs during rest and/or an irresistible urge to move the legs. This typically occurs in the evening or at night, especially when sitting or lying down. The sensations are only relieved with movement. The discomfort of RLS can interfere with sleep onset and make it more difficult to fall back to sleep when awake during the night. PLMD and RLS are currently treated with medications that either target the leg movements directly or reduce the arousal threshold. Dopaminergic agents are the most commonly prescribed class of medications (see Chapter 18).

A third sleep disorder common in the older adult is advanced sleep phase (ASP), as described above. Patients with ASP get sleepy early in the evening and awaken early in the morning hours. Two scenarios are likely to occur. In the first scenario, the older adult, although sleepy, may force himself/herself to stay awake to a more "acceptable" bedtime, yet still awaken between 3:00 AM and 5:00 AM. This results in daytime sleepiness and perhaps daytime napping. In the second scenario, the older patient falls asleep after dinner while reading or watching television and then has a difficult time falling asleep when going to bed later in the evening. That patient still awakens early in the morning. These patients then complain of both difficulty falling asleep and difficulty staying asleep, both of which really result form the advanced phase and poor sleep habits. This type of "insomnia" is best treated with light therapy (see below).

Medications and Substances

With the high rates of medical and psychiatric disorders in older adults it is not surprising that they also have a higher rate of both prescription and over the counter medication use. Although most medications do not have wake-promotion as their primary clinical effect, many have alerting side effects that can interfere with sleep. The timing of dosing and pharmacokinetic properties of a medication will determine its potential impact on sleep. Medications taken at night and those with long half-lives have the greatest potential to impact sleep. Some of the classes of medications known to negatively affect sleep include: β-blockers, bronchodilators, corticosteroids, decongestants, diuretics, and other cardiovascular, neurological, psychiatric, and gastrointestinal medications. A number of medications can have sedating effects and promote sleep when taken at night, but can have a negative impact when taken during the day. Daytime dosing of sedating medications can produce intentional or unintentional sleep episodes during the day and disrupt both homeostatic and circadian process (see section on napping). Despite the well known alerting or sedating effects of many medications, many prescribers fail to take this into consideration when determining the appropriate dosing strategy. With polypharmacy often the norm for older adults, the chances of medications having a negative impact on sleep are high.

The effects of alcohol on sleep are well documented. Although alcohol can facilitate sleep onset, there is often a disruption of sleep later in the night (68). Many individuals are unaware of this negative effect and use alcohol to self-medicate for disturbed sleep. Studies have found that older adults are more likely than their younger counterparts to use alcohol for this purpose (69).

TREATMENT OF INSOMNIA IN THE ELDERLY

There are several options for the treatment of insomnia in the elderly. These treatments are covered in more detail in other chapters but each will be described here with emphasis on application with elderly patients.

Pharmacologic

The first line treatment of insomnia has traditionally been pharmacologic. A wide range of medications has been used to treat insomnia including sedative-hypnotics, antihistamines, antidepressants, antipsychotics, and anticonvulsants. Commonly used medications include those that are indicated for the treatment of insomnia or off-label medications, used due to their sedating side-effects. There are no data available in the elderly to support the use of agents other than sedative-hypnotics so those medications should be used cautiously, if at all. The 2005 State of the Science Conference on Insomnia concluded that antihistamines, antidepressants, antipsychotics and anticonvulsants all have more risks than benefits associated with them and should not be used for the treatment of insomnia (70).

Sedative-hypnotic medications can be classified as benzodiazepines (e.g., temazepam), nonbenzodiazepine receptor agonists (i.e., zaleplon, zolpidem, zolpidem MR, eszopiclone), or melatonin receptor agonists (i.e., ramelteon). Pharmacologic treatment has the advantage of rapid treatment response but there are important disadvantages including potential residual daytime sedation, dependence, tolerance, and withdrawal. Daytime sedation is especially important to consider in the elderly who may be at increased risk of falls. Several studies have found an association between use of benzodiazepines and other psychotropic drugs and an increased risk of falls (71) although there are limited data regarding the use of the newer sedative-hypnotic medications. Brassington and colleagues attempted to separate the risks posed by medications from those due to disturbed sleep in a large sample of community-dwelling elderly (2). Their results suggested that sleep problems rather than the medications was associated with an increased risk of falls. A recent study by Formiga et al followed adults older than age 89 years and found no difference in use of benzodiazepines between those that fell and those that did not (72). These mixed results suggest that caution is warranted when prescribing sedative-hypnotic medications for the elderly, especially with the older benzodiazepines and longer-acting agents. Other factors that need to be factored into decisions for pharmacologic treatment in the elderly are drug interactions given the high prevalence of polypharmacy, and possible age-related changes in drug metabolism and excretion that may narrow the therapeutic index. While there have been few studies of the effect of the older benzodiazepines or sedating antidepressants in older adults, the newer sedative hypnotics have been shown to be safe and effective in older patients with insomnia.

Given some of the problems associated with sedative-hypnotic medications, there has been interest in the use of exogenous melatonin as a treatment for insomnia, particularly in the elderly. There have been a number of randomized trials of melatonin in the elderly, both with and without dementia, including a large multisite trial of 157 patients with Alzheimer's disease (42). Although some studies have found beneficial effects on sleep (ex. 73), a 2005 NIH Consensus Conference on Insomnia concluded that there was not sufficient evidence of efficacy (74). Melatonin receptor agonists, such as the drug ramelteon, may have more potent hypnotic properties because they selectively bind to MT_1/MT_2 receptors with a 1,000-fold greater affinity than melatonin (75).

Cognitive-Behavioral Treatment

Although pharmacologic management is the most commonly employed treatment option, the risks of side effects and potential need for long-term use suggest that alternative approaches may be desirable, either alone or in combination with hypnotic medications. Cognitive-behavioral treatment of insomnia (CBT-I) is a nonpharmacologic approach that uses a collection of strategies to break the cycle of insomnia and reestablish a healthy sleep/wake pattern. The first component of CBT-I is *sleep hygiene*, a set of habits and practices in which patients can engage in order to promote healthy sleep. Some sleep hygiene guidelines that are particularly relevant for older adults include reducing daytime napping and engaging in regular physical activity. For many patients with insomnia, the bed and bedroom are not a cue for sleep because nonsleep activities such as reading and watching TV takes place in bed. McCrae and colleagues assessed sleep hygiene practices in community-dwelling older adults and found that those with insomnia did not engage in a greater number of poor sleep hygiene practices, but may have been more susceptible to their sleep-disrupting effects (76). *Stimulus control* is designed to reestablish an association between the bed and sleep by eliminating sleep-incompatible activities in bed (77). Often, patients with insomnia believe they can achieve a reasonable amount of sleep by spending excessive time in bed, but this results in a low sleep efficiency. The technique of *sleep restriction* has patients curtail time spent in bed in order to increase sleep efficiency (78). The rationale behind this approach is that reducing time in bed will lead to an acute reduction in total sleep time and hence an accumulation of homeostatic sleep drives. Over the course of several weeks the increased sleep drive leads in increase in sleep efficiency. As sleep efficiency improves, the patient is allowed to increase time in bed. There has been concern about using sleep restriction in the elderly due to the potential sleep-deprivation related increased risk of falls. To minimize this risk, a variant of sleep restriction, called *sleep compression* (79), can be used that reduces time in bed more gradually. Patients with insomnia often report that they have difficulty in sleeping because of excessive mental activity. *Cognitive strategies* are designed to alter both the content and process of mental activity in order to facilitate sleep (80). Although there are several cognitive techniques available, a commonly-used approach is to help patients identify distorted beliefs about sleep that are strongly held (ex: "I must get 8 hours of sleep in order to function the next day.") During the night when there is difficulty with sleep initiation, these thoughts are activated and exacerbate the disturbance. Patients are taught to challenge these distorted patterns of thinking, which, over time, can lead to changes in patterns of sleep-related thinking.

Meta-analyses of studies testing the efficacy of CBT-I have demonstrated significant improvement in symptoms comparable to pharmacotherapy (81,82) including an analysis limited to studies in the elderly (83). A particularly noteworthy study by Morin and colleagues compared CBT-I with temazepam in older adults with insomnia with a follow-up of two years (84). Outcomes were comparable across treatment groups by the end of the active treatment phase. However, CBT-I produced more durable improvements that were significantly better than pharmacotherapy alone on follow-up assessment. This study also raises the question of whether pharmacotherapy and CBT-I should be combined in order to capitalize on the quicker treatment response of mediation and the long-lasting effects of CBT-I. They found, however, that the combined treatment group had worse outcomes long-term than CBT-I alone (84). More research is needed to determine if a combined treatment approach can be an efficacious option.

Light Therapy

Aging is associated with changes in the circadian system, as described previously. Treatment strategies that target the circadian system may therefore improve insomnia in the elderly. Given that bright light is the most potent zeitgeber, exposure to bright light, (ie, *light therapy*) should strengthen rhythms. There have been a number of studies of light therapy in elderly with insomnia related to circadian rhythm disturbance. The specific timing of light therapy can produce a phase delay, phase advance, or no shift in phase. The advanced sleep phase commonly seen with aging can be treated with evening light exposure (85). Bright light should be avoided in the morning in these individuals, which may necessitate wearing sunglasses when outside. Although a delayed sleep phase is less common in the elderly, morning bright light exposure is effective for producing a phase advance (85).

SUMMARY

In summary, many older adults suffer from insomnia. There is an increased vulnerability to insomnia due to changes in basic sleep/wake processes, as well as a number of factors that can contribute to disturbed sleep. Treatment options are generally consistent with those used in younger adults, but there are additional considerations when working with the elderly.

REFERENCES

1. Foley D, Monjan A, Brown S, et al. Sleep complaints among elderly persons: An epidemiologic study of three communities. Sleep 1995; 18:425–432.
2. Brassington GS, King AC, Bliwise DL. Sleep problems as a risk factor for falls in a sample of community-dwelling adults aged 64–99 years. J Am Geriatr Soc 2000; 48:1234–1240.
3. Goldman SE, Stone KL, Ancoli-Israel S, et al. Poor sleep is associated with poorer physical performance and greater functional limitations in older women. Sleep 2007; 30:1317–1324.
4. Tinetti ME, Williams CS. Falls, injuries due to falls, and the risk of admission to a nursing home. N Engl J Med 1997; 337:1279–1284.
5. Crenshaw MC, Edinger JD. Slow-wave sleep and waking cognitive performance among older adults with and without insomnia complaints. Physiol Behav 1999; 66:485–492.
6. Dew MA, Hoch CC, Buysse DJ, et al. Healthy older adults' sleep predicts all-cause mortality at 4 to 19 years of follow-up. Psychosom Med 2003; 65:63–73.
7. APA. Diagnostic and Statistical Manual of Mental Disorders, 4th ed. Washington, D.C.: American Psychiatric Association, 1994.
8. American Academy of Sleep Medicine. International Classification of Sleep Disorders, 2nd ed. American Academy of Sleep Medicine, Westchester, IL 2005.
9. Fichten CS, Creti L, Amsel R, et al. Poor sleepers who do not complain of insomnia: Myths and realities about psychological and lifestyle characteristics of older good and poor sleepers. J Behav Med 1995; 18:189–223.
10. Bliwise DL. Sleep in normal aging and dementia. Sleep 1993; 16:40–81.

11. Ohayon MM, Carskadon MA, Guilleminault C, et al. Meta-analysis of quantitative sleep parameters from childhood to old age in healthy individuals: Developing normative sleep values across the human lifespan. Sleep 2004; 27:1255–1273.
12. Ancoli-Israel S. Sleep problems in older adults: Putting myths to bed. Geriatrics 1997; 52:20–30.
13. Ancoli-Israel S, Martin JL. Insomnia and daytime napping in older adults. J Clin Sleep Med 2006; 2:333–342.
14. Metz ME, Bunnell DE. Napping and sleep disturbances in the elderly. Fam Pract Res J 1990; 10:47–56.
15. Goldman SE, Hall M, Boudreau R, et al. Association between nighttime sleep and napping in older adults. Sleep 2008; 31:733–740.
16. Monk TH, Buysse DJ, Carrier J, et al. Effects of afternoon "siesta" naps on sleep, alertness, performance, and circadian rhythms in the elderly. Sleep 2001; 24:680–687.
17. Borbely AA. A two process model of sleep regulation. Hum Neurobiol 1982; 1:195–204.
18. Pigeon WR, Perlis ML. Sleep homeostasis in primary insomnia. Sleep Med Rev 2006; 10:247–254.
19. Finelli L, Baumann H, Borbely A, et al. Dual electroencephalogram markers of human sleep homeostasis: Correlation between theta activity in waking and slow-wave activity in sleep. Neuroscience 2000; 3:523–529.
20. Breslau J, Starr A, Sicotte N, et al. Topographic EEG changes with normal aging and SDAT. Electroencephalogr Clin Neurophysiol 1989; 72:281–289.
21. Samis HV. Aging: The loss of temporal organization. Perspect Biol Med 1968; 12:95–102.
22. Pittendrigh CS, Daan S. A functional analysis of circadian pacemakers in nocturnal rodents I. The stability and lability of spontaneous frequency. J Comp Physiol 1976; 106:223.
23. Weitzman ED, Moline ML, Czeisler CA, et al. Chronobiology of aging: Temperature, sleep-wake rhythms and entrainment. Neurobiol Aging 1982; 3:299–309.
24. Klerman EB, Dijk D-, Kronauer RE. Simulations of effects of light on the human circadian pacemaker: Implications for assessment of intrinsic period. Am J Physiol 1996; 270:R271–R282.
25. Czeisler CA, Duffy JF, Shanahan TL, et al. Stability, precision, and near-24-hour period of the human circadian pacemaker. Science 1999; 284:2177–2181.
26. Czeisler CA, Dumont M, Duffy JF, et al. Association of sleep-wake habits in older people with changes in output of circadian pacemaker. Lancet 1992; 340:933–936.
27. Girardin J-, Kripke DF, Ancoli-Israel S, et al. Circadian sleep, illumination, and activity patterns in women: Influences of aging and time reference. Physiol Behav 2000; 68:347–352.
28. Van Coevorden A, Mockel J, Laurent E. Neuroendocrine rhythms and sleep in aging men. Am J Physiol 1991; 260:E651–661.
29. Van Cauter E, Leproult R, Kupfer DJ. Effects of gender and age on the levels and circadian rhythmicity of plasma cortisol. J Clin Endocrinol Metab 1996; 81:2468–2473.
30. Wever RA. The Circadian System of Man: Results of experiments under temporal isolation. Berlin: Springer-Verlag, 1979.
31. Cahn HA, Folk GEJ, Huston PE. Age comparison of human day-night physiological differences. Aerosp Med 1968; 39:608.
32. Swaab DF, Fliers E, Partiman TS. The suprachasmatic nucleus of the human brain in relation to sex, age and senile dementia. Brain Res 1985; 342:37–44.
33. Eastman CI, Mistlberger RE, Rechtschaffen A. Suprachiasmatic nuclei lesions eliminate circadian temperature and sleep rhythms in the rat. Physiol Behav 1984; 32:357–368.
34. Malatesta M, Fattoretti P, Baldelli B, et al. Effects of ageing on the fine distribution of the circadian CLOCK protein in reticular formation neurons. Histochem Cell Biol 2007; 127:641–647.
35. Harper DG, Stopa EG, McKee AC, et al. Differential circadian rhythm disturbances in men with Alzheimer Disease and frontotemporal degeneration. Arch Gen Psychiatry 2001; 58:353–360.
36. Sanchez R, Ge Y, Zee PC. A comparison of the strength of external zeitgebers in young and older adults. Sleep Res 1993; 22:416.
37. Espiritu RC, Kripke DF, Ancoli-Israel S, et al. Low illumination by San Diego adults: Association with atypical depressive symptoms. Biol Psychiatry 1994; 35:403–407.
38. Kennaway DJ, Lushington K, Dawson D, et al. Urinary 6-sulfatoxymelatonin excretion and aging: New results and a critical review of the literature. J Pineal Res 1999; 27:210–220.
39. Pandi-Perumal SR, Zisapel N, Srinivasan V, et al. Melatonin and sleep in aging population. Exp Gerontol 2005; 40:911–925.
40. von Gall C, Weaver DR. Loss of responsiveness to melatonin in the aging mouse suprachiasmatic nucleus. Neurobiol Aging 2008; 29:464–470.
41. Lushington K, Lack L, Kennaway DJ, et al. 6-Sulfatoxymelatonin excretion and self-reported sleep in good sleeping controls and 55–80-year-old insomniacs. J Sleep Res 1998; 7:75–83.
42. Singer C, Tractenberg RE, Kaye J, et al. A multicenter, placebo-controlled trial of melatonin for sleep disturbance in Alzheimer's disease. Sleep 2003; 26:893–901.

43. Kornhauser JM, Nelson DE, Mayo KE, et al. Photic and circadian regulation of c-fos gene expression in the hamster suprachiasmatic nucleus. Neuron 1990; 5:127–134.
44. Sutin EL, Dement WC, Heller HC, et al. Light-induced gene expression in the suprachiasmatic nucleus of young and aging rats. Neurobiol Aging 1993; 14:441–446.
45. Spielman A, Caruso L, Glovinsky P. A behavioral perspective on insomnia treatment. Psychiatr Clin North Am 1987; 10:541–553.
46. Foley D, Ancoli-Israel S, Britz P, et al. Sleep disturbances and chronic disease in older adults: Results of the 2003 National Sleep Foundation Sleep in America Survey. J Psychosom Res 2004; 56:497–502.
47. Wilcox S, Brenes GA, Levine D, et al. Factors related to sleep disturbance in older adults experiencing knee pain or knee pain with radiographic evidence of knee osteoarthritis. J Am Geriatr Soc 2000; 48:1241–1251.
48. Klink ME, Quan SF, Kaltenborn WT, et al. Risk factors associated with complaints of insomnia in a general adult population. Influence of previous complaints of insomnia. Arch Intern Med 1992; 152:1634–1637.
49. Quan SF, Katz R, Olson J, et al. Factors associated with incidence and persistence of symptoms of disturbed sleep in an elderly cohort: The Cardiovascular Health Study. Am J Med Sci 2005; 329:163–172.
50. Garcia-Borreguero D, Larrosa O, Bravo M. Parkinson's disease and sleep. Sleep Med Rev 2003; 7:115–129.
51. Benca RM, Obermeyer WH, Thisted RA, et al. Sleep and psychiatric disorders: A meta-analysis. Arch Gen Psychiatry 1992; 49:651–670.
52. Riemann D, Voderholzer U. Primary insomnia: A risk factor to develop depression? J Affect Disord 2003; 76:255–259.
53. Regier DA, Boyd JH, Burke JD Jr, et al. One-month prevalence of mental disorders in the United States. Based on five Epidemiologic Catchment Area sites. Arch Gen Psychiatry 1988; 45: 977–986.
54. Stepanski EJ, Rybarczyk B. Emerging research on the treatment and etiology of secondary or comorbid insomnia. Sleep Med Rev 2006; 10:7–18.
55. McCurry SM, Reynolds CF, Ancoli-Israel S, et al. Treatment of sleep disturbance in Alzheimer's disease. Sleep Med Rev 2000; 4:603–628.
56. Pat-Horenczyk R, Klauber MR, Shochat T, Ancoli-Israel S. Hourly profiles of sleep and wakefulness in severely versus mild-moderately demented nursing home patients. Aging Clin Exp Res 1998; 10:308–315.
57. Pollak CP, Perlick D. Sleep problems and institutionalization of the elderly. J Geriatr Psychiatry Neurol 1991; 4:204–210.
58. Dauvilliers Y. Insomnia in patients with neurodegenerative conditions. Sleep Med 2007; 8(suppl 4):S27–S34.
59. Uchida K, Okamoto N, Ohara K, et al. Daily rhythm of serum melatonin in patients with dementia of the degenerate type. Brain Res 1996; 717:154–159.
60. Van Someren EJW, Hagebeuk EEO, Lijzenga C, et al. Circadian rest-activity rhythm disturbances in Alzheimer's Disease. Biol Psychiatry 1996; 40:259–270.
61. Campbell S, Kripke DL, Gillin JC, et al. Exposure to light in healthy elderly subjects and Alzheimer's patients. Physiol Behav 1988; 42:141–144.
62. Ancoli-Israel S, Klauber MR, Jones DW, et al. Variations in circadian rhythms of activity, sleep, and light exposure related to dementia in nursing-home patients. Sleep 1997; 20:18–23.
63. McCurry S, Ancoli-Israel S. Sleep dysfunction in Alzheimer's disease and other dementias. Curr Treat Options Neurol 2003; 5:261–272.
64. Ancoli-Israel S, Kripke DF, Klauber MH. Sleep disordered breathing in community-dwelling elderly. Sleep 1991; 14:486–495.
65. Gooneratne NS, Gehrman PR, Nkwuo JE, et al. Consequences of comorbid insomnia symptoms and sleep-related breathing disorder in elderly subjects. Arch Intern Med 2006; 166:1732–1738.
66. Ancoli-Israel S, Kripke DF, Klauber MR. Periodic limb movements in sleep in community-dwelling elderly. Sleep 1991; 14:496–500.
67. Hornyak M, Trenkwalder C. Restless legs syndrome and periodic limb movement disorder in the elderly. J Psychosom Res 2004; 56:543–548.
68. Stein MD, Friedmann PD. Disturbed sleep and its relationship to alcohol use. Subst Abus 2005; 26: 1–13.
69. National Sleep Foundation/WB&A Market Research. Sleep in American Survey. Washington, D.C.: National Sleep Foundation, 2005.
70. NIH State-of-the-Science Conference Statement on manifestations and management of chronic insomnia in adults. NIH Consens State Sci Statements 2005; 22(2):1–30.

71. Kelly KD, Pickett W, Yiannakoulias N, et al. Medication use and falls in community-dwelling older persons. Age Ageing 2003; 32:503–509.
72. Formiga F, Ferrer A, Duaso E, et al. Falls in Nonagenarians Living in their Own Homes: The Nonasantfeliu Study. J Nutr Health Aging 2008; 12:273–276.
73. Dowling GA, Mastick J, Colling E, et al. Melatonin for sleep disturbances in Parkinson's disease. Sleep Med 2005; 6:459–466.
74. National Institutes of Health. National Institutes of Health State of the Science Conference statement on Manifestations and Management of Chronic Insomnia in Adults, June 13–15, 2005. Sleep 2005; 28:1049–1057.
75. Kato K, Hirai K, Nishiyama K, et al. Neurochemical properties of ramelteon (TAK-375), a selective MT1/MT2 receptor agonist. Neuropharmacology 2005; 48:301–310.
76. McCrae CS, Rowe MA, Dautovich ND, et al. Sleep hygiene practices in two community dwelling samples of older adults. Sleep 2006; 29:1551–1560.
77. Bootzin RR, Nicassio PM. Behavioral treatments for insomnia. In: Hersen M, Eisler RM, Miller PM, eds. Progress in Behavior Modification, Vol. 6. New York, NY: Academic Press, Inc, 1978:1–45.
78. Spielman AJ, Saskin P, Thorpy MJ. Treatment of chronic insomnia by restriction of time in bed. Sleep 1987; 10:45–56.
79. Lichstein KL, Riedel BW, Wilson NM, et al. Relaxation and sleep compression for late-life insomnia: A placebo-controlled trial. J Consult Clin Psychol 2001; 69:227–239.
80. Harvey AG, Tang NK, Browning L. Cognitive approaches to insomnia. Clin Psychol Rev 2005; 25:593–611.
81. Morin CM, Culbert JP, Schwartz MS. Non-pharmacological interventions for insomnia: A meta-analysis of treatment efficacy. Am J Psychiatry 1994; 151:1172–1180.
82. Smith MT, Perlis ML, Park A, et al. Comparative meta-analysis of pharmacotherapy and behavior therapy for persistent insomnia. Am J Psychiatry 2002; 159:5–11.
83. Montgomery P, Dennis J. Cognitive behavioural interventions for sleep problems in adults aged 60+. Cochrane Database Syst Rev 2003; (1):CD003161.
84. Morin CM, Colecchi C, Stone J, et al. Behavioral and pharmacological therapies for late-life insomnia: A randomized controlled trial. JAMA 1999; 281:991–999.
85. Sack RL, Auckley D, Auger RR, et al. Circadian rhythm sleep disorders: Part II, advanced sleep phase disorder, delayed sleep phase disorder, free-running disorder, and irregular sleep-wake rhythm. An American Academy of Sleep Medicine review. Sleep 2007; 30:1484–1501.

21 Pediatric Insomnia

Bobbi Hopkins and Daniel Glaze

Baylor College of Medicine, Texas Children's Hospital Children's Sleep Center, Houston, Texas, U.S.A.

INTRODUCTION

Pediatric insomnia is defined as a "repeated difficulty with sleep initiation, duration, consolidation, or quality that occurs despite age appropriate time and opportunity for sleep and results in some form of daytime functional impairment for the child and/or the family" (1). The etiology of the insomnia varies based on age and is frequently multifactorial. Factors contributing to insomnia in children vary, but include bedtime resistance, inability to fall asleep easily, frequent or prolonged night awakenings, early morning awakenings, circadian rhythm disorders, parasomnias, sleep-related movement disorders, and sleep-related breathing disorders (2,3).

Children with insomnia and decreased sleep duration are more likely to have difficulties with attention, hyperactivity, excessive daytime sleepiness, interpersonal relationships, and health (4,5). Tantrums and behavior issues are more likely to occur in young children with sleep problems compared to those without sleep problems. Up to 20% of school-aged children with sleep difficulties have failed at least one year of school (6). Depression and anxiety are increased in children with sleep problems (7). When children do not sleep well, their families do not sleep well. Mothers of infants with sleep problems are more likely to report depression (8). For every one-hour reduction in the number of hours of sleep per night, the odds of childhood obesity increase by 41% (9). Unfortunately, children with early sleep difficulties are more likely to have problems sleeping when they are older (2). Therefore, early diagnosis and treatment is paramount to a child's success.

THE DEVELOPMENT OF NORMAL SLEEP

Identification and diagnosis of insomnia in children requires knowledge about the normal development of sleep in children. Pediatric sleep patterns evolve with age. The average number of hours of sleep in a 24-hour period decreases from 14.2 hours as an infant to 8.1 hours as an adolescent (10).

Infants and Toddlers (0–2 Years)

During the first three months of life, infants typically sleep three to four hours at a time, achieving between 16 to 17 hours of sleep in a 24 hour period (11). However, over the course of the first year, most infants develop a diurnal sleep pattern with the majority of their sleep being consolidated during the night with an accumulated two to three hours of napping during the day (12). By nine months of age, 70% of children sleep throughout the night (13). At one year of age, most children sleep between 13 to 16 hours in a 24-hour period with the majority of the sleep consolidated during the night and with two daytime naps (12). By 18 months of age, children change from two daytime naps to one daytime nap (10).

Parents of infants report frequent nighttime awakenings and early morning awakenings (14). Observational studies have shown that normally developing infants wake intermittently throughout the night and most will vocalize with the awakenings (15). Infants who are put into their beds awake are more likely to be able to self-regulate or "self-soothe" themselves back to sleep without intervention following an awakening and this skill increases with age (15). Self-soothers have longer periods of consolidated sleep and an increased amount of quiet sleep than non self-soothers (15).

Parent-infant interaction, environment, and childhood illnesses all impact the development of the infant's sleep habits. The presence of parents at sleep onset and provision of food or drink at a nighttime awakening are associated with a greater likelihood of sleep difficulties in infants (16,17). Maternal separation anxiety is associated with increased night waking (18). Frequent nocturnal awakenings are associated with increased accidental injury in toddlers (19).

Young Children (3–6 Years)

At three years of age a child sleeps approximately 12 hours in a 24 hour period decreasing to approximately 11 hours in a 24 hour period by three years of age (10). The majority of the sleep is consolidated during the night. Although 50% of children take a daytime nap at three years of age, daytime naps become shorter and less frequent with age with only 8% of children napping at five years of age (10).

In this age range many children experience bedtime issues, including refusal to go to bed or to sleep. In a study of children four to six years of age, 17.3% were reported to take more than 30 minutes to fall asleep and 10.1% were reported to have "too much energy to sleep" at least once per week (2). Night awakenings tend to decrease with age, but 15.6% of parents report night awakenings to be at least a weekly problem for their children (2).

School-Aged Children (7–12 Years)

The total number of hours a child sleeps in a 24-hour period decreases further from an average of 10.6 hours at 7 years of age to approximately 9.3 hours at 12 years of age (10). Children in this age range no longer take routine naps (10). The frequency of problematic night awakenings continues to decline with under 10% of children 11 to 12 years of age experiencing difficulties more than one time per week (2). However, sleep initiation insomnia remains problematic with 13.1% of 7 to 10 year olds and 15.3% of 11 to 12 year old children taking more than 30 minutes to fall asleep at least one time per week (2). Inadequate sleep hygiene starts to contribute to insomnia in this age group. Television decreases sleep efficiency and computer games prolong the time to go to sleep in school-aged children (20). Adjustment and psychophysiologic insomnia as well as insomnia secondary to other medical or mental disorders become more prevalent at this age.

Adolescents (13–18 Years)

Adolescents typically require between eight to nine hours of sleep per night, but in reality, many achieve less than 8 hours of sleep per night (10,21). Adolescents tend to go to bed and sleep at later times, but are obligated to rise early for school (21). In a large population study of adolescents aged 15 to 18 years, 14.1% reported difficulty initiating sleep, 10.5% reported early morning awakenings, and 8.4% reported disrupted sleep (22). Insufficient sleep syndrome and sleep onset insomnia in adolescents are associated with lower school performance (21,23). A significantly increased number of adolescent girls 11 to 14 years of age report difficulties initiating and maintaining sleep compared to boys of the same age or younger children (24). Adolescent somatic, interpersonal, and psychological function are negatively influenced by insomnia (25).

EPIDEMIOLOGY

Insomnia is a common problem for children and the etiology tends to vary based on age. Up to 40% of infants and up to 50% of preschool aged children have difficulty initiating sleep or frequent night awakenings (26–30). Of school-aged children 4 to 12 years, 15% take longer than 30 minutes to fall asleep and 12% experience frequent nighttime awakenings more than once per week (2). Approximately one quarter of adolescents have symptoms of insomnia (31).

Family history plays a role in the development of insomnia. Of persons with childhood-onset insomnia, 55% have a positive family history (32). Persons with mood disorders who are homozygous for the Clock 3111C variant are more likely to have difficulties initiating and maintaining sleep and are more likely to have early morning awakenings (33).

Insomnia occurs more frequently in children with neurological and psychiatric disorders. More than 40% of toddlers with developmental delays or autism suffer from insomnia (34). Children with autism and sleep difficulties have more affective problems compared to those children with autism who were considered to be good sleepers (35). Children with attention-deficit/hyperactivity disorder and sleep onset insomnia have delayed sleep phase and delayed melatonin release compared to children with attention deficit and hyperactivity disorder (ADHD) and no difficulties initiating sleep (36).

CLASSIFICATION OF PEDIATRIC INSOMNIA

Since the publication of the second edition of the International Classification of Sleep Disorders, there have been no large scale studies examining the prevalence of the different classifications of insomnia in the pediatric population. Table 1 summarizes the various types of insomnia and provides information as it pertains to children. Children are susceptible to the same types of insomnia reported in adults, but behavioral insomnia of childhood is unique to these age groups.

Behavioral Insomnia of Childhood

Up to 30% of infants, toddlers, and preschool aged children have difficulties going to bed or with frequent night awakenings (29). When these issues are persistent and significant enough to affect the child and/or the family, and are related to a behavioral etiology, this is referred to as behavioral insomnia of childhood. The condition may be the result of several factors. First, sleep difficulties in young children may be related to neurodevelopmental maturation or an underlying genetic predisposition to insomnia (64). Second, the parent-child interaction as well as the parents' personal characteristics play a role in the child's ability to learn "self soothing" techniques (16–18,64). Third, the environment (e.g., cosleeping in some cultures) in which the child sleeps may contribute to sleep difficulties (64).

Children may display one of two types of behavioral insomnia: sleep onset association type or limit-setting type (37). The two types may occur independently, but frequently occur together. Children with *sleep-onset association type* of behavioral insomnia have significant difficulty falling asleep without a specific routine, environment, or object (37). Common routines include rocking, feeding, or massaging to go to sleep. Some children learn to go to sleep only in their parents' room or when riding in the car. Certain objects, such as blankets, can be used to help develop a positive sleep association. However, some object associations may become problematic if the object is not available at all times for sleep or if the object is easily lost during the night (e.g., pacifiers). Sleep onset association often results in frequent nighttime awakenings requiring parental intervention (37).

Children with *limit setting type* of behavioral insomnia refuse to go to bed either at the initial bedtime or following nighttime awakenings (37). Children may bargain with their parents, citing a variety of reasons including thirst, hunger, or fear to avoid going to bed. Insufficient or variable limit setting by parents in the face of these challenges results in persistent and progressive resistance to sleep on the part of the child (37).

DIFFERENTIAL DIAGNOSIS

Before diagnosing a patient with a specific type of insomnia it is important to evaluate the patient for other sleep disorders which could present in a similar fashion.

Delayed sleep phase syndrome is a common disorder, which typically presents during adolescence. It is characterized by difficulty falling asleep until later than the desired bedtime. Once asleep, the patient sleeps for normal durations, if allowed, often waking late in the day (37). Teenagers may experience problems initiating sleep at conventional hours and insufficient sleep because of early awakening to meet school start times. Treatment for delayed sleep phase syndrome may include chronotherapeutic approaches to reset the circadian clock, use of bright light upon awakening and dim light prior to bed, melatonin, and/or pharmacotherapy (65). (Chapter 18)

Restless leg syndrome and periodic limb movement disorders are increasingly recognized in children. Children with restless leg syndrome may have difficulty initiating and maintaining sleep. Older children and adolescents may have sleep disturbances dating back to infancy (66). Periodic limb movements in sleep may contribute to decreased REM sleep and increased arousals (67). Because of the chronic nature of both of these disorders, they may mimic idiopathic insomnia if left untreated. These disorders have been associated with low serum ferritin (68). Treatment strategies are poorly studied in children, but may include dietary (iron supplement, decrease caffeine), sleep hygiene, and pharmacologic agents (68).

Obstructive sleep apnea is associated with snoring, gasping and coughing during sleep, and early morning headaches. It can contribute to frequent arousals from sleep and night awakenings, mimicking insomnia. First line treatment is often tonsillectomy and

Table 1 Summary of ICSD Second Edition Classification of Insomnia: Pediatric Associations

All forms of insomnia share basic criteria:(37)

- Difficulty initiating or maintaining sleep, early morning awakenings, or nonrestorative sleep
- The patient has an age appropriate opportunity to sleep
- Sleep difficulties contribute to daytime impairment
- Sleep difficulties are not better explained by a sleep disorder, psychiatric, or medical condition.

Insomnia Classification (37)	**Pediatric Associations**
Adjustment Insomnia • Symptoms present for less than 3 mo • Identifiable stressor • Symptoms resolve after removal of or adaptation to the stressor	• Pediatric prevalence unknown • Not well studied in children • Potential stressors for children: ○ Change in family (divorce, death, move) ○ School-related challenges (tests, tryouts, big game) ○ Relationships (difficulty with friends, bullies, children who are abused)
Psychophysiologic Insomnia • Symptoms present for > 1 mo • Anxiety associated with sleep • Trouble sleeping in bed, but able to fall asleep in other places not typically meant for sleep or away from home • Heightened arousal when trying to go to sleep	• Not well studied in children • 46% of adults with chronic insomnia cite adverse events in childhood with persisting insomnia (38) • Anecdotally, children frequently present with longstanding difficulty initiating sleep accompanied by anxiety associated with sleep and hyperarousal when in bed. These children (and their families) become excessively focused on their inability to sleep. • Can give rise to multiple problems involving sleep hygiene including sleeping during class or taking an afternoon nap, use of media, and use of substances both to stay awake and to promote sleep.
Paradoxical Insomnia • Symptoms present for at least 1 mo • Report of chronic, severe, almost nightly sleep deprivation • Increased awareness of environmental stimuli and/or conscious thoughts • Daytime impairment is less than expected given the severity of the reported sleep deprivation • There may be a discrepancy between subjective sleep logs and objective measures (actigraphy, polysomnography)	• Pediatric prevalence unknown, but thought to be rare (37) • Be aware of discrepancies between parent and child sleep time reporting. • If this diagnosis is considered, sleep diaries combined with actigraphy may be helpful.
Idiopathic Insomnia • Persistent unremitting insomnia starting during infancy or childhood • Diagnosis of exclusion, no cause identified	• Prevalence for 15–18 yr = 0.7%; In younger ages, the prevalence is unknown (22) • In a small sample of adults reporting onset of insomnia as a child, more reported neurological conditions including dyslexia, hyperkinesis, abnormal electroencephalograms, or "minimal brain damage" compared to persons with adult onset insomnia (32). • Consider behavioral insomnia of childhood in younger children. • Older children may develop inadequate sleep hygiene, medication dependence, or features of psychophysiologic insomnia (39).

Table 1 Summary of ICSD Second Edition Classification of Insomnia: Pediatric Associations (*Continued*)

Insomnia Because of Mental Disorder • Symptoms present for > 1 mo • A mental disorder is present. • The insomnia is associated with the mental disorder • The insomnia is significant enough that it requires treatment separate from the treatment for the mood disorder	• Prevalence in the pediatric population is > 50% in children presenting to a sleep disorders clinic (40) • Children with a comorbid psychiatric disorder present with insomnia an average of two years earlier than children without psychiatric disorders (41). • Children with anxiety and depression have prolonged sleep latencies (7). • Children with bipolar disorder have decreased sleep efficiency, more frequent nocturnal awakenings, and a decreased need for sleep (42,43). • Almost 30% of unmedicated children with ADHD have difficulties with sleep onset (44,45).
Inadequate Sleep Hygiene • Symptoms present > 1 mo • At least one: ○ Developmentally inappropriate sleep schedule ○ Use of substances (caffeine, alcohol, nicotine, illicit drugs, or supplements prior to bed) ○ Mentally or physically stimulating activity prior to bedtime ○ Activities other than sleep in the bed ○ Uncomfortable sleeping environment	• Prevalence in the pediatric population is 1%–2% (22) • Parents may have developmentally inappropriate expectations for sleep times. In addition, children who do not sleep well at night, may fall asleep in class during the day or take developmentally inappropriate naps after school making it harder to fall asleep at night. • Media: including television, computers, video games, and cell phones. Use of media is associated with decreased sleep duration, less time in bed, and feeling sleepier the next day (46,47). • Environment (cosleeping, noise, room temperature (should be < 75°F), pets, allergens) (48)
Behavioral Insomnia of Childhood • Sleep onset association type: ○ Sleep initiation requires special circumstances ○ Without the special conditions, sleep is delayed and/or interrupted ○ Sleep associations are problematic for the family ○ Awakenings require the caregiver to intervene • Limit-setting type ○ Difficulty initiating or maintaining sleep ○ Child refuses to go to bed or stay in bed ○ The caregiver is not able to adequately set limits for the child	• Prevalence in infants, toddlers, and preschoolers: 20%–30% (49) • Common sleep associations: ○ Feeding, pacifiers, blankets, stuffed animals, parental presence during sleep • Common limit-setting difficulties: ○ Children come out of their room and bargain: i.e., need a drink, hungry, monsters, need a hug, need the light readjusted, one more book ○ Look for limit setting difficulties at other times of the day as well
Insomnia Due to Drug or Substance • Symptoms present for > 1 mo • Dependence on, abuse of, or exposure to a drug, substance, medication, food, or toxin that results in sleep disturbances • Insomnia relates to the ingestion of the drug or substance	• Prevalence in children 12–17 yr old: 17.8% (50) • Prescription Medications: steroids, stimulants (44,51,52) • Caffeine: Adolescents with a high caffeine intake are 1.9 times more likely to report difficulty sleeping than adolescents with a very low caffeine intake. Additionally, students with a high caffeine intake were more likely to report being tired during the day (53). • Of 13,831 adolescents 12–17 yr of age surveyed, alcohol, nicotine, and illicit drug use were all associated with a higher rate of reported sleep difficulties (50).

(Continued)

Table 1 Summary of ICSD Second Edition Classification of Insomnia: Pediatric Associations (*Continued*)

Insomnia Due to A Medical Condition	
• Symptoms present for > 1 mo • Medical condition known to result in sleep disturbances • Insomnia fluctuates with changes in condition severity or activity	• Pediatric prevalence unknown • Discomfort during sleep ○ asthma (54), reflux (55,56), juvenile rheumatoid arthritis (57,58) • Neurological disorders ○ seizures (59), autism spectrum disorders (60,61), cerebral palsy (62), and Angelman's syndrome (63).

This table was paraphrased in part from the ICSD 2nd Edition Classification of Insomnia. (37) For a full discussion of the criteria for the various types of insomnia, please see this resource.
Source: From Ref. 37.

adenoidectomy, but treatment of allergies, weight loss, and positive airway pressure are options as well (69).

Disorders of arousal include confusional arousals, sleep terrors, and sleepwalking (37). Parents may believe that their child is fully aroused and describe the children as having insomnia. However, children with disorders of arousal usually appear confused during the event and do not remember the event of the next day. Management of disorders of arousal usually involves reassuring the parents, ensuring that the child has an age appropriate amount of sleep, taking appropriate steps to ensure safety, and screening for other primary sleep disorders, which may provoke events. However, in some cases, children require behavioral or pharmacologic therapies (70).

EVALUATION

In general, all children should be screened for sleep problems. A parent report or a child or adolescent's self- report of sleep difficulties requires a thorough characterization of the sleep problem and related factors (Table 2). This should include determination that the child or adolescent has a developmentally and age appropriate opportunity to sleep. The history should include details about the bedtime routine and the parent's and the child's response to night awakening. Evaluation of the quality of sleep is also important. The clinician should determine if the child awakes refreshed, if there are additional sleep disorders such as obstructive sleep apnea and periodic limb movement disorder, and if there are medical or psychiatric conditions that may disrupt sleep. Because some medications contribute to insomnia, a list of over-the-counter, prescription, and illicit drugs should be obtained. In addition, identification of previous treatment techniques, medications, and the duration of the time that they were used are necessary. The clinician should also characterize significant daytime symptoms including excessive daytime sleepiness, irritability, hyperactivity, and difficulty with concentration. Older children should be interviewed separately from their parents to discuss safety at home and at school, exposure to nicotine, alcohol, and illicit drugs, and to determine if there is an underlying psychiatric disorder.

The general physical examination should screen for medical disorders such as reflux, asthma, and pain that may contribute to insomnia. Polysomnography is not typically indicated unless there is concern for obstructive sleep apnea or periodic limb movement disorder contributing to insomnia. A two-week sleep diary or actigraphy can help to better delineate bedtimes, sleep times, and wake times. These tools can help distinguish between delayed sleep phase syndrome and paradoxical insomnia.

MANAGEMENT

Management of pediatric insomnia depends on the underlying etiology. A discussion regarding realistic developmentally appropriate bedtime, wake time, naptime, and sleep hygiene (Table 3) should be considered for all children. The majority of cases of behavioral insomnia of childhood are best managed through behavioral interventions including teaching new positive sleep habits (49). In select cases, pharmacologic treatment may be used on a short-term basis in combination with the behavioral interventions. For example, if a child's insomnia is severe

Table 2 Patient History

Ensure that the patient has a developmentally appropriate number of hours of sleep in a 24 hr period	• What time does your child go to bed? • What time does your child go to sleep? • What time does your child wake for the day? • Does your child take any naps? • How many hours of sleep does your child receive in a 24 hour period? • How many awakenings does your child have per night? • How long are the awakenings?
Bedtime resistance	• What is the prebed routine? • Does your child require the presence of a parent to go to sleep? • Does your child feed prior to going to sleep? • Does your child bargain to avoid going to bed? • What is the parent's response to refusal to go to bed or nighttime awakening?
Is there evidence for adjustment or psychophysiologic insomnia?	• Does the patient lay awake at night worrying about going to sleep? • Does the patient appear tired, but have difficulty going to sleep once he/she goes to bed? • Does the patient sleep better when not sleeping in his/her own bed? • Was the sleep difficulty provoked by a stressful event?

Screen for primary sleep disorders	• OSA
	  ○ Snoring or pauses in breathing during sleep?
	• RLS
	  ○ Abnormal feelings in the legs or feet that are relieved with rest?
	• Restless sleep?
	• Delayed sleep phase syndrome
	• If allowed to go to bed when you want, will you go right to sleep? If so, how long do you sleep until you wake up on your own?

Screen for medical disorders	• Asthma • Gastroesophageal reflux disease • Seasonal allergies • Pain • Other disorders
Screen for mental disorders	• Anxiety • Depression • Bipolar disorder • Post traumatic stress disorder (previous or current history of trauma, child abuse, bullying)
Medications/Substances	• Does the child take any medications known to result in insomnia? • Does the child take any medications to treat insomnia? • Does the child use nicotine, alcohol, or illicit drugs?
Diet	• Caffeine? • Eating prior to going to bed
Daytime symptoms	• Excessive daytime sleepiness • Attention difficulties • Hyperactivity • Mood changes

Table 3 Sleep Hygiene for Children

Sleep Routine

- Determine the latest time the child can wake up and still get to school on time. Make this the wake up time. This should be observed consistently even on weekends until the sleep problem resolves.
- Determine the developmentally appropriate number of hours of sleep and count backwards from the wake up time. This is the new bedtime. This should be observed consistently even on weekends until the sleep problem resolves.
- Schedule developmentally appropriate nap times if indicated.
- Create a calm prebedtime routine that fits with the child and the family. This should be started 30–60 min prior to the expected bedtime.
- Children should be allowed to fall asleep alone to avoid sleep-onset association with parents.
- Expose the child to bright light upon awakening and dim light for one hour prior to bedtime.
- Discontinue use of all media (TV, computer, video games, cell phones, texting) 30 min prior to bed. Media may need to be removed from the child's room.
- Discuss the parents' response to night awakening (young children) and the child's response to night awakening (older children).

Lifestyle Changes

- The child should get plenty of exercise during the day. However, vigorous activity should be limited during the hour prior to bedtime.
- Some children take a bath directly prior to bed. This is acceptable if it is a warm, calming bath. However, if the child is young and the bath is fun and exciting, the parents should consider moving the bath to earlier in the evening or in the morning.
- Keep the child's bedroom temperature below 75°F.
- Remove environmental barriers to sleep if possible (i.e., pets, other siblings, noise, potential sources for allergens).

Dietary and Medication Changes

- Eliminate caffeine from the diet or at least curtail consumption in the hours prior to bed.
- Children may have a snack prior to bed if hungry.
- Limit fluid intake 30 min prior to bedtime.
- Unless medically indicated, from 7 mo of age on, children should not eat or drink after bedtime to avoid symptoms of gastroesophageal reflux and bladder distention that can result in arousal of the child. If a child is still drinking from the bottle, wean down the amount and the frequency until the bottle can be discontinued.
- Ensure that the child is not receiving medications containing alcohol or caffeine that could interfere in the child's sleep.
- Consider adjustment of other medications the child is receiving if they are contributing to insomnia (i.e., stimulants for ADHD).

Source: Adapted from Ref. 48.

enough to significantly affect the family's ability to implement the recommended behavioral interventions, medication may be used to improve the patient's sleep and bring about behavioral changes sooner (3). Additionally, there are some children with neurological or medical disorders who require long-term pharmacologic treatment for insomnia. Unfortunately, research evaluating the safety and efficacy of pharmacologic agents in the treatment of pediatric insomnia is lacking (71).

Behavioral Interventions

Behavioral Insomnia of Childhood

Because of the serious impact sleep disorders can have on a child's daytime functioning and the potential for long term difficulties with sleep, The American Academy of Sleep Medicine set forth practice parameters for the treatment of behavioral insomnia of childhood (49). These parameters are based on the combined results from 52 studies evaluating the effectiveness of behavioral interventions for behavioral insomnia of childhood in children primarily five years of age and younger. Almost all (94%) of the studies reveal that behavioral interventions including unmodified extinction, graduated extinction, positive routine, faded bedtime with response cost,

Table 4 Treatment of Behavioral Insomnia of Childhood

Unmodified Extinction	• The child is placed in their bed at a prescribed bedtime. • The parent leaves the room and does not respond to signaling. However, parents must respond to illness or danger. • The child is allowed out of their bed/room at a prescribed wake time.
Modified extinction	• The child is placed in their bed at a prescribed bedtime. • The parent remains in the room but does not interact with the child. • The child is allowed out of their bed/room at a prescribed wake time.
Graduated extinction	• The child is placed in their bed at a prescribed bedtime. • The parents respond to signaling after a set period of time. • The parental response should be brief and the parent should leave the room immediately after evaluating the child. • The duration between the parental responses should be gradually extended (5, 10, 15 minutes).
Positive routines	• Provide the patient with a specific bedtime and wake time. • Prior to bed the family should develop a brief, calm routine to be performed every night prior to bed.
Faded bedtime with response cost	• The child is put to bed close to the time of their current sleep onset. • After the child starts to go to sleep easily at this time, the bedtime is advanced (moved earlier) by 15 min. Once the child is falling asleep easily the bedtime is advanced again. • This process is repeated until the desired bedtime is achieved. • If the child is not falling asleep easily, the child is removed from the bed briefly and then placed back in bed.
Scheduled awakenings	• The patient is awakened 15–30 min prior to their nocturnal awakenings. • The time between scheduled awakenings should be increased over time. • Parents respond to their children during these awakenings with their typical routine.
Parental education	• Help families establish age appropriate consistent bedtimes, wake times, and nap times. • Remind families to avoid creating an association that requires parental Involvement.

Source: Adapted from Ref. 49.

scheduled awakenings, and parental education are effective in correcting bedtime resistance and night wakings (64). (Table 4)

Extinction techniques are designed to decrease unwanted behaviors (49). Unmodified extinction involves putting the child to bed at a prescribed time and leaving the child in the room, ignoring the child's signaling (crying) until it is time to wake in the morning. The parents should remain extremely consistent in their responses to bargaining and night waking and avoid positive reinforcement for unwanted behaviors. However, if the parent is concerned that the child is ill or hurt, he/she is encouraged to investigate. Parents should be aware that once positive sleep habits are established, illness or a change in routine (i.e., vacation) may result in reemergence of the unwanted behavior. Consistently ignoring the child's signaling will help the child reestablish self-sufficient sleep. Some families find listening to the signaling (crying) of their child stressful and may be unable to ignore their child for a sufficient amount of time to allow the technique to work. A modification of the extinction technique involves the family staying in the room with the child, but not interacting with the child (64,72). Graduated extinction is another technique that may decrease parental stress. This technique involves the parent ignoring the child's behavior for a predetermined period of time (i.e., 5 minutes) and then checking on the child. When the parent checks on the child, the interaction should be minimal and last less than 15 seconds to avoid reinforcing negative behavior. The periods of time between checking on the child are gradually increased (i.e., 5 minutes, 10 minutes, 15 minutes) (64).

Difficulty with the extinction techniques may be encountered when the child does not stay in his/her room. This can be counteracted by confining the children to a space using the crib or closing the door of the room. Parents should ensure that the rooms are safe by covering electrical outlets and removing hard toys and climbable surfaces. If the parent is concerned about the child being in the room alone, securely attached stacked baby gates, half doors, or cameras will allow parents to be able to see in the child's room. Extinction techniques are effective if performed with consistency and result in decreased bedtime problems, decreased night awakenings, and improved sleep continuity (64).

Positive bedtime routines help to encourage appropriate behaviors. The family should create a positive, but calm prebed routine. This routine may consist of a warm relaxing bath, reading books, listening to music, etc. Dim light during the prebed routine is recommended (48). The goal of this technique is to help the child slowly decrease their activity and to create a positive association with bedtime (64).

For those children who have difficulty initiating sleep, the faded bedtime with response cost may be beneficial. The child is put to bed close to the time when they typically fall asleep. Once the child is going to sleep easily at the later time, the bedtime is advanced by 15 minutes until the goal bedtime is reached. If the child does not fall asleep, the child is removed from bed for a specific period of time and then placed back in bed. Children should wake up at a specific time each morning. Naps, other than developmentally appropriate prescribed naps, should be avoided (64).

Children with frequent night awakenings may benefit from scheduled night awakenings to ultimately improve the amount of consolidated sleep. Children are put to bed at their usual time, but are awakened by the parent about 15 to 30 minutes prior to the typical time of the nighttime awakening. Parents are allowed to respond to the awakening with their usual routine. Over time, the period between the scheduled awakenings is increased (64).

Parental education has been used in several studies starting as early as the prenatal period. This technique focuses on educating parents on appropriate bedtimes, parental role in sleep initiation, and response to nocturnal awakenings and is geared toward preventing the development of unwanted behaviors (64). Early maternal sleep education is associated with long-term decreased incidence of maternal depression and decreased sleep problems in their children (73).

One behavioral technique has not been proven to be more effective than another in the treatment of behavioral insomnia of childhood (64). Unmodified extinction may produce results faster than scheduled awakenings (74). More than 80% of children treated with behavioral techniques improved and had lasting effects for three to six months (64). No adverse secondary effects have been identified in participating children and parental energy and mood are reported to improve following the implementation of the behavioral interventions (64,75,76). The practitioner should consider the unique situation for the child and the family before prescribing a particular technique and many practitioners combine techniques for maximum efficacy (64).

Behavioral Interventions for Other Types of Insomnia

Children with insomnia not related to behavioral insomnia of childhood may respond to other behavioral techniques that have classically been used to treat adult insomnia (65). Stimulus control is a highly effective technique that is used to develop specific stimuli for sleep (77,78). Children are asked to use their bed only for sleeping and to avoid staying in bed when they are unable to go to sleep (65). This technique helps children identify their bed and bedroom with sleep and decrease the association with other things, which preclude sleep (78). Sleep restriction is often used in conjunction with stimulus control (65). This technique involves decreasing the amount of time a child spends in bed to the amount of time the family estimates that the child actually sleeps (but no less than six hours in children). The morning wake time remains constant and the initial bedtime is later, in order to produce the appropriate time in bed. When the child falls asleep easily, the bedtime is then advanced by 15 minutes every four to seven days. This process continues until the child achieves a developmentally appropriate amount of sleep.

Parents may wish to incorporate positive reinforcement (i.e. sticker chart) to encourage children to participate in the various treatment techniques. Children with mood disorders or ADHD often complain that they cannot stop thinking when they go to bed. Relaxation techniques have also been found helpful to decrease physiologic arousal as well as provide a focus for their attention as they try to go to sleep (78). Combinations of these techniques along with sleep education and sleep hygiene are reported to result in significant improvement in sleep latency, night awakenings, and sleep duration in adolescents receiving treatment for substance abuse (78).

Pharmacologic Interventions

Despite a lack of research support and FDA approval for pharmacologic treatment of pediatric insomnia, multiple medications have been used by both physicians as well as parents without physician guidance to help children sleep. Up to 25% of children 0 to 18 months of age have been prescribed medication to help them sleep (79). In a large cross-sectional study between 1993 and 2004, 18,640,820 pediatric patient visits (aged 0 to 17 years) for sleep related difficulties were evaluated (80). Physicians prescribed nutritional counseling for 7% and behavioral therapy for 22%. However, 81% of patients were prescribed a medication (33% antihistamines, 26% α_2 agonists, 15% benzodiazepines, 6% nonbenzodiazepines, 6% antidepressants). Nineteen percent of patient visits received both pharmacological and behavioral treatment (80). In a separate study, more than 75% of practitioners had recommended nonprescription medications at least once for pediatric insomnia. Antihistamines were the most frequently recommended over the counter medication. Fifteen percent of practitioners reported prescribing melatonin or herbal remedies (81).

Due to the lack of controlled, well-powered studies evaluating the safety and efficacy of hypnotics in children, pharmacotherapy should be reserved for those children who experience significant negative consequences as a result of their chronic sleep difficulties, children requiring a rapid solution to their insomnia, and/or children who have a disorder (e.g., neurological condition) that precludes appropriate response to behavioral interventions (71). Pharmacotherapy should be paired with a behavioral intervention for maximum efficacy (48). Choice of the medication is guided by whether the patient has trouble initiating or maintaining sleep, comorbid conditions, and the individual characteristics of the medication (Table 5). Caution is advised with regard to the use of any agents which promote sleep in children. These agents should not be combined with other central nervous system depressants or used in high doses due to concern for respiratory depression. Commonly prescribed medications are discussed below. This discussion is not meant to be a comprehensive review of these medications and readers are encouraged to check manufacturer prescribing guidelines for dose recommendations, cautions, and potential side effects prior to recommending these medications.

Antihistamines

Antihistamines including diphenhydramine hydrochloride and hydroxyzine are the most commonly prescribed agents in the treatment of pediatric insomnia (80). These medications compete with histamine at H_1-receptors, promoting mild sedation at the prescribed dosing (82). They have been reported to decrease sleep latency and nighttime awakenings (83). However, in a randomized placebo controlled trial evaluating sleep disturbance in infants aged 6 to 15 months, diphenhydramine hydrochloride showed no improvement compared to placebo (97). In addition, antihistamines may lead to insomnia in some children, may interfere with sleep quality, and may contribute to daytime drowsiness (82). These medications are not recommended for children less than two years of age (98). Persons taking antihistamines regularly develop tolerance resulting in decreased effectiveness of the medication with chronic use (99).

α_2-adrenergic receptor agonists

Clonidine, a α_2-adrenergic receptor agonist, acts at the brainstem and decreases noradrenergic output (85). This decreased activity is thought to be responsible for sedation, but the exact role

Table 5 Pharmacotherapy

Antihistamines (48,71,82)	Mechanism of action • H_1-receptor blocker • ↓ sleep latency Side effects • May impair sleep quality • Paradoxical insomnia in children • Morning sedation • Daytime sleepiness • Anti-cholinergic side effects
Diphenhydramine (83)	Pharmocodynamics and pharmacokinetics • Maximum sedation: 1–3 hr • Duration: 4–7 hr Pediatric dosing • Oral dosing 30 min prior to bed: • 2–12 yr: oral: 1 mg/kg/dose (max 50 mg), • $>$ 12 yr: 50 mg Available formulations • Chewable tablet • Strip • Liquid • Capsule • Injection (for in hospital use without alternative administration)

Hydroxyzine (48,84)	Pharmacodynamics and pharmacokinetics
	• Time to peak concentration: 2 hr
	• Half life increases with increasing age:
	  ○ 1 yr old = 4 hr
	  ○ 14 yr old = 11 hr
	  ○ adults = 3 hr
	Pediatric dosing
	Oral dosing for preoperative sedation
	• Children: oral 0.5 mg/kg 30 min prior to bed
	Available formulations
	• Capsule
	• Tablet
	• Syrup
	• Suspension
	• Injection

α_2-adrenergic receptor agonists (48,71,85,86)	Mechanism of action • Central acting • Stimulates α_2-adreno receptors • Decreased noradrenergic activity • Results in decreased REM sleep Side effects • Sedation • Hypotension • Bradycardia • Rebound hypertension if discontinued abruptly • Insomnia • Dizziness • Fatigue

Clonidine (85)	Pharmacodynamics and pharmacokinetics
	• Onset of action: 30–60 min
	• Serum half-life:
	  ○ Infants: 44–72 hr
	  ○ Children: 8–12 hr
	  ○ Adults: 6–20 hr

Table 5 Pharmacotherapy (*Continued*)

	Pediatric dosing • No recommendations are available for pediatric sedation • Study in children with ADHD: 50–800 μg (mean 157 μg) (87) Available formulations • Tablet • Transdermal patch
Melatonin (88)	Mechanism of action and effects on sleep • Phase shift • Hypnotic Side effects • Morning sedation • Dysphoria • Regulation of growth hormone and gonadotropic hormone secretion Pharmacokinetics and pharmacodynamics • Rapid absorption • Peak plasma level at 1 hr Pediatric dosing • No recommendations for dosing in children are available. • Start with low dose 0.5 or 1 mg 1–5 hr prior to bedtime and increase q 1–2 wk up to a maximum of 10 mg. • Consider controlled release formulations for night awakenings Available formulations • Rapid release ○ Tabs ○ Spray ○ Sublingual ○ Liquid • Controlled release ○ Tabs
Benzodiazepines (48,71)	Mechanism of action: • GABA agonist Sido Effects • Drowsiness • Confusion • Paradoxical excitement • Decreased respiratory rate • Apnea • Hypotension • Bradycardia • Abrupt discontinuation is associated with seizures
Diazepam (48,89)	Pharmacodyndamics and pharmacokinetics • Half-life ○ Infants: 40–50 hr ○ Children: 15–21 hr ○ Adults: 20–50 hr Pediatric dosing • 0.04–0.25 mg/kg at bedtime Available formulations • Oral • Rectal

(*Continued*)

Table 5 Pharmacotherapy (*Continued*)

Clonazepam (48,90)	Pharmacodynamics and pharmacokinetics • Onset of action: 20–60 min • Half-life: ○ Children: 22–33 hr ○ Adults: 30–40 hr Pediatric dosing • Initial dose: 0.01 mg/kg at bedtime • Max dose: 0.025 mg/kg Available formulations • Tablet • Wafers
Lorazepam(71,91)	Pharmacodynamics and pharmacokinetics • Onset of action: oral: within 60 min • Duration of action: 8–12 hr • Half-life: ○ Infants: 8–73 hr ○ Children: 6–17 hr ○ Adults: 10–16 hr Pediatric dosing • 0.05 mg/kg at bedtime Available formulations • Tablet • Solution • Injection
Nonbenzodiazepine hypnotics (92)	Mechanism of action • Enhances GABA activity at the benzodiazepine$_1$-receptor. Side effects • Paradoxical effects if dose is too low or high • Dizziness • Headaches • Somnolence
Zolpidem (93)	Pharmacokinetics and pharmacodynamics • Time to maximum concentration: 1.1 hr • Half-life: 2.1 hr Pediatric dosing • 0.25 mg/kg prior to bedtime with max dose of 20 mg Available formulations • Regular • Controlled release
Antidepressants Tricyclic Antidepressants (71,94)	Mechanism of action • Increases presynaptic serotonin and norepinephrine by blocking their reuptake Side effects • Cardiovascular side effects requiring cardiac evaluation prior to prescribing these medications • Anticholinergic effects
Imipramine (94)	Pharmacokinetics and pharmacodynamics • Peak serum concentration: 1–2 hr • Mean half-life: ○ Children: 11 hr ○ Adults: 16–17 hr

Table 5 Pharmacotherapy (*Continued*)

	Pediatric dosing
	• No recommendations are available for pediatric sedation
	• For enuresis > 6 yr
	  ○ 10–25 mg PO at bedtime
	• For depression
	  ○ 1.5 mg/kg/day with max dose of 5 mg/kg/d divided 1–4 times/day
	  ○ Monitor carefully doses > 3.5 mg/kg/day
	Available formulations
	• Capsule
	• Tablet

Amitriptyline (95)	Pharmacokinetics and pharmacodynamics
	• Peak serum concentration: 4 hr
	• Half-life in adults: 9–25 hr with mean of 15 hr
	Pediatric dosing
	• No recommendations are available for pediatric sedation
	• For depression
	  ○ Children: 1 mg/kg/day divided in 3 doses
	  ○ Adolescents: 25–50 mg/day

Trazodone (96)	Mechanism of action
	• Inhibits reuptake of serotonin
	• α-adrenergic blockade
	Side effects
	• Blurred vision
	• Prolonged priaprism
	• Postural hypotension
	• Drowsiness
	Pharmacokinetics and pharmacodynamics
	• Peak serum concentration: 1–2 hr
	• Half-life: 5–9 hr
	Pediatric Dosing
	• Not FDA approved for depression or sedation in children
	• Children 2–18 yr of age
	  ○ 1.5–2 mg/kg/day in 3 divided doses
	  ○ Max dose 6 mg/kg/day
	• Adolescents
	  ○ 25–50 mg/day with max of 150 mg/day in divided doses
	• Adults
	  ○ 150 mg/day in 3 divided doses with max of 600 mg/day

This table serves as an outline of medications that have been used to treat pediatric insomnia. It is not comprehensive and providers are encouraged to look at manufacturer prescribing information for side effects, and cautions prior to recommending any of these medications to a patient.

in sedation is unclear (71). Clonidine has primarily been used to promote sedation in children with ADHD (71). The benefit in this patient population is thought to relate to clonidine's effect on both ADHD symptoms as well as the side effect of sedation (87). One study found that the degree of drowsiness decreases with time, which may mean that the dose required inducing sedation, will increase over time (100).

Clonidine has also been found to reduce sleep latency and night awakening in children with autism spectrum disorders (101). Despite the fact that clonidine has not been studied in healthy children without comorbid disorders, general pediatricians commonly prescribe clonidine for children with difficulty initiating sleep (102). Some children will experience insomnia with this medication (85). Anecdotally, rebound insomnia appears to occur approximately four to six hours following administration of the medication. Caution is recommended when prescribing clonidine due to adverse effects such as dysphoria, bradycardia, hypotension, and rebound hypertension (71). The FDA recommends a thorough cardiac evaluation prior to the initiation of this medication due to concern regarding sudden cardiac death (85). Because of the side effect profile and lack of research in normal healthy children, clonidine is not recommended for insomnia in healthy children (71).

Melatonin

Melatonin has been used to treat insomnia in adults as well as children. In vivo, levels increase with darkness and decrease with light, playing a role in the circadian rhythm of sleep and wakefulness (71). As with many medications used to treat insomnia in children, large studies have not been performed to determine efficacy or safety. In a small randomized double blind placebo controlled trial, short term use of melatonin was reported to be effective for phase advancement, decreasing sleep latency, and increasing total sleep duration in children with chronic insomnia (103). It has also been found to be efficacious in special patient populations including children with blindness, intellectual disabilities, Angelman syndrome, Rett syndrome, and autism (63,104–107). Although many studies evaluating the short-term efficacy in various pediatric populations are available, studies evaluating the pharmocokinetics and long-term safety and efficacy have not been performed in children. Significant adverse effects have not been documented, but daytime somnolence has been reported (88). In addition, several children have reported vivid dreams, but this warrants further study. There is an association between melatonin and regulation of growth hormone and gonadotropic hormone (88,108). Therefore, the practitioner should inform families of the theoretical risk of affecting these hormones in children. Recommended dosing for children is not available. Based on studies in children, doses of 0.5 mg up to 10 mg have been reported to be effective (48). Melatonin can be used prior to bedtime as a hypnotic or up to four hours prior to bedtime as treatment for delayed sleep phase. Controlled release melatonin is available for children with difficulties with both sleep initiation and maintenance (109).

Benzodiazepines

Benzodiazepines bind to the γ-aminobutyric acid (GABA) receptor complex and modulate action of GABA at the receptor site. As a result, benzodiazepines not only induce sleep and decrease partial arousals during sleep transitions, but also contribute to decreased muscle tone and decreased anxiety (71,110). Choosing a specific benzodiazepine depends on the patient's specific sleep disturbance. Patients with difficulty initiating sleep may benefit from a benzodiazepine that is rapidly absorbed with a short half-life. A benzodiazepine with a longer half-life may be chosen to treat nighttime or early morning awakenings (71). Although effective in treating insomnia, benzodiazepines may be associated with tolerance, rebound partial arousals, and daytime somnolence (71). In addition, discontinuation following longer-term use in children may result in increased insomnia in addition to anxiety, agitation, diarrhea, fever, sweating, and tachypnea (111). In children, benzodiazepines have primarily been used to treat disorders of arousal such as sleep terrors and confusional arousals (71). However, controlled clinical trials using benzodiazepines in children do not exist. They are not approved for sedation in children (71). Due to the significant side effects associated with benzodiazepines, these medications are not recommended for patients with preexisting CNS depression, decreased pulmonary function, apnea, or those patients taking medications that contribute to CNS depression (48).

Other benzodiazepine receptor agonists (BzRAs)

BzRA hypnotics are selective GABA agonistic modulators that effect the benzodiazepine$_1$-receptor resulting primarily in sedation, with presumably less muscle relaxant, anti-anxiety and other effects of nonselective benzodiazepines (71,92). Previously, these hypnotics such as zolpidem have not been well studied in children. However, a recent study evaluated the pharmacokinetics of zolpidem in children (93). The effect on sleep was variable and included paradoxical effects when the dose was too low or too high. Zolpidem has been reported to increase the proportion of stage 3 NREM sleep as well as REM sleep without increasing the total sleep time in pediatric burn patients (112). In children, short-term side effects are considered to be mild and self-limited (93). Common side effects in adults include dizziness, headaches, and somnolence (92).

Antidepressants

Antidepressants have been prescribed for insomnia associated with depression or anxiety in adults (113). Studies evaluating the safety and efficacy of antidepressants in children are not available. Caution is advised when prescribing antidepressants to children due to the black box warning regarding increase risk of suicide in children taking these medications (114).

Tricyclic antidepressants are thought to decrease arousal from sleep but may also impair deep sleep as well as REM sleep (71,113). Most studies in adults have not found lasting sleep associated benefits from treatment with tricyclic antidepressants (113). In children, imipramine hydrochloride is prescribed most frequently for control of nocturnal enuresis and it has been reported to be beneficial in decreasing disorders of arousal such as sleep terrors and confusional arousals in children (71). Side effects include dry mouth, orthostatic hypotension, and cardiac dysrhythmias (71).

Trazodone is a 5-HT_2-receptor antagonist with weak α_2-receptor antagonism (113). It is associated with an increase in total sleep time, increase in the percentage of slow wave sleep, and a decrease in arousals in adults (115). In a group of adolescents with depression it was found to minimally decrease the time for insomnia resolution compared to fluoxetine alone (116). Side effects of trazodone include sedation, dizziness, psychomotor impairment, and priaprism (117).

Selective serotonin reuptake inhibitors (SSRIs) or serotonin-norepinephrine reuptake inhibitors (SNRIs) are not generally used as primary sleep-promoting agents (113). Positive effects on insomnia may result as part of the treatment of an underlying mood disorder.

SUMMARY

Pediatric insomnia is common and the etiology is often multifactorial. It has significant consequences for children as well as their families. Behavioral insomnia of childhood is the most common etiology of sleep disturbance in young children. Older children are susceptible to the other types of insomnia seen in adults. In adolescents, delayed sleep phase is an especially common cause of sleep initiation problems and morning sleepiness. A comprehensive history and evaluation is important to determine the exact etiology for a child's insomnia. Treatment is based on parental education, a discussion of sleep hygiene, and behavioral techniques. For select children who need pharmacologic intervention, medications are available, but must be used with caution.

REFERENCES

1. Mindell JA, Emslie G, Blumer J, et al. Pharmacologic management of insomnia in children and adolescents: Consensus statement. Pediatrics 2006; 117(6):e1223–e1232.
2. Stein MA, Mendelsohn J, Obermeyer WH, et al. Sleep and behavior problems in school-aged children. Pediatrics 2001; 107(4):E60.
3. Glaze DG. Childhood insomnia: Why Chris can't sleep. Pediatr Clin North Am 2004; 51(1):33–50, vi.
4. Nixon GM, Thompson JM, Han DY, et al. Short sleep duration in middle childhood: Risk factors and consequences. Sleep 2008; 31(1):71–78.
5. Roberts RE, Roberts CR, Duong HT. Chronic insomnia and its negative consequences for health and functioning of adolescents: A 12-month prospective study. J Adolesc Health 2008; 42(3):294–302.
6. Kahn A, Van de Merckt C, Rebuffat E, et al. Sleep problems in healthy preadolescents. Pediatrics 1989; 84(3):542–546.
7. Forbes EE, Bertocci MA, Gregory AM, et al. Objective sleep in pediatric anxiety disorders and major depressive disorder. J Am Acad Child and Adolesc Psychiatry 2008; 47(2):148–155.
8. Hiscock H, Wake M. Infant sleep problems and postnatal depression: A community-based study. Pediatrics 2001; 107(6):1317–1322.
9. Ievers-Landis CE, Storfer-Isser A, Rosen C, et al. Relationship of sleep parameters, child psychological functioning, and parenting stress to obesity status among preadolescent children. J Dev Behav Pediatr 2008; 29(4):243–252.
10. Iglowstein I, Jenni OG, Molinari L, et al. Sleep duration from infancy to adolescence: Reference values and generational trends. Pediatrics 2003; 111(2):302–307.

11. Parmelee AH Jr., Schulz HR, Disbrow MA. Sleep patterns of the newborn. J Pediatr 1961; 58:241–250.
12. Anders TF, Keener M. Developmental course of nighttime sleep-wake patterns in full-term and premature infants during the first year of life. I. Sleep 1985; 8(3):173–192.
13. Adair RH, Bauchner H. Sleep problems in childhood. Curr Probl Pediatr 1993; 23(4):147–170; discussion 2.
14. Anders TF, Halpern LF, Hua J. Sleeping through the night: A developmental perspective. Pediatrics 1992; 90(4):554–560.
15. Goodlin-Jones BL, Burnham MM, Gaylor EE, et al. Night waking, sleep-wake organization, and self-soothing in the first year of life. J Dev Behav Pediatr 2001; 22(4):226–233.
16. Simard V, Nielsen TA, Tremblay RE, et al. Longitudinal study of preschool sleep disturbance: The predictive role of maladaptive parental behaviors, early sleep problems, and child/mother psychological factors. Arch Pediatr Adolesc Med 2008; 162(4):360–367.
17. Touchette E, Petit D, Paquet J, et al. Factors associated with fragmented sleep at night across early childhood. Arch Pediatr Adolesc Med 2005; 159(3):242–249.
18. Scher A. Maternal separation anxiety as a regulator of infants' sleep. J Child Psychol Psychiatry 2008; 49(6):618–625.
19. Schwebel DC, Brezausek CM. Nocturnal awakenings and pediatric injury risk. J Pediatr Psychol 2008; 33(3):323–332.
20. Dworak M, Schierl T, Bruns T, et al. Impact of singular excessive computer game and television exposure on sleep patterns and memory performance of school-aged children. Pediatrics 2007; 120(5):978–985.
21. Wolfson AR, Carskadon MA. Sleep schedules and daytime functioning in adolescents. Child Dev 1998; 69(4):875–887.
22. Ohayon MM, Roberts RE. Comparability of sleep disorders diagnoses using DSM-IV and ICSD classifications with adolescents. Sleep 2001; 24(8):920–925.
23. Pagel JF, Forister N, Kwiatkowki C. Adolescent sleep disturbance and school performance: The confounding variable of socioeconomics. J Clin Sleep Med 2007; 3(1):19–23.
24. Camhi SL, Morgan WJ, Pernisco N, et al. Factors affecting sleep disturbances in children and adolescents. Sleep Med 2000; 1(2):117–123.
25. Roberts RE, Roberts CR, Chen IG. Impact of insomnia on future functioning of adolescents. J Psychosom Res 2002; 53(1):561–569.
26. Richman N. A community survey of characteristics of one- to two- year-olds with sleep disruptions. J Am Acad Child Psychiatry 1981; 20(2):281–291.
27. Bernal JF. Night waking in infants during the first 14 months. Dev Med Child Neurol 1973; 15(6):760–769.
28. Carey WB. Night waking and temperament in infancy. J Pediatr 1974; 84(5):756–758.
29. Lozoff B, Wolf AW, Davis NS. Sleep problems seen in pediatric practice. Pediatrics 1985; 75(3):477–483.
30. Ottaviano S, Giannotti F, Cortesi F, et al. Sleep characteristics in healthy children from birth to 6 years of age in the urban area of Rome. Sleep 1996; 19(1):1–3.
31. Ohayon MM, Roberts RE, Zulley J, et al. Prevalence and patterns of problematic sleep among older adolescents. J Am Acad Child Adolesc Psychiatry 2000; 39(12):1549–1556.
32. Hauri P, Olmstead E. Childhood-onset insomnia. Sleep 1980; 3(1):59–65.
33. Serretti A, Benedetti F, Mandelli L, et al. Genetic dissection of psychopathological symptoms: Insomnia in mood disorders and CLOCK gene polymorphism. Am J Med Genet B Neuropsychiatr Genet 2003; 121B(1):35–38.
34. Goodlin-Jones BL, Sitnick SL, Tang K, et al. The Children's Sleep Habits Questionnaire in toddlers and preschool children. J Dev Behav Pediatr 2008; 29(2):82–88.
35. Malow BA, Marzec ML, McGrew SG, et al. Characterizing sleep in children with autism spectrum disorders: A multidimensional approach. Sleep 2006; 29(12):1563–1571.
36. Van der Heijden KB, Smits MG, Van Someren EJ, et al. Idiopathic chronic sleep onset insomnia in attention-deficit/hyperactivity disorder: A circadian rhythm sleep disorder. Chronobiol Int 2005; 22(3):559–570.
37. American Academy of Sleep Medicine. Insomnia. In: Sateia M, ed. The International Classification of Sleep Disorders : Diagnostic and Coding Manual, 2nd ed. Westchester, IL.: American Academy of Sleep Medicine, 2005:1–31.
38. Bader K, Schafer V, Schenkel M, et al. Adverse childhood experiences associated with sleep in primary insomnia. J Sleep Res 2007; 16(3):285–296.
39. Hon KL, Lam MC, Leung TF, et al. Are age-specific high serum IgE levels associated with worse symptomatology in children with atopic dermatitis? Int J Dermatol 2007; 46(12): 1258–1262.

40. Ivanenko A, Barnes ME, Crabtree VM, et al. Psychiatric symptoms in children with insomnia referred to a pediatric sleep medicine center. Sleep Med 2004; 5(3):253–259.
41. Johnson EO, Roth T, Schultz L, et al. Epidemiology of DSM-IV insomnia in adolescence: Lifetime prevalence, chronicity, and an emergent gender difference. Pediatrics 2006; 117(2):e247–e256.
42. Mehl RC, O'Brien LM, Jones JH, et al. Correlates of sleep and pediatric bipolar disorder. Sleep 2006; 29(2):193–197.
43. Kowatch RA, Youngstrom EA, Danielyan A, et al. Review and meta-analysis of the phenomenology and clinical characteristics of mania in children and adolescents. Bipolar Disord 2005; 7(6): 483–496.
44. Corkum P, Panton R, Ironside S, et al. Acute impact of immediate release methylphenidate administered three times a day on sleep in children with attention-deficit/hyperactivity disorder. J Pediatr Psychol 2008; 33(4):368–379.
45. Corkum P, Moldofsky H, Hogg-Johnson S, et al. Sleep problems in children with attention-deficit/hyperactivity disorder: Impact of subtype, comorbidity, and stimulant medication. J Am Acad Child Adolesc Psychiatry 1999; 38(10):1285–1293.
46. Van den Bulck J. Television viewing, computer game playing, and Internet use and self-reported time to bed and time out of bed in secondary-school children. Sleep 2004; 27(1):101–104.
47. Hitze B, Bosy-Westphal A, Bielfeldt F, et al. Determinants and impact of sleep duration in children and adolescents: Data of the Kiel Obesity Prevention Study. Eur J Clin Nutr 2009; 63(6):739–746.
48. Sheldon S. Disorders of initiating and maintaining sleep. In: Sheldon S, Ferber R, Kryger M, eds. Principles and Practice of Pediatric Sleep Medicine. Elsevier Saunders, USA, 2005:127–160.
49. Morgenthaler TI, Owens J, Alessi C, et al. Practice parameters for behavioral treatment of bedtime problems and night wakings in infants and young children. Sleep 2006; 29(10):1277–1281.
50. Johnson EO, Breslau N. Sleep problems and substance use in adolescence. Drug Alcohol Depend 2001; 64(1):1–7.
51. Scadding GK. Corticosteroids in the treatment of pediatric allergic rhinitis. J Allergy Clin Immunol 2001; 108(suppl 1):S59–S64.
52. Hinds PS, Hockenberry MJ, Gattuso JS, et al. Dexamethasone alters sleep and fatigue in pediatric patients with acute lymphoblastic leukemia. Cancer 2007; 110(10):2321–2330.
53. Orbeta RL, Overpeck MD, Ramcharran D, et al. High caffeine intake in adolescents: Associations with difficulty sleeping and feeling tired in the morning. J Adolesc Health 2006; 38(4): 451–453.
54. Strunk RC, Sternberg AL, Bacharier LB, et al. Nocturnal awakening caused by asthma in children with mild-to-moderate asthma in the childhood asthma management program. J Allergy Clin Immunol 2002; 110(3):395–403.
55. Carr MM, Brodsky L. Severe non-obstructive sleep disturbance as an initial presentation of gastroesophageal reflux disease. Int J Pediatr Otorhinolaryngol 1999; 51(2):115–120.
56. Bandla H, Splaingard M. Sleep problems in children with common medical disorders. Pediatr Clin North Am 2004; 51(1):203–227, viii.
57. Bloom BJ, Owens JA, McGuinn M, et al. Sleep and its relationship to pain, dysfunction, and disease activity in juvenile rheumatoid arthritis. J Rheumatol 2002; 29(1):169–173.
58. Zamir G, Press J, Tal A, Tarasiuk A. Sleep fragmentation in children with juvenile rheumatoid arthritis. J Rheumatol 1998; 25(6):1191–1197.
59. Byars AW, Byars KC, Johnson CS, et al. The relationship between sleep problems and neuropsychological functioning in children with first recognized seizures. Epilepsy Behav 2008; 13(4):607–613.
60. Allik H, Larsson JO, Smedje H. Sleep patterns of school-age children with Asperger syndrome or high-functioning autism. J Autism Dev Disord 2006; 36(5):585–595.
61. Allik H, Larsson JO, Smedje H. Insomnia in school-age children with Asperger syndrome or high-functioning autism. BMC Psychiatry 2006; 6:18.
62. Newman CJ, O'Regan M, Hensey O. Sleep disorders in children with cerebral palsy. Dev Med Child Neurol 2006; 48(7):564–568.
63. Braam W, Didden R, Smits MG, et al. Melatonin for chronic insomnia in Angelman syndrome: A randomized placebo-controlled trial. J Child Neurol 2008; 23(6):649–654.
64. Mindell JA, Kuhn B, Lewin DS, et al. Behavioral treatment of bedtime problems and night wakings in infants and young children. Sleep 2006; 29(10):1263–1276.
65. Owens JA, Palermo TM, Rosen CL. Overview of current management of sleep disturbances in children: II–Behavioral Interventions. Curr Ther Res 2002; 63(suppl B):B38–B52.
66. Picchietti DL, Stevens HE. Early manifestations of restless legs syndrome in childhood and adolescence. Sleep medicine 2008; 9(7):770–781.
67. Crabtree VM, Ivanenko A, O'Brien LM, et al. Periodic limb movement disorder of sleep in children. J Sleep Res 2003; 12(1):73–81.

68. Mindell J, Owens J. Restless leg syndrome and periodic limb movement disorder. In: Mindell J, Owens J, eds. A Clinical Guide to Pediatric Sleep: Diagnosis and Management of Sleep Problems. Philadelphia, PA: Lippincott Williams & Wilkins, 2003:123–134.
69. Capdevila OS, Kheirandish-Gozal L, Dayyat E, et al. Pediatric obstructive sleep apnea: Complications, management, and long-term outcomes. Proc Am Thorac Soc 2008; 5(2):274–282.
70. Hopkins B, Glaze D. Disorders of arousal in children. Pediatr Ann 2008; 37(7):481–487.
71. Reed MD, Findling RL. Overview of Current Management of Sleep Disturbances in Children: I–Pharmacotherapy. Curr Ther Res 2002; 63(suppl B):B18–B37.
72. Williams CD. The elimination of tantrum behavior by extinction procedures. J Abnorm Soc Psychol 1959; 59:269.
73. Hiscock H, Bayer JK, Hampton A, et al. Long-term mother and child mental health effects of a population-based infant sleep intervention: Cluster-randomized, controlled trial. Pediatrics 2008; 122(3):e621–e627.
74. Rickert VI, Johnson CM. Reducing nocturnal awakening and crying episodes in infants and young children: A comparison between scheduled awakenings and systematic ignoring. Pediatrics 1988; 81(2):203–212.
75. Eckerberg B. Treatment of sleep problems in families with young children: Effects of treatment on family well-being. Acta Paediatr 2004; 93(1):126–134.
76. Hiscock H, Wake M. Randomised controlled trial of behavioural infant sleep intervention to improve infant sleep and maternal mood. BMJ (Clinical research ed 2002; 324(7345):1062–1065.
77. Morin CM, Culbert JP, Schwartz SM. Nonpharmacological interventions for insomnia: A meta-analysis of treatment efficacy. Am J Psychiatry 1994; 151(8):1172–1180.
78. Bootzin RR, Stevens SJ. Adolescents, substance abuse, and the treatment of insomnia and daytime sleepiness. Clin Psychol Rev 2005; 25(5):629–644.
79. Ounsted MK, Hendrick AM. The first-born child: Patterns of development. Dev Med Child Neurol 1977; 19(4):446–453.
80. Stojanovski SD, Rasu RS, Balkrishnan R, et al. Trends in medication prescribing for pediatric sleep difficulties in US outpatient settings. Sleep 2007; 30(8):1013–1017.
81. Owens JA, Rosen CL, Mindell JA. Medication use in the treatment of pediatric insomnia: Results of a survey of community-based pediatricians. Pediatrics 2003; 111(5 Pt 1):e628–e635.
82. Diphenhydramine, Lexi-Comp Online™, Pediatric Lexi-Drugs Online™. Hudson, Ohio: Lexi-Comp, Inc; 2008. Accessed September 18, 2008.
83. Russo RM, Gururaj VJ, Allen JE. The effectiveness of diphenhydramine HCI in pediatric sleep disorders. J Clin Pharmacol 1976; 16(5–6):284–288.
84. Hydroxyzine, Lexi-Comp Online™, Pediatric Lexi-Drugs Online™. Hudson, Ohio: Lexi-Comp, Inc;2008. Accessed September 18, 2008.
85. Clonidine, Lexi-Comp Online™, Pediatric Lexi-Drugs Online™. Hudson, Ohio: Lexi-Comp, Inc; 2008. Accessed September 18, 2008.
86. Guanfacine, Lexi-Comp Online™, Pediatric Lexi-Drugs Online™. Hudson, Ohio: Lexi-Comp, Inc;2008. Accessed September 18, 2008.
87. Prince JB, Wilens TE, Biederman J, et al. Clonidine for sleep disturbances associated with attention-deficit hyperactivity disorder: A systematic chart review of 62 cases. J Am Acad Child Adolesc Psychiatry 1996; 35(5):599–605.
88. Melatonin, Lexi-Comp Online™, Poisoning and Toxicology. Hudson, Ohio: Lexi-Comp, Inc; 2008. Accessed September 18, 2008.
89. Diazepam, Lexi-Comp Online™, Pediatric Lexi-Drugs Online™. Hudson, Ohio: Lexi-Comp, Inc; 2008. Accessed September 18, 2008.
90. Clonazepam, Lexi-Comp Online™, Pediatric Lexi-Drugs Online™. Hudson, Ohio: Lexi-Comp, Inc; 2008. Accessed September 18, 2008.
91. Lorazepam, Lexi-Comp Online™, Pediatric Lexi-Drugs Online™. Hudson, Ohio: Lexi-Comp, Inc; 2008. Accessed September 18, 2008.
92. Zolpidem, Lexi-Comp Online™, Pediatric Lexi-Drugs Online™. Hudson, Ohio: Lexi-Comp, Inc; 2008. Accessed September 18, 2008.
93. Blumer JL, Reed MD, Steinberg F, et al. Potential pharmacokinetic basis for zolpidem dosing in children with sleep difficulties. Clin Pharmacol Ther 2008; 83(4):551–558.
94. Imipramine, Lexi-Comp Online™, Pediatric Lexi-Drugs Online™. Hudson, Ohio: Lexi-Comp, Inc; 2008. Accessed September 18, 2008.
95. Amitriptyline, Lexi-Comp Online™, Pediatric Lexi-Drugs Online™. Hudson, Ohio: Lexi-Comp, Inc; 2008. Accessed September 18, 2008.
96. Trazodone, Lexi-Comp Online™, Pediatric Lexi-Drugs Online™. Hudson, Ohio: Lexi-Comp, Inc; 2008. Accessed September 18, 2008.

97. Merenstein D, Diener-West M, Halbower AC, et al. The trial of infant response to diphenhydramine: The TIRED study–a randomized, controlled, patient-oriented trial. Arch Pediatr Adolesc Med 2006; 160(7):707–712.
98. Public Health Advisory: FDA recommends that over-the-counter (OTC) cough and cold products not be used for infants and children under 2 years of age. 2010. http://www.fda.gov/drugs/drugsafety/publichealthadvisories/ucm051137.html. Accessed March 5, 2010.
99. Richardson GS, Roehrs TA, Rosenthal L, et al. Tolerance to daytime sedative effects of H1 antihistamines. J Clin Psychopharmacol 2002; 22(5):511–515.
100. Daviss WB, Patel NC, Robb AS, et al. Clonidine for attention-deficit/hyperactivity disorder: II. ECG changes and adverse events analysis. J Am Acad Child Adolesc Psychiatry 2008; 47(2):189–198.
101. Ming X, Gordon E, Kang N, et al. Use of clonidine in children with autism spectrum disorders. Brain Dev 2008; 30(7):454–460.
102. Schnoes CJ, Kuhn BR, Workman EF, et al. Pediatric prescribing practices for clonidine and other pharmacologic agents for children with sleep disturbance. Clin Pediatr 2006; 45(3):229–238.
103. Smits MG, Nagtegaal EE, van der Heijden J, et al. Melatonin for chronic sleep onset insomnia in children: A randomized placebo-controlled trial. J Child Neurol 2001; 16(2):86–92.
104. Palm L, Blennow G, Wetterberg L. Long-term melatonin treatment in blind children and young adults with circadian sleep-wake disturbances. Dev Med Child Neurol 1997; 39(5):319–325.
105. Braam W, Didden R, Smits M, et al. Melatonin treatment in individuals with intellectual disability and chronic insomnia: A randomized placebo-controlled study. J Intellect Disabil Res 2008; 52(Pt 3):256–264.
106. Andersen IM, Kaczmarska J, McGrew SG, et al. Melatonin for insomnia in children with autism spectrum disorders. J Child Neurol 2008; 23(5):482–485.
107. Miyamoto A, Oki J, Takahashi S, et al. Serum melatonin kinetics and long-term melatonin treatment for sleep disorders in Rett syndrome. Brain Dev 1999; 21(1):59–62.
108. Karasek M, Stawerska R, Smyczynska J, et al. Increased melatonin concentrations in children with growth hormone deficiency. J Pineal Res 2007; 42(2):119–124.
109. Wasdell MB, Jan JE, Bomben MM, et al. A randomized, placebo-controlled trial of controlled release melatonin treatment of delayed sleep phase syndrome and impaired sleep maintenance in children with neurodevelopmental disabilities. J Pineal Res 2008; 44(1):57–64.
110. Dahl RE. The pharmacologic treatment of sleep disorders. Psychiatr Clin North Am 1992; 15(1):161–178.
111. Ista E, van Dijk M, Gamel C, et al. Withdrawal symptoms in critically ill children after long-term administration of sedatives and/or analgesics: A first evaluation. Crit Care Med 2008; 36(8):2427–2432.
112. Armour A, Gottschlich MM, Khoury J, et al. A randomized, controlled prospective trial of zolpidem and haloperidol for use as sleeping agents in pediatric burn patients. J Burn Care Res 2008; 29(1):238–247.
113. Wilson S, Argyropoulos S. Antidepressants and sleep: A qualitative review of the literature. Drugs 2005; 65(7):927–947.
114. US Food and Drug Administration.Safety Alerts for Drugs, Biologics, Medical Devices, and Dietary Supplements: Antidepressant Medication Products. 2007. http://www.fda.gov/medwatch/safety/2007/safety07.htm#Antidepressant. Accessed September 18, 2008.
115. Kaynak H, Kaynak D, Gozukirmizi E, et al. The effects of trazodone on sleep in patients treated with stimulant antidepressants. Sleep Med 2004; 5(1):15–20.
116. Kallepalli BR, Bhatara VS, Fogas BS, et al. Trazodone is only slightly faster than fluoxetine in relieving insomnia in adolescents with depressive disorders. J Child Adolesc Psychopharmacol 1997; 7(2): 97–107.
117. Mendelson WB. A review of the evidence for the efficacy and safety of trazodone in insomnia. J Clin Psychiatry 2005; 66(4):469–476.

22 Overview of Treatment Considerations

Daniel J. Buysse

Neuroscience Clinical and Translational Research Center, University of Pittsburgh School of Medicine, Pittsburgh, Pennsylvania, U.S.A.

As reviewed in the first two sections of this volume, insomnia is a prevalent health problem in the general population and in medical practice. Advances in our understanding of the origins and evaluation of insomnia have been paralleled by advances in clinical treatment, reviewed in this final section.

The treatment of insomnia falls into two major categories; psychological-behavioral treatments, and pharmacologic treatments. Other treatments that do not fall into these categories, such as bright light, exercise, and various somatic treatments, have also been examined. However, these are far less developed than the psychological-behavioral and pharmacologic treatments, and for that reason are not reviewed in this volume.

The efficacy of psychological-behavioral treatments and pharmacological treatments has been well established. Published reviews have systematically evaluated the evidence for efficacy of psychological-behavioral treatments, and suggest that standard treatments such as multicomponent cognitive behavioral therapy lead to both statistically and clinically significant improvements in patients with primary and comorbid insomnias (1,2). Similarly, published metaanalyses regarding benzodiazepine receptor agonist therapy demonstrate the efficacy of this approach (3,4). Greater variability is evident in reviews of the efficacy of pharmacologic treatments; some of these have suggested more limited benefits relative to observed adverse effects, particularly among the elderly (5). Although it is often difficult to compare behavioral and pharmacologic treatment studies because of differences in study design, available evidence suggests that the two types of treatment are broadly comparable in their efficacy (4). Individual studies have sometimes indicated larger treatment effects for behavioral versus pharmacologic treatments (e.g., 6,7), but small sample sizes and methodologic features that favor one treatment or another make such studies difficult to conduct and interpret.

Despite the proven efficacy of behavioral and pharmacologic treatments for insomnia, a number of important questions remain. Early studies have begun to address some of these questions, as indicated in subsequent chapters. These questions fall into four general areas.

INSOMNIA AND ITS MEASUREMENT

What is the etiology and pathophysiology of insomnia? As described in previous chapters in this volume, significant advances have been made in our understanding of the psychological and neurobiological underpinnings of insomnia. However, there is no definitive evidence that supports any single theory of insomnia. Likewise, no biological or neurophysiological markers have demonstrated adequate sensitivity and specificity. Improving our understanding of the causes of insomnia can only lead to more specific treatments for this condition.

What are the most appropriate outcome measures to use in the treatment of insomnia? Insomnia symptoms can be assessed in a variety of ways, including patient report instruments, diaries, polysomnography, and actigraphy. Even self-report outcomes have typically focused on "quantitative" outcomes such as sleep latency, wakefulness after sleep onset, and total sleep time. Whether these measures adequately capture the core insomnia experience is open to question. The development of patient report outcomes is increasingly using qualitative research methods to ensure that insomnia assessment instruments capture those dimensions most salient to patients themselves. Thus, more qualitative self-report outcomes may complement polysomnography and other objective sleep outcomes in the future. Another important trend in insomnia outcome measures is increasing emphasis on both sleep and waking aspects of the disorder. As exemplified in the Research Diagnostic Criteria for Insomnia (8) and the International Classification of Sleep Disorders, Second Edition (ICSD-2) (9), increased emphasis has been placed on the measurement of waking symptoms of insomnia, including objective measurement of neuropsychological impairments. Thus, greater sophistication in both self-report and objective indicators of sleep and wake function in insomnia may lead to a better understanding of treatment effects.

BEHAVIORAL TREATMENTS

What are the effective elements of multimodal cognitive behavioral therapy for insomnia (CBT-I)? Although the efficacy of CBT-I is now well demonstrated, treatments can be made more efficient if they focus on those elements that have the greatest efficacy. In order to identify these elements, dismantling trials are needed to compare the various components of CBT-I.

What is the minimal effective "dose" of behavioral treatment? One objection sometimes raised to the more widespread use of CBT-I and other behavioral treatment is the effort required to provide six to eight individual treatment sessions. Some evidence already suggests that a smaller number of treatments may have similar efficacy (10,11). Although the ideal number of sessions is likely to vary for different individuals, further evidence is needed to clarify the range of effective treatment duration.

How can we most effectively disseminate behavioral treatments for insomnia? Recognizing the efficacy of behavioral treatments for insomnia, we must also confront the mismatch between the number of trained behavioral sleep medicine specialists and the number of individuals in the population who experience insomnia. As outlined in this section, early evidence suggests that alternate forms of treatment and treatment delivery may be part of the answer. Briefer, more focused treatments, the use of group therapy, and the use of self-guided treatments such as internet-based therapy may all provide useful methods for dissemination. These methods must also be accompanied by additional efforts toward education of other health professionals and building the workforce of trained behavioral sleep medicine practitioners.

PHARMACOLOGIC TREATMENT

What are the viable targets for new pharmacotherapies? Sleep–wake regulation is complex, and the number of neurotransmitters and neuromodulators involved is large. The good news is that this creates a number of viable targets for insomnia therapy; the bad news is that no single neurochemical is sufficient to reliably alter sleep–wake balance and treat insomnia. Nevertheless, the long standing reliance on benzodiazepine receptor agonists is likely to give way to a greater variety of treatments, including those affecting targets such as histamine, orexin, and serotonin receptors.

What are the ideal delivery systems? Insomnia pharmacotherapy has been provided only in the form of oral tablets or capsules. Alternate delivery systems, including transdermal systems, sublingual, and nasal delivery systems may all be feasible for insomnia treatments. These systems are currently under investigation; their place in the pharmacotherapy armamentarium remains to be seen.

What is the optimal duration of treatment? Until the last five to ten years, the widespread assumption was that insomnia pharamacotherapy should be restricted to short term. As evidence is accumulated regarding the longer term efficacy of pharmacotherapy agents, as well as the chronic nature of insomnia, reasonable questions emerge regarding the optimal length of pharmacotherapy. Although it seems undesirable to consign a patient to lifelong pharmacologic treatment, there is currently very little evidence suggesting how to optimize the duration of treatment.

GENERAL TREATMENT CONSIDERATIONS

How can we match treatments to specific patients? Very little evidence currently guides practitioners in terms of selecting behavioral or pharmacologic treatments for a specific patient, much less the specific treatment within these broad categories. Understanding how to match treatments in patients requires studies with large numbers of subjects, and well-characterized treatments and patients. Nonetheless, such efforts are important in order to reduce the time and expense of treatment in real-world clinical settings.

What are the optimal forms of combination and sequenced treatments? Although the efficacy of behavioral and pharmacologic treatments is well established, the circumstances under which

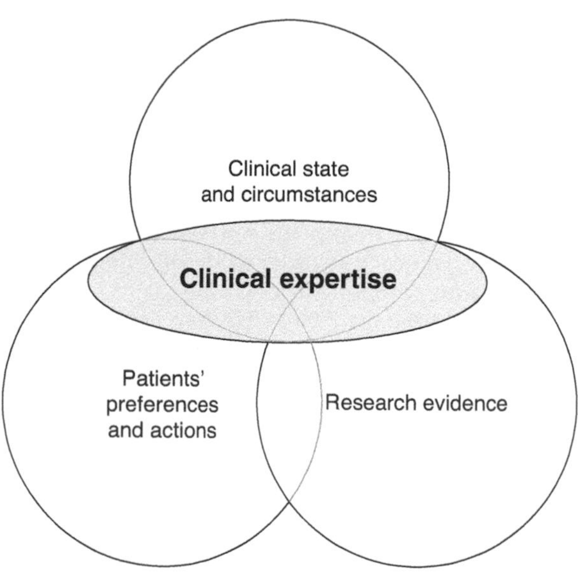

Figure 1 The optimal management of insomnia patients depends on research evidence, the patient's clinical state, circumstances, and preferences, and the practitioner's clinical expertise. *Source:* From Refs. 12 and 13.

these treatments should be combined, or when patients should be treated sequentially with the different modalities is largely unknown. Identifying the most effective treatment sequences will help to address the problem of treatment nonresponse and residual symptoms, which have heretofore received little attention.

How does treatment affect insomnia and its comorbidities? Convincing evidence indicates that insomnia is a risk factor for mental disorders, and newer evidence suggests that insomnia may be a risk factor for, or worsen the experience, of medical conditions such as hypertension and chronic pain. An important question for future research is whether treating insomnia leads to reduced risk for adverse health outcomes, and whether it actually improves the symptoms of comorbid medical and psychiatric disorders.

Can we develop effective evidence-based treatment guidelines for insomnia? Basic evidence regarding treatment efficacy is available for behavioral and pharmacologic treatments, although more sophisticated evidence, such as treatment matching and optimal sequencing strategies, is not. Initial treatment guidelines have been developed for insomnia, but a larger empirical database is clearly needed to make these guidelines more meaningful and effective in clinical practice. While there is clearly a need for evidence-based guidelines in insomnia, it is also important to consider patients' preferences in the selection of treatments as well. As Haynes wrote, "the term evidence based medicine was developed to encourage practitioners and patients to pay due respect—no more no less—to current best evidence in making decisions" (12) or, as stated even more succinctly by DaCruz, "evidence does not make decisions, people do" (13).

SUMMARY

Many components of the effective treatment of insomnia have been addressed by previous research, as presented in detail in this section. However, many other questions remain. The optimal treatment of insomnia patients will depend on the continued collection of new research evidence, as well as understanding and respect for the patient's clinical state, preferences and actions, and the practitioner's expertise (Fig. 1).

ACKNOWLEDGMENT

Supported in part by NIH grants MH024652, AG020677 and AR052155.

REFERENCES

1. Morin CM, Bootzin RR, Buysse DJ, et al. Psychological and behavioral treatment of insomnia: An update of recent evidence (1998–2004). Sleep 2006; 29(11):1398–1414.

2. Morgenthaler T, Kramer M, Alessi C, et al. Practice parameters for the psychological and behavioral treatment of insomnia: An update. An american academy of sleep medicine report. Sleep 2006; 29(11):1415–1419.
3. Nowell PD, Mazumdar S, Buysse DJ, et al. Benzodiazepines and zolpidem for chronic insomnia: A meta-analysis of treatment efficacy. JAMA 1997; 278(24):2170–2177.
4. Smith MT, Perlis ML, Park A, et al. Comparative meta-analysis of pharmacotherapy and behavior therapy for persistent insomnia. Am J Psychiatry 2002; 159(1):5–11.
5. Glass J, Lanctot KL, Herrmann N, et al. Sedative hypnotics in older people with insomnia: Meta-analysis of risks and benefits. BMJ 2005; 331(7526):1169.
6. Jacobs GD, Pace-Schott EF, Stickgold R, et al. Cognitive behavior therapy and pharmacotherapy for insomnia: A randomized controlled trial and direct comparison. Arch Intern Med 2004; 164(17):1888–1896.
7. Sivertsen B, Omvik S, Pallesen S, et al. Cognitive behavioral therapy vs zopiclone for treatment of chronic primary insomnia in older adults: A randomized controlled trial. JAMA 2006; 295(24):2851–2858.
8. Edinger JD, Bonnet MH, Bootzin RR, et al. Derivation of research diagnostic criteria for insomnia: Report of an American Academy of Sleep Medicine Work Group. Sleep 2004; 27(8):1567–1596.
9. American Academy of Sleep Medicine. International classification of sleep disorders, 2nd ed: Diagnostic and coding manual, American Academy of Sleep Medicine, Westchester, IL 2005.
10. Edinger JD, Means MK. Cognitive-behavioral therapy for primary insomnia. Clin Psychol Rev 2005; 25(5):539–558.
11. Germain A, Moul DE, Franzen PL, et al. Effects of a brief behavioral treatment for late-life insomnia: Preliminary findings. J Clin Sleep Med 2006; 2(4):403–406.
12. Haynes RB, Devereaux PJ, Guyatt GH. Physicians' and patients' choices in evidence based practice. BMJ 2002; 324(7350):1350.
13. DaCruz D. Good governance must be introduced globally. BMJ 2002; 324(7333):364.

23 Role of Healthy Sleep Practices: Alcohol/Caffeine/Exercise/Scheduling

Leah Friedman
Department of Psychiatry and Behavioral Sciences, Stanford University, Stanford, California, U.S.A.

Jamie M. Zeitzer
Department of Psychiatry and Behavioral Sciences, Stanford University, Stanford, and Psychiatry Service, VA Palo Alto Health Care System, Palo Alto, California, U.S.A.

Martin S. Mumenthaler
Department of Psychiatry and Behavioral Sciences, Stanford University, Stanford, California, U.S.A.

INTRODUCTION

Everyday behaviors can have a profound impact on sleep and modification of these behaviors is considered a useful nonpharmacologic approach in treating many manifestations of insomnia. Four behaviors commonly targeted in such treatments are the amount and daily timing of alcohol and caffeine consumption, the nature, amount and timing of physical exercise, and the scheduling of sleep and wake.

Most codified nonpharmacologic treatments for insomnia have included regulation of some or all of these behaviors as treatment components [e.g., scheduling in stimulus control (1)] or bundled with other recommended daily health practices as an independent behavioral treatment called "sleep hygiene" [e.g., (2)]. Sleep hygiene has also been used as a control treatment for other nondrug approaches [e.g., (3,4)]. The components of sleep hygiene vary but the basic paradigm is consistent: the prescription of some practices thought to improve sleep and the limitation or prohibition of others thought to harm sleep.

Although there have been studies of sleep hygiene as a package, it is difficult to test the validity of sleep hygiene as a stand-alone treatment because there is no formal consensus as to what components should be included nor have the instructions for these components been standardized (5). Stepanski and Wyatt (5) have suggested that given the inconsistency in the components of sleep hygiene treatments, evidence for specific health practices should be reviewed independent of one another. Thus, we will review the extant research on the effects of alcohol, caffeine, exercise and scheduling on sleep quality and quantity and, when available, the effects of modifying these behaviors on disturbed sleep. In this chapter, the impact of routine alcohol and caffeine use as components of inadequate sleep hygiene is discussed. Abuse of these substances, and others, as primary causative factors in insomnia is discussed in detail in Chapter 17.

ALCOHOL

Most nonpharmacologic treatments for insomnia advise patients to limit alcohol intake or abstain from alcohol before bedtime. In some of the published techniques, the instructions are vague [e.g., the patient is advised to "moderate alcohol consumption and eliminate 'night caps'" (6) or "practice light to moderate use of alcoholic beverages" (7)] though some are more specific, such as those endorsed by a recent American Academy of Sleep Medicine wellness booklet: "Do not drink alcoholic beverages within four to six hours of bedtime" (8).

The soporific effects of alcohol have long been known; witness the drunken sleep of Noah in Genesis. Because of its initial sleep-inducing effects, alcohol is frequently used to self-medicate insomnia. Alcohol is a global depressant of the central nervous system (CNS) and acts through the inhibitory GABA-A receptor complex to increase the length of time it is opened after its chloride channel is activated by GABA. Notably, this same receptor complex is also modulated by barbiturates and benzodiazepines, though these act at receptor complex sites distinct from those at which alcohol acts (9).

Alcohol is undoubtedly the most commonly used sleep-promoting substance (10), but the worm in this apple is that the sedative effects are transient. After intake before bedtime, even in healthy individuals without insomnia, alcohol reduces sleep onset, increases nonrapid eye movement (NREM) and reduces rapid eye movement (REM) sleep early in the night. This seeming immediate benefit of alcohol vanishes relatively quickly since alcohol is metabolized rapidly (at the approximate rate of one glass of wine or a half-pint of beer per two hours). The second part of the night after evening alcohol ingestion is characterized by light, disturbed sleep, with more REM sleep and associated increased dream or nightmare recall and sympathetic arousal, including tachycardia and sweating (11). Gastric irritation, headache, and a full bladder may also be among the effects that interrupt sleep in the latter part of the night. The negative impact of alcohol on sleep can continue long after blood alcohol concentrations reach zero, and lead to the so-called "hangover effect" (7). This may reduce overall vigor and daytime alertness, leading to daytime sleep and a subsequent disruption of nighttime sleep due to sleep fragmentation. In addition to the sleep-specific effects, alcohol increases the risk of nocturnal falling (10) that may lead to an increase in injuries in certain vulnerable populations (e.g., older individuals).

A further complication of alcohol intake late in the day is its impact on breathing, particularly during sleep, in those who have compromised ventilation (7). In individuals with mild or moderate sleep apnea, even moderate blood alcohol levels (0.07 gms/dL) can increase the frequency of obstructive apneas and the mean sleep heart rate (12). In addition to the acute effects of alcohol on sleep, chronic alcohol intake is likely to affect sleep as well. The amplitude and incidence of K-complexes are reduced in older alcoholics (13) and this effect may be reversible through extended alcohol abstinence. Although the incidence and prevalence of chronic alcohol use as a factor contributing to insomnia is not known, a community-based survey found that those who met insomnia criteria reported more than twice as much use of alcohol over the course of a week than age and sex-matched controls not meeting criteria (14).

In sum, while alcohol is often used as both a short- and long-term self-treatment for insomnia, in addition to being used in an unrelated recreational fashion, it has overall detrimental effects on sleep as it changes both the timing and nature of sleep-related physiology, the consequence of which for long-term health is unknown.

CAFFEINE

If alcohol is the most widely used substance to self-medicate nocturnal sleeplessness, caffeine is the most commonly used substance to self-medicate excessive sleepiness. While not quite antediluvian, Chinese folklore dating from the third century reports a tale regarding the alerting effects of caffeine (in tea). According to the tale, a Chinese general cut off his eyelids in order to stay awake and a tea tree sprang up from the site where the eyelids fell to the ground (15).

Although the specific details vary, almost all behavioral insomnia treatments caution against drinking caffeinated beverages late in the day. Some narrowly address coffee and tea while others include chocolate and caffeinated soft drinks (16). Hygiene directions for limiting caffeine intake vary from very stringent instructions (e.g., avoid caffeine use completely for four weeks, followed by limiting caffeine use to three cups of coffee prior to 10 AM) (7) to more liberal approaches [e.g., caffeine (should) be discontinued four to six hours before bedtime] (17).

Caffeine is a mild CNS stimulant that acts through the inhibition of A1 and A2A adenosine receptors (18). As adenosine receptors are present throughout the brain, it has been difficult to specify the location or locations at which caffeine inhibition acts to induce wakefulness. While still controversial, the cholinergic basal forebrain is likely one such locus (19). Both coffee and tea are beverages with high caffeine content; a standard cup of coffee has approximately 80 mg of caffeine while a similar sized drink of tea contains approximately 40 mg of caffeine (20). There is, however, very large variation in the caffeine content of coffees and teas, ranging from <0.05 mg/mL in decaffeinated coffees and teas to more than 3.5 mg/mL in some espressos (21,22). Caffeine is also present in carbonated colas, pepper drinks, citrus drinks, root beers, cold teas, and the growing market segment of energy drinks. The caffeine content of these drinks can range from 0 (these are naturally uncaffeinated—the caffeine is added as a supplement) to

120 mg in some energy drinks (23). Other less commonly imagined sources of caffeine include chocolate (~10–30 mg/43 g bar) and both sleepiness-specific (e.g., caffeine pills, ~200 mg) and nonspecific medications (e.g., migraine and diet medication, ~30 mg) (24,25). Worldwide, tea is, however, second only to water as the most widely consumed beverage (26). Because of its utility as a stimulant, and no doubt because of its relatively low cost, near ubiquitous availability, and apparent health safety both acutely and chronically, (18) caffeine is used extensively as a benign drug to maintain alertness. The per capita consumption in the United States has been estimated at 200 mg/day (20).

Contrary to alcohol, caffeine delays sleep initiation. Caffeine also increases the proportion of sleep spent in lighter stages (N1 and N2), while reducing both slow wave sleep (N3) and total sleep time, increases the time to first REM period, and increases the number of changes between sleep stages (18). Caffeine ingestion even early in the day can have objectively quantifiable effects on nocturnal sleep (27) possibly by disrupting the effects of adenosine, one hypothesized mechanism underlying homeostatic sleep pressure (19). Individuals may be unaware of these nocturnal effects as ingestion of low doses of caffeine during the daytime may fail to induce an increase in subjective alertness during the day, but can still disrupt sleep at night (26). Daytime caffeine ingestion can also lead to significant amounts of caffeine being present in the blood when attempting to initiate sleep, as the half-life of caffeine is approximately 4.5 hours (25) and its metabolites, notably theophylline, have potent inhibitory effects on the same A1 and A2A adenosine receptors as does caffeine (18).

There is wide inter-individual variability in sleep responses to caffeine, with some individuals being more sensitive to the effects of caffeine than others (28,29). There is likely a genetic component to this variability as a common genetic polymorphism in the adenosine A2A receptor is related to both the subjective and objective effects of caffeine on sleep (29). The issue of caffeine sensitivity, however, is complex as a number of studies have shown that individuals both with and without insomnia self-regulate caffeine intake such that those who rated themselves as 'caffeine sensitive' would drink fewer caffeinated beverages (29,30). A further complexity is that the change in sleep onset behavior that can be associated with mild caffeine intake may be innately more worrisome, and therefore be perceived as more disruptive of sleep, for some individuals than for others (31). The anxiety or worry associated with a delayed sleep onset may exacerbate the mild sleep disruption that would have otherwise occurred after exposure to a low dose of caffeine. Caffeine use is also associated with a subjective increase in tolerance to the alerting effects of caffeine that is not accompanied by a change in metabolism or objective effects on performance (32–34). This can lead to increasing caffeine intake during the day in an effort to increase subjective alertness, which will secondarily increase caffeine levels during the night, potentially disrupting sleep.

Given the complexities of interindividual difference in caffeine metabolism and sensitivity, as well as issues of tolerance and subjective response to caffeine-induced alertness, it is not surprising that there are no specific consensus instructions related to moderating caffeine intake in individuals with insomnia. It should be noted that the International Classification of Sleep Disorders, second edition (ICSD-2) makes diagnostic distinctions regarding both caffeine and alcohol use. Persons whose use of either alcohol or caffeine is *inappropriate* in relation to their sleep would be diagnosed as having insomnia due to inadequate sleep hygiene; whereas those who are *dependent* on caffeine or alcohol or use them excessively would be assigned a diagnosis of insomnia due to substance abuse (35). Education about the sources and possible long-lasting effects of caffeine should be part of any nonpharmacologic treatment of insomnia.

EXERCISE

For more than 25 years, regular, daily exercise has been suggested as a component of nonpharmacologic methods for treating insomnia (2). Exercise is still promoted widely as a nonpharmacologic method for improving the quality and quantity of sleep (8,36).

One metaanalysis of the acute effects of exercise on sleep, found support for small to moderate effects of acute exercise on slow wave sleep, REM sleep latency, total time spent in REM sleep, and total time asleep (37). Despite these findings, as Driver and Taylor note, the sleep-promoting effect of exercise in both normal and clinical populations has not yet been conclusively demonstrated (38).

One hypothesized mechanism of the effects of exercise on sleep involves the production of heat during exercise and subsequent cooling. In theory, this exercise-induced cooling could enhance the normal sleep onset related cooling mechanisms that appear essential for normal sleep induction and maintenance (39). The temperature-sensitive neurons in the hypothalamus (40) that can respond to cooling and are sleep active may be the ultimate physiologic mechanism responsible for exercise-induced changes in sleep. This would also help explain why exercise that increases core temperature, when scheduled too close to the onset of sleep, can lead to sleep disruption (41). Even passive forms of cooling (e.g., hot bath followed by evaporative cooling several hours before intended bedtime) have been suggested as being beneficial to sleep onset (42).

Another hypothetical mechanism underlying the effects of exercise on sleep is exercise induction of cytokines, notably interleukin-6 (43). Low concentrations of cytokines, associated with mild to moderate exercise, can promote drowsiness while elevated concentrations are associated with intense exercise and increased wake. There are many other changes in endocrine activity associated with exercise that may also underlie the changes associated with sleep (e.g., endorphins, cortisol).

One of the problems in assessing the effects of exercise on sleep is the variation in the length, intensity, and timing of exercise, as well as the efficacy of acute and chronic exercise routines. Each of these, as well as sex, age, and overall fitness level are likely to impact the effects of exercise on sleep (44). Understanding the specific mechanism, by which exercise improves sleep in individuals with insomnia, as well as in individuals without insomnia, will be a critical step in understanding how to maximize its effects. The timing of exercise may also lead to an indirect effect, which is greater exposure to daylight when the exercise intervention is scheduled to take place outdoors (e.g., tennis, walking, jogging) (45). In older individuals whose reduced daytime light exposure may lead to circadian-associated sleep problems (see below), outdoor exercise may be especially important.

While there is yet to be a definitive link established between exercise and improved sleep, there is sufficient evidence to suggest that there is a likely connection. A better understanding of the mechanistic connection between the two will lead to an improved, more thoughtful recommendation of exercise as a nonpharmacologic treatment of insomnia.

SCHEDULING

Bon vivant that he was, it is questionable whether Ben Franklin followed his own "early to bed, early to rise" advice but he certainly was on to something important as chronic insomnia is often associated with irregular sleep timing (30). Regularity in time-in-bed scheduling supports the entrainment of sleep and wake to the basic daily alternation of day and night. Regular sleep and wake patterns lead to regular exposure to light. Light is the primary zeitgeber (Gm., time cue) of the circadian timing system. Thus, regular sleep and wake patterns lead to regular dark and light exposure that leads to a regular position of the circadian clock relative to sleep and wake. Such a pattern leads to circadian timing that is maximally supportive of proper sleep and wake (46,47). Not only does regularly timed light exposure lead to a proper entrainment of the circadian system, but it also maximizes circadian amplitude (48), which may be especially important in older individuals who may have an innately decreased amplitude of their circadian clock (49,50).

Given the nature of agricultural work in pre-industrial times, an inherent tie existed between the daily alternation of light and dark and peoples' work and sleep schedules. The invention of the electric light likely accelerated our movement away from a natural light/dark exposure and highly regular entraining signals for the circadian system. In our advanced technological society, there are fewer built-in factors that support a consistently followed daily schedule. Advances in science and technology have led to great latitude in the timing of work and play, much of which can theoretically occur now at any time of the day. Twenty-four hour access to supermarkets and computers and businesses maximizing utilization of equipment and space by scheduling work around the clock are just a few examples of infrastructure changes that weaken the practice of fixed day/night schedules. This circumstance is thought to contribute to the high prevalence of insomnia in modern societies and is also likely linked to decreased daytime alertness (51,52).

Scheduling or timing is in some sense at the core of the other health practices discussed in this chapter. As seen above, a major concern regarding the consumption of alcohol, and caffeine, and exercise practices is their timing in relation to sleep. Notably, the question is not necessarily *how much*, but *when*. From its earliest formulations [e.g., (53)] to the most recent formulation of approved guidelines for treatment of insomnia (54), the admonition to keep a regular schedule has been included in nonpharmacological treatments for insomnia. An important caveat is that regularity or scheduling alone is not sufficient, however, for patients to get adequate amounts of sleep. It is necessary for them to allocate sufficient time in bed to get an adequate amount of sleep (52). The various nonpharmacologic methods used for treating insomnia have different instructions relating to regular sleep schedules. Stimulus control, given its goal of strengthening the association between bed and sleep, has a very flexible into bedtime. A central stimulus control instruction is to get into bed "only when sleepy." On the other hand, the morning instruction is to set a standard fixed wake-up time (1). Cognitive behavioral therapy for the treatment of insomnia also prescribes adherence to a standard rise time (55). The essential treatment mechanism in sleep restriction therapy involves scheduling. The time allotted in bed is manipulated in order to build up sufficient sleep debt so that there will be adequate homeostatic pressure for sleep during the scheduled time in bed. Although the restriction of time in bed to the amount of time the individual actually sleeps is the central mechanism of sleep restriction therapy, the regularity of sleep schedules is intrinsic to this therapy, even if not emphasized (56). Sleep restriction therapy, along with some of the other nonpharmacologic treatments for insomnia, also proscribe daytime napping. Not only does this increase the likelihood of being able to maintain a regular nocturnal sleep schedule, but it also reduces daytime exposure to darkness. The human circadian system is sensitive to light during the daytime (57) and the change in light exposure through napping may also deleteriously influence the position of the circadian clock.

CONCLUSION

The benefit of each specific health practice described above remains to be definitively answered. The most recent consensus guidelines for the treatment of insomnia concluded that "although there is insufficient evidence of the effectiveness of sleep hygiene as an insomnia treatment the general principles of sleep hygiene should be included in other behavioral treatments," and for the most part they have been (54).

Although the effectiveness and determination of the optimal parameters of the four health practices described in this chapter are still in question, the overall evidence from our reading of the research literature and our clinical experience is sufficient for us to suggest following the four basic health practices discussed above. At worst, the suggested practices appear to do no harm. At best, if any or all of these health practices have been the source of an individual's sleep problem or have exacerbated it, correcting these practices may help. Finally, they are all supportive of good general mental and physical health independent of their effects on sleep and this indirectly supports good sleep.

We suggest the following:

1. The collection of baseline sleep logs, which is widely recommended as a first step in behavioral treatments, can generate helpful information as to what should be treatment targets. For example, when patient information reveals regular late afternoon and evening use of caffeine, this should be explored as a source of sleep disruption and insomnia complaints (58). Many who have used these techniques have noted that in the process of collecting these self-report data, individuals often become aware that some of their behavior is antithetical to good sleep. This awareness helps increase compliance.
2. Limit evening drinking of alcoholic beverages to ONE alcoholic drink with dinner and NO alcoholic drinks within three hours of bedtime. Information about alcohol and its paradoxical effects on sleep initiation and sleep maintenance should be disseminated.
3. Limit caffeine (tea, coffee, cola, caffeinated soft drinks, chocolate) use no more than two cups taken no later than lunchtime. The impact of caffeine metabolism should be explained such that individuals with insomnia understand that what is a great boost in the daytime is a negative at night. There are decaffeinated drinks that many have substituted for that habitual beverage that people reflexively take throughout the day.

4. Schedule some form of moderate (or greater) physical activity (walking, swimming, jogging, gardening) for at least 30 min every day to be completed no later than four hours before bedtime. Most people are aware of the importance of exercise for their general health, and if only because exercise improves health it should contribute to good sleep. This exercise is also likely to synergistically support circadian variation in core body temperature and contribute to good sleep.
5. Set a sleep schedule that fits with usual habits as recorded by two weeks of sleep log information. Once a realistic schedule is determined, the alarm should be set for the same time, seven days a week. The evening into-bed-time can be scheduled within a one-hour time frame to allow for that essential phone call or must-see TV program. If there are special events that result in delayed bedtime, keep the alarm set at its regular time and wake as usual. Keeping the same wake time instead of sleeping-in ensures the buildup of sufficient homeostatic sleep pressure to maintain sleep the next evening and does not disrupt the normal light exposure in the morning that is critical for keeping sleep rhythm coupled to circadian rhythm.

Two parting thoughts: "Bad sleep hygiene is seldom the sole cause of any sleep problem, but rare is the sleep problem that is not partially maintained by poor sleep hygiene," (2) and, as another early sleep hygiene investigator noted, "...removing the [sleep hygiene] abuses from the daily routines of abusers is...probably...a good idea" (59).

REFERENCES

1. Bootzin RR. Nicassio P. Behavioral treatments for insomnia. In: Hersen M, Eisler RM, Miller PM, eds. Progress in Behavior Modification, Vol 6. New York, NY: Academic Press, 1978:1–45.
2. Hauri PJ. Current Concepts: The Sleep Disorders, 2nd ed. Kalamazoo, MI: The Upjohn Company, 1982.
3. Friedman L, Benson K, Noda A, et al. An actigraphic comparison of sleep restriction and sleep hygiene treatments for insomnia in older adults. J Geriatr Psychiatry Neurol 2000; 13:17–27.
4. Friedman L, Zeitzer JM, Kushida CA, et al. Scheduled bright light for treatment of insomnia in older adults. J Am Geriatr Soc 2009; 57:441–452.
5. Stepanski EJ. Wyatt JK. Use of sleep hygiene in the treatment of insomnia. Sleep Med Rev 2003; 7:215–225.
6. Espie CA, MacMahon KM, Kelly HL, et al Randomized clinical effectiveness trial of nurse-administered small-group cognitive behavior therapy for persistent insomnia in general practice. Sleep 2007; 30:574–584.
7. Zarcone V. Sleep hygiene. In: Kryger, MH, Roth T, Dement WC, eds. Principles and Practice of Sleep Medicine, 3rd ed. Philadelphia: W.B. Saunders Company, 2000:657–661.
8. American Academy of Sleep Medicine. Sleep Hygiene: Behaviors that help promote sound sleep. Westchester, IL: American Academy of Sleep Medicine, 2005.
9. Hevers W, Luddens H. The diversity of GABAA receptors. Pharmacological and electrophysiological properties of GABAA channel subtypes. Mol Neurobiol 1998; 18:35–86.
10. Gillin JC, Drummond SPA, Clark CP, et al. Medication and substance abuse. In: Kryger MH, Roth T, Dement WC, eds. Principles and Practice of Sleep Medicine, 4th ed. Philadelphia, PA: Elsevier Saunders, 2005:1345–1358.
11. Kobayashi T, Misaki K, Nakagawa H, et al. Alcohol effect on sleep electroencephalography by fast Fourier transformation. Psychiatry Clin Neurosci 1998; 52:154–155.
12. Scanlan MF, Roebuck T, Little PJ, et al. Effect of moderate alcohol upon obstructive sleep apnoea. Eur Respir J 2000; 16:909–913.
13. Colrain IM, Crowley KE, Nicholas CL, et al. The impact of alcoholism on sleep evoked delta frequency responses. Biol Psychiatry 2009; 66:177–184.
14. Jefferson CD, Drake CL, Scofield HM, et al. Sleep hygiene practices in a population-based sample of insomniacs. Sleep 2005; 28, 611–615.
15. Yü L. The Classic of Tea (Ch'a Ching). Boston, MA: Little, Brown, and Company, 1974.
16. Hauri PJ. Sleep hygiene, relaxation therapy, and cognitive interventions. In: Hauri PJ, ed. Case Studies in Insomnia. New York, NY: Plenum Publishing Corp, 1991.
17. Morin CM. Insomnia: Psychological Assessment and Management. New York, NY: Guilford, 1993.
18. Fredholm BB, Battig K, Holmen J, et al. Actions of caffeine in the brain with special reference to factors that contribute to its widespread use. Pharmacol Rev 1999; 51:83–133.

19. Porkka-Heiskanen T, Strecker RE, McCarley RW. Brain site-specificity of extracellular adenosine concentration changes during sleep deprivation and spontaneous sleep: An in vivo microdialysis study. Neuroscience 2000; 99:507–517.
20. Barone JJ. Roberts HR. Caffeine consumption. Food Chem Toxicol 1996; 34:119–129.
21. McCusker RR, Fuehrlein B, Goldberger BA, et al. Caffeine content of decaffeinated coffee. J Anal Toxicol 2006; 30:611–613.
22. McCusker RR, Goldberger BA, Cone EJ. Caffeine content of specialty coffees. J Anal Toxicol 2003; 27:520–522.
23. McCusker RR, Goldberger BA, Cone EJ. Caffeine content of energy drinks, carbonated sodas, and other beverages. J Anal Toxicol 2006; 30:112–114.
24. Durrant,KL. Known and hidden sources of caffeine in drug, food, and natural products. J Am Pharm Assoc (Wash) 2002; 42:625–637.
25. Somani SM, Gupta P. Caffeine: A new look at an age-old drug. Int J Clin Pharmacol Ther Toxicol 1988; 26:521–533.
26. Hindmarch I, Rigney U, Stanley N, et al. A naturalistic investigation of the effects of day-long consumption of tea, coffee and water on alertness, sleep onset and sleep quality. Psychopharmacology (Berl) 2000; 149:203–216.
27. Landolt HP, Werth E, Borbely AA, et al. Caffeine intake (200 mg) in the morning affects human sleep and EEG power spectra at night. Brain Res 1995; 675:67–74.
28. Drake CL, Jefferson C, Roehrs T, et al. Stress-related sleep disturbance and polysomnographic response to caffeine. Sleep Med 2006; 7:567–572.
29. Retey JV, Adam M, Khatami R, et al. A genetic variation in the adenosine A2A receptor gene (ADORA2A) contributes to individual sensitivity to caffeine effects on sleep. Clin Pharmacol Ther 2007; 81:692–698.
30. Cheek RE, Shaver JL. Lentz MJ. Variations in sleep hygiene practices of women with and without insomnia. Res Nurs Health 2004; 27:225–236.
31. Omvik S, Pallesen S, Bjorvatn B, et al. Night-time thoughts in high and low worriers: Reaction to caffeine-induced sleeplessness. Behav Res Ther 2007; 45:715–727.
32. Parsons WD. Neims AH. Effect of smoking on caffeine clearance. Clin Pharmacol Ther 1978; 24: 40–45.
33. George J, Murphy T, Roberts R, et al. Influence of alcohol and caffeine consumption on caffeine elimination. Clin Exp Pharmacol Physiol 1986; 13:731–736.
34. Kalow W. Variability of caffeine metabolism in humans. Drug Res 1985; 35:319–324.
35. American Academy of Sleep Medicine. International Classification of Sleep Disorders: Diagnostic and Coding Manual, 2nd ed. Westchester, IL: American Academy of Sleep Medicine, 2005.
36. American Sleep Disorders Association. Sleep hygiene: Behaviors that help promote sound sleep. Rochester, MN: American Sleep Disorders Association, 1997.
37. Youngstedt SD, O'Connor PJ, Dishman RK. The effects of acute exercise on sleep: A quantitative synthesis. Sleep 1997; 20:203–214.
38. Driver HS, Taylor SR. Exercise and sleep. Sleep Med Rev 2000; 4:387–402.
39. Krauchi K, Cajochen C, Werth E, et al. Warm feet promote the rapid onset of sleep. Nature 1999; 401:36–37.
40. McGinty D, Szymusiak R. Keeping cool: A hypothesis about the mechanisms and functions of slow-wave sleep. Trends Neurosci 1990; 13:480–487.
41. Edinger JD, Morey MC, Sullivan RJ, et al. Aerobic fitness, acute exercise and sleep in older men. Sleep 1993; 16:351–359.
42. Hauri PJ, Linde SM. No More Sleepless Nights. New York, NY: John Wiley & Sons, 1990.
43. Santos RV, Tufik S, De Mello MT. Exercise, sleep and cytokines: Is there a relation? Sleep Med Rev 2007; 11:231–239.
44. Kubitz KA, Landers DM, Petruzzello SJ, et al.The effects of acute and chronic exercise on sleep. A meta-analytic review. Sports Med 1996; 21:277–291.
45. Montgomery P, Dennis J. A systematic review of non-pharmacological therapies for sleep problems in later life. Sleep Med Rev 2004; 8:47–62.
46. Dijk DJ. Czeisler CA. Contribution of the circadian pacemaker and the sleep homeostat to sleep propensity, sleep structure, electroencephalographic slow waves, and sleep spindle activity in humans. J Neurosci 1995; 15:3526–3538.
47. Dijk DJ, Duffy JF, Czeisler CA. Circadian and sleep/wake dependent aspects of subjective alertness and cognitive performance. J Sleep Res 1992; 1:112–117.
48. Jewett ME, Kronauer RE, Czeisler CA. Phase-amplitude resetting of the human circadian pacemaker via bright light: A further analysis. J Biol Rhythms 1994; 9:295–314.

49. Dijk DJ, Duffy JF, Riel E, et al. Ageing and the circadian and homeostatic regulation of human sleep during forced desynchrony of rest, melatonin and temperature rhythms. J Physiol 1999; 516 (Pt 2):611–627.
50. van Someren EJ, Mirmiran M. Swaab DF. Non-pharmacological treatment of sleep and wake disturbances in aging and Alzheimer's disease: Chronobiological perspectives. Behav Brain Res 1993; 57:235–253.
51. Billiard M, Alperovitch A, Perot C, et al. Excessive daytime somnolence in young men: Prevalence and contributing factors. Sleep 1987; 10:297–305.
52. Manber R, Bootzin RR, Acebo C, et al. The effects of regularizing sleep-wake schedules on daytime sleepiness. Sleep 1996; 19:432–441.
53. Hauri P. The Sleep Disorders. Current Concepts. Upjohn, Kalamazoo MI: Scope Publications, 1977.
54. Schutte-Rodin S, Broch L, Buysse D, et al. Clinical guideline for the evaluation and management of chronic insomnia in adults. J Clin Sleep Med 2008; 4:487–504.
55. Edinger JD, Means MK. Cognitive-behavioral therapy for primary insomnia. Clin Psychol Rev 2005; 25:539–558.
56. Spielman AJ, Saskin P, Thorpy MJ. Treatment of chronic insomnia by restriction of time in bed. Sleep 1987; 10:45–56.
57. Khalsa SB, Jewett ME, Cajochen C, et al. A phase response curve to single bright light pulses in human subjects. J Physiol 2003; 549:945–952.
58. Mitler MM, O'Malley MB. Wake-promoting medications: Efficacy and adverse effects. In: Kryger MH, Roth T, Dement WC, eds. Principles and Practice of Sleep Medicine, 4th ed. Philadelphia, PA: Elsevier Saunders, 484–498.
59. Lacks P, Rotert M. Knowledge and practice of sleep hygiene techniques in insomniacs and good sleepers. Behav Res Ther 1986; 24:365–368.

24 Stimulus Control Therapy

Richard R. Bootzin

Departments of Psychology and Psychiatry, University of Arizona, Tucson, Arizona, U.S.A.

Leisha J. Smith

Department of Psychology, University of Arizona, Tucson, Arizona, U.S.A.

Peter L. Franzen

Sleep Medicine Institute and Department of Psychiatry, University of Pittsburgh School of Medicine, Pittsburgh, Pennsylvania, U.S.A.

Shauna L. Shapiro

Department of Counseling Psychology, Santa Clara University, Santa Clara, California, U.S.A.

Stimulus control therapy (SCT) for insomnia is based primarily upon an operant conditioning model of the development and maintenance of insomnia in which falling asleep is conceptualized as an instrumental act emitted to produce the reinforcement, sleep. Difficulty in falling asleep, then may be due to inadequate stimulus control (1). This could be either because of the lack of discriminative stimuli that facilitate sleep or the presence of stimuli that are associated with activities that interfere with sleep.

The role of stimuli in facilitating or interfering with sleep is not the only learning principle that affects sleep. Pavlovian conditioning is also important in that the bed and bedroom can become cues for the anxiety and frustration associated with trying to fall asleep (1). Internal cues, such as mind racing, anticipatory anxiety, and physiological arousal can become cues for further arousal and sleep disruptions (2). SCT aims to reduce cues associated with arousal as well as cues that are discriminative stimuli for activities that are incompatible with sleep.

Stimulus control therapy was designed to help individuals suffering from insomnia to strengthen the bed and bedroom as cues for sleep, to weaken the bed and bedroom as cues for arousal, and to develop a consistent sleep–wake schedule to help maintain improvement. Stimulus control therapy for the treatment of insomnia was proposed by Bootzin in 1972 (3). The instructions were expanded during the next few years (1,4) and have remained unchanged to the present. The six instructions that comprise SCT are as follows:

1. Lie down to go to sleep only when you are sleepy.
2. Do not use your bed for anything except sleep; that is, do not read, watch television, eat, or worry in bed. Sexual activity is the only exception to this rule. On such occasions, the instructions are to be followed afterward when you intend to go to sleep.
3. If you find yourself unable to fall asleep, get up and go into another room. Stay up as long as you wish and then return to the bedroom to sleep. Although we do not want you to watch the clock, we want you to get out of bed if you do not fall asleep immediately. Remember the goal is to associate your bed with falling asleep *quickly*! If you are in bed more than 10 minutes without falling asleep and have not gotten up, you are not following this instruction.
4. If you still cannot fall asleep, repeat step 3. Do this as often as is necessary throughout the night.
5. Set your alarm and get up at the same time every morning irrespective of how much sleep you got during the night. This will help your body acquire a consistent sleep rhythm.
6. Do not nap during the day.

While the instructions are concerned mainly with sleep onset, they may also be used with individuals with sleep maintenance problems by repeating instructions three and four during mid-night awakenings. Each of the instructions stated above is important in reestablishing the bed and bedroom as cues for sleep rather than wakefulness. It is important that the rationale for each instruction be described to patients in detail. Although the instructions seem straightforward, they may be difficult for patients to follow, and if the reasons behind the instructions are unclear, compliance may be even more challenging.

Instruction 1: The first instruction is designed to help individuals become more aware of their bodies' cues for sleepiness. Frequently, individuals with insomnia decide to go to bed because of clock time as a result of a calculation of how much sleep they feel they must have before awakening in the morning. This may produce increasing anxiety as sleeplessness persists coupled with excessive time in bed for the amount of sleep that is obtained.

Initially, individuals with insomnia may rarely use internal cues of sleepiness. Thus, instruction one should be viewed as a goal to be achieved gradually over the first few weeks rather than as an imperative to be started immediately. Becoming sensitive to internal cues of sleepiness will aid patients in determining an appropriate time to go to bed based on sleepiness, not on the clock. Going to bed when sleepy will also make it easier for patients to fall asleep more quickly.

Instruction 2: Instruction two is intended to help strengthen the cues of the bed and bedroom with sleep and weaken the cues of bed and bedroom with arousal and wakefulness. Often individuals with insomnia will engage in activities in bed that interfere with falling asleep, such as reading, watching television, talking on the phone, text-messaging, or working. This behavior establishes the bed and bedroom as conditioned stimuli for wakefulness. By prohibiting any activity associated with arousal, other than sexual activity, from taking place in the bed and bedroom, the second instruction of SCT serves to reduce the bed and bedroom as cues for wakefulness, and reestablish them as cues for sleep.

Patients are typically asked to engage in activities associated with arousal in a different room in the house. For example, if a patient typically thinks about and plans the following day's activities as they are lying in bed, he or she would be asked to do this planning in another room *before* going into the bedroom. This may help individuals with insomnia create a new bedtime routine that is better suited to facilitate sleep onset.

Instructions 3 and 4: The third and fourth instructions are core elements of SCT. Instructing patients to get out of bed, if they are not sleeping, limits them from being awake in bed and further strengthens the association between the bed and bedroom and sleep. While SCT is focused primarily on sleep onset problems, instruction four is incorporated for use with sleep maintenance issues. Getting out of bed to engage in other activities when unable to sleep can also give individuals a sense of control over their insomnia. This makes the problem less distressing and more manageable for the patient.

There are a few important issues in successfully implementing these instructions. First, how long should someone with insomnia be in bed before getting out of bed? The instructions place a premium on getting out-of-bed quickly, within 10 minutes. However, some individuals with insomnia become anxious by such a recommendation and will constantly check the clock to see if it is time to get out of bed. To avoid that, patients are typically instructed to turn the face of the clock away from them, so that clock checking does not occur. If time-pressure produces increased anxiety, the third instruction is often modified to put emphasis on the internal cues of frustration and anxiety rather than on how much time has passed. Thus, while it is permissible to be in bed while in the process of falling asleep, the patient should get out of bed at the first signs of frustration with not falling asleep.

Importantly, however, it is not permissible to stay in bed for long periods of time waiting to fall asleep (such as 45, 60 minutes, or longer) even if not frustrated. The goal of the SCT instructions remains to associate the bed and bedroom with falling asleep quickly. Research has indicated a quarter-hour rule (staying in bed before falling asleep no more than 15 minutes) is manageable and effective in producing improved sleep in those with insomnia (5).

Second, once up, how long should the patients stay awake and what should they do? A good clinical rule of thumb is that patients should stay out-of-bed long enough to feel that they might successfully be able to fall asleep if they return to bed. This is an opportunity to practice paying attention to internal cues of sleepiness and using them as a guide. Generally, this means staying awake at least 15 or more minutes before trying to go to sleep again. As for the activities to be engaged in, patients should be encouraged to do something relaxing and enjoyable.

Because of the increasing evidence that even room light can alter sleep-wake circadian schedules (e.g., 6), we have placed additional emphasis on keeping lights dim when out-of-bed during the night. Reading with a reading light and watching television from a distance are acceptable. We discourage patients from doing anything on the computer, even checking email, since the amount of light from the monitor when sitting close to it is brighter than most individuals realize and activities done on the computer are usually arousing.

Finally, many adults with sleep maintenance problems elect to start the day at 4 AM or 5 AM rather than return to the bed for additional sleep. This is not a wise strategy since even 30 or 60 minutes of additional sleep increases alertness and reduces fatigue during the day. As long as the usual final wake-up time is maintained, returning to bed is recommended when there is 45 minutes or more until wake-up time.

Instruction 5: One of the goals of instruction five is to set a more consistent wake-up time for all seven days of the week, with less than one hour of discrepancy between days off and workdays. Keeping a consistent wake time helps establish a more regular sleep schedule. Many people with insomnia stay in bed later in the morning in hopes of catching up on the sleep they missed the night before. However, irregular schedules weaken the association between the cues of the bed and bedroom and sleep. Maintaining regular sleep schedules has been found to reduce daytime fatigue and sleepiness (7). Consequently, a regular schedule helps both strengthen cues for sleep and reduce daytime problems associated with sleep disturbance.

Instruction 6: The final instruction encourages patients to maintain more regular sleep patterns by not napping during the day. In addition, the lack of daytime naps after a poor night's sleep when following SCT allows the homeostatic drive for sleep to build throughout the day, making it more likely that the patient will successfully fall asleep faster the next night. This strengthens the cues of the bed and bedroom with falling asleep and provides a success experience for the patient to help maintain compliance with the instruction.

It should be emphasized that we are not opposed to all naps. Instruction six is intended to increase the likelihood that SCT will successfully change a dysfunctional sleep pattern. With some individuals, such as the elderly, however, it may be wise to have a brief nap (30 min or less) scheduled at the same time every day. It is the irregularity of napping that produces and maintains irregular sleep schedules.

EFFECTIVENESS OF STIMULUS CONTROL THERAPY

There have been numerous reviews and meta-analyses of the effectiveness of cognitive behavioral treatments for insomnia. In 1999, a review (8) and practice guidelines (9) identified SCT as the only psychological and behavioral treatment to meet the highest standard for recommendation. In 2006, the American Academy of Sleep Medicine (AASM) published an update of both the review of the literature (10) and evidence-based practice parameters for psychological and behavioral treatment of insomnia (11). While most of the newly added studies included in the review investigated multicomponent cognitive behavioral treatments for treating insomnia, the AASM recommendations maintained that SCT is an "effective and recommended therapy in the treatment of chronic insomnia" (11, p.1417) and endorsed some additional single-treatments as well.

MULTICOMPONENT TREATMENTS CONTAINING STIMULUS CONTROL THERAPY

A commonly employed multicomponent package combines stimulus control instructions, sleep restriction, sleep education, and cognitive therapy. This combination of interventions lends itself well to clinical settings in which adults of all ages are seen. Case series studies have found this combination to be as effective in clinical settings as in controlled outcome studies (12–15). Despite differences in which specific variables improve, as well as the degree of improvement, all case series studies have reported significant improvement in primary sleep variables.

For example, Morin, and colleagues (13) reported that improvement ranged from 42% to 50% on the main target symptoms of sleep onset latency, wake after sleep onset, and early morning awakening. There was a statistically significant, but modest 8%, gain on total sleep time (from 325 minutes at baseline to 350 minutes after therapy). In contrast to the small improvement in total sleep time found by Morin and colleagues (13) Perlis, and colleagues (15) found a 29% improvement in total sleep time along with a 56% reduction in wake after sleep onset and a 34% reduction in sleep onset latency.

Other studies have focused on the comparison of cognitive behavioral treatment for insomnia (CBTi) with pharmacotherapy and for patients who have poor sleep despite using medication. One study compared a CBTi intervention (including stimulus control instructions) to zopiclone and placebo for the treatment of insomnia in older adults (16). Participants who received CBTi improved on measures of sleep efficiency, amount of slow wave sleep, and time spent awake during the night at both posttreatment and six-month follow-up assessments. Participants in the drug and placebo groups did not show similar improvements. Another study evaluated the effectiveness of CBTi for continuing insomnia in older adults who were dependent on sedative-hypnotic medications (17). Participants were assigned to either a CBT group, which included stimulus control instructions, or a placebo group. The group that received CBTi showed clinically significant and subjective improvement on measures of sleep quality, whereas the placebo group did not.

In multicomponent treatment studies, it is difficult to identify which components are most effective. Harvey, Inglis, & Espie (18) surveyed 90 participants at the one year follow-up to determine which of 10 components of their cognitive-behavioral insomnia treatment were associated with changes in sleep measures. The combination of stimulus control and sleep restriction was the best predictor of improved sleep latency and total sleep time, and cognitive restructuring, a form of cognitive therapy, significantly predicted a reduction in wakefulness. Relaxation, although most commonly endorsed by patients, did not predict improvement on any variable. Likewise, sleep hygiene was unrelated to changes in sleep.

It should be stressed that it is important to include components in multicomponent treatments that have been evaluated and found effective as single interventions. All of the multicomponent treatments discussed here used SCT as a core element. From a theoretical perspective it is easy to see how different components might cover a broader range of problems, but it is desirable to empirically test that proposition by comparing a single component, such as SCT, against a multiple component intervention.

NEW TREATMENT DIRECTIONS INVOLVING STIMULUS CONTROL THERAPY

New directions in insomnia treatment include ways of delivering treatment so that more patients can be helped more quickly, bringing treatments into the bedroom, developing new treatments that can accelerate improved sleep, and integrating mindfulness meditation with SCT and other cognitive-behavioral treatments.

Reaching More Patients

Among the methods that have been evaluated are the use of group treatments (19,20), the internet (21), the telephone (22), mass media including television (23), and self-help tapes and books (24,25). Multicomponent treatments are almost always used and the specific treatment components vary from study to study.

Although improvement on sleep measures has been demonstrated, there appears to be a trade-off between the number of insomniacs who might be reached and the magnitude of treatment effects (26). For example, individual and group treatments tend to produce larger effects than mass media treatments. An additional problem when self-help methods such as tapes, books, and television are employed is that there is no professional assessment of the sleep problems. Consequently, comorbid disorders may go untreated resulting in potentially less effective treatment for the sleep problem as well. It may be more effective to include self-help materials within the context of professional care so that a thorough assessment can be completed.

Because insomnia has been associated with increased future risk for physical and psychiatric disorders, there has been increased interest in extending insomnia treatment to primary care facilities where professional assessment can be provided (e.g., 27). Baillargon, Demers, and Ladouceur (28) reported that stimulus control instructions could be used effectively by family physicians. Eighty percent of the patients who completed the treatment for insomnia reduced their sleep onset latency and six of seven who had been on hypnotics reduced or stopped taking hypnotics.

In a thorough study incorporating treatment of insomnia as part of a local health service in Scotland, visiting nurses were trained to provide a multicomponent CBTi for insomnia (29). One hundred and thirty-nine insomniacs participated in a clinical trial that compared multicomponent CBTi with a self-monitoring control condition. CBTi produced significantly reduced sleep latency and wakefulness during the night. These improvements were maintained at a one-year follow-up. Total sleep increased significantly during follow-up and 84% of patients initially using hypnotics remained medication-free.

An example of an attempt to develop abbreviated treatment using self-help materials and professional assessment was reported by Edinger and Sampson (30). They designed two 25-minute sessions combined with take-home pamphlets and audiotapes that reinforced the information provided during the sessions. The abbreviated CBTi intervention produced 50% improvement in WASO in 52% of the patients and produced substantial improvement on more than half of the patients on an insomnia symptom questionnaire.

Following Edinger and Sampson, there have been a number of investigations that have reported improved sleep as a result of abbreviated multicomponent treatment, in which SCT was one of the core components, with different populations of individuals with sleep disturbances. They include an evaluation of a two session and two telephone follow-up multicomponent behavioral treatment (combining SCT with sleep restriction, another behavioral intervention for insomnia) in older adults with insomnia who have psychiatric and medical comorbidities of aging (31,32), a three session multicomponent insomnia treatment in a family medicine clinical setting (33), a brief (two individual sessions and two telephone follow-ups) multicomponent intervention for older adults provided by rural care providers who were trained in a two-day workshop (34), and a brief multicomponent intervention of family caregivers of cancer patients (35).

The abbreviated treatments produced improved sleep comparable to that found in longer studies. An advantage of these abbreviated treatments is that they all involve individual contact between the clinician and the patient that allows for the tailoring of treatment to the individual problems of the patients. Many of these brief CBTi interventions are discussed in greater detail elsewhere in this section

Bringing Treatment into the Bedroom

Cognitive-behavioral treatments for insomnia are fundamentally self-help treatments. Clinicians provide a thorough assessment of the nature of the sleep problems and prescribe changes in activities and life-style at home. Although both subjective and objective measures of sleep can be obtained, there is not usually any means of providing an objective measure of whether the patients are adhering to the treatment recommendations.

As an example, consider the stimulus control instruction to get out-of-bed quickly if the individual with insomnia has not yet fallen asleep. Many individuals with insomnia are not good judges of whether or not they have been asleep. Would they be helped by a monitor on the bed-table that would provide a signal about when to get out-of-bed? Due to advances in the technologies of sleep-wake detection, there are a number of alternatives available to provide feedback to patients in the bedroom including using auditory signals to which the sleeper responds if awake, actigraphy, or single-channel electroencephalographic-based sleep-wake detection. The sleep-wake detection monitor can be combined with algorithms to provide feedback about when to get out-of-bed when following stimulus control or other cognitive-behavioral instructions. Although there are preliminary data to indicate that systems like this can be helpful in the treatment of insomnia (e.g., 36), randomized control treatment outcome studies have yet to be published.

Accelerating Improvement

In the previous section, we discussed how technology might be used to accelerate improvement. In this section, we describe an entirely new approach to help the individual with insomnia to relearn to fall asleep quickly. In Intensive Sleep Retraining, individuals with insomnia were invited into the sleep laboratory during which participants received 40 hours of sleep deprivation and were given 50 opportunities, one each half hour, to fall asleep for no more than four minutes (37). These sleep opportunities began two hours before the participants usual bedtimes and continued for 25 hours. The idea being evaluated was whether those who had difficulty falling asleep quickly could learn to do so when given 50 trials at falling asleep when sleep deprived.

On average, across the 50 trials, the participants were able to fall asleep quickly and fell asleep in 6.9 minutes as measured by polysomnography. Posttreatment assessment indicated substantial improvements in sleep onset latency, wake after sleep onset, and total sleep time, as well as on broader measures of fatigue and vigor, cognitive anticipatory anxiety, and self-efficacy for sleep. These improvements were maintained at the six week follow-up assessment.

In a subsequent clinical trial, 68 insomnia participants were randomly assigned to four treatment conditions: (1) Sleep hygiene control, (2) Intensive Sleep Retraining, (3) Four-week SCT, and (4) Combined Intensive Sleep Retraining and SCT (38). Preliminary analyses indicate that the three active treatment conditions were all more effective than the sleep hygiene control. ISR produced improvement faster than SCT but both reached the same degree of improvement. The combined treatment provided both faster initial treatment gains plus additional improvement that led to trends for the best overall outcomes.

Integrating Mindfulness Meditation with Stimulus Control Therapy

Mindfulness meditation has been a recently added component in multicomponent treatments for insomnia. Mindfulness is defined as the awareness that arises out of intentionally attending in an open, accepting and discerning way (39), and involves formal meditation practices to cultivate this awareness, as well as principles for applying this awareness to one's moment to moment experience.

In the first systematic study for insomnia in adolescents, we developed a manualized, small-group treatment to improve sleep, daytime sleepiness, and emotional distress (40) in teens with a substance-abuse treatment history. In this population, and more generally in clinical practice with adults, we have found mindfulness-based principles and practices to be effective for reducing mind-racing and other arousal associated symptoms of insomnia. Our multicomponent treatment consisted of six 90 minute weekly small group sessions, with the first session dedicated to sleep education and sessions two to six split each session into cognitive-behavioral sleep intervention and a modified Mindfulness-Based Stress Reduction (MBSR) program.

The cognitive-behavioral sleep treatment consisted of SCT, special emphasis on regularizing sleep–wake schedules across both school and weekend days, the use of bright light therapy to advance circadian sleep-wake schedules, and cognitive therapy. The MBSR treatment consisted of instruction in meditation practices and application of mindfulness into one's daily life. The teens who completed at least four of the six treatment sessions were considered completers and showed pre to posttreatment improvement ($p < 0.05$) in daily sleep diary variables including sleep onset latency, number of awakenings, wake after sleep onset, total sleep time, sleep efficiency, and ratings of sleep quality (40) as well as in emotional regulation, e.g., reductions in aggressive ideation and actions (41).

Although reductions in substance use were not a primary target of this treatment development study, improvement in substance use through the three month follow-up was seen in female completers, but not in female noncompleters, or male completers or noncompleters. In our study, the multicomponent sleep treatment was instituted after the outpatient substance abuse treatment was completed. This was done to separate the effects of the sleep treatment from those of the substance abuse treatment. It is possible, however, that combining the two treatments would enhance the effectiveness of the substance abuse treatment since the additional cognitive and emotional resources available to the teens as a result of improved sleep are likely to enhance resources available for comorbid problems, including substance abuse. In this regard, recent research has found that CBTi produces improvement in comorbid depression even in the absence of direct treatment for depression (42). The same emotional benefit that occurs from CBTi for depression may also occur for those with substance abuse problems.

Another multicomponent development study that integrated mindfulness principles and practices with SCT with cognitive-behavioral treatment components has shown similarly encouraging results for adults with insomnia (43). Twenty-seven adults with insomnia completed a multicomponent group treatment that consisted of SCT, sleep restriction, sleep education, sleep hygiene, and MBSR in an integrative framework. The treatment was delivered in 6 weekly sessions lasting 90 to 120 minutes.

There were statistically significant changes in both sleep measures (total wake time, sleep onset latency, wake after sleep onset, number of awakenings, sleep efficiency, and ratings of sleep quality) and measures of arousal (cognitive and somatic presleep arousal and the Hyperarousal Scale). Overall clinical significance was demonstrated using intent-to-treat analyses of the 30 participants who attended the first session. At posttreatment, 87% of the sample would no longer meet the inclusion criteria and 15 of the 30 participants showed a 50% or greater reduction in the primary sleep outcome measure of total wake time.

In the study of substance-abusing adolescents, frequency of mindfulness meditation practice, but not duration of practice, was significantly related to improvement in total sleep time and to improvement in self-efficacy about sleep problems (44). Similarly, in the adults with insomnia study, frequency of meditation practice, but not duration, was significantly related to reductions in the Hyperarousal Scale (43). Both studies suggest that emphasis should be placed more on the frequency than the duration of mindfulness meditation practice. Further, both studies indicate that mindfulness meditation may make a contribution to improvement of sleep problems and reduction in arousal in multicomponent treatment studies for insomnia.

CONCLUSION

Stimulus control therapy for insomnia is a behavioral treatment that has been consistently documented to be effective in the treatment of insomnia, whether delivered as a single-component treatment or part of a multicomponent behavioral or cognitive-behavioral intervention. Although the six instructions of SCT are relatively straightforward, individuals fare better when a rationale is provided.

Recent studies have focused on multicomponent treatments and new components such as the use of bright light to change circadian rhythms and the use of mindfulness meditation to reduce symptoms of arousal are strong additions. Recent studies have also suggested that even brief interventions that include SCT improve insomnia, which may be important for treating the vast numbers of people with insomnia symptoms. Some method for helping patients find the appropriate level of care will need to be considered.

The development of entirely new treatments based on SCT such as Intensive Sleep Retraining and using technology to bring treatment into the bedroom is exciting. We can be justifiably proud of how much progress has been made in developing and evaluating cognitive and behavioral treatments for insomnia. Nevertheless, many challenges in prevention, public policy, as well as treatment, remain. Effective treatments and new directions are very welcome.

REFERENCES

1. Bootzin RR, Nicassio P. Behavioral treatments for insomnia. In: Hersen M, Eisler R, Miller P, eds. Progress in Behavior Modification, Vol. 6. New York, NY: Academic Press, 1978:1–45.
2. Bootzin RR, Epstein DR. Stimulus control instructions. In: Lichstein KL, Morin CM, eds. Treatment of Late-Life Insomnia. Thousand Oaks, CA: Sage 2000:167–187
3. Bootzin RR. Stimulus control treatment for insomnia. Proceedings of the 80th Annual Convention of the American Psychological Association 1972; 7:395–396.
4. Bootzin R. Effects of self-control procedures for insomnia. In: Stuart R, ed. Behavioral Self-Management: Strategies and Outcomes. New York, NY: Brunner/Mazel, 1977.
5. Malaffo M, Espie CA. Insomnia: The quarter of an hour rule (QHR), a single component of stimulus control, improves sleep. Sleep 2006; 29:A257.
6. Zeitzer JM, Dijk DJ, Kronauer RE, et al. Sensitivity of the human circadian pacemaker to nocturnal light: Melatonin phase resetting and suppression. J. Physiol 2000; 526(Pt.3): 695–702.
7. Manber R, Bootzin RR, Acebo C, et al. The effects of regularizing sleep-wake schedules on daytime sleepiness. Sleep 1996; 19:432–441.
8. Morin CM, Hauri PJ, Espie CA, et al. Nonpharmacologic treatment of chronic insomnia: An American Academy of Sleep Medicine Review. Sleep 1999; 22:1134–1156.
9. Chesson AL, McDowell WA, Littner M, et al. Practice parameters for the nonpharmacologic treatment of chronic insomnia. Standards of Practice Committee of the American Academy of Sleep Medicine. Sleep 1999; 22(8):1128–1133.

10. Morin CM, Bootzin RR, Buysse DJ, et al. Psychological and behavioral treatment of insomnia: Update of the recent evidence (1998–2004). Sleep 2006; 29(11):1398–1414.
11. Morgenthaler T, Kramer M, Alessi C, et al. Practice parameters for the psychological and behavioral treatment of insomnia: An update. An american academy of sleep medicine report. Sleep 2006; 29(11):1415–1419.
12. Chambers MJ, Alexander SD. Assessment and prediction of outcome for a brief behavioral insomnia treatment program. J Behav Ther Exp Psychiatry 1992; 23:289–297.
13. Morin CM, Stone J, McDonald K, et al. Psychological management of insomnia: A clinical replication series with 100 patients. Behavior Therapy 1994; 25:291–309.
14. Perlis M, Aloia M, Millikan A, et al. Behavioral treatment of insomnia: A clinical case series study. J Behav Med 2000; 23:149–161.
15. Perlis ML, Sharpe M, Smith MT, et al. Behavioral treatment of insomnia: Treatment outcome and the relevance of medical and psychiatric morbidity. J Behav Med 2001; 24:281–296.
16. Sivertsen B, Omvik S, Pallesen S, et al. Cognitive behavioral therapy vs zopiclone for treatment of chronic primary insomnia in older adults: A randomized controlled trial. JAMA 2006; 295(24):2851–2858.
17. Soeffing JP, Lichstein KL, Nau SD, et al. Psychological treatment of insomnia in hypnotic-dependant older adults. Sleep Med 2008; 9(2):165–171.
18. Harvey L, Inglis SJ, Espie CA. Insomniacs' reported use of CBT components and relationship to long-term clinical outcome. Behav Res Ther 2002; 39:45–60.
19. Backhaus J, Hohagen F, Voderholzer U, et al. Long-term effectiveness of a short-term cognitive-behavioral group treatment for primary insomnia. Eur Arch Psychiatry Clin Neurosci 2001; 251(1): 35–41.
20. Epstein DR. A Behavioral Intervention to Enhance the Sleep-Wake Patterns of Older Adults with Insomnia. Unpublished dissertation. Tucson, AZ: University of Arizona, 1994.
21. Ström L, Pettersson R, Andersson G. Internet-based treatment for insomnia: A controlled evaluation. J Consult Clin Psychol 2004; 72:113–120.
22. Verbeek I, Declerck G, Neven AK, et al. Sleep information by telephone: Callers indicate positive effects on sleep problems. Sleep and Hypnosis 2002; 4:47–51.
23. Oosterhuis A, Klip EC. The treatment of insomnia through mass media: The results of a televised behavioural training programme. Soc Sci Med 1997; 8:1223–1229.
24. Mimeault V, Morin CM. Self-help treatment of insomnia: Bibliotherapy with and without professional guidance. J Consult Clin Psychol 1999; 67:511–519.
25. Morawetz D. Behavioral self-help treatment for insomnia: A controlled evaluation. Behavior Therapy 1989; 20:365–379.
26. Bootzin RR. Is brief behavioral treatment for insomnia effective? Invited editorial commentary on Germain A, Moul DE, Franzen PL, et al. Effects of a brief behavioral ent for late-life insomnia: Preliminary findings. J Clin Sleep Med 2006; 2:403–406.
27. Smith MT, Neubauer DN. Cognitive behavior therapy for chronic insomnia. Clinical Cornerstone 2003; 5:28–40.
28. Baillargeon L, Demers M, Ladouceur R. Stimulus-control: Nonpharmacologic treatment for insomnia. Can Fam Physician 1998; 44:73–79.
29. Espie CA, Inglis SJ, Tessier S, et al. The clinical effectivenss of cognitive behaviour therapy for chronic insomnia: Implementaion and evaluation of a sleep clinic in general medical practice. Behav Res Ther 2001; 39:45–60.
30. Edinger JD, Sampson WS. A primary care "friendly" cognitive behavioral insomnia therapy. Sleep 2003; 26:177–182.
31. Germain A, Moul DE, Franzen PL, et al. Effects of a brief behavioral treatment for late-life insomnia: Preliminary findings. J Clin Sleep Med 2006; 2(4):407–408.
32. Buysse DJ, Germain A, Moul DE, et al. Efficacy of brief behavioral treatment for insomnia (BBTI) in older adults with insomnia. Sleep 2009; 32:A282.
33. Goodie JL, Isler WC, Hunter C, et al. Using behavioral health consultants to treat insomnia in primary care: A clinical case series. J Clin Psychol 2009; 65(3):294–304.
34. McCrae CS, McGovern R, Lukefahr R, et al. Research Evaluating Brief Behavioral Sleep Treatments for Rural Elderly (RESTORE): A preliminary examination of effectiveness. Am J Geriatr Psychiatry 2007; 15(11):979–982.
35. Carter PA. A brief behavioral sleep intervention for family caregivers of persons with cancer. Cancer Nurs 2006; 29(2):95–103.
36. Kaplan R, Wang Y, Loparo K, et al. Evaluation of an automated system for in-home behavioral treatment of chronic insomnia: Part III. Sleep 2007; 30:A346.

37. Harris J, Lack L, Wright H, et al. Intensive Sleep Retraining treatment for chronic primary insomnia: A preliminary investigation. J Sleep Res 2007; 16(3):276–284.
38. Harris J, Lack L, Bootzin R. Randomized controlled trial of an accelerated insomnia therapy. Sleep 2007; 30:A261.
39. Shapiro SL, Carlson LE. The Art and Science of Mindfulness. Washington, DC: American Psychology Association Books 2009.
40. Bootzin RR, Stevens SJ. Adolescents, substance abuse, and the treatment of insomnia and daytime sleepiness. Clin Psychol Rev 2005; 25(5):629–644.
41. Haynes PL, Bootzin RR, Smith L, et al. Sleep and aggression in substance abusing adolescents: Results from an integrative, behavioral sleep treatment pilot program. Sleep 2006; 29:512–520.
42. Manber R, Edinger JD, Gress JL, et al. Cognitive behavioral therapy for insomnia enhances depression outcome in patients with comorbid major depressive disorder and insomnia. Sleep 2008; 31:489.
43. Ong JC, Shapiro SL, Manber R. Combining mindfulness meditation with cognitive-behavior therapy for insomnia: A treatment-development study. Behavior Therapy 2008; 29:171–182.
44. Britton WB, Bootzin RR, Cousins JC, et al. The contribution of mindfulness practice to a multi-component behavioral sleep intervention following substance abuse treatment in adolescents: A pilot study. Substance abuse. In press.

25 Insomnia: Sleep Restriction Therapy

Arthur J. Spielman

Cognitive Neurosciences Doctoral Program, Department of Psychology, The City College of New York, City University of New York, New York; Center for Sleep Medicine, Department of Neurology, New York Presbyterian Hospital, Weill Cornell Medical College, New York; and Center for Sleep Disorders Medicine and Research, Department of Pulmonary Medicine, New York Methodist Hospital, Brooklyn, New York, U.S.A.

Chien-Ming Yang

Department of Psychology, The Research Center for Mind, Brain & Learning, National Cheng-Chi University, Taipei, Taiwan

Paul B. Glovinsky

Cognitive Neurosciences Doctoral Program, Department of Psychology, The City College of New York, City University of New York, New York, and Department of Medicine, Section of Psychology, St. Peter's Hospital, St. Peter's Sleep Center, Albany, New York, U.S.A.

THE DEVELOPMENT OF SLEEP RESTRICTION THERAPY

The practical and theoretical roots underlying the development of sleep restriction therapy (SRT) in 1987 (1) are readily traced: foremost, two decades of research into the physiological and cognitive consequences of sleep deprivation under various paradigms had led to solid findings regarding the effects of deprivation or restriction on sleep itself. These findings suggested that disturbed sleep might in some instances benefit from restricted bedtime. Second, psychological theories of the genesis and persistence of emotional distress provided a framework for understanding how attitudes and anxieties about sleep might harden into chronic insomnia. This work suggested that an intervention able to break the vicious cycle of anticipatory anxiety leading to sleeplessness leading to increased anticipatory anxiety could be of great benefit even if it could only be tolerated in the short term. Third, the new field of chronobiology was burgeoning, and its findings beginning to find clinical application. There was much greater appreciation of how the timing of bedtime affects the ability to fall and stay asleep. Finally, while pharmacologic treatment for insomnia with benzodiazepines and other medications was gaining wide acceptance, pitfalls and inadequacies associated with such treatment were becoming apparent, fueling the search for effective behavioral interventions.

In the early 1970s, two behavioral approaches specifically formulated for the management of insomnia took their place alongside progressive muscle relaxation (2), hypnosis and other therapies that had long been employed to alleviate various anxiety disorders. At a time when learning theory was ascendant, stimulus control instructions (3) introduced proscriptions and prescriptions designed to foster the association of bedroom cues with rapid sleep onset. Sleep hygiene (4) shared a focus on concrete behaviors, attempting to shape common-sense practices that strengthen mechanisms regulating sleep. SRT was clearly influenced by the direct, prescriptive and behavior-focused nature of these two pioneering therapies.

With regard to basic research, many studies had explored the effects of sleep deprivation and partial sleep deprivation (also known as sleep restriction). These studies followed a long tradition in the biological sciences, one that sought to better understand a particular function by removing or restricting access to it. The consequences of depriving organisms of sleep were analogous to depriving them of the objects of other "drive behaviors" such as food and water. Just as increased hunger and thirst led to greater efforts to find food and water, increased sleepiness led to greater efforts to find a safe place in which to sleep. Sleep regulation was therefore conceptualized as under homeostatic control. In this view, under conditions of deprivation a negative feedback system is activated that produces an increase in appetitive features. Consummatory behaviors such as eating, drinking, and sleeping restore the homeostatic balance.

The SRT instruction to spend less time in bed (TIB) effectively reduces total sleep time. This partial sleep deprivation in turn activates a homeostatic response (5). The composition of sleep stages across the night known as "sleep architecture" is changed; sleep becomes deeper as it becomes more compact (6,7). Light NREM stage 1 sleep and wakefulness are reduced under the pressure of sleep restriction. The amount of deep NREM slow wave sleep (currently designated stage N3) remains the same but increases as a proportion of total sleep time. REM sleep changes are more inconsistent. Some studies show a decrease in REM % of total sleep time and REM minutes while other studies show REM% remains the same. The heightened homeostatic response triggered by reducing sleep time also leads to shorter sleep latencies. All of these changes recommended sleep restriction as a means of addressing both sleep-onset and sleep-maintenance insomnia.

The near immediacy of SRT's initial effects provides another boon to treatment: it interrupts the circular, self-fulfilling prophecies concerning the prospects for sleep that ultimately maintain chronic insomnia. At the time SRT was developed theorists were beginning to understand how psychological dynamics could account for both the appearance of distress and its perpetuation. Within the realm of sleep, for example, individuals who tend to internalize psychological problems were seen to have heightened emotional arousal, which in turn produces trouble sleeping (8). The poor sleep provides a new focus for concern, increasing emotional distress and further exacerbating the sleep disturbance. This circularity of cause and effect, called cyclical psychodynamics, represented a major theoretical integration of behavior therapy and psychodynamics and captured the imagination of clinicians (9). Responding to this insight, SRT attempted to short-circuit the apprehensive worry about poor sleep that served to maintain that very condition.

By the late 1970s human circadian rhythm organization was under intense investigation. The importance of a habitual wake-up time and morning exposure to temporal cues for purposes of entrainment were widely appreciated. In an early clinical application of chronobiology, individuals with severe difficulty falling asleep reported much shorter sleep latencies when they went to bed later than usual on weekends (10). Going to bed later and setting a fixed wake-up time, staples of SRT, are in line with this chronobiological understanding that sleep onset is typically more rapid later at night, and that providing regular temporal cues helps stabilize the sleep–wake cycle.

The improved safety and effectiveness of the benzodiazepines over earlier hypnotic medications encouraged more individuals to seek treatment for chronic sleep disturbance. While helpful in reducing sleep latency and promoting sustained sleep, these agents were not without significant limitations especially when used chronically and upon discontinuation (11). Chronic use of hypnotics with long elimination half-lives was prone to produce daytime hangover while agents with short half-life were associated with morning anxiety or early morning awakening. Memory problems and moodiness were reported as well. Finally, the development of drug tolerance and dependence were of concern.

Thus by the early 1980s, the time was ripe for new approaches to insomnia treatment. Behavioral therapies for a wide range of psychological problems were showing much promise. A deepening understanding of the circadian organization of life was starting to shape clinical interventions. There was much room for improvement in the pharmacological management of insomnia. Finally, the nascent specialty of behavioral sleep medicine, fostered in newly established sleep disorders centers as well as academic departments, was for the first time conceiving of insomnia as not merely the symptom of various underlying problems, but as a worthy target for systematic treatment trials. SRT drew upon all of these developments.

In the years since its introduction, SRT has been deployed as a stand alone treatment in a number of studies (Table 1), often in a form slightly modified from its original description. It was quickly incorporated into the multicomponent treatment known as cognitive behavior therapy for insomnia (CBT-I; Table 2). The effectiveness of CBT-I for a wide range of insomnias has been consistently demonstrated; it is now considered the frontline treatment for insomnia (12). The 2006 American Academy of Sleep Medicine's Practice Parameters for the treatment of insomnia rates SRT as a Guideline (13). The Practice Parameters deemed CBT-I a Standard, describing its behavioral components as follows:

3.6 Cognitive behavior therapy, with or without relaxation therapy is effective and recommended therapy in the treatment of chronic insomnia. [4.2, 4.6] (Standard) ... The behavioral

Table 1 Studies of SRT and modified SRT: Summary of methods and results

Author(s)	Treatment condition	N	Mean Age	Treatment Format	No. of Sessions	Measures	Med.	F/U	Results
Spielman et al. (1,14)	SRT (no control condition)	35	46	Individual	8 weekly sessions	Call-ins Sleep log ISQ	Hypnotics: 12 Antidep: 1 Anxiolytic:1 Alcohol: 2 No med: 19	36 wks	Both post-treatment & F/U: TST↑, SOL↓, TWT↓, SE↑, ISQ↓
Morin et al. (15)	SRT	1 case (depressed patient with chronic pain)	49	Inpatient individual	12 days inpatient	Sleep log	No med.	4 mons	Post-treatment: TST from 2.5 h to 6:23 h F/U: 7 h
Friedman et al. (16)	1: Modified SRT 2: Relaxation therapy (RT)	SRT:10 RT:12	69.7	Individual	4 weekly sessions	Call-ins	BZD: 4 No med: 18	3 mons	SRT: Post-treatment: TST↑, SOL↓, WASO↓, SE↑; F/U: maintain treatment effects except for SOL RT: TST↑ & SOL↓, but no effect in the other variables
Brooks et al. (17)	Nap mod. SRT (no control condition)	9	67.7	Individual	4 weekly sessions	Actigraph Sleep log	No med	N/A	Actigraph: TST↑, SOL = , WASO↓, SE↑ Sleep log: TST = , SOL↓, WASO↓, SE↑
Riedel et al. (18)	1: Self-help Video (Modified SRT-sleep compression + Sleep Education) 2: VIDEO + therapist guidance 3:Waiting- list control	25 subjects for each groups	67.4	1:Self-help Video 2:Video + Individual	1:2 Video viewing sessions 2:4 weekly sessions	Sleep log Rating scale SSS	No med	2 mons	1: TST↑, SOL = , WASO↓, SE↑, sleep satisfaction↑, SSS↓; all effects maintained at F/U 2: TST = , SOL↓, WASO↓, SE↑, sleep satisfaction↑, SSS↓; all effects maintained and TST↑ at F/U 3: TST = , SOL↓, WASO↓, SE↑, SSS↓
Bliwise et al. (19)	1: Modified SRT 2: Relaxation Therapy (RT)	16 subjects for both groups	68.7	Individual	4 weekly sessions + a wrap-up session	Call-ins	N/A	3 mons	1: Post-treatment: TST = , SOL↓; F/U: TST↑ 2: Similar to SRT, but TST improved less at F/U
Friedman et al. (20)	1: Modified SRT + sleep hygiene 2: Nap mod. SRT + sleep hygiene 3:Sleep hygiene	1:12 2:12 3:13	64.2	Individual	4 weekly session + a wrap-up session	Actigraph Sleep log	No med.	3 mons	Actigraph: Post-treatment: no sig. effects, TST↓; F/U: TST = Sleep log: Post-treatment: SE↑ for both SRT conditions; F/U: SE↑ for all conditions

(Continued)

Table 1 Studies of SRT and modified SRT: Summary of methods and results (*Continued*)

Author(s)	Treatment condition	N	Mean Age	Treatment Format	No. of Sessions	Measures	Med.	F/U	Results
Riedel & Lichstein (21)	Modified SRT	22	67.96	Individual	6 weekly sessions	Sleep log ESS	No med.	N/A	TST = , SOL↓, No. awakening↓, WASO↓, SE↑, ESS =
Lichstein et al. (22)	1:SRT (sleep compression) 2:Relaxation (RT) 3:Placebo desensitization (PL)	1: 24 2: 27 3: 23	68.03	Individual	6 weekly sessions	Sleep log	No med.	1 year	SOL: decreased for all conditions, maintained for SRT only No. of awakenings: decreased for both treatment groups, maintained for SRT only WASO: decreased for all groups both post-treatment and at F/U TST: interact w/ fatigue level High fatigue: increased at post-treatment and F/U for RT, at F/U for PL; no diff for SRT Low fatigue: increased at post-treatment for RT, at F/U for SRT; no diff for PL SE: interact w/ fatigue level High fatigue: increased at post-treatment and F/U for RT & SRT; increased at F/U for PL Low fatigue: increased at F/U for SRT; increased at post-treatment for PL; no diff for RT

Abbreviations: TST, total sleep time; TWT, total waking time; SOL, sleep onset latency; WASO, wake after sleep onset; No. Awakening, Number of awakenings; SE, sleep efficiency; ISQ, Insomnia Symptom Questionnaire; SSS, Stanford Sleepiness Scale; ESS, Epworth Sleepiness Scale; post-tx, post treatment; F/U, follow-up.

Friedman et al. (16): The SRT was modified. Subject tolerance was weighed heavily in the assignment of the allowed TIB at start of treatment. TIB was not reduced for failure to reach criterion.

Friedman et al. (20): Modified SRT-Subject tolerance was weighed heavily in the assignment of the allowed TIB at start of treatment. TIB was not reduced for failure to reach criterion. Patients were given weekly increments of TIB according to a fixed algorithm based on their initial TST. TIB is only increased by getting into bed earlier at the beginning of the sleep period. The algorithm for determining increased TIB was based on patients' reported sleepiness and their initial TIB. All patients received seven-hours TIB by the end of the 4th treatment week.

Nap modification SRT-Optional daytime naps were included. Patients were encouraged to take a 30-min nap daily within a 1:00 to 3:00 PM window.

Brooks et al. (17) : Mandatory daytime naps were included in the protocol because some subjects object to SRT due to daytime sleepiness.

Riedel et al. (18): Sleep compression allows patients to gradually reduce TIB to more closely match TST, and the prescribed TIB is not increased in response to higher SE. During the first session, patients were advised to reduce TIB by one-half of the difference between baseline TIB and baseline TST. During session 2 and 3, TIB was further reduced by one-fourth of the difference between baseline TIB and baseline TST.

Bliwise et al. (19): TIB was extended when the floating mean SE over the preceding five days equaled or exceeded 85%. Flexibility in the procedure was employed in the assignment of initial TIB.

Riedel & Lichstein (21): During the first session, patients were recommended to reduce TIB by one-fifth of the difference between baseline TIB and TST. Over the next four sessions, gradual reductions of TIB were recommended to approach baseline TST.

Table 2 Studies of Insomnia Utilizing Sleep Restriction Therapy as Part of Cognitive Behavior Therapy (a partial list)

Authors	Techniques	Patient
Morin et al. (23)	CBT (Cognitive Therapy, *Sleep Restriction,* Stimulus Control)	Late-life insomnia
Morin et al. (24)	CBT (Cognitive Therapy, *Sleep Restriction,* Sleep Hygiene, Stimulus Control)	Primary late life insomnia
Mimeault & Morin (25)	CBT (Cognitive Therapy, *Sleep Restriction,* Stimulus Control)	Primary insomnia
Verbeek et al. (26)	CBT (Cognitive Therapy, *Sleep Restriction,* Sleep Hygiene, Relaxation Therapy, Stimulus Control)	Chronic insomnia
Currie et al. (27)	CBT (Cognitive Therapy, *Sleep Restriction,* Relaxation, Stimulus Control,)	Secondary insomnia
Perlis et al. (28)	CBT (Cognitive Restructuring, *Sleep Restriction,* Sleep Hygiene, Relapse Prevention, Stimulus Control)	Primary insomnia
Espie et al. (29)	CBT (Cognitive Restructuring, *Sleep Restriction,* Sleep Information, Sleep Hygiene, Relaxation, Stimulus Control)	Chronic insomnia
Perlis et al. (30)	CBT (Cognitive Restructuring, *Sleep Restriction,* Sleep Hygiene, Relapse Prevention Stimulus Control)	Primary and secondary insomnia
Edinger et al.. (31)	CBT (Cognitive Therapy, *Sleep Restriction,* Sleep Education, Relaxation, Stimulus Control)	Chronic primary insomnia
Harvey et al. (32)	CBT (Cognitive Restructuring, *Sleep Restriction,* Relaxation, Sleep Hygiene, Stimulus Control,)	Nonspecified insomnia
Currie SR, et al. (33)	CBT (Cognitive Restructuring, *Sleep Restriction,* Relaxation, Sleep Hygiene, Stimulus Control,)	Comorbid Insomnia and pain
Rybarczyk et al. (34)	CBT (Cognitive Therapy, *Sleep Restriction,* Relaxation, Stimulus Control,)	Secondary insomnia (geriatric)
Edinger & Sampson (35)	CBT (Cognitive Therapy, *Sleep Restriction,* Seep Hygiene, Stimulus Control)	Primary insomnia
Ouellet & Morin (36)	CBT (Cognitive Therapy, *Sleep Restriction,* Sleep Hygiene, Stimulus Control)	Insomnia associated (TBI)
Morin et al. (37)	CBT (Cognitive Therapy, *Sleep Restriction,* Stimulus Control)	Benzodiazepine withdrawal, older insomnia
Morgan et al. (38)	CBT (Cognitive Treatments, *Sleep Restriction,* Sleep Hygiene, Relaxation, Stimulus Control)	Chronic insomnia, long-term hypnotic drug users
Currie et al. (39)	CBT (Cognitive Therapy, *Sleep Restriction,* Sleep Hygiene, Stimulus Control)	
Perlis et al. (40)	CBT (Cognitive Restructuring, *Sleep Restriction,* Sleep Hygiene, Relapse Prevention, Stimulus Control)	Primary insomnia
Jacobs et al. (41)	CBT (Cognitive Therapy, *Sleep Restriction,* Relaxation, Stimulus Control)	Primary Insomnia
Dopke et al. (42)	CBT (Cognitive Therapy, *Sleep Restriction,* Sleep Hygiene, Relaxation, Stimulus Control)	Insomnia associated with psychiatric disorders
Stiefel& Stagno (43)	CBT (Cognitive Therapy, *Sleep Restriction,* Imagery Training, Relaxation, Stimulus Control)	Insomnia with chronic pain
Rybarczyk et al. (44)	CBT (Cognitive Therapy, *Sleep Restriction,* Stimulus Control)	Comorbid, older insomnia
Savard et al. (45)	CBT (Cognitive Therapy, *Sleep Restriction,* Sleep Hygiene, Stimulus Control)	Insomnia secondary to breast cancer
Sivertsen et al. (46)	CBT (Cognitive Therapy, *Sleep Restriction,* Sleep Hygiene, Relaxation, Stimulus Control)	Chronic primary Insomnia (older adults)
Ouellet & Morin (47)	CBT (Cognitive Restructuring, *Sleep Restriction,* Sleep Hygiene, Fatigue Management, Stimulus Control)	Insomnia associated (TBI)
Dirksen & Epstein (48)	CBT (Cognitive Therapy, *Sleep Restriction,* Sleep Hygiene, Stimulus Control)	Insomnia secondary to breast cancer

component may include therapies such as stimulus control therapy, sleep restriction, or relaxation training.

The review paper (49) accompanying the Practice Parameter paper highlights a dozen key treatment studies supporting the efficacy of CBT-I. Only six of these studies incorporated Relaxation Therapy as part of the multicomponent therapy, whereas in all twelve of the studies SRT was a component.

THE RATIONALE FOR SLEEP RESTRICTION THERAPY

Restricting TIB, the cornerstone of SRT, is certainly counterintuitive to the expectations of most insomnia sufferers, who generally believe they need more sleep, not less. Patients with chronic insomnia tend to respond to SRT prescriptions with a mixture of disbelief and curiosity—a mindset which turns out to be surprisingly open to fair appraisal of the rationale for treatment (Table 3).

A key component of this rationale involves the well-known effects of mild sleep loss as well as the less appreciated ramifications of extending time in bed. From experience, most patients will understand that the drive to sleep is increased by partial sleep deprivation. Most have encountered the occasional night of "recovery sleep" when a chain of poor nights is finally broken with a night of deeper and more satisfying sleep. The problem is typically that once the accrued sleep debt is paid off, poor sleep begins anew. SRT modulates this haphazard pattern. It restricts sleep over a sufficient span of nights and precludes recovery sleep so as to promote more consistently shorter sleep latencies, as well as more consolidated, deeper sleep. These gains are of course delivered along with the likelihood of increased daytime sleepiness and fatigue. Patients are forewarned of this sleepiness, but reassured that sleep generally becomes more reliable within a few weeks of SRT, and that as TIB is increased in response to increasing sleep efficiency, daytime functional deficits will diminish.

While the deepening and consolidating of sleep produced by SRT are clearly advantageous, even the increased daytime sleepiness that typically results from this intervention has its benefits. People who contend with chronic insomnia commonly report that they "never feel sleepy" or "have lost the ability to sleep". The welling up of sleepiness during the day, even if ill-timed, provides evidence that the sleep system is not irrevocably broken, and holds out promise that it may soon be harnessed in the service of sleeping well at night.

The scientific literature also provides information about what might be expected when individuals extend their TIB, as opposed to restricting it. This knowledge can be used to counter the tendency of many poor sleepers to increase their time in bed, thinking as they do that by "casting a wide net" they will catch as much sleep as possible. This literature also sheds light on how insomnia can persist for years after it first appears when triggering events have long since resolved. It should be noted these studies primarily examined the effects of increasing TIB in noncomplaining individuals, as opposed to people with insomnia. In general, when noncomplaining subjects are confined to bed for longer than usual periods of time, they do in fact accumulate more sleep, and their daytime sleepiness is decreased. However, their sleep becomes more fragmented or even biphasic; it begins to resemble in this respect the disturbed sleep of insomnia.

Table 3 Rationale Offered to Patients for the Effectiveness of SRT

- The sleep loss entailed by SRT increases sleep drive, which in turn is manifest as
  a. More rapid sleep onset,
  b. Increased depth of sleep,
  c. Fewer or briefer awakenings during the night,
  d. Increased daytime sleepiness and fatigue. (Taken as evidence that the sleep drive has in fact increased. As sleep improves over the first few weeks, TIB will be increased and fatigue reduced.)
- Reducing TIB addresses factors that perpetuate insomnia:
  a. More predictable sleep (few very poor or very good nights) reduces anticipatory anxiety over what each night will bring.
  b. Less time spent tossing and turning in bed repairs the broken association between the bed and sleep.
  c. More consistently timed sleep rebuilds an attenuated circadian sleep/wake cycle.

One early study asked subjects to remain in bed for nearly 24 hours. Sleep broke into fragments, but the duration of these stints of sleep summed up to more than 14 hours or about 60% of TIB (50). In another study of prolonged bed rest, this time to sixty hours, sleep expanded to fill nearly 50% of TIB; once again sleep was frequently interrupted by awakenings (51). Whether the greater percentage of time given over to sleep in these studies reflected the effects of prior sleep restriction or merely the opportunity presented by extra time in bed is open to interpretation.

Another study (51) looked at the effects of chronic rather than acute extension of bedtime. Normal control subjects were exposed to a conventional photoperiod (16 hours, followed by 8 hours in bed) for one week and a short photoperiod (10 hours, followed by 14 hours in bed) for four weeks. Sleep duration increased by about one hour a night under conditions of prolonged bed rest. As seen in the studies of acute bedtime extension, sleep efficiency was reduced and sleep fragmentation increased. However, a distinct pattern emerged with repeated 10:14 light/dark cycles: Sleep was split into two equal bouts, the first on the "evening" end of the prolonged bed rest period, the second on the "morning" end, separated by one to three hours of wakefulness. The author suggests that this biphasic sleep pattern may be more representative of sleep in humans over hundreds of thousands of years until the recent past, when artificial light became available to produce a fixed, prolonged photoperiod across the seasons, resulting in the monophasic, highly efficient sleep we think of as "normal."

Another protocol employed prolonged bed rest to investigate the presence of objective sleepiness [a sleep latency less than or equal to six minutes on a multiple sleep latency test (MSLT)] in individuals with no subjective sleepiness complaint (52). One group of subjects spent 10 hours in bed and the other spent their habitual time in bed (averaging about 8 hours) for 14 days. Nocturnal sleep recordings followed by daytime MSLTs occurred periodically across the two weeks. Consistent with the studies cited above, the group following an extended TIB schedule showed increased sleep time and reduced sleep efficiency at night, as well as reduced objective sleepiness during the day, compared to those following a self-selected TIB schedule. It is interesting to note with regard to the present discussion that a subgroup of individuals in this study did not demonstrate reduced objective sleepiness after extending TIB. Sleep efficiency plummeted immediately after TIB was increased for these subjects. This response is similar to the experience of individuals with insomnia, who try to accumulate additional sleep by spending more time in bed and wind up instead with more frequent or longer awakenings.

A second component of the rationale for SRT is that it focuses on practices perpetuating insomnia that are more amenable to treatment. According to our conceptualization of insomnia (known as the 3P Model, Figure 1 53,14) the factors that predisposed a particular patient to

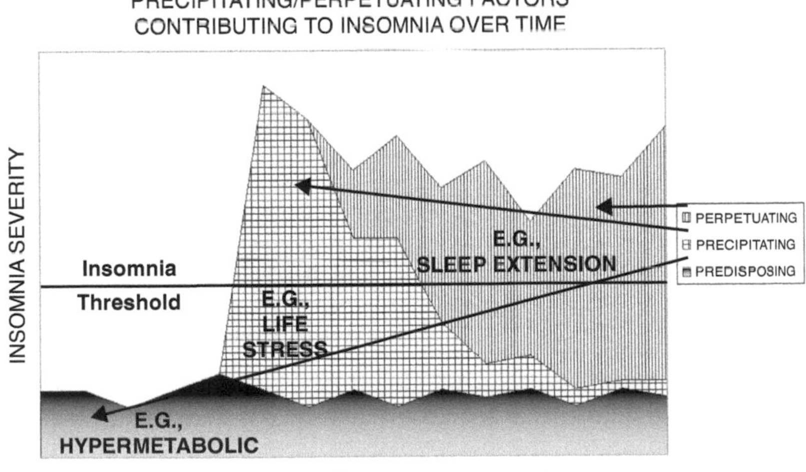

Figure 1 The 3P model of insomnia depicting changing influences during the course of insomnia. *Source:* From Ref. (53, Adapted from 14; modified by Max Hirschkowitz and Michael Perlis).

insomnia as well as those that precipitated the disturbance may be too remote or too entrenched to serve as fruitful targets for short-term treatment. However, insomnia can still be effectively treated by addressing factors, which perpetuate the sleep disturbance. Compensating for sleep loss by spending an excessive amount of time in bed is, as discussed above, a frequently encountered factor maintaining chronic insomnia—one that is directly targeted by SRT.

In some cases patients may readily concur that the factors that originally triggered their sleep disturbance are not operative at present. For example, insomnia may have appeared in the midst of a patient's bitter divorce, yet his sleeplessness persists in the context of a successful new relationship. Or it may have followed the arrival of a colicky newborn, who three years later, is now sleeping through the night while her mother still struggles with frequent awakenings.

Even when the original trigger of insomnia still looms large as a source of distress, it may be advantageous to target seemingly secondary perpetuating factors to achieve rapid improvement. For example, a woman's sleeplessness may be clearly related to the ongoing stress of contending with a tyrannical boss who never appears satisfied with her performance. A holistic approach to this problem may include advocating changes in behavior (such as negotiating clearly defined benchmarks that will serve as the basis of regular reviews) as well as attitude (such as challenging the idea that any shortfalls in meeting objectives necessarily reflect incompetence). While these changes are being supported, it still may make clinical sense to take steps that directly impact sleep. It may not be easy to adhere to an early alarm, but at least this is an action that is fully under the patient's control, and one that should yield predictable results. It counters the loss of efficacy that can prove so corrosive to self confidence, regardless of whether that sense of helplessness is encountered on the job or when trying to sleep.

The 3P Model also posits that patients may, over the course of a chronic insomnia, become sensitized to potential sources of sleep disruption. Prior to the onset of the disturbance, sleep is often seen as more resilient, and behaviors such as drinking caffeinated or alcoholic beverages at dinner or oversleeping on weekends could apparently be engaged in with impunity. Seven and a half hours in bed would hardly be deemed generous. We explain that "that was then" and that now, at least for the time being, a patient in a sensitized or hyperaroused state may not be capable of consistently sustaining seven or more hours of sleep. It is better under these conditions to more closely match bedtime with expected total sleep time, even if that is currently six hours. While we do not guarantee that seven and a half hours of sleep will eventually be attained on a nightly basis, we do hold out the reasonable expectation that both bedtime and sleep time will gradually increase over the course of treatment, and invite patients to partner with us in determining what the optimal balance between sleep restriction and sleep quality is for them.

A third major benefit of SRT is that it improves the experience of going to bed. Tossing and turning for hours on end is not pleasant. The bed starts to be dreaded as a place of torment rather than as a haven from waking concerns. A self-fulfilling prophecy is set in motion, one in which the expectation of another miserable night and the prospects of having to muddle through the next day increases anxiety and arousal, thereby leading to that very result. By contrast, with SRT patients come to expect that bedtime will be short—and sweet, in the sense that a greater proportion of it will be spent in blissful oblivion. They may actually look forward to the designated time when they can "finally get into bed."

A fourth reason why SRT benefits people with insomnia is that it strengthens the circadian sleep–wake cycle. It replaces a welter of short stints of sleep occurring at various times around the clock with a single nocturnal period that is more predictably filled with sleep. Patients are more likely to be awoken by an alarm when under this treatment, leading to consistently timed exposure to morning light and the various demands of waking life. These cues help keep sleep synchronized with other biological rhythms, which in turn leads to the more reliable appearance of sleep shortly after bedtime, and deeper sleep once it arrives.

Offering a considered and detailed rationale for the effectiveness of SRT satisfies patients' 'need to know' while acknowledging the counterintuitive nature of the treatment. Taking the time to thoroughly prepare patients for this therapy will motivate them for the difficulties ahead. Hopefully they will begin to think differently about their prospects for sleep, about what it means to be awake and out of bed later into the night or earlier in the morning, and more generally about their ability to shape their nocturnal experience over the long term. These cognitive changes are critical therapeutic components that work in concert with behavioral change to foster improved sleep.

IMPLEMENTING SLEEP RESTRICTION THERAPY

SRT begins with a two-week sleep diary. The average subjective sleep time over the course of this diary is calculated. This value is then prescribed, as the amount of time in bed (TIB) patients should spend at the start of treatment. Changes in sleep efficiency (SE, calculated as subjective sleep time/time in bed X 100%) more than a five day moving window trigger increases and decreases in TIB (see Table 4) (1).

Setting specific times of retiring and rising to delimit an initial time in bed requires thoughtful analysis. The patient's sleep diary may offer clues as to what period would be most likely to maximize sleep at the start of treatment. In the case of a patient who has no difficulty falling asleep but who awakens too early in the morning, with difficulty falling back to sleep, TIB should start at the habitual time of retiring at night. As a result the wake-up time will be earlier than usual. In patients who typically get their best sleep in the middle of the night, or whose sleep is quite broken with awakenings scattered haphazardly across the night, the assigned sleep schedule should start later and end earlier than usual. Finally, if a patient's primary difficulty is one of falling asleep, the assigned retiring and rising times should be later than usual, within the constraint of meeting starting time for work.

Some patients will have obligations such as variable work shifts or shared childcare responsibilities that necessitate rising early on an intermittent basis. In the interests of entraining a robust circadian sleep–wake cycle, the clinician may take the opportunity to set a fixed early morning rising time as part of the initial SRT instructions. The choice of retiring and rising times should also take various practical concerns into account such as possible disturbance of bed partners or nighttime needs of pets.

It should be stressed that although SRT can be summarized with a few quantitatively based prescriptions, this does not relieve the clinician of the need to exercise judgment. Patients' forbearance for the challenges posed by the treatment is typically limited to one good effort, and this chance for improvement may be squandered if the clinician's approach is too rigid. Some individuals become so concerned at the prospect of a limited bedtime (". . .but I always sleep so much worse when I know I have to get up early") that clinical judgment trumps strict adherence to the SRT method. Negotiation with such patients is required to come up with an acceptable level of sleep restriction. In anticipation of their difficulties adhering to even modified SRT schedules, it is recommended that the clinician 'go on record' as follows: "OK, we will permit a bit more time in bed for you, but it may take longer for your sleep to improve. Therefore, for this to work it is imperative that you limit your time in bed to the specific hours we have agreed on."

A number of variations on the original SRT procedure have emerged in the two decades since the therapy was introduced. Some investigators and clinicians set the initial TIB equal to the average sleep obtained from the sleep diary plus half-hour, since even good sleepers do not have 100% sleep efficiency. The extra bedtime therefore allows a more realistic possibility of garnering the targeted amount of sleep. Another method called sleep compression (54) restricts TIB minimally at first. As treatment proceeds time in bed is further reduced. This approach is easier for patients to adhere to at the start of treatment. We have employed an SRT variation that runs in the opposite direction, with initial TIB initially quite restricted as in standard SRT, followed by weekly extension of TIB in 15 or 30 minute increments, continued so long as TIB contains less than 45 minutes of wakefulness (15). This method avoids the dispiriting effect of having to reduce TIB repeatedly—the patient knows that "the worst is over" in terms of bedtime restriction after the first week or so.

Table 4 Sleep Restriction Therapy Method (1)

- Determine average time asleep from sleep diary
- Set time in bed = time asleep
- Set a consistent wake-up time
- No daytime naps
- If 5 day average sleep efficiency $\geq$ 90% ($\geq$ 85% in > 65 yr olds) then increase time in bed (15–30 min)
- If 5 day average sleep efficiency < 85% (< 80% in > 65 yr olds) then decrease time in bed (15–30 min)

Patient characteristics should be taken into account before prescribing SRT. There is little reason, for example, to recommend SRT to individuals whose sleep is already compact. (These individuals may still present with insomnia, typically complaining of insufficient sleep due to early morning awakenings.) Consider the patient who can fall asleep soon after getting into bed at 11 PM and obtain a solid five hours of sleep, but who then awakens around 4 AM and ruminates on the day ahead for two hours before getting out of bed. Her sleep efficiency is low at 71% and she is complaining of daytime fatigue. Restricting bedtime to about five hours via SRT is not likely to significantly heighten her sleep drive, because it will not appreciably reduce total sleep time. She is likely to continue to have a compact but short sleep period of five hours on SRT. Employing stimulus control instructions may present the better option here, with the aim of weakening the association between this patient's early morning awakenings and the opportunity they present to obsess in bed. It would allow the possibility of "resetting" her frame of mind through a period of distracting activity such as reading and then returning to bed and to sleep. If, on the other hand, you deduce that a patient is in fact flitting in and out of sleep for the last two hours in bed, perhaps understandably not counting this as "really sleeping," SRT offers an appropriate treatment choice.

When conducting SRT in patients with Paradoxical Insomnia (previously called Sleep State Misperception) the original rules for increasing time in bed do not work well. It is true that sleep efficiency can be marginally increased when the assigned time in bed of patients who report, say, one hour of sleep is decreased well below the minimum duration of about five hours we typically employ. However, their sleep efficiency will rarely approach even a relaxed criterion for increasing time in bed, as these patients typically do not perceive and report any increases in sleep time (unpublished data). In these patients, weekly increases in time in bed following a severe initial reduction, one of the SRT variants discussed above, may improve daytime functioning although nighttime complaints will likely persist.

A COST/BENEFIT MODEL OF SLEEP RESTRICTION THERAPY UTILIZING SLEEP EFFICIENCY AND DAYTIME FUNCTIONING AS MARKERS OF SLEEP NEED

SRT is predicated on the use of sleep efficiency as a means to constrain TIB. Sleep efficiency is a particularly useful index on which to base adjustments to TIB because it is a single ratio that is derived from measures of both sleep and wakefulness. It can be conceived of as a measure of the density of sleep, and is affected by both voluntary choices regarding times of retiring and rising, as well as involuntary experiences such as difficulties encountered in falling and/or staying asleep. While it cannot serve as a surrogate for sleep sufficiency—a two-hour bedtime will likely be both highly efficient and grossly insufficient—it does neatly convey a sense of the quality of the sleep that has been obtained.

Sleep efficiency, when combined with an evaluation of daytime functioning, may serve as a marker within the ill-defined territory of sleep need. Changes in sleep efficiency and daytime functioning over the course of SRT can be construed as reflecting the degree to which sleep need is being satisfied by a given sleep/wake pattern, and at what cost. We have modeled the changing ratio of benefits and costs as tracked by sleep efficiency and daytime functioning in Figure 2. Benefits in this model are nocturnal sleep duration and daytime functional capacity while costs are time spent in bed and vulnerability to insomnia.

Prior to the start of SRT treatment costs are high. Much time is "spent" in bed and there is high vulnerability to sleep disturbance. Benefits are relatively low in this pretreatment phase. Sleep time is reduced or variable, while fatigue, poor concentration, irritability and/or other daytime impairments are present. The daytime deficits suggest that sleep need is nowhere near being satisfied despite sleep efficiency being low—that is, despite the potential for extra sleep afforded at least in theory by the extended bedtime.

At the start of SRT costs are dramatically reduced. Not much time is "spent" in bed and there is little vulnerability to sleep disturbance, given the substantial increase in sleep propensity that occurs as a result of accruing sleep loss. However, benefits are also further reduced as a result of the severe curtailment of TIB dictated at the start of treatment. Less sleep is accumulated than had been present at baseline, and functional capacity is even further diminished. While sleep efficiency has now risen markedly, the exacerbation of daytime functional deficits testifies to continuing unsatisfied sleep need.

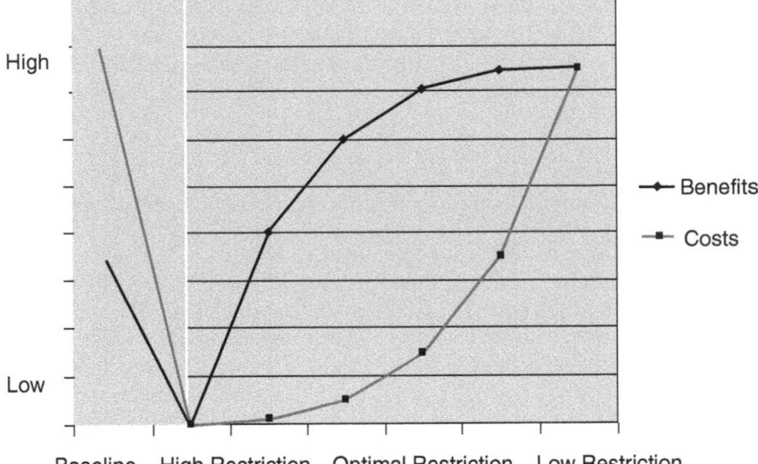

Figure 2 A cost/benefit model of sleep restriction therapy utilizing sleep efficiency and daytime functioning as markers of sleep need. Costs are indexed by time spent in bed and vulnerability to insomnia while benefits are reflected by duration of sleep time and daytime function.

As treatment proceeds levels of TIB are gradually increased while maintaining sleep efficiency near an optimal level. Both costs and benefits rise, but initially the rate of beneficial change greatly outpaces the rise in costs. Consistent accumulation of well-consolidated sleep, even if of modest duration, yields better daytime performance than had short stints of sleep scattered haphazardly across the clock. Relatively few hours are being spent in bed, while residual sleep loss guards against the resurgence of insomnia. Through a process of bedtime titration, a point is reached where both sleep efficiency and daytime functioning are at relatively high levels, where sleep need has been satisfied, but not sated to the point of inviting the reappearance of insomnia. The benefit/cost ratio will be highest on this bedtime schedule. It should be maintained going forward at least until such time that other salient factors which had predisposed, precipitated and/or perpetuated insomnia have changed. For example, once anticipatory anxiety over what each night will bring has subsided, a slightly longer TIB may be indulged in without courting harm to sleep.

As TIB approaches baseline levels, the slope of the curve representing incurred costs accelerates. A relatively large amount of time is again being spent in bed. More critically, the potential for sleep disturbance rises disproportionately at higher levels of TIB. There is little residual sleep loss at this point that may be counted upon to quickly induce and sustain sleep. Meanwhile, benefits plateau when TIB is minimally restricted. Neither sleep time nor functional capacity can be expected to continue to rise much, if at all, as sleep efficiency begins to ebb. Thus sleep need may still be partially unmet after successful treatment. Optimally balancing sleep efficiency and daytime functioning does not mean that either nocturnal sleep or daytime capacity alone will be maximized. There are many intransigent aspects of insomnia (typically categorized in the 3P Model as predisposing factors, such as hyperarousal) that may require concessions of benefits received from sleep, both by night and day, in the interest of maximizing the overall sleep/wake experience.

CONCLUSION

In the 21 years since SRT was first introduced, awareness of the health, economic and public safety issues raised by sleep disturbance has crystallized. Insomnia is no longer exclusively confined to the role of symptom or side effect, but rather recognized as at times a primary complaint, with its own course and indications for treatment (55). A new generation of hypnotic medication has been developed to remedy sleep initiation and maintenance difficulties, and a new paradigm of long-term reliance on such medication has gained adherents. In this context, the role played by psychological factors such as anticipatory anxiety and drug dependence in perpetuating insomnia looms large. CBT-I, with SRT now firmly ensconced among its cornerstones, is uniquely positioned to address the psychophysiological, behavioral and cognitive challenges posed by chronic insomnia. A multitude of patients stand to benefit as their physicians and clinicians gain a stronger appreciation of these demonstrably effective treatments.

REFERENCES

1. Spielman AJ, Saskin P, Thorpy MJ. Treatment of chronic insomnia by restriction of time spent in bed. Sleep 1987; 10(1):45–56.
2. Jacobson E. You Must Relax. New York, NY: McGraw-Hill Book, Co, 1934:201.
3. Bootzin RR. Stimulus control treatment for insomnia. Proc Am Psychol Assoc 1972; 7:395–396.
4. Hauri PJ. The Sleep Disorders: Current Concepts, 2nd ed. Kalamazoo, MI: Upjohn, 1982.
5. Borbely AA, Achermann P. Sleep homeostasis and models of sleep regulation. In: Kryger M, Roth T, Dement W, eds. Principles and Practices of Sleep Medicine, 4th, ed. Toronto, Canada: W.B. Saunders Co, 2005: 405–417.
6. Webb WB, Agnew HW. The effects of a chronic limitation of sleep length. Psychophysiology. 1974; 11:265–274.
7. Mullaney DJ, Johnson LC, Naitoh JP, et al. Sleep during and after gradual sleep reduction. Psychophysiology 1977; 14:237–244.
8. Kales A, Caldwell AB, Preston TA, et al. Personality patterns in insomnia. Theoretical implications. Arch Gen Psychiatry 1976; 33(9):1128–1124.
9. Wachtel P. Psychoanalysis and Behavior Therapy: Toward an Integration. New York, NY: Basic Books, Inc, 1977.
10. Weitzman ED, Czeisler C, Coleman R, et al. Delayed sleep phase syndrome: A chronobiological disorder with sleep onset insomnia. Arch Gen Psychiatry 1981; 38:737–746.
11. Mendelson WB, Roth T, Cassella J, et al. The treatment of chronic insomnia: Drug indications, chronic use and abuse liability. Summary of a 2001 new clinical drug evaluation unit meeting symposium. Sleep Med Rev 2004; 8:7–17.
12. Morgenthaler T, Kramer M, Alessi C, et al. Practice parameters for the psychological and behavioral treatment of insomnia: An update. an american academy of sleep medicine report standards of practice. Sleep 2006; 29(11):1415–1419.
13. Morin CM, Bootzin RR, Buysse DJ. Psychological and behavioral treatment of insomnia: Update of the recent evidence (1998–2004). Sleep 2006; 29(11):1398–1414 .
14. Spielman AJ, Caruso L, Glovinsky P. A behavioral perspective on insomnia treatment. Psychiatr Clin North Am 1987; 10(4):541–553.
15. Morin CM, Kowatch RA, O'Shanick G. Sleep Restriction for the inpatient treatment of insomnia. Sleep 1990; 13(2):183–186.
16. Friedman L, Bliwise DL, Yesavage JA, et al. A preliminary study comparing sleep restriction amd relaxation treatment for insomnia in older adults. J Gerontol 1991; 46:1–8.
17. Brooks JO 3rd,Friedman L, Bliwise DL, et al. Use of the wrist actigraph to study insomnia in older adults. Sleep 1993; 16(2):51–55.
18. Riedel BW, Lichstein KL, Dwyer WO. Sleep compression and sleep education for older insomniacs: Self-help versus therapist guidance. Psychol Aging 1995; 10:54–63.
19. Bliwise DL, Friedman L, Nekich JC, et al. Prediction of outcome in behaviorally based insomnia treatments. J Behav Ther Exp Psychiatry 1995; 26(1):17–23.
20. Friedman L, Benson K, Noda A, et al. An actigraphic comparison of sleep restriction and sleep hygiene treatments for insomnia in older adults. J Geriatr Psychiatry Neurol 2000; 13(1):17–27.
21. Riedel BW, Lichstein KL. Strategies for evaluating adherence to sleep restriction treatment for insomnia. Behav Res Ther 2001; 39:201–212.
22. Lichstein KL, Riedel BW, Wilson NM, et al. Relaxation and sleep compression for late-life insomnia: A placebo-controlled trial. J Consult Clin Psychol 2001; 69 (2): 227–239.
23. Morin CM, Kowatch RA, Barry T, et al. Cognitive-behavior therapy for late-life insomnia. J Consult Clin Psychol 1993; 61 (1):137–146.
24. Morin CM, Colecchi C, Stone J, et al. Behavioral and pharmacological therapies for late-life insomnia: A randomized controlled trial. JAMA 1999; 281 (11):991–999.
25. Mimeault V, Morin CM. Self-help treatment for insomnia: Bibliotherapy with and without professional guidance. J Consult Clin Psychol 1999; 67 (4):511–519.
26. Verbeek I, Schreuder K, Declerck G. Evaluation of short-term nonpharmacological treatment of insomnia in a clinical setting. J Psychosom Res 1999; 47 (4):369–383.
27. Currie SR, Wilson KG, Pontefract AJ, et al. Cognitive-behavioral treatment of insomnia secondary to chronic pain. J Consult Clin Psychol 2000; 68 (3): 407–416.

28. Perlis M, Aloia M, Millikan A. et al. Behavioral treatment of insomnia: A clinical case series study. J Behav Med 2000; 23(2):149–161.
29. Espie CA, Inglis SJ, Tessier S, et al. The clinical effectiveness of cognitive behaviour therapy for chronic insomnia–implementation and evaluation of a sleep clinic in general medical practice. Behav Res Ther 2001; 39(1):45–60.
30. Perlis ML, Sharpe M, Smith MT, et al. Behavioral treatment of insomnia: Treatment outcome and the relevance of medical and psychiatric morbidity. J Behav Med 2001; 24(3):281–296.
31. Edinger JD, Wohlgemuth WK, Radtke RA, et al. Cognitive behavioral therapy for treatment of chronic primary insomnia: A randomized controlled trial. JAMA 2001; 285(14):1856–1864.
32. Harvey L, Inglis SJ, Espie CA. Insomniacs' reported use of CBT components and relationship to long-term clinical outcome. Behav Res Ther 2002; 40(1):75–83.
33. Currie SR, Wilson KG, Curran D. Clinical significance and predictors of treatment response to cognitive-behavior therapy for insomnia secondary to chronic pain. J Behav Med 2002; 25 (2):135–153.
34. Rybarczyk B, Lopez M, Schelble K, et al. Home-based video CBT for comorbid geriatric insomnia: A pilot study using secondary data analyses. Behav Sleep Med 2005; 3 (3):158–175.
35. Edinger JD, Sampson WS. A primary care "friendly" cognitive behavioral insomnia therapy. Sleep 2003; 26:177–182.
36. Ouellet MC, Morin CM. Cognitive behavioral therapy for insomnia associated with traumatic brain injury: A single-case study. Arch Phys Med Rehabil 2004; 85(8):1298–1302.
37. Morin CM, Bastien C, Guay B, et al. Randomized clinical trial of supervised tapering and cognitive behavior therapy to facilitate benzodiazepine discontinuation in older adults with chronic insomnia. Am J Psychiatry 2004; 161 (2):332–342.
38. Morgan K, Dixon S, Mathers N, et al. Psychological treatment for insomnia in the regulation of long-term hypnotic drug use. Health Technol Assess (Rockv) 2004; 8(8):iii–iv, 1–68.
39. Currie SR, Clark S, Hodgins DC, El-Guebaly N. Randomized controlled trial of brief cognitive-behavioural interventions for insomnia in recovering alcoholics. Addiction 2004; 99:1121–1132.
40. Perlis ML, Smith MT, Orff H, et al. The effects of modafinil and cognitive behavior therapy on sleep continuity in patients with primary insomnia. Sleep 2004; 27 (4):715–725.
41. Jacobs GD, Pace-Schott EF, Stickgold R, et al. Cognitive behavior therapy and pharmacotherapy for insomnia: A randomized controlled trial and direct comparison. Arch Intern Med 2004; 164 (17):1888–1896.
42. Dopke CA, Lehner RK, Wells AM. Cognitive behavioral group therapy for insomnia in individuals with serious mental illnesses: A preliminary evaluation. Psychiatr Rehabil J 2004; 27:235–242.
43. Stiefel F, Stagno D. Management of insomnia in patients with chronic pain conditions. CNS Drugs 2004; 18(5);285–296.
44. Rybarczyk B, Stepanski E, Fogg L, et al. A placebo-controlled test of cognitive-behavioral therapy for comorbid insomnia in older adults. J Consult Clin Psychol 2005; 73 (6):1164–1174.
45. Savard J, Simard S, Ivers H, et al. Randomized study on the efficacy of cognitive-behavioral therapy for insomnia secondary to breast cancer, part I: Sleep and psychological effects. J Clin Oncol 2005; 23(25):6083–6096.
46. Sivertsen B, Omvik S, Pallesen S, et al. Cognitive behavioral therapy vs. zopiclone for treatment of chronic primary insomnia in older adults: A randomized controlled trial. JAMA 2006; 295(24):2851–2858.
47. Ouellet MC, Morin CM. Efficacy of cognitive-behavioral therapy for insomnia associated with traumatic brain injury: A single-case experimental design. Arch Phys Med Rehabil 2007; 88(12):1581–1592.
48. Dirksen SR, Epstein DR. Efficacy of an insomnia intervention on fatigue, mood and quality of life in breast cancer survivors. J Adv Nurs 2008; 61(6):664–675.
49. Nakagawa Y. Continuous observation of EEG patterns at night and daytime of normal subjects under restrained conditions. I. Quiescent state when lying down. Electroencephalogr Clin Neurophysiol 1980; 49 (5–6):524–537.
50. Campbell SS. Duration and placement of sleep in a "disentrained" environment. Psychophysiology 1984; 21 (1):106–113.
51. Wehr TA. In short photoperiods, human sleep is biphasic. J Sleep Res 1992; 1 (2):103–107.
52. Roehrs T, Shore E, Papineau K, et al. A two-week sleep extension in sleepy normals. Sleep 1996; 19 (7):576–582.
53. Spielman AJ. Assessment of insomnia. Clin Psychol Rev 1986; 6:11–25.
54. Glovinsky PB, Spielman AJ. The Insomnia Answer. New York, NY: A Perigee Book, division of The Penguin Group, 2006.
55. National Institutes of Health. National institutes of health state of the science conference statement on manifestations and management of chronic insomnia in adults, June 13–15, 2005. Sleep 2005; 28:1049–1057.

26 Other Nonpharmacological Treatments of Insomnia

Daniel J. Taylor, Emily A. Grieser, and JoLyn I. Tatum
Department of Psychology, University of North Texas, Denton, Texas, U.S.A.

There are a wide variety of nonpharmacological treatments for insomnia including stimulus control, sleep restriction, and cognitive therapy (1,2), which are all covered extensively elsewhere in this volume. There are also "other" types of nonpharmacological treatments sometimes used to treat insomnia discussed within this chapter. Some of these methods, such as progressive muscle relaxation and paradoxical intention, are commonly used, have significant empirical backing, and have been listed as "effective and recommended therapies" by the Standards of Practice Committee of the American Academy of Sleep Medicine (3). Others (e.g., exercise, acupuncture, aromatherapy) have less rigorous empirical backing, often consisting of case studies or case-series designs without control conditions, but were deemed worthy of review because they are used by some practitioners and have not received adequate review elsewhere. The current chapter addresses these "other" nonpharmacological treatments of insomnia with a description of efficacy/effectiveness studies. In terms of description of efficacy/effectiveness studies, more focus was given to those treatments which have received less systematic review in the current literature.

RELAXATION TECHNIQUES

Relaxation techniques are some of the most frequently used treatments of insomnia (2,4,5). The rationale and proposed mechanisms of action underlying the use of relaxation methods in the treatment of insomnia stem from the hypothesis that people with insomnia suffer from increased somatic and cognitive arousal. Relaxation methods serve to reduce somatic arousal and/or cognitive arousal, thereby increasing the likelihood that patients will fall asleep. Although a variety (e.g., breathing retraining, imagery, meditation, biofeedback) of relaxation interventions have been tested as treatments for insomnia, progressive muscle relaxation (PMR) (6,7) has the most evidence as a treatment for insomnia (3).

Progressive Muscle Relaxation (PMR)

The Standards of Practice Committee of the American Academy of Sleep Medicine identified PMR as an "empirically supported treatment" because four studies demonstrated that relaxation was better at treating insomnia than a placebo control (highest level of evidence) (3). Progressive muscle relaxation involves alternately tensing and relaxing different muscle groups throughout the body (8). Homework involves practicing the relaxation at home during the day, just prior to bedtime, and sometimes during nighttime awakenings. Patients are trained to focus and compare feelings of relaxation with the tension that was present before the relaxation procedure. This technique typically takes 10 to 30 minutes. Multiple scripts for progressive muscle relaxation are available both online and within treatment texts (e.g., 9–11). A copy of the script used in our laboratory, developed from the text of Lichstein (9), is reproduced in Appendix A.

Other Relaxation Methods

As mentioned, many other relaxation techniques exist, but to date only meditation, imagery, and autogenic training have been assessed for the treatment of insomnia. Although these treatments have shown effectiveness in at least one clinical trial, other studies found no benefit, and the overall evidence did not support a recommendation of these techniques as single treatments (1). Other relaxation methods such as diaphragmatic breathing, hypnosis, and transcendental meditation, may be used clinically, but they have no empirical backing as treatments of insomnia.

Few studies have compared relaxation procedures, so the fact that PMR has the greatest evidence may be due to a greater interest in this procedure during the early days of insomnia treatment research, with little subsequent research focusing on single methods of treatment. It is possible that other relaxation treatments are equally efficacious, but have not been rigorously evaluated. In practice, many if not most clinicians actually combine multiple forms of relaxation treatment (e.g., progressive relaxation, breathing retraining, and autogenics). Detail about the actual techniques of the various relaxation treatments available and the myriad of issues (e.g., variants, therapist issues, common factors) involved in each are covered in much greater depth in numerous texts (e.g., 9–11).

Biofeedback

Because only one placebo-controlled trial has been performed to date, the Standards of Practice Committee of the American Academy of Sleep Medicine did not identify this treatment as "empirically supported," instead listing it as "probably efficacious" because two studies have shown it was better than wait-list control and one study showed it was better than no treatment.

Biofeedback is a specific form of relaxation treatment that differs from those mentioned above in that it actually provides sensory feedback (usually visual or auditory), either mechanically (i.e., thermometers) or more frequently with computers and amplifiers, to help patients learn how to control physiological parameters such as finger temperature or muscle tension, in order to reduce somatic arousal (3). For instance, frontalis electromyography (EMG) biofeedback, the most commonly studied, teaches subjects to reduce muscle tension in the muscles of the forehead and face. Biofeedback seems to help patients attain states of mental and physical relaxation and become more aware of their own bodily sensations and responses to stressors. Biofeedback actively involves the patient in the therapeutic process and provides immediate measures of progress. One difficulty with evaluating the effectiveness of biofeedback is that it is often paired with some form of relaxation exercise, making it difficult to parse out the independent effects of each. In addition, improvements appear to be comparable to PMR, which takes less time for the patient to learn and requires no expensive equipment. Therefore, this method is not recommended over stimulus control, sleep restriction, or PMR, unless the patient fails to benefit from those other methods.

Other Biofeedback Methods

Neurofeedback (EEG biofeedback) may offer an alternative treatment for insomnia (12). Thus far, one case study and two case-series studies have shown that some form of neurofeedback was effective in improving self-report insomnia measures (13,14). The results were somewhat mixed for the one study that evaluated objective sleep with overnight polysomnography (14).

Yoga

Kundalini Yoga was popularized by Yogi Bhajan in the late 1960s as a means of general life enhancement and to explore altered states of consciousness without the use of drugs. Yoga involves the awareness of breath (pranayama) and thought processes in addition to a series of postures (asanas) designed to stretch and strengthen the body. Yoga as traditionally practiced is often combined with aspects of PMR (especially in "corpse pose") and meditation. As one can see, many of these elements overlap with the relaxation techniques already discussed.

There is growing evidence supporting yoga as an alternative treatment for insomnia, and yoga research has recently received funding from the National Institute of Complementary and Alternative Medicine at the National Institutes of Health (15). So far, many trials investigating the use of yoga for the purpose of improving sleep have been limited by small sample size and lack of replication (16). One randomized controlled trial found that yoga was more effective than wait-list control in reducing self-reported sleep disturbance in elderly residents in a care facility. To date, the majority of the data concerning the efficacy of yoga consists of case series designs using mainly self-report measures of improvement (17,18). This is less than optimal because these forms of assessment are more susceptible to social desirability and placebo effects. It is also unknown how much of the benefit gleaned from Yoga in these previous studies would have been found by just using traditional relaxation procedures, due to the lack of comparison groups.

PARADOXICAL INTENTION

Paradoxical intention aims to reduce the patient's performance anxiety about falling asleep through instructions to get in bed and passively remain awake rather than try to fall asleep. This persuasion to engage in a feared behavior (staying awake) is thought to alleviate performance anxiety, thereby allowing sleep to come more easily (2).

All research on this technique has focused on patients with sleep-onset insomnia, with two studies showing it to be more effective than placebo control, and one study showing it to be better than wait-list control. Because the effects of this intervention are generally smaller than the single treatments of stimulus control, sleep restriction, and PMR, it is rarely recommended over those interventions, but may be useful to those who do not benefit from other methods (2,4,5).

BRIGHT LIGHT THERAPY

Many companies sell phototherapy devices to the public, usually made of full-spectrum or cool white fluorescent light bulbs emitting on average 2500 lux (19). These devices simulate bright sunlight via indirect exposure to the eyes, and use is recommended while reading, eating meals, or during similar activities.

Studies show bright light therapy can be used to realign the circadian rhythms through effects on the Suprachiasmatic Nucleus (SCN) (20). The proposed mechanism of action for the treatment of insomnia is that some insomnias may be due in part to a circadian misalignment, such as advanced sleep phase syndrome (early bedtime and early awakening) and delayed sleep phase syndrome (late bedtime and late awakening) (19). Past studies have shown that bright light therapy was useful in treating these two circadian rhythm disorders (20). The use of bright light in the treatment of specific sleep–wake schedule disorders is discussed in detail elsewhere in this text. In milder forms, phase shifts could present as terminal or onset insomnia. Therefore, it stands to reason that in those cases of insomnia where a circadian component is at work, bright light therapy (BLT) might be a useful treatment. In addition, it could be that BLT works even in those without a strong circadian component, simply by increasing sleep propensity during the nighttime hours.

Three placebo controlled studies have now been performed examining the effect of *varying intensities* (i.e., lux and duration) of BLT, on the sleep of *different types* of insomnia, with mixed results. One trial of half-hour exposure to 2000 to 2500 lux in the morning for five days in patients with "winter" insomnia (occurring during the "dark period" above Arctic Circle), resulted in shorter sleep latency and increased drowsiness compared to a wait-list control (21). In a randomized placebo-controlled trial of older adults (age 62–81) with sleep-maintenance insomnia, 12 days of BLT (4000 lux) improved both maintenance insomnia and sleep quality over the dim red light control (50 lux) (22). These results were not replicated in a more recent case-series design by these same researchers (23). The most rigorous of these trials was a more recent single-blind, placebo-controlled, 12-week, parallel-group randomized design comparing four treatment groups representing a factorial combination of two lighting conditions (~ 4000 lux vs. ~65 lux) for 45 minutes with two different times of light administration (morning vs. evening), in a mixed sample of insomnia types (i.e., onset, maintenance, terminal, nonrestorative) (24). These authors found "Scheduled light exposure was able to shift the circadian phase predictably but was unrelated to changes in objective or subjective sleep measures."

Clearly, before specific recommendations can be made about the use of BLT to treat specific types of insomnia, more efficacy research is needed. This research might focus on other specific types of insomnia (i.e., onset and terminal insomnia) and be more strategic in administration (i.e., morning administration for onset insomnia and evening administration for terminal insomnia). It is important to note that side effects of bright light therapy can include jumpiness or jitteriness, headache, and nausea (25).

EXERCISE

Exercise and physical activity have known benefits on health (e.g., improved cardiovascular fitness, weight loss, increased maximal oxygen uptake) (26). There is also a known relationship between physical activity and sleep, although the exact nature of that relationship is unknown. The strongest theoretical basis for this relationship comes from the *thermodynamic hypothesis of sleep*. This theory is founded on the drop in body temperature that accompanies the onset of sleep, and which may serve as a signal to the body that it is time for sleep. If the rapid decrease in temperature that precedes sleep serves as a signal for sleep onset, it is possible that by raising the body temperature (e.g., via exercise), the internal signal will either be enhanced (i.e., if exercise occurs at the right time to have the resultant cooling of the body coincide with sleep onset), or delayed (i.e., if exercise occurs too close to sleep) (27,28).

Generally, research shows that moderate to high intensity exercise sessions four to eight hours before bedtime results in improved sleep quality in a normal population (29–31). There is also evidence that discrete episodes of physical activity either less than four or more than eight hours before bed time can actually be detrimental to sleep (29). Unfortunately, there is little information regarding the effects of physical activity on insomnia. Most of the research that has examined these two variables has been epidemiological in nature. For example, a longitudinal study in older adults found lower levels of physical activity consistently predicted insomnia status, along with depressed mood and lower physical health, over an eight-year period (32). Another epidemiological study found that regular exercise was associated with a lower prevalence of insomnia (33).

One intervention study, in older adults with moderate sleep complaints, showed that a 16-week moderate intensity exercise program was better than a wait-list control at improving global Pittsburg Sleep Quality Index (PSQI) (34) scores as well as sleep onset latency, sleep duration, and rated sleep quality, as assessed by the PSQI and sleep diaries (31). Another study that did not specifically target insomnia, but whose sample met the research diagnostic criteria for insomnia at baseline, also found positive results following a four-week moderate intensity exercise intervention (35). However, this was a very small study that also included an afternoon nap as part of the intervention; thus, the results are not as easily interpreted.

While epidemiologic research provides some information regarding the relationship between insomnia and physical activity, there is a definite need for additional randomized controlled trials examining the effects of a physical activity intervention in a population with insomnia and on the specific sleep parameters that make up insomnia.

ACUPUNCTURE

Based in Traditional Chinese Medicine, acupuncture involves the insertion of very fine needles into the skin at specific points to influence the body's functioning. These points are considered to rest on 'meridians', or channels of a network of energy called 'chi' that flows throughout the body. Each meridian is thought to be related to specific internal functions and imbalances in the flow of chi are thought to lead to disease processes in whichever internal function the imbalanced meridian governs. Acupuncture is thought to correct this imbalance, thereby alleviating the disease process. The neurological mechanisms of acupuncture are beyond the scope of this chapter, and are more thoroughly covered in other texts (e.g., 36,37).

One open clinical trial of 18 anxious adult subjects found that acupuncture significantly increased nighttime endogenous melatonin secretion, as well as improving PSG measures of SOL, TST, and SE (38). Although this was not a group of people with insomnia, we do know that insomnia and anxiety are closely related (39,40), and it is reasonable to assume that if acupuncture can improve sleep in those without a diagnosed insomnia disorder, then it may produce similar or greater changes in those with insomnia. To date, very little efficacy data exists on the effects of acupuncture on insomnia. Almost all of the data come from case-series studies showing improvement of sleep in individuals with disorders other than insomnia (e.g., HIV, stress) (41,42). In addition, many have publication or location biases (43).

Alternate Forms

Acupuncture is sometimes used in combination with other forms of traditional Eastern medicine, such as moxibustion. Moxibustion is the combustion of mugwort herb that has been ground into a powder; it is either applied directly to the skin or held over acupuncture points and is thought to warm and stimulate the circulation and chi. Electroacupuncture is the application of a pulsating electrical current to acupuncture needles. This is thought to provide stronger and more prolonged stimulation to the acupuncture point than could be attained via finger stimulation alone. Acupressure involves the application of finger pressure, not needles, to acupuncture sites. Auriculotherapy involves stimulation of specific acupoints on the auricle of the ear in order to treat various disorders of the body. To date, none of these alternate forms of acupuncture have been adequately assessed in patients with insomnia.

MASSAGE

Massage is manipulation of the body's soft tissues (muscles, connective tissue, lymphatic vessels, etc.) either manually or with aids such as rollers or rocks. Various types of massage exist, from Swedish "relaxation" massage to deep tissue "shiatsu" massage. Each can be applied to various parts of the body, including feet, back, shoulders, and face. Among the many goals of massage (physical, therapeutic, psychological) it has the potential to improve sleep by reducing somatic arousal and/or cognitive arousal, similar to the previously reviewed relaxation methods (44).

To date, no studies have specifically examined the effects of massage on insomnia. Several case-series studies have been performed which examine the effect of various types of massage on sleep in populations without insomnia. For instance, a back massage technique similar to Effleurage (i.e., skim or lightly touch the skin) has been shown to improve sleep in elderly hospital patients. One technique of massage combined with sesame oil, increased post-massage sleep time versus no-treatment control in healthy infants versus control group (45).

AROMATHERAPY

Aromatherapy is a rapidly growing subfield of Complementary and Alternative Medicine (46), but little evidence exists for the efficacy of aroma alone. Aromatic essential oils reported to have calming, relaxing or sedating effects include: Bergamot *(Citrus bergamia)*, Roman Chamomile (*Chamomelium nobilis*), Jasmine (*Jasminum grandiflorum*), Lavender (*Lavandula angustifolia*), Mandarin (*Citrus deliciosa*), Marjoram (*Origanum majorana*), Melissa (*Melissa officinalis*), Neroli (*Neroli bigarade*), Patchouli (*Pogostemon cabin*), Egypt Rose (*Rosa damascene*), Ylang-ylang (*Cananga odourata*), and Vetiver (*Vetivera zizanoides*) (47). Aromatherapy is dispersed via mists or a specialized misting machine, sprayed on pillows, placed in sachets, potpourri, or scented oil warmers, or combined with massage. As with herbal therapies, the exact "mechanisms of action are speculative and unclear "(48).

Lavender

One small (N = 10) randomized controlled trial using a cross-cover design showed a trend ($p = 0.07$) for Lavender oil (*Lavandula angustifolia*) to improve scores on the PSQI (48). Another small (N = 12) study of children aged 12 to 15 with autism and learning difficulties showed no benefit on sleep patterns of aromatherapy massage with lavender oil (49). In a single-blind repeated measures study of 42 female college students, diluted lavender fragrance had a beneficial effect on several sleep parameters—sleep latency, insomnia severity, and sleep quality (50). Other studies have shown some improvements in sleep of "healthy" sleepers, but these have not been translated to insomnia patients (51). Effective proportions of lavender oil/carrier oil have yet to be confirmed through further studies.

Sandalwood

A study using inhaled diluted sandalwood oil in sleep-disturbed rats showed significant decreases in total wake time and an increase in total nonrapid eye movement sleep (52). This method of aromatherapy may be useful in individuals with difficulty maintaining sleep, but human replication of this study is lacking.

Aromatherapy is not recommended in critically ill patients due to the unclear research on safety and efficacy in this population (53). Contraindications to the use of aromatherapy include pregnancy, recent surgery, thrombosis, fractures/wounds, and some medications (54).

SUMMARY

There are a wide variety of "other" types of nonpharmacological treatments used to treat insomnia, not including stimulus control, sleep restriction, and cognitive therapy (1,2), which are covered elsewhere in this volume. Progressive muscle relaxation and paradoxical intention both have significant empirical backing, and have been listed as "efficacious" by the Standards of Practice Committee of the American Academy of Sleep Medicine, while biofeedback has good empirical backing and is listed as "probably efficacious" (3). Other forms of relaxation therapy, yoga, bright light therapy, exercise, acupuncture, massage, and aromatherapy, all show some promise as treatments for insomnia, but do not have sufficient empirical support to be recommended as treatments. Future studies are needed to more effectively evaluate these alternate treatments of insomnia.

APPENDIX A
RELAXATION PROCEDURE

Please close your eyes and get as comfortable as possible. Keep your eyes closed throughout the procedure and listen to my instructions. **(If legs or arms are crossed ask them to uncross them.)** I am going to help you achieve a deeper level of relaxation with the following procedures. Most people find this is an enjoyable experience. It is not hypnosis. You will not lose consciousness and will not lose control.

I am going to ask you to tense different muscles of your body. When I do, I want you to focus all your attention on those muscles until I say, "relax". As soon as I say, "relax" I want you to relax muscles immediately. Throughout the tensing and relaxing phases it is very important for you to focus all of your attention on the sensation coming from your muscles. It is also important to only tense the one muscle group at a time while leaving the others as relaxed as possible. Even if this means you cannot fully tense the target muscle group.

FOREHEAD

This time when I say "now", I want you to tense the muscles of your forehead by raising your eyebrows as high as they will go and wrinkling your forehead. "NOW" Keep your muscles tight... I want you to feel the strain and tension... "RELAX" Relax immediately... Just give up control of the muscles... Smooth out the muscles on your forehead letting all tension slip away... Feel the muscles relax and become loose and limp... The more carefully you focus your attention on calmness and tranquility, the greater the relaxation effect you will enjoy...

(Relax phase should take 45 seconds).

EYES AND NOSE

This time when I say "now", tense the muscle in the middle part of your face by closing your eyes tightly and wrinkling your nose. "NOW" Keep your muscles tight... feel the strain and tension as your muscles work. "RELAX." Relax immediately... Just let those muscles go loose and limp... soft and calm... Compare in your mind the feeling of tension you were feeling just a few seconds ago in your eye and nose muscles to the restful feeling that is now gradually emerging...

(Relax phase should take 45 seconds).

MOUTH

This time when I say "now", I want you to tense the lower part of your face by pursing your lips, pressing your teeth together and pressing your tongue against the roof of your mouth. "NOW" Keep the muscles tight... The muscles are working very hard. "RELAX." Relax immediately and completely... Let your teeth part, and let all the muscles in your jaw and around your mouth relax... Let the tension in those muscles melt away... Let your muscles go loose and limp... Soft and calm...

(Relax phase should take 45 seconds).

SHOULDERS AND MIDDLE BACK

This time when I say "now" I want you to tense the large muscle groups in your shoulders and the middle of your back by pulling your shoulders up and back as though you were trying to touch your shoulder blades behind your ears. Do this "NOW". Tense your muscles... Feel the burning. "RELAX" Relax completely... Feel the tightness in your muscles going away... Feel the stillness and peacefulness... Just give up control of the muscles and then let them lie there quietly. This is an area where a lot of people hold tension during the day. Just let these muscles go loose and limp... Soft and calm...

(Relax phase should take 45 seconds).

RIGHT BICEP

This time when I say "NOW," go ahead and tense the bicep of your right arm, by bending your arm at the elbow and flexing. Remember, I want you to try to keep your hand and forearm relaxed, as well as your shoulder. Make sure not to make a fist with your hand. "NOW". Keep it tight... feel the strain... feel the tension. (wait 7 seconds) "RELAX." Relax completely and immediately...

Think about how relaxed your muscles feel... Imagine the tightness and pain flowing out of your bicep... Let your muscles go loose and limp... Soft and calm...

(relax phase should take 45 seconds).

RIGHT HAND AND FOREARM

When I say "now" I want you to go ahead and tense the muscles of your right hand and forearm by clenching your fists. Remember to only tense this muscle group while leaving the others as relaxed as possible. "NOW" Keep it tight... feel the strain... feel the tension. (7 seconds) "RELAX." Relax completely and immediately.

Just give up control of the muscles and then let them lie there quietly... Compare in your mind the feeling of tension you were feeling just a few seconds ago in your right hand and forearm to the restful feeling that is now gradually emerging...

(Relax phase should take 45 seconds).

LEFT BICEP (See RIGHT BICEP above)

LEFT HAND AND FOREARM (see RIGHT HAND AND FOREARM above)

RIGHT UPPER LEG

When I say "now", tense the muscles in your upper right leg. The thigh has many muscles that work in opposition to each other. You can tense all of these at the same time by raising your leg about an inch and making your thigh hard. "NOW" Feel the strain and tension in your muscles... Keep the muscles tight... "RELAX" Relax completely... Feel the peacefulness... Focus on this peacefulness... Give up the control of your muscles and focus on the feelings of peace and tranquility... Feel the muscles relax and become loose and limp, tension flowing away like water out of a faucet... Focus on and notice the difference between the tension and the relaxation. (Relax phase should take 45 seconds)

RIGHT CALF

When I say "now", tense your right calf by pointing your foot and toes forward. Don't strain too hard, this muscle has a tendency to cramp. "NOW" Tighten the muscle... (only 3 seconds here). "RELAX" Relax completely... Focus on the stillness... Just give up control of the muscles and then let them lie there quietly... Compare in your mind the feeling of tension you were feeling just a few minutes ago to the restful feeling that is now gradually emerging... Let the comfortable feelings of tranquility grow deeper and deeper...deeper and deeper. Feel the peaceful... calm sensations. (Relax phase should take 45 seconds).

LEFT UPPER LEG (see RIGHT UPPER LEG above)

LEFT CALF (see RIGHT CALF above) (tense for only 3 seconds)

REFERENCES

1. Chesson AL Jr, Anderson WM, Littner M, et al. Practice parameters for the nonpharmacologic treatment of chronic insomnia. An American Academy of Sleep Medicine report. Standards of Practice Committee of the American Academy of Sleep Medicine. Sleep 1999; 22(8):1128–1133.
2. Morin CM, Hauri PJ, Espie CA, et al. Nonpharmacologic treatment of chronic insomnia. An American Academy of Sleep Medicine review. Sleep 1999; 22(8):1134–1156.
3. Morgenthaler T, Kramer M, Alessi C, et al. Practice parameters for the psychological and behavioral treatment of insomnia: An update. An american academy of sleep medicine report. Sleep 2006; 29(11):1415–1419.

4. Morin CM, Culbert JP, Schwartz SM. Nonpharmacological interventions for insomnia: A meta-analysis of treatment efficacy. Am J Psychiatry 1994; 151(8):1172–1180.
5. Murtagh DR, Greenwood KM. Identifying effective psychological treatments for insomnia: A meta-analysis. J Consult Clin Psychol 1995; 63(1):79–89.
6. Jacobson E. Progressive relaxation. Chicago, IL: University of Chicago Press, 1929.
7. Wolpe J. Psychotherapy by reciprocal inhibition. Stanford, CA: Stanford University Press, 1958.
8. Jacobson E. Progressive relaxation; a physiological and clinical investigation of muscular states and their significance in psychology and medical practice. Chicago, IL: The University of Chicago Press, 1929.
9. Lichstein KL. Clinical relaxation strategies. New York, NY: Wiley, 1988.
10. Morin CM, Espie CA. Insomnia : A clinical guide to assessment and treatment. New York, NY: Kluwer Academic/Plenum Publishers, 2003.
11. Smith JC. Relaxation, meditation and mindfulness. New York, NY: Springer Pub Co, 2005.
12. Hammond DC. What is neurofeedback? J Neurother 2007; 10(4):25–36.
13. Bell JS. The use of EEG theta biofeedback in the treatment of a patient with sleep-onset insomnia. Biofeedback Self Regul 1979; 4(3):229–236.
14. Hauri PJ, Percy L, Hellekson C, et al. The treatment of psychophysiologic insomnia with biofeedback: A replication study. Biofeedback self Regul 1982; 7(2):223–235.
15. Shannahoff-Khalsa DS. Kundalini Yoga Meditation Techniques for the Treatment of Obsessive-Compulsive and OC Spectrum Disorders. Brief Treat Crisis Interv 2003; 3(3):369–382.
16. Gooneratne NS. Complementary and alternative medicine for sleep disturbances in older adults. Clin Geriatr Med 2008; 24(1):121–138, viii.
17. Chen KM, Tseng WS. Pilot-testing the effects of a newly-developed silver yoga exercise program for female seniors. J Nurs Res 2008; 16(1):37–46.
18. Khalsa SB. Treatment of chronic insomnia with yoga: A preliminary study with sleep-wake diaries. Appl Psychophysiol Biofeedback 2004; 29(4):269–278.
19. Rajput V, Bromley SM. Chronic insomnia: A practical review. Am Fam Physician 1999; 60(5):1431–1438, discussion 41–42.
20. Sack RL, Auckley D, Auger RR, et al. Circadian rhythm sleep disorders: Part II, advanced sleep phase disorder, delayed sleep phase disorder, free-running disorder, and irregular sleep-wake rhythm: An American academy of sleep medicine review. Sleep 2007; 30(11):1484–1501.
21. Lingjaerde O, Bratlid T, Hansen T. Insomnia during the "dark period" in northern Norway. An explorative, controlled trial with light treatment. Acta Psychiatr Scand 1985; 71(5):506–512.
22. Campbell SS, Dawson D, Anderson MW. Alleviation of sleep maintenance insomnia with timed exposure to bright light. J Am Geriatr Soc 1993; 41(8):829–836.
23. Suhner AG, Murphy PJ, Campbell SS. Failure of timed bright light exposure to alleviate age-related sleep maintenance insomnia. J Am Geriatr Soc 2002; 50(4):617–623.
24. Friedman L, Zeitzer JM, Kushida C, et al. Scheduled bright light for treatment of insomnia in older adults. J Am Geriatr Soc 2009; 57(3):441–452.
25. Terman M, Terman JS. Bright light therapy: Side effects and benefits across the symptom spectrum. J Clin Psychiatry 1999; 60(11):799–808, quiz 9.
26. Fletcher GF, Balady G, Blair SN, et al. Statement on exercise: Benefits and recommendations for physical activity programs for all Americans. A statement for health professionals by the Committee on Exercise and Cardiac Rehabilitation of the Council on Clinical Cardiology, American Heart Association. Circulation 1996; 94(4):857–862.
27. Horne JA, Moore VJ. Sleep EEG effects of exercise with and without additional body cooling. Electroencephalogr Clin Neurophysiol 1985; 60(1):33–38.
28. Horne JA, Staff LH. Exercise and sleep: Body-heating effects. Sleep 1983; 6(1):36–46.
29. Youngstedt SD, O'Connor PJ, Dishman RK. The effects of acute exercise on sleep: A quantitative synthesis. Sleep 1997; 20(3):203–214.
30. Singh NA, Clements KM, Fiatarone MA. A randomized controlled trial of the effect of exercise on sleep. Sleep 1997; 20(2):95–101.
31. King AC, Oman RF, Brassington GS, et al. Moderate-intensity exercise and self-rated quality of sleep in older adults. A randomized controlled trial. JAMA 1997; 277(1):32–37.
32. Morgan K. Daytime activity and risk factors for late-life insomnia. J Sleep Res 2003; 12(3):231–238.
33. Sherrill DL, Kotchou K, Quan SF. Association of physical activity and human sleep disorders. Arch Intern Med 1998; 158(17):1894–1898.
34. Buysse DJ, Reynolds CF III, Monk TH, et al. The Pittsburgh Sleep Quality Index: A new instrument for psychiatric practice and research. Psychiatry Res 1989; 28(2):193–213.
35. Tanaka H, Taira K, Arakawa M, et al. Effects of short nap and exercise on elderly people having difficulty in sleeping. Psychiatry Clin Neurosci 2001; 55(3):173–174.

36. Stux G, Pomeranz B. Acupuncture textbook and atlas with 98 figures and an acupuncture selector. Berlin, Germany: Springer-Verlag, 1987.
37. Baldry P. Acupuncture, Trigger Points, and Musculoskeletal Pain: A Scientific Approach to Acupuncture for use by Doctors and Physiotherapists in the Diagnosis and Management of Myofascial Trigger Point Pain, 2nd ed. Edinburgh, New York, NY: Churchill Livingstone, 1993.
38. Spence DW, Kayumov L, Chen A, et al. Acupuncture increases nocturnal melatonin secretion and reduces insomnia and anxiety: A preliminary report. J Neuropsychiatry Clin Neurosci 2004; 16(1): 19–28.
39. Taylor DJ, Lichstein KL, Durrence HH. Insomnia as a Health Risk Factor. Behav Sleep Med 2003; 1(4):227–247.
40. Taylor DJ, Lichstein KL, Durrence HH, et al. Epidemiology of insomnia, depression, and anxiety. Sleep 2005; 28(11):1457–1464.
41. Phillips KD, Skelton WD. Effects of individualized acupuncture on sleep quality in HIV disease. J Assoc Nurses AIDS Care 2001; 12(1):27–39.
42. Sommers E, Porter K, DeGurski S. Providers of complementary and alternative health services in Boston respond to September 11. Am J Public Health 2002; 92(10):1597–1598.
43. Vickers A, Goyal N, Harland R, et al. Do certain countries produce only positive results? A systematic review of controlled trials. Control Clin Trials 1998; 19(2):159–166.
44. Soden K, Vincent K, Craske S, et al. A randomized controlled trial of aromatherapy massage in a hospice setting. Palliat Med 2004; 18(2):87–92.
45. Agarwal KN, Gupta A, Pushkarna R, et al. Effects of massage & use of oil on growth, blood flow & sleep pattern in infants. Indian J Med Res 2000; 112:212–217.
46. Zollman C, Vickers A. ABC of complementary medicine. BMJ 2000; 319(7216):1050–1053.
47. Perry N, Perry E. Aromatherapy in the management of psychiatric disorders: Clinical and neuropharmacological perspectives. CNS Drugs 2006; 20(4):257–280.
48. Lewith GT, Godfrey AD, Prescott P. A single-blinded, randomized pilot study evaluating the aroma of Lavandula augustifolia as a treatment for mild insomnia. J Altern Complement Med 2005; 11(4): 631–637.
49. Williams TI. Evaluating effects of aromatherapy massage on sleep in children with autism: A pilot study. Evid Based Complement Alternat Med 2006; 3(3):373–377.
50. Lee IS, Lee GJ. Effects of lavender aromatherapy on insomnia and depression in women college students. Taehan Kanho Hakhoe Chi 2006; 36(1):136–143.
51. Goel N, Kim H, Lao RP. An olfactory stimulus modifies nighttime sleep in young men and women. Chronobiol Int 2005; 22(5):889–904.
52. Ohmori A, Shinomiya K, Utsu Y, et al. Effect of santalol on the sleep-wake cycle in sleep-disturbed rats. Nihon Shinkei Seishin Yakurigaku Zasshi 2007; 27(4):167–171.
53. Richards K, Nagel C, Markie M, et al. Use of complementary and alternative therapies to promote sleep in critically ill patients. Crit Care Nurs Clin North Am 2003; 15(3):329–340.
54. Long L, Huntley A, Ernst E. Which complementary and alternative therapies benefit which conditions? A survey of the opinions of 223 professional organizations. Complement Ther Med 2001; 9(3):178–185.

27 Cognitive Therapy for Insomnia

Colin A. Espie

University of Glasgow Sleep Centre, Sackler Institute of Psychobiological Research, Southern General Hospital, Glasgow, Scotland, U.K.

Jason Ellis

Northumbria Centre for Sleep Research, School of Psychology and Sports Science, Northumbria University, Newcastle upon Tyne, U.K.

INTRODUCTION

Cognitive therapy is a generic term, referring to a broad set of therapeutic techniques designed to address the maladaptive thought processes associated with a specific disease or disorder. As the term *cognition* encompasses all aspects of thinking (i.e., perception, attention, memory, problem solving, attitudes, beliefs, attributions, and expectations), the breadth and range of cognitive therapies is extensive, and most certainly has not yet been exhausted. It should also be acknowledged that even predominantly behavioral interventions (Chapter 24) should be considered within a cognitive context, in that, behavior is often determined, and as such challenged and changed, through cognitive processes. However, the aim of this chapter is to examine the contribution of cognitive therapies to the management of insomnia, and therefore the focus will be on interventions that are predominantly cognitively orientated.

COGNITIVE-ATTENTIONAL PROCESSES IN INSOMNIA

Before describing and evaluating these cognitive interventions in turn, two issues merit consideration. First, it remains rather unclear what terminology is best applied to these cognitive 'treatments'. Does each constitute a distinct cognitive therapy? Are they better regarded as cognitive techniques or as cognitive strategies? Certainly at this point we would advocate caution in any claim that there is a well-tested cognitive therapy for insomnia, in the traditional sense. With this caveat in mind, we will inevitably use terms somewhat interchangeably in this chapter, but we will always be referring to intervention upon some aspect of the cognitive-attentional system. Second, however, and perhaps in contrast to the above, we do actually have several well-argued cognitive theoretical frameworks for understanding insomnia. It is beyond the scope of this chapter to review these in detail, but three well articulated and empirically supported models converge in recognizing the importance of cognitive-attentional systems in the aetiology and maintenance of insomnia. These are Perlis' neurocognitive model (1), Harvey's cognitive model (2), and Espie's psychobiological inhibition model which incorporates the attention-intention-effort pathway (3,4) [for a comprehensive review, see Perlis et al, 5].

COGNITIVE THERAPEUTIC APPROACHES FOR INSOMNIA

Each of the cognitive interventions outlined in this chapter aim to address one or more of seven potential cognitive-attentional mechanisms that either fuel or are a causal pathway to insomnia. In Table 1 these have been brought together under three cognitive domains each having two or three associated therapeutic mechanisms. The types of thoughts that, in our opinion, are most likely to respond to each cognitive intervention have also been outlined.

Probably the best known approaches are those that can be termed *active rational*. Sleep education is seldom a stand-alone therapy, but can provide, along with data gathered from personal sleep diaries, observations and experiments, the raw material upon which formal cognitive restructuring can operate. Thus these corrective and appraisal actions may ameliorate the cognitive component of insomnia. Consequently, these will be considered together in the same section.

We suggest that there is also a *protective-preventative* domain of cognitive action. Three cognitive therapies are linked here because they have in common a focus upon avoiding or curtailing sleep-interfering mental processes. Cognitive control is viewed as a preemptive strike

Table 1 Cognitive Therapies for Insomnia and their Proposed Action Upon Cognitive Attentional Mechanisms (After 6)

Cognitive domain	Specific action upon cognitive attentional mechanisms	Thought content most likely to respond	Specific cognitive therapy
Active-rational			
	Corrective	Misunderstanding of sleep processes and needs	Sleep education
	Appraisal	Intrusive, irrational but compelling negative thinking	Cognitive restructuring
Protective-preventative			
	Preemptive	Rehearsal, planning, self-evaluative reflections	Cognitive control
	Blocking	Repetitive but nonaffect laden thoughts	Articulatory suppression
	Distraction	Agitated, unfocused, flitting thoughts, mental tension	Imagery training
Passive-paradoxical			
	Acceptance	Persistent worry about lack of control over sleep	Mindfulness meditation
	Disengagement	Rumination about sleeplessness and its consequences, sleep effort	Paradoxical intention

against thought content that would otherwise occupy quiet wakefulness; and imagery training and the lesser known articulatory suppression technique distract or block unwanted intrusive thinking.

Finally, we suggest that there are useful *passive-paradoxical* techniques. Unlike the cognitive therapies, which at some level emphasize control or at least active management of thoughts and behaviors, paradoxical intention is a disengagement method and mindfulness an acceptance-based approach. Indeed paradox might even be regarded as the extreme/ultimate end of the acceptance dimension.

COGNITIVE RESTRUCTURING AND SLEEP EDUCATION

Cognitive restructuring was developed as part of Beck's (7,8) Cognitive Behavioral Therapy and Ellis' (9) Rational Emotive Therapy. The rationale behind cognitive restructuring suggests that negative thoughts have the potential to create a negative schema, through an interpretative bias. In other words, a particular problem or issue (e.g. perception of poor sleep) will stimulate the activation and refinement of distal attitudes, beliefs, and expectations about that problem and these will be evaluated against any thoughts, feelings, or behaviors believed to be a result of the problem (irrespective of whether they are or not), further maintaining a catastrophic schema. As such, cognitive restructuring involves eliciting and discussing the responses to six main questions (Table 2) in order to identify, appraise and correct any and all forms of dysfunctional thought.

Table 2 The Process of Cognitive Restructuring

1. Are these attitudes and beliefs about the problem accurate?
2. What evidence is there to support these attitudes and beliefs?
3. Are there alternative explanations for these attitudes and beliefs?
4. Do I underestimate my ability to cope with the current problem?
5. What is the worst that can happen if these attitudes and beliefs are true?
6. What can I do to address the problem?

Dysfunctional sleep-related attitudes and beliefs are generally accepted to be a central feature of insomnia. For example, Morin, Stone, Trinkle et al (10) found that people with insomnia endorsed more dysfunctional beliefs about sleep compared to controls. However, the extent to which they mediate the relationship between perceptions of sleep, catastrophic interpretations about the consequences of poor sleep, and attributions for insomnia is still unclear, but thought to be significant (11). In addition, it has been shown that the endocrine system reacts negatively when there is a discrepancy between what is expected and what really exists (12). Although Eriksen et al's (12) study related to stress, it has been shown that subjective sleep quantity and quality are better indicators of insomnia reporting than objective sleep measures (13). Additionally, researchers have found that irrespective of the actual sleep obtained, those who scored highly on the Dysfunctional Beliefs and Attitudes to Sleep Scale (DBAS) were also those who were more likely to complain of disrupted sleep (14,15).

The primary mechanism by which dysfunctional beliefs affect sleep is thought to be through the relationship between attitudes and sleep-incompatible behaviors. An individual who believes that they need eight hours of sleep is more likely to reduce their sleep efficiency by attempting to obtain sleep during the day, lying in bed when not asleep, or going to bed earlier, all of which are sleep incompatible behaviors and are likely to exacerbate the problem.

Dysfunctional beliefs may be particularly pertinent for older adults, whose sleep patterns can change as a function of normal ageing. Changes in the timing of the circadian rhythm, as well as structural changes in sleep architecture, can render the belief that eight hours of consolidated sleep is essential for normal functioning as even more unrealistic (16) and the dissonance between this expectation and perceived reality becomes greater and more anxiety provoking.

The notion of general sleep education falls within the remit of cognitive restructuring in so far as its intention is to provide information about a) what constitutes 'normal', or more likely, 'typical' sleep over the life span and the intra-individual differences therein, b) what sleep disruption is, c) an exploration of the factors which exacerbate or increase the likelihood of sleep disruption, and d) an exploration of the factors which increase the likelihood of good sleep occurring. In this instance, exploring the individuals' constructs of 'sleep' and 'sleep disorder' can offer a platform for identifying sleep-related dissonance and provide the beginnings of an intervention aimed at reducing this dissonance.

The Efficacy of Cognitive Restructuring in the Management of Insomnia

Unfortunately, cognitive restructuring has not been evaluated as a stand-alone therapy, however, Edinger, Wohlgemuth, Radtke, Marsh & Quillian (17) found that Cognitive Behavior Therapy for Insomnia (CBT-I), which specifically targeted sleep-related dysfunctional beliefs, resulted in both improvements to objectively measured sleep parameters and subjective sleep satisfaction. Likewise, Espie et al (18) reported that many item scores on the DBAS reduced, following CBT. Indeed, interventions that have incorporated cognitive restructuring tend to routinely use this measure as a secondary index of treatment efficacy (19). In these respects, the evidence for incorporating cognitive restructuring within CBT-I is good. However, one of the main issues with cognitive restructuring is that it is difficult to deliver in a self-help or remote format (e.g. manualized CBT-I), because a therapist is usually needed to help people identify and challenge current negative schemas and develop new positive ones.

COGNITIVE CONTROL

It is well documented that intrusive, unwanted thoughts and images are a prominent feature of most psychological disorders (20) and that attempts to suppress intrusive thoughts usually result in a rebound effect. Clark and Rhyno (21) define intrusive thoughts as *'any distinct, identifiable cognitive event that is unwanted, unintended, and recurrent. It interrupts the flow of thoughts, interferes in task performance, is associated with negative affect, and is difficult to control.'* (p. 4)

The role of intrusive thoughts, and the subsequent use of thought control strategies to deal with them in insomnia, is well documented (22–24). In addition, when the suppression of presleep cognitive activity has been experimentally manipulated, those told to suppress had longer sleep-onset latencies than nonsupressors (25).

Table 3 Cognitive Control ("putting the day to rest") instructions

You may find this technique particularly useful for thoughts that have to do with the past day and planning for the following day. The aim is to put the day to bed, along with your plans for the next day . . . so that you can get to sleep!. If you can manage to stop the thinking you usually do in bed, before it happens, then you should sleep better.

To put the day to rest:-

1. *Set aside 20 minutes in the early evening (say around 7 pm.) and sit down with a pen and a notebook*
2. *Think of what has happened during the day, how it has gone, and how you feel about it – evaluate things*
3. *Write down anything you need to do on a 'to do' list, and any steps that you can take to complete any loose ends*
4. *Try to use your 20 minutes to leave you feeling more organized and in control and close the notebook when you are done*
5. *When it comes to bedtime remind yourself that you have already dealt with things when they come to your mind*
6. *If new thoughts come up note them down on a piece of paper at your bedside, to be dealt with the next day*

Source: From Ref. 33, pp. 97–98.

Harvey (26) examined the individual contributions of the different forms of thought control in insomnia; namely distraction (focusing away from the thought), punishment (self-chastisement for the thought), reappraisal (logical interpretation of the thought), worry (worrying about the thought), and social control (seeking support about the thought's validity). She found that poor sleepers were more likely to use distraction, reappraisal, and worry, as opposed to punishment and social control. However, to explain paradoxical effects, Harvey makes a distinction between suppression and replacement when distraction is used as a thought control strategy, believing suppression to be a negatively toned thought control strategy and replacement to be a positive one.

Perhaps surprisingly, Ellis and Cropley (27) found that distraction (not separated into suppression and replacement) was related to not developing chronic insomnia, and that the main strategies used by people with chronic insomnia were worry and punishment, with punishment being associated with a longer reported duration of insomnia. This pattern of thought control use conforms to findings from research on other anxiety related disorders (28). Further support for the role of thought control in the maintenance of insomnia comes from Watts, Coyle and East (29). They found the presleep cognitions of nonworrying people with insomnia focused on not sleeping, whereas worrying insomniacs focused on a diversity of topics. In a more recent study, intrusive thoughts and avoidance behaviors were not strongly related to subjective sleep quality, only objective sleep latency (30) suggesting that the outcome measures used may be an important factor in determining the importance of cognitive intrusions. Similarly, Bonnet and Arand (31) found no increases in subjective anxiety after a period of poor sleep in 10 patients with insomnia. These findings together suggest that thought control does play a role in insomnia but may not lead to, or exacerbate further, cognitive activity directly.

The only specific cognitive control procedure used in the treatment of insomnia was initially outlined in a case study first described some 20 years ago (32). It is really an extension of the idea of stimulus control (Chapter 24), but recognizes that it may be primarily thoughts and worries that seem to be incompatible with successful sleep. The great majority of people with insomnia report excessive mental arousal in bed. They complain of difficulty in emptying their minds and of racing thoughts. Cognitive control comprises a simple set of procedures to remove mental activity from the bed and bedroom environment, or at least to reduce the influence of cognitive activity upon sleep. The instructional set is provided in Table 3.

The Efficacy of Cognitive Control in the Management of Insomnia

Although there are no interventions solely related to cognitive control within insomnia populations cognitive control does fall within the broader premise of sleep stimulus control, which is highly efficacious for insomnia (34–36), and cognitive control procedures are routinely used within multicomponent CBT (33).

Table 4 Instructions for Using Articulatory Suppression

1. *While lying in bed with your eyes closed*
2. *Repeat the word 'the' once or twice every second in your head*
3. *Don't say it out loud, but it may help if you 'mouth it'*
4. *Keep up these repetitions for about 5 minutes or until sleep ensues*

ARTICULATORY SUPPRESSION

As the review of cognitive factors in the previous section might suggest 'thought-blocking' techniques have obvious intuitive appeal in insomnia. Although, there is some evidence that thought suppression may be a counterproductive strategy employed by poor sleepers (37), Morin & Espie (33) report that there is one form of thought-blocking that might be recommended.

Articulatory suppression is a technique widely used in studies of working memory. The phonological component of the central executive is referred to as the articulatory loop, which serves to hold in store the verbal elements required in any cognitive task. Levey et al. (38) applied articulatory suppression techniques to the treatment of insomnia. They thought that by blocking up this short-term store with semantically meaningless phonemes no other mental information would be processed. They presented an interesting case series supporting this contention, particularly for sleep maintenance insomnia (i.e. using the technique at any wakening from sleep). The instructions for articulatory suppression are summarized in Table 4.

The Efficacy of Articulatory Suppression in the Management of Insomnia

As for cognitive control, there is only case study material supporting the efficacy of articulatory suppression (and other thought blocking techniques) as single component therapy.

IMAGERY TRAINING

Harvey (39) suggests that unwanted cognitive activity can be visual as well as verbal, and controlling or replacing these images, using distraction techniques, has been shown to result in reduced arousal in several anxiety-related disorders (40–42). It has been demonstrated that poor sleepers report more negative images than normal sleepers and the imagery of poor sleepers tends to be catastrophic (envisioning the worst possible outcome), in that it is usually distressing and related to physical sensation (43). They also showed that levels of visual imagery in poor sleepers related to an increased subjective Sleep Onset Latency (43). Using replacement distraction visual imagery when faced with a visually catastrophic stimulus has been shown to be effective in samples of poor sleepers (44,45).

The aim of imagery training is to block or distract the individual from intrusive and preoccupying sleep-related thoughts, using visualization techniques. Imagery techniques are useful for some but not all patients, probably because there are individual differences in the ability to visualize. First, there is need to establish the patient's ability to visualize, and their degree of comfort with the process. This can be achieved by asking them to close their eyes and try to picture some objects (a boat under sail in a gentle breeze, a clock face with a ticking second hand). Second, it is better to get patients to decide upon an imaginable scene for them to use rather than to leave it literally to their imagination at the time. For example, if it is something like walking through a favorite piece of parkland and gardens, they should prepare the scene and the sequence in advance, so it is like 'rolling the tape' when it comes to using the imagery. Finally, practice is crucial to train the imagery if it is going to be useful (33).

The Efficacy of Imagery Training in Managing Insomnia

Studies examining the efficacy of imagery training as a sole intervention are rare and this is reflected in AASM being unable to recommend it is a discrete management strategy. Morin & Azrin (46,47) found that stimulus control was more efficacious than imagery training but that the imagery training component was associated with shorter awakening durations. What is worth noting is that both of Morin and Azrin's studies showed an increase in efficacy at follow-up, suggesting that with increased use, the intervention may become more powerful. Whether this finding relates to increased sophistication and skill in the use of images to block unwanted thoughts over time or whether this is artefact remains to be seen. Commonly imagery is used alongside (other) relaxation techniques in clinical practice, and is used in some multicomponent CBT-I interventions.

MINDFULNESS & ACCEPTANCE-BASED THERAPIES

Although 'mindfulness' techniques have been around for a long time, (Buddhism is believed to originate in 6th Century BC), in one form of another, their incorporation into clinical research is recent. Mindfulness-Based Stress Reduction (MBSR) was developed in 48 by Kabatzin with the aim of reducing both cognitive and somatic arousal. This program consists of teaching the individual mindfulness principles, namely; nonjudging, patience, beginner's mind, trust, nonstriving, acceptance, and letting go. The premise behind mindfulness suggests that there are three stages which result in negative action towards a given event or object; a latency stage containing a deeper understanding of the self and its capabilities, a conscious stage whereby both internal and external stimuli are processed affectively in response to a threat to this latent self, and a reactive stage whereby actions 'spill out' as a result of this processing, creating emotional arousal. Mindfulness teaches the individual to attend to and manage both latency thoughts and conscious thoughts, thus avoiding negative actions, through practiced meditation and acceptance.

In insomnia, instead of attempting to suppress or control intrusive thoughts, a common occurrence presented by people with insomnia (49), which generally results in rumination or thought rebound, this intervention teaches the patient to acknowledge the thought, feeling or sensation, but not to dwell on it (i.e. to create cognitive deactivation) (50).

The Efficacy of Mindfulness in the Management of Insomnia

Although a relatively new area of investigation with regard to insomnia, the results from uncontrolled studies to date are promising. Lundh and Hindmarsh (51) asked 40 people with insomnia to monitor their presleep-onset thoughts, feelings, and bodily sensations, without any attempt to change them, over the period of one week, and compared sleep diaries before and afterward. The results showed reductions in sleep latency and increased sleep time. However, because there was no control group and no measure of treatment adherence, these results should be viewed cautiously. In another study, Ong, Shapiro & Manber (52) combined CBT with MBSR and found a relationship between meditation practice and reduced trait arousal. However, meditation adherence was only 57%, suggesting a problem with uptake. Finally, Yook and colleagues (53) showed significant improvements in sleep after eight weeks of mindfulness-based cognitive therapy for sleep problems in a sample of patients with anxiety disorders.

A better understanding of mindfulness is clearly warranted but whether it remains an adjunct to other therapies or can be utilized as a strategy in its own right remains to be seen.

PARADOXICAL INTENTION

Although it could be argued that paradoxical intention is not exclusively a cognitive therapy, in that it was not developed within a cognitive framework being more grounded in learning theory, throughout its refinement it has applied cognition to its existing elements.

The term *paradox* was termed long before the intention part was introduced by Frankl (54,55). Dubois (56), for example, suggested humor 'paradoxically' should be advocated for patients to help them in dealing with their symptoms. Furthermore, Dunlap (57,58) suggested one method that could be utilized to break a bad habit was to repetitively perform that particular habit. Frankl (59), who was also a proponent of humor in the therapeutic encounter, refined these early ideas, suggesting that in order to break vicious cycles of anticipatory anxiety surrounding a thought or behavior, individuals must focus in on that particular problem or perform that particular behavior repeatedly. Alongside paradoxical intention Frankl also outlined another therapeutic technique; dereflection. Because Frankl believed the roots of most psychological problems were caused by an overemphasis on the self, shifting attention away from the self might also be used to alleviate the problem (an early version of thought blocking/distraction).

The main advocate of paradoxical intention, since its inception, has been Ascher, who with various colleagues demonstrated its effectiveness in areas as diverse as urinary retention and agoraphobia (60,61). In each case, the use of paradoxical intention has lead to a reduction in symptom reporting, and in some cases, increases in self-efficacy.

Table 5 Suggested Rationale and Instructions for Using Paradoxical Intention Therapy in Insomnia

≪If you can't get to sleep it might seem reasonable to ask someone who is a good sleeper how he/ she manages it. What do you think they would say? Something like ≪I just fall asleep . . . it just happens . . . I don't do anything really?≪ You might think this is not very helpful, but the secret is right there – they do precisely nothing!≫

≪Sleep is a natural process which happens involuntarily. The good sleeper doesn't make it happen, or have some kind of method that you don't know about it. You are the one with all the methods and tactics, and none of them works! To become a good sleeper you need to learn to abandon all your efforts to sleep because they simply get in the way of the natural process. They make you too self-conscious about your sleep and about your sleep failures. You know how sometimes you lie awake for ages or toss and turn until it's getting close to morning time? And you feel some relief as you think that soon you can get up? Why do you sometimes fall asleep at that point? That's because you give up trying then and you give up being concerned. How about having that as a general approach. Try this:-

1. *When you are in bed lie in a comfortable position and put the light out*
2. *In the darkened room, keep your eyes open, and try to keep them open 'just for just a little while longer'. That's your catch phrase*
3. *As time goes by congratulate yourself on staying awake but relaxed*
4. *Remind yourself not to try to sleep but to let sleep overtake you, as you gently try to resist it*
5. *Keep this mind set going as long as you can, and if you get worried at staying awake remind yourself that that is the general idea, so you are succeeding*
6. *Don't actively prevent sleep by trying to rouse yourself. Be like the good sleeper, let sleep come to you*

Source: From Ref. 33.

Within the framework of insomnia, paradoxical intention aims to reduce the anxiety and frustration often experienced by people with insomnia at sleep-onset by recommending that the individual do the opposite of their normal behavior (Table 5). In this case, to lie down with their eyes open and attempt to stay awake for as long as possible. This strategy operates on the premise that, in insomnia, sleep onset is prevented because the patient is attempting to place sleep under voluntary control, resulting in arousal of the autonomic nervous system. In other words, the more effortful monitoring that is employed to sleep, the more likely it is to keep the individual awake, creating performance anxiety which then leads to catastrophic interpretations about daytime functioning, fuelling a vicious cycle of performance anxiety. Evidence for this comes from the use of measures such as the Glasgow Sleep Effort Scale, Sleep Associated Monitoring Index and Sleep Preoccupation Scale which, independently, have identified people with insomnia as being more effortful in their attempts to sleep, spending more time self-monitoring, and becoming increasingly anxious and sleep preoccupied when these efforts fail (62–64). As such, sleep may be facilitated by breaking the pathway between attention to sleep-related cues – increased intention to sleep – and increased effort to sleep (4).

The Efficacy of Paradoxical Intention in the Management of Insomnia

One of the first reports on the efficacy of paradoxical intention for insomnia came from Ascher and Efran (65) who demonstrated a significant reduction in SOL (from 40 minutes to 10 minutes). Although this was a very small sample, subsequent uncontrolled studies (66–69) and randomized controlled trials (70,71) suggested this to be a robust effect. On the other hand, three other studies have questioned the use of paradoxical intention, finding that it did not result in decreased sleep-onset latencies (72,73,74).

Overall, paradoxical intention appears to be effective and retains a 'guideline' rating according to the American Academy of Sleep Medicine (34). Recently, Broomfield & Espie (75) found that those who used paradoxical intention had lower levels of sleep performance anxiety and reduced their sleep effort compared to controls.

COGNITIVE THERAPY WITHIN COGNITIVE-BEHAVIORAL-THERAPY FOR INSOMNIA (CBT-I)

As is discussed in chapter 29, the main framework under which cognitive therapies are delivered and have been evaluated is within studies of multicomponent CBT-I. Cognitive therapies have taken various forms ranging from sleep education and low-level cognitive interventions, to in depth cognitive restructuring and paradoxical intention. Although this creates a difficulty when attempting to determine the relative value of cognitive therapy within CBT-I, there is undoubtedly very strong evidence that CBT-I as a "package" is an effective treatment for persistent insomnia. Cognitive components are perhaps integral to this success.

To date, there has been only one study that has formally examined cognitive therapy as a stand-alone treatment (76). Based on Harvey's (2) cognitive model, and using a mainly Socratic questioning approach, this therapy involved three phases (case formulation, personalized experiments with guided discovery, and planning for continued success whilst preventing against relapse). The therapeutic aim was to reverse the five main cognitive processes thought to maintain insomnia; namely, worry and rumination, attentional bias and monitoring for sleep-related threat, unhelpful beliefs about sleep, the use of safety behaviors that maintain unhelpful beliefs, and misperception of sleep and daytime deficits, (77). In terms of efficacy, significant improvements in sleep diary measures as well as significant reductions in anxiety and depression scores were obtained and maintained at 12 months follow up.

Although the lack of a control group or comparable intervention and the small sample size limit the reliability and generalizability of the Harvey et al. (76) study, it represents emerging evidence that cognitive therapy may prove to be effective for persistent insomnia. Whether it would outperform CBT-I as a standard therapy, however, remains questionable.

Another welcome development in the literature has been the examination of cognitive processes in insomnia beyond the actual intervention itself. Recently, interpersonal aspects surrounding the patient/therapist interaction have come under scrutiny. For example, one study has suggested that increased levels of perceived therapeutic alliance may provide additive efficacy to CBT-I (52). As such it may not be just the intervention itself, but the mode of delivery that can increase the chances of treatment success.

SUMMARY AND FUTURE DIRECTIONS

Clearly, cognitive therapies warrant further attention both as a stand-alone treatment and within the broader framework of CBT-I. What is clear is that there is a range of cognitive interventions to choose from. However, the evidence base is rather limited, relative to other CBT strategies (78). With increasing interest in addressing daytime cognitions of patients with chronic insomnia as well as their night-time symptoms, coupled with a broadening of cognitive models and therapies to include all aspects of cognition (both proximal and distal), an improved understanding of the impact cognitive therapies may not be far away. Another area, yet to be addressed, where cognitive therapies may prove beneficial, is in the domain of adjustment or acute insomnia (27). The two main factors that may differentiate acute insomnia from its chronic presentation are the absence of a conditioned response to the bedroom or pre-sleep routine and the presence of an identifiable stressor. Cognitive approaches may be appropriate to circumvent the establishment of poor sleep as a conditioned response, thus a therapeutic focus upon the perception of stress (rather than the actual stressor) may also be beneficial.

REFERENCES

1. Perlis ML, Giles DE, Mendelson WB, et al Psychophysiological insomnia: The behavioural model and a neurocognitive perspective. J Sleep Res 1997; 6:179–188.
2. Harvey AG. A cognitive model of insomnia. Behav Res Ther 2002; 40:869–893.
3. Espie CA. Insomnia: Conceptual issues in the development, persistence, and treatment of sleep disorder in adults. Annu Rev Psychol 2002; 53:215–243.
4. Espie CA, Broomfield NM, MacMahon KMA,et al. The attention-intention-effort pathway in the development of Psychophysiologic Insomnia: An invited theoretical review. Sleep Med Rev 2006; 10:215–245.
5. Perlis ML, et al. Etiology and pathophysiology of insomnia. In: Kryger MH, Roth T, Dement WC, eds. Principles and Practice of Sleep Medicine, 4th ed. Philadelphia, PA: WB Saunders, 2005.
6. Espie CA. The Psychological Treatment of Insomnia. England, Chichester: John Wiley and Sons Ltd., 1991.
7. Beck AT. Depression: Causes and Treatment. Philadelphia, PA: University of Pennsylvania Press, 1972.
8. Beck A. Cognitive therapy: Nature and relation to behavior therapy. Behav Ther 1970; 1(2):184–200.
9. Ellis A. Rational psychotherapy and individual psychology. J Individ Psychol 1957; 13:38–44.
10. Morin CM, Stone J, Trinkle D, et al. Dysfunctional Attitudes about Sleep Among Older Adults With and Without Insomnia Complaints. Psychol Aging 1993; 8(3):463–467.

11. Ellis J, Hampson SE, Cropley M. The role of sleep preoccupation in attributions for poor sleep. Sleep Med 2007; 8(3):277–280.
12. Eriksen HR, Olff M, Murison R, et al. The Time Dimension in Stress Responses: Relevance for Survival and Health. Psychiatry Res 1999; 85(1):39–50.
13. Riedel BW, Lichstein KL. Objective Sleep Measures and Subjective Sleep Satisfaction: How do Older Adults with Insomnia Define a Good Night's Sleep. Psychol Ageing 1998; 13(1):159–163.
14. Edinger JD, Glenn DM, Bastian LA, et al. Slow-wave sleep and waking cognitive performance II: Findings among middle-aged adults with and without insomnia complaints. Physiol Behav 2000; 70(1–2):127–134.
15. Edinger JD, Glenn DM, Bastian LA, et al. The roles of dysfunctional cognitions and other person factors in mediating insomnia complaints. Sleep 21:S144.
16. Lichstein KL, Fischer SM. Insomnia: In: Hersen M, Bellack AS, eds. Handbook of Clinical Behavior Therapy with Adults. New York, NY: Plenum Press, 1985:319–352.
17. Edinger JD, Wohlgemuth WK, Radtke RA, et al. Does Cognitive Behaviour Therapy alter dysfunctional beliefs about sleep? Sleep 2001; 24(5):591–599.
18. Espie CA, Inglis SJ, Harvey L, et al. Insomniacs' attributions: Psychometric properties of the Dysfunctional Beliefs and Attitudes about Sleep scale and the Sleep Disturbance Questionnaire. J Psychosom Res 2000; 48:141–148.
19. Morin CM, Blais F, Savard J. Are Changes in Beliefs and Attitudes about Sleep Related to Sleep Improvements in the Treatment of Insomnia. Behav Res Ther 2002; 40:741–752.
20. Wenzlaff RM, Wegner DM, Roper D. Depression and mental control: The resurgence of unwanted negative thoughts. J Pers Soc Psychol 1988; 55:882–892.
21. Clark DA. Rhyno S. Unwanted intrusive thoughts in nonclinical individuals. In: Clark's DA, eds. Intrusive Thoughts in Clinical Disorders: Theory, research, and Treatment. New York, NY: Guilford Press, 2004:1–29.
22. Borkovec TD. Insomnia. J Consult Clin Psychol 1982; 50:880–895.
23. Gendron L, Blais FC, Morin CM. Cognitive activity among insomniac patients. Sleep 1998; 21:130.
24. Lichstein KL, Rosenthal TL. Insomniacs' perceptions of cognitive versus somatic determinants of sleep disturbance. J Abnorm Psychol 1980; 89(1):105–107.
25. Gross RT, Borkovec TD. Effects of Cognitive Intrusion Manipulation on the Sleep-Onset Latency of Good Sleepers. Behav Ther 1982; 13:112–116.
26. Harvey AG. I Can't Sleep, My Mind is Racing! An Investigation of Strategies of Thought Control in Insomnia. Behav Cogn Psychother 2001; 29:3–11.
27. Ellis J, Cropley M. An examination of thought control strategies employed by acute and chronic insomniacs. Sleep Med 2002; 3(5):393–400.
28. Warda G, Bryant RA. Cognitive Bias in Acute Stress Disorder. Behav Res Ther 1998; 36(12):1177–1184.
29. Watts FN, Coyle K, East MP. The Contribution of Worry to Insomnia. Br J Clin Psychol 1994; 33:211–220.
30. Hall M, Buysse DJ, Dew MA, et al. Intrusive Thoughts and Avoidance Behaviours are Associated with Sleep Disturbances in Bereavement-Related Depression. Depress Anxiety 1997; 6(3):106–112.
31. Bonnet MH, Arand DL. The Consequences of a Week of Insomnia II: Patients with Insomnia. Sleep 1998; 21(4):359–368.
32. Espie CA, Lindsay WR. Cognitive strategies for the management of severe sleep-maintenance insomnia: A preliminary investigation. Behav Psychother 1987; 15:388–339.
33. Morin CM, Espie CA. Insomnia: A Clinical Guide to Assessment and Treatment. New York, NY: Kluwer Academic/Plenum Publishers, 2003.
34. Morgenthaler T, Kramer M, Alessi C, et al. Practice parameters for the psychological and behavioral treatment of insomnia: An update. An american academy of sleep medicine report. Sleep 2006; 29(11):1415–1419.
35. Morin CM, Bootzin RR, Buysse DJ, et al. Psychological and behavioural treatment of insomnia. Update of the recent evidence (1998–2004) prepared by a Task Force of the American Academy of Sleep Medicine. Sleep 2006; 29:1398–1414
36. Morin CM, Hauri P, Espie CA, et al. Nonpharmacologic treatment of chronic insomnia: An American Academy of Sleep Medicine Review. Sleep 1999; 22:1134–1156.
37. Harvey AG. Attempted suppression of pre-sleep cognitive activity in insomnia. Cognit Res Ther 2001.
38. Levey AB, Aldaz JA, Watts FN, et al. Articulatory suppression and the treatment of insomnia. Behav Res Ther 1991; 29:85–89.
39. Harvey AG. Pre-sleep cognitive activity: A comparison of sleep-onset insomniacs and good sleepers. Br J Clin Psychol 2000; 39:275–286.
40. Borkovec TD, Hu S. The effect of worry on cardiovascular response to phobic imagery. Behav Res Ther 1990; 28(1):69–73.

41. Borkovec TD, Ray WJ, Stober J. Worry: A cognitive phenomenon intimately linked to affective, physiological, and interpersonal behavioral processes. Cognit Ther Res 1998; 22:561–576.
42. Freeston MH, Dugas MJ, Ladouceur R. Thoughts, Images, Worry and Anxiety. Behav Res Ther 1996; 20:265–273.
43. Nelson J, Harvey AG. Pre-sleep imagery under the microscope: A comparison of patients with insomnia and good sleepers. Behav Res Ther 2003; 41(3):273–284.
44. Harvey AG, Payne S. The management of unwanted pre-sleep thoughts in insomnia: Distraction with imagery versus general distraction. Behav Res Ther 2002; 40(3):267–277.
45. Means MK, Lichstein KL, Epperson MT, et al. Relaxation Therapy for Insomnia: Nighttime and Day Time Effects. Behav Res Ther 2000; 38:665–678.
46. Morin CM, Azrin NH. Stimulus Control and Imagery Training in Treating Sleep-Maintenance Insomnia. J Consult Clin Psychol 1987; 55(2):260–262.
47. Morin CM, Azrin NH. Behavioral and cognitive treatments of geriatric insomnia. J Consult Clin Psychol 1988; 56:748–753.
48. Kabat-Zinn J. Full Catastrophe Living: Using the wisdom of your body and mind to face stress, pain and illness. London: Piatkus, 1990.
49. Wicklow A, Espie CA. Intrusive Thoughts and their Relationship to Actigraphic Measurement of Sleep: Towards a Cognitive Model of Insomnia. Behav Res Ther 2000; 38:679–693.
50. Lundh L. The role of acceptance and mindfulness in the treatment of insomnia. J Cogn Psychother 2005; 19:29–39.
51. Lundh L, Hindmarsh I. Can meta-cognitive observation be used in the treatment of insomnia? A pilot study of cognitive-emotional self-observation task. Behav Cogn Psychother 2002; 30:233–236.
52. Ong J, Shapiro C, Manber R. Combining mindfulness meditation with cognitive-behavior therapy for insomnia: A treatment-development study. Behav Ther 2008; 39(2):171–182.
53. Yook K, Lee SH, Ryu M, et al. Usefulness of mindfulness-based cognitive therapy for treating insomnia in patients with anxiety disorders: A pilot study. J Nerv Ment Dis 2008; 196(6):501–503.
54. Frankl VE. The Doctor and the Soul. Berlin: Knopf, 1955.
55. Frankl VE. Paradoxical intention: A logotherapueutic technique. Am J Psychother 1960; 14:520–535.
56. DuBois (1908) Cited In: Frankle VE, DuBois JM, eds On the Theory and Therapy of Mental Disorders: An Introduction to Logotherapy and Existential Analysis op.cit. London: Routledge, 2004:
57. Dunlap K. Repetition in the breaking of habits. Sci Mon 1930; 30:66–70.
58. Dunlap K. Habits Their Making and Unmaking. New York, NY: Liveright, 1932.
59. Frankl VE. (1963). (I. Lasch, Trans.) *Man's Search for Meaning: An Introduction to Logotherapy.* New York: Washington Square Press.
60. Ascher LM. Paradoxical intention in the treatment of urinary retention. Behav Res Ther 1979; 17(3):267–270.
61. Turner RM, Ascher LM. Controlled comparison of progressive relaxation, stimulus control, and paradoxical intention therapies for insomnia. J Consult Clin Psychol 1979; 47(3):500–508.
62. Broomfield NM, Espie CA. Towards a valid, reliable measure of sleep effort. J Sleep Res 2005; 14(4):401–407.
63. Ellis J, Mitchell K, Hogh H. Sleep preoccupation in poor sleepers: Psychometric properties of the Sleep Preoccupation Scale. J Psychosom Res 2007; 63(6):579–585.
64. Neitzert Semler C, Harvey AG. Monitoring for sleep-related threat: A pilot study of the Sleep Associated Monitoring Index. Psychosom Med 2004; 66:242–250.
65. Ascher LM, Efran JS. Use of paradoxical intention in a behavioral program for sleep onset insomnia. J Consult Clin Psychol 1978; 46(3):547–550.
66. Espie CA, Lindsay WR. Paradoxical intention in the treatment of chronic insomnia: six case studies illustrating variability in therapeutic response. Behav Res Ther 1985; 23(6):703–709.
67. Ladouceur R, Gros-Louis Y, Paradoxical intention vs stimulus control in the treatment of severe insomnia. J Behav Ther Exp Psychiatry.1986; 17(4):267–269.
68. Ott BD, Levine BA, Ascher LM. Manipulating the explicit demand of paradoxical intention instructions. Behav Psychother 1983; 11:25–35.
69. Relinger H, Bornstein PH. Treatment of Sleep Onset Insomnia by Paradoxical Instruction. Behav Modif 1979; 3(2):203–222.
70. Ascher LM, Turner R. Paradoxical intention and insomnia: An experimental investigation. Behav Res Ther 1979; 17(4):408–411.
71. Espie CA, Lindsay WR, Brooks DN, et al. A controlled comparative investigation of psychological treatments for chronic sleep-onset insomnia. Behav Res Ther 1989; 27(1):79–88.
72. Lacks P, Bertelson AD, Gans I, et al. The effectiveness of three behavioural treatments for different degrees of sleep-onset insomnia. Behav Ther 1983; 14:593–605.

73. Lacks P, Bertelson AD, Sugerman J, et al. The treatment of sleep-maintenance insomnia with stimulus-control techniques. Behav Res Ther 1983; 21(3):291–295.
74. Turner RM, Ascher LM. Therapist factor in the treatment of insomnia. Behav Res Ther1982; 20(1): 33–40.
75. Broomfield NM, Espie CA. Initial insomnia and paradoxical intention: An experimental investigation of putative mechanisms using subjective and actigraphic measurement of sleep. Behav Cogn Psychother 2003; 31:313–324
76. Harvey AG, Sharpley AL, Ree MJ, et al. An open trial of cognitive therapy for chronic insomnia. Behav Res Ther 2007; 45(10):2491–2501.
77. Harvey AG. Toward a cognitive theory and therapy for chronic insomnia. J Cogn Psychother 2005; 19:41–59.
78. Belanger L, Savard J, Morin CM. Clinical management of insomnia using cognitive therapy. Behav Sleep Med 2006; 4(3):179–198.

28 Short-Term and Group Treatment Approaches

Christina S. McCrae
Department of Clinical and Health Psychology, University of Florida, Gainesville, Florida, U.S.A.

Natalie D. Dautovich
Department of Psychology, University of Florida, Gainesville, Florida, U.S.A.

Joseph M. Dzierzewski
Department of Clinical and Health Psychology, University of Florida, Gainesville, Florida, U.S.A.

INTRODUCTION

The efficacy of cognitive behavioral treatments of insomnia has been well-documented in adults of all ages (1). A major challenge facing behavioral sleep medicine experts is how to best disseminate cognitive behavioral treatments to patients in primary care settings. A major barrier to the routine provision of such interventions in primary care settings is the length of the time required for treatment. Cognitive behavioral interventions have traditionally been administered over the course of 6 to 10 sessions lasting 50 to 90 minutes each (1). Another barrier is the common approach of providing treatment on a one-to-one basis. It is not difficult to see how lengthy intervention periods and individually administered treatment combine to consume a great deal of clinician time--a valuable and often limited resource in primary care settings. As a result, access to cognitive behavioral treatments for insomnia is frequently limited outside of a few select academic medical settings and specialized sleep treatment centers. Both of the intervention approaches presented in this chapter represent methods of treatment administration that offer potential solutions to these barriers. For example, shortened protocols and group treatment (treating more than one patient at a time) can make the best use of available healthcare provider resources by reducing demands on clinician time. Importantly, evidence suggests that these alternative approaches to administering cognitive behavioral treatment of insomnia can be adopted without compromising treatment quality. As will be presented in this chapter, research indicates that both brief and group approaches can be as efficacious in the treatment of insomnia as traditional cognitive behavioral protocols. Additionally, although the majority of research on these approaches has examined their *efficacy*, a smaller body of evidence provides promising preliminary support for their *effectiveness* as well. The first half of this chapter provides an overview of brief interventions, while the second half focuses on group therapy.

BRIEF INTERVENTIONS

A growing number of researchers have examined briefer approaches to insomnia treatment using cognitive behavioral therapy. The majority of studies have contrasted multicomponent cognitive behavioral approaches to 'usual care' treatment (typically consisting of sleep hygiene/sleep education). The number of sessions examined has ranged from one to five sessions. In a review of psychological and behavioral treatments for insomnia, Morin and colleagues (2006) described the average number of treatment sessions as 5.7 meetings (1). Consequently, for the purpose of this chapter, therapies not exceeding five treatment sessions will be reviewed and designated as 'brief approaches'.

Brief Interventions (4–5 Sessions)

Brief behavioral interventions of a longer length (i.e., 4–5 sessions) will be examined first. The effectiveness of brief behavioral treatments was examined within a rural elderly sample (2). Sleep treatments were administered to rural elderly within the framework of an existing service delivery system. Two brief approaches were compared: multicomponent behavioral treatment (MBT; stimulus control, sleep restriction, and passive relaxation) and sleep hygiene education

(SHE). Treatment was primarily administered in two in-person sessions and two telephone sessions. Results indicated that the MBT approach resulted in greater improvements as measured by sleep diary for sleep-onset latency and sleep efficiency compared to SHE (Table 1). Additionally, the results for MBT had greater clinical significance with 10 participants no longer meeting the criteria for insomnia after receiving the MBT versus three for the SHE treatment.

The efficacy of four treatment sessions for alleviating sleep complaints was examined in a sample of older adults with secondary insomnia (10). The treatment package consisted of sleep hygiene, stimulus control, and relaxation exercises. Compared to the delayed treatment condition, participants receiving the treatment showed significant improvement at posttreatment for the sleep diary measures of wake time after sleep onset, sleep efficiency, and sleep quality. The results appeared durable at three months with improvements maintained for wake time after sleep onset, sleep efficiency, and sleep quality.

Another study also examined the efficacy of four treatment sessions for treating insomnia in older adults but compared various components of behavioral treatments (12). One treatment group received a combination of sleep hygiene and relaxation exercises while another treatment involved sleep hygiene and stimulus control components. There were significant differences in pre/post scores for the treatment groups compared to the waitlist controls. The sleep hygiene/relaxation group and the sleep hygiene/stimulus control group significantly improved on the sleep diary measures of sleep-onset latency, total sleep time, and sleep efficiency compared to the control group. The significant improvement for the two treatment groups was maintained at follow-up. There were no significant differences between the two treatment groups suggesting that both approaches were efficacious.

The efficacy of a four session brief treatment approach was assessed in an older adult sample using one of three treatment conditions (sleep hygiene education, sleep restriction and sleep hygiene, and a nap restriction condition) (7). The nap restriction condition encouraged participants to partake in a daily 30 minute nap between 1 PM and 3 PM. Results indicated significant improvement at posttreatment for the sleep and nap restriction conditions for actigraphically measured total sleep time and for sleep diary sleep efficiency and time in bed.

Finally, two studies by Perlis and colleagues (38,39) examined the behavioral treatment for insomnia using a case based approach in which the number of sessions ranged from three to nine. Due to the variability in the number of sessions, these studies are not reviewed in depth here.

Brief Interventions (~2 Sessions)

Two to three session brief behavioral treatments were investigated by a number of authors (3,4,6,8,9,11,14). These approaches either delivered treatment across two sessions or delivered treatment primarily in one session while using the second session to follow-up with participants. A brief behavioral treatment of insomnia (BBTI) was compared to an information-only control (IC) in a sample of older adults who had normal psychiatric and medical comorbidities associated with aging (8). Both treatments consisted of two sessions. The BBTI treatment consisted of sleep education, sleep hygiene, stimulus control, and sleep restriction. The results indicated that in terms of sleep diary outcomes, the BBTI treatment resulted in significantly greater pre/post improvements in overall sleep quality, sleep latency, and wake time after sleep onset compared to the IC group. Additionally, there were moderate improvements in depression for the BBTI group.

A one-session CBT approach to treating insomnia showed significant improvements in sleep (4). A unique aspect to this approach included a cognitive restructuring component in the CBT regimen. The authors assessed sleep using the Sleep Questionnaire and Assessment of Wakefulness (37) and did a pre/post comparison with the postassessment occurring approximately 222 days after treatment. The results suggest that the brief CBT approach significantly decreased sleep-onset latency, wake time after sleep onset, and increased total sleep time. Although some of the participants received one to two follow-up sessions after the initial therapy, treatment was primarily delivered in one session, and there were not significant differences in treatment outcomes across the treatment lengths.

A two session, abbreviated cognitive-behavioral intervention (ACBT) produced significantly better improvement over baseline as measured by sleep diaries compared to a usual care

(*text continues on page 324.*)

Table 1 Summary of Research Employing Brief Treatment Approaches for Insomnia

Study	#, Format of sessions, & length of intersession interval	Content of sessions	Therapist qualifications	Population	Exclusionary criteria	Measures	Results	Durability of Effects	Effect Size*
Carter (3)	2 in-person sessions intersession interval of 2 wks	(Caregiver Sleep Intervention – CASI) – 1st session: stimulus control, relaxation therapies, cognitive therapy, sleep hygiene (60 min) – 2nd session: review and rates goal attainment (60 min)	– Master's level nurses – trained during $^{1}/_{2}$ day intensive training session	– 19 women, 11 men – age ($m = 53$, range 21–85)	– major depressive disorder – sleep disorder other than insomnia	PSQI actigraphy sleep diary CES-D CQOLC	(sleep diary) – significantly greater decrease in SOL for CASI vs. control (14 min) at wk 5 (one wk after second session) No significant differences between intervention and control for CES-D or CQOLC	(PSQI) – significantly lower PSQI for CASI vs. control (decrease of 4.5) after 4mo (actigraphy) – significantly lower SOL (decrease of 5.4 min) after 2 mo and higher TST (increase of 1.1hr) after 4mo for CASI vs. control	overall large effect sizes (sleep diary) – SOL $d = 0.84$ for CASI vs. control at week 5 – (PSQI) - PSQI for CASI vs. control, $d = 1.03$ after 4mths (actigraphy) – SOL $d = 0.79$ after 2mths and TST $d = 1.15$ after 4mths for CASI vs. control
Chambers & Alexander (4)	1–3 in-person sessions Unable to ascertain intersession interval	– included stimulus control, sleep restriction, sleep hygiene, & cognitive restructuring (typically delivered in one 2—3 hr session) – follow-up sessions (1–2) were used for some to monitor progress and encourage compliance – no differences in treatment outcome for number of sessions	– clinical psychologist	– 69 women, 34 men – age ($m = 39.9$, range 19–75)	– organic sleep disorders – poor physical health – acute psychiatric conditions – required prescription of anxiolytics, antidepressant or neuroleptic med	SQAW	SOL ↓30 min, TST ↑68 min, WASO ↓23 min Secondary outcomes: Significant improvement in daytime sleepiness, daytime fatigue, alertness during the day, & general well-being following treatment	postassessment was conducted at follow-up (on average 222 days later; see results section for post-assessment findings)	overall small/ medium to large effect sizes SOL $d = 0.42$ TST $d = 0.75$ WASO $d = 0.57$

Edinger, et al. (5)	1, 2, 4, & 8 sessions Sessions were conducted in-person with a taped recording of sleep education and a pamphlete describing stimulus control & sleep restriction provided Intersession intervals: – 2 sessions (3 wk) – 4 sessions (2 wks) – 8 sessions (no interval between sessions)	1st session: sleep education, stimulus control, & sleep restriction (45—60 min) Follow-up session: troubleshoot & modify TIB prescription as needed (15—30 min)	– 2 Clinical Psychologists – 5–17 yr experience working with sleep-disordered patients	– 43 women, 43 men – age ($m = 55.4 \pm 9.7$)	– pregnancy – med condition affecting sleep – major psychiatric disorder – <27 MMSE – substance abuse / sleep medication – anxiolytics / antidepres-sants – PLM – primary sleep disorder other than PI - PSG sleep time ≥ 2 x higher than sleep diary sleep time	sleep diaries actigraphy ISQ BDI STAI POMS SES	– 1 and 4 sessions: – ↑12% and 10% for sleep diary SE – WASO min ↓53.6 and 52.4 for sleep diary – TWT min ↓64.3 and 58.5 for sleep diary – TWT min ↓21.3 and 29.9 for actigraphy 4 sessions: – ↑4.7% for actigraphy SE ISQ scores improved from baseline to posttreatment for 1,4, & 8 sessions and from baseline to follow-up for 1 & 4 sessions	6 month follow-up 1,2, 4 sessions: – ↑9.3%, 6.9%, and 11.9% for sleep diary SE – TST min ↑34.7, 44, and 40.6 for sleep diary – TWT min ↓46.5, 28.9 and 60.1 for sleep diary 4 sessions: – ↓52.7 min for sleep diary WASO – ↑6.1% for actigraphy SE – TWT min ↓30.1 for actigraphy	Overall medium to large effect sizes Posttreatment: – 1 and 4 sessions: – $d = 1.13$ and $d = 1.16$ for sleep diary SE – WASO $d = 1.07$ and $d = 1.28$ for sleep diary – TWT $d = 1.24$ and $d = 1.24$ for sleep diary – TWT min $d = 0.41$ and $d = 0.80$ for actigraphy 4 sessions: – $d = 0.60$ for actigraphy SE Follow-up: – 1,2, 4 sessions: – $d = 0.92$, $d = 1.00$, and $d = 1.52$ for sleep diary SE – TST $d = 0.70$, $d = 1.11$ and $d = 0.87$ for sleep diary – TWT $d = 0.86$, $d = 0.78$ and $d = 1.24$ for sleep diary 4 sessions: – $d = 1.39$ for sleep diary WASO – $d = 0.59$ for actigraphy SE – TWT $d = 0.60$ for actigraphy

(Continued)

Table 1 Summary of Research Employing Brief Treatment Approaches for Insomnia (*Continued*)

Study	#, Format of sessions, & length of intersession interval	Content of sessions	Therapist qualifications	Population	Exclusionary criteria	Measures	Results	Durability of Effects	Effect Size*
Edinger & Sampson (6)	2 in-person sessions pamphlet with behavioral recommendations & audio cassette with treatment guidelines provided 2 wk intersession interval	(ACBT) – 1st session: review of sleep logs, sleep education, stimulus control, sleep restriction – 2nd session: review instructions, trouble shoot – sessions ~ 25 min (SHC) – 1st session: review of sleep logs (no problem solving), sleep education, sleep hygiene – 2nd session: review instructions, trouble shoot – sessions ~ 25min	– beginning-level clinical psychologist – received training and monthly supervision from 1st author	2 women, 18 men – age ($m = 51.0 \pm 13.7$)	– sleep-disruptive med condition – terminal illness – other primary sleep disorder – Axis I disorder – use of hypnotics / alcohol as sleep aid	sleep diary ISQ SES DBAS	Sleep diaries: – ACBT: WASO ↓43 min, SE ↑9%, SQ ↑.3/5 – SHC: WASO ↑1min, SE ↑1%, SQ no change Secondary outcome measures: ACBT group showed significant improvement compared to SCH group on ISQ, DBAS	3mo after treatment Sleep diaries: – ACBT: WASO ↓51 min, SE ↑12%, SQ ↑.2/5 – SHC: WASO ↑8min, SE ↑3%, SQ.1/5 Secondary outcome measures: ACBT group showed significant improvement compared to SCH group on ISQ, sleep-related self-efficacy, DBAS	Insufficient information to calculate effect sizes

Friedman et al. (7)	4 in-person treatment sessions 1 wrap-up session at end of treatment Brief meeting at 3mth follow-up No intersession intervals between 4 in-person sessions	Control condition (CC): Sleep hygiene education provided except for information on napping or regular bed/wake times. Sleep Restriction (SR): In addition to education received by CC, sleep restriction therapy as described in Friedman et al. (1991) was provided Nap Restriction (NR): Identical protocol to SR group except were encouraged to take a 30 min daily nap between 1–3 *pm*	Not able to ascertain	24 women, 11 men – age ($m = 64.2 \pm 7.4$) Participants met criteria for insomnia	– sleep apnea – periodic limb movements – acute, unstable medical or psychiatric illness – chronic illness associated with insomnia – use of stimulating or sedating medications – not free of sleeping medications for 3 wk – MMSE	actigraphy sleep logs polysomnography MSLT SSS Urine toxicology	Actigraphy – Significant improvement at posttreatment for NR and SR condition for TST ↑24 min & 26 min Sleep diary: – significant improvement at posttreatment for NR and SR condition for SE ↑8.6% & 15.2%, ↓TIB 55min & 95min	3mths after treatment Unable to ascertain	overall medium to large effect sizes Posttreatment: Actigraphy – Significant improvement at posttreatment for NR and SR condition for TST $d = 0.47$ & $d = 0.77$ Sleep diary: – significant improvement at posttreatment for NR and SR condition for SE $d = 0.80$ & $d = 1.07$, ↓TIB $d = 0.92$ & $d = 2.04$

(*Continued*)

Table 1 Summary of Research Employing Brief Treatment Approaches for Insomnia (*Continued*)

Study	#, Format of sessions, & length of intersession interval	Content of sessions	Therapist qualifications	Population	Exclusionary criteria	Measures	Results	Durability of Effects	Effect Size*
Germain et al. (8)	2 sessions with 2 wk intersession interval (BBTI) – in-person – wkbook (IC) – in-person – telephone follow-up – pamphlets	(BBTI) – 1st session: sleep education, sleep hygiene, stimulus control, sleep restriction (45min) – 2nd session: review sleep education, treatment adherence, modify sleep schedule as needed (30 min) (IC) – 1st session: given 3 AASM brochures	– Masters-level adult psychiatric and primary care nurse practitioner – trained in BBTI intervention	(BBTI) – 12 women, 5 men – age ($m = 70.9 \pm 5.3$) (IC) – 13 women, 5 men – age ($m = 69.6 \pm 7.3$) – 33 participants were Caucasian – 14 participants were using hypnotics	PSQI sleep diary HRSD HRSA	Significant differences between the two groups were reported for the following: (sleep diaries) – BBTI: SOL ↓22 min, WASO ↓33 min – IC: SOL ↓3 min, WASO ↓12 min (PSQI) – BBTI: ↓ 3.94 – IC ↑.06 (clinical significance) 53% BBTI, 17% IC met criteria for remission Moderate improvement in depression (HRSD) for BBTI group	n/a	overall medium to large effect sizes (sleep diaries) SOL $d = 0.80$ WASO $d = 0.67$ (PSQI) $d = 1.37$	

Germain, et al. (9)	1 in-person session & follow-up telephone call (3 wk later) Materials provided: wkbook with educational materials	– session consisted of a combination of imagery rehearsal therapy (IRT) a CBT to reduce post-traumatic nightmares and CBT for insomnia – session included education about sleep & nightmares, rationale & practice of imagery rescripting & rehearsal, stimulus control, sleep restriction – 90 min session – follow-up phone call was scheduled 3wks later to asses time in bed prescription	– delivered by doctoral-level practitioner	– participants met diagnostic criteria for PTSD – 4 women, 3 men age ($m = 33.93 \pm 5.67$)	– substance abuse – psychotic /bipolar disorder, major depression – sleep apnea diagnosis	PSQI PSQI-A Pittsburgh Sleep Diary	– small improvements for PSQI ($p<0.10$) – marked improvements in PTSD symptoms	post-assessment was conducted 6–8 wk post-intervention (see results section)	overall medium effect size PSQI $d = 0.66$

(*Continued*)

Table 1 Summary of Research Employing Brief Treatment Approaches for Insomnia (*Continued*)

Study	#, Format of sessions, & length of intersession interval	Content of sessions	Therapist qualifications	Population	Exclusionary criteria	Measures	Results	Durability of Effects	Effect Size*
Lichstein, et al. (10)	4 in-person sessions (1 h) No intersession interval (sessions occurred on a weekly basis) Participants were assigned to either a treatment group or delayed treatment condition	Treatment package was composed of sleep hygiene instructions, stimulus control, and relaxation	4 graduate students in clinical psychology Training included studying a detailed treatment manual, mock therapy sessions, observation, discussion, and weekly supervision provided by 1st author	– 21 women, 23 men age (treatment group $m = 67.1 \pm 6.1$; control group $m = 70.1 \pm 6.8$)	– medication taken specifically for sleep – presence of other sleep disorders (e.g., sleep apnea, periodic limb movement, narcolepsy) – irregular sleep schedule due to shift work	sleep diary IIS GDS STAI adherence logs	Sleep Diary: Treatment group showed significant improvement at posttreatment for WASO↓26min, SE ↑11%, SQ↑0.5 No significant differences were observed for secondary measures	Follow-up was conducted at 3mos Sleep Diary: Treatment group showed significant improvement at follow-up relative to baseline for WASO↓31min, SE ↑11%, SQ↑0.5 No significant differences were observed for secondary measures	overall small to large effect sizes Sleep Diary: Treatment group at posttreatment for WASO $d = 0.42$, SE $d = 0.69$, SQ $d = 0.71$ Sleep Diary: Treatment group at follow-up for WASO $d = 0.59$, SE $d = 0.77$, SQ $d = 0.77$
Means, et al. (11)	3 in-person sessions Intersession interval (sessions occurred 3–7 days apart) Treatment group was compared to a waitlist control group Authors also assessed sleep and daytime functioning of a subset of participants not complaining of insomnia	Treatment consisted of a 16 muscle group relaxation	3 graduate students Students received performed at least 3 practice sessions, had competence assessed by 2nd author, and therapy was supervised by 2nd author	– 85 women, 33 men age ($m = 21.2 \pm 5.2$)	– medication taken specifically for sleep – presence of other sleep disorders (e.g., sleep apnea, periodic limb movement, narcolepsy) – irregular sleep schedule due to shift work – chronic illness – persistent anxiety or depression	sleep diary IIS DBAS ESS FSS PSWQ	Sleep Diary: Treatment group had significantly better WASO ↓9min, SE ↑3.6%, and SQ ↑0.3 than control group at posttreatment No group differences were observed for daytime measures	No follow-up assessment	overall medium to large effect sizes Sleep Diary: Treatment group WASO $d = 0.58$, SE $d = 0.52$, and SQ $d = 0.75$ at posttreatment

McCrae, et al. (2)	2 in-person sessions 2 telephone sessions Materials provided: wk book & audio tape of passive relaxation provided No intersession interval (sessions were conducted on weekly basis)	– MBT 1st session: stimulus control, sleep restriction (~50mins) – 2nd session: passive relaxation – 2 telephone follow-ups: progress review & troubleshooting – SHE initial session: sleep education & sleep hygiene – 2nd session: sleep education – 2 telephone follow-ups: progress review & troubleshooting	– mental health counselor – social worker – provisionally licensed counselor – training was provided by McCrae during 2-day workshop	– 13 women, 7 men – age ($m = 77.2 \pm 8.0$)	– significant med condition affecting sleep – major psychopathology – other sleep disorders – MMSE ≤ 23	sleep diary	(Sleep diaries) – MBT: SOL ↓25 min, SE ↑16% (significantly greater than SHE) – SHE: SOL ↓0 mins, SE ↑6% (clinical significance) 10 MBT, 3 SHE no longer met insomnia criteria	n/a	overall large effect size for treatment group (Sleep diaries) – MBT: SOL $d = 1.12$, SE $d = 2.12$ – SHE: SOL $d = 0.02$, SE $d = 0.99$

Table 1 Summary of Research Employing Brief Treatment Approaches for Insomnia (*Continued*)

Study	#, Format of sessions, & length of intersession interval	Content of sessions	Therapist qualifications	Population	Exclusionary criteria	Measures	Results	Durability of Effects	Effect Size*
Pallesen et al. (12)	4 in-person sessions (~30 min) No intersession interval (sessions were conducted on a weekly basis) Immediate Treatment groups: – Sleep hygiene and relaxation tape – Sleep hygiene and stimulus control Waitlist control	– Sleep hygiene and relaxation tape (SH+R): – advice based on standard sleep treatment – relaxation tape involved oral instructions with components consisting of progressive relaxation, passive focal attention, and active expiration. Sleep hygiene and stimulus control (SH+SC): – consisted of sleep hygiene advice described above – stimulus control consisted of 6 standard stimulus control instructions	Not able to ascertain	– 46 women, 9 men – age ($m = 69.8 \pm 6.53$)	– MMSE<25 – primary goal to stop taking hypnotics – participants with affective and anxiety disorders, patients who used hypnotics, and those with restless legs syndrome were included to increase external validity	sleep diary life satisfaction (13) intervention log	Sleep Diary: Significant differences between immediate and delayed treatment groups (no difference between treatment groups) SH+R: SOL ↓20 mins, TST ↑26mins, SE↑7% SH+SC: SOL ↓31 mins, TST ↑30mins, SE↑12% There were no significant differences between the immediate and delayed treatment groups for daytime measures	Follow-up was conducted 6mths post-intervention Significant differences at posttreatment were maintained at follow-up	overall small to large effect size for immediate treatment group Sleep Diary: pre to post difference SH+R: SOL $d = 0.57$ mins, TST $d = 0.50$, SE $d = 0.79$ SH+SC: SOL $d = 0.49$ mins, TST $d = 0.39$, SE $d = 0.89$ Sleep Diary: pre to follow-up difference SH+R: SOL $d = 0.53$ mins, TST $d = 0.69$, SE $d = 1.00$ SH+SC: SOL $d = 0.52$ mins, TST $d = 0.42$, SE $d = 0.94$

Riedel et al. (14)	4 groups: – stimulus control with medication withdrawal – stimulus control alone – medication withdrawal alone – waitlist control Those receiving stimulus control met with therapist for 2 one-hour in-person sessions for stimulus control treatment There was no intersession interval (sessions were held on consecutive weeks) The two groups undergoing medication withdrawal participated in a sleep medication withdrawal program (1 session)	Stimulus control sessions: – consisted of standard recom-mendations Sleep medication withdrawal program: – education on short and long-term effects of sleep medication on sleep and side effects – provided instructions for gradual withdrawal from sleep medication	– graduate psychology students – therapists were trained by first author and a supervising faculty member – supervision was provided through weekly meetings	– 11 women, 10 men – age ($m = 56.6 \pm 13.8$) – individuals were included in the study who had hypnotic-dependent insomnia and primary insomnia	– current nonpharmaco-logical treatment for insomnia – alcohol use close to bedtime – self-report of medical conditions affecting sleep – other sleep disorders (e.g., sleep apnea or periodic limb movement)	sleep diaries use of hypnotic medication ESS BDI STAI-T stimulus control compliance	No significant improvement for stimulus control participants from pre to post Significantly less daytime sleepiness for stimulus control participants at posttreatment	Follow-up was conducted 8wks after posttreatment Significant improvement for stimulus control participants from pre to follow-up for TST, SE, and SQ Medicated stimulus control participants: – TST ↑33 mins, SE ↑6%, SQ ↑0.3 Nonmedicated stimulus control participants: – TST ↑60 mins, SE ↑14.5%, SQ ↑0.6 Significantly less daytime sleepiness for stimulus control participants at follow-up	overall small to large effect size for stimulus control treatment Stimulus control participants from pre to follow-up Medicated stimulus control participants: – TST $d = 0.39$, SE $d = 0.47$, SQ $d = 0.59$ Nonmedicated stimulus control participants: – TST $d = 0.75$, SE ↑ $d = 1.23$, SQ $d = 0.57$

(*Continued*)

Table 1 Summary of Research Employing Brief Treatment Approaches for Insomnia (*Continued*)

Study	#, Format of sessions, & length of intersession interval	Content of sessions	Therapist qualifications	Population	Exclusionary criteria	Measures	Results	Durability of Effects	Effect Size*
Strom et al. (15)	Treatment duration consisted of 5 consecutive wks No intersession treatment intervals Two groups: Treatment group (sleep management program) and waitlist control All information was presented via the internet.	Treatment consisted of sleep restriction, stimulus control, information about sleep hygiene, cognitive restructuring, information about medication withdrawal, and applied relaxation	2 clinical psychologists	– 71 women, 38 men – age ($m = 44.1 \pm 12.0$)	– young (<18yrs) – sleep apnea or related self-reported respiratory problems – restless legs syndrome – depression or anxiety – sleep difficulties explained by physical symptoms – night-shift work or regular daytime sleep – previous or ongoing CBT for insomnia – insomnia being a minor problem	sleep diary HADS medication index DBAS treatment credibility	Sleep Diary: – greater pre/post improvement in TWT (↓55 mins), TST (↑34mins), and SE (↑10%) for treatment group compared to control group – improvements in SOL, NWAK, WASO, early morning awakening, TIB, and SQ were noted for both treatment and control group – control group also saw improvements	Treatment group (follow-up conducted after 9mths) saw improvements maintained over pretreatment for Sleep Diary: – SE (↑10%), TST (↑51min), TWT (↓47 min), SQ (↑0.54) Waitlist control group (follow-up conducted 6mths after completing treatment): – SE improved compared to pretreatment (↑7%) and	Sleep Diary: – pre/post improvement in TWT $d = 0.79$, TST $d = 0.46$, and SE $d = 0.71$ for treatment group Treatment group (follow-up) improvements over pretreatment for: – SE $d = 0.86$, TST $d = 0.87$, TWT $d = 0.82$, SQ $d = 1.39$ Waitlist control group for follow-up: – SE improved compared to

Strom et al. (15)	Questions, questionnaires, and diaries were submitted through the internet Psychologists would prompt participants to complete their sleep diaries if they were late to do so and also responded to questions	on TWT, TST, and SE – greater reduction of DBAS and medication use for treatment compared to control group	posttreatment (↑3%), TST improved compared to pretreatment (↑30min) and posttreatment (↑23min), TWT improved compared to pretreatment (↓39 min) and posttreatment (↓23 min), SOL improved compared to pretreatment (↓12min), SQ improved compared to pretreatment (↑0.64)	pretreatment $d = 0.72$ and posttreatment $d = 0.35$, TST improved compared to pretreatment $d = 0.57$ and posttreatment $d = 0.46$, TWT improved compared to pretreatment $d = 0.73$ and posttreatment $d = 0.51$, SOL improved compared to pretreatment $d = 0.41$, SQ improved compared to pretreatment $d = 1.77$

Notes: ∗Effect Size Estimates represent Cohen's *d*.

Abbreviations: BDI, Beck Depression Inventory (16); CES-D, Center for Epidemiological Studies Depression Scale (17); CQOLC, Caregiver Quality of Life Index-Cancer (18); DBAS, Dysfunctional Beliefs and Attitudes about Sleep Scale (19); ESS, Epworth Sleepiness Scale (20); FSS, Fatigue Severity Scale (21); GDS, Geriatric Depression Scale (22); HADS, Hospital Anxiety and Depression Scale (23); HRSA, Hamilton Rating Scale for Anxiety (24); HRSD, Hamilton Rating Scale for Depression (25); IIS, Insomnia Impact Scale (26); ISQ, Insomnia Symptom Questionnaire (27); MSLT, Multiple Sleep Latency Test (28); POMS, Profile of Mood States (29); PSWQ, Penn State Worry Questionnaire (30); PSQI, Pittsburgh Sleep Quality Index (31); PSQI-A, PSQI addendum for PTSD (32); SES, sleep related Self-Efficacy Scale (33); SII, Sleep Impairment Index (34); SSS, Stanford Sleepiness Scale (35); STAI, State-Trait Anxiety Inventory (36); SQAW, Sleep Questionnaire and Assessment of Wakefulness (37);

sleep hygiene/education treatment (6). Participants in the ACBT group experienced decreased wake time after sleep onset, improved sleep efficiency, and higher sleep quality ratings. The authors also compared the two groups at a three-month follow-up period. The results indicate the durability of ACBT intervention with the significant gains of the ACBT group maintained over time.

Significant improvements in sleep were seen for college students diagnosed with insomnia using a three-session treatment approach (11). Treatment consisted of a 16-muscle group progressive relaxation exercise. The group receiving the relaxation treatment showed significantly better improvement at posttreatment compared to the waitlist control for the sleep diary variables of wake time after sleep onset, sleep efficiency, and sleep quality.

A brief approach of two to four sessions was used to reduce sleep medication use and improve insomnia among individuals with hypnotic dependent insomnia and primary insomnia (14). Three treatment groups (stimulus control with medication withdrawal, stimulus control alone, medication withdrawal alone) were compared to a waitlist control. The results suggested that while there was no significant improvement for the groups at posttreatment, follow-up testing conducted eight weeks after treatment indicated significant improvement for both stimulus control groups in terms of the sleep diary variables. The stimulus control with medication withdrawal group experienced an increase in total sleep time, an increase of sleep efficiency, and an increase in sleep quality. The nonmedicated stimulus control group experienced an increase in total sleep time, an increase in sleep efficiency, and an increase in sleep quality. Additionally, in terms of secondary outcome measures, the groups receiving stimulus control experienced significantly less daytime sleepiness at posttreatment and follow-up.

Brief Approaches with post-traumatic stress disorder (PTSD) Patients and Caregivers

The applicability of brief cognitive behavioral intervention for insomnia to different populations was demonstrated in two studies. A brief, one session, cognitive behavioral intervention was developed to treat individuals diagnosed with post-traumatic stress disorder (PTSD) and poor sleep (9). The cognitive behavioral intervention included a combination of imagery rehearsal therapy (IRT), CBT to reduce posttraumatic nightmares, and CBT for insomnia. The results suggested small ($p<0.10$) improvements in self-reported sleep quality as measured by the Pittsburgh sleep quality index (PSQI) (31) and marked improvements in PTSD symptoms (9).

Second, the effectiveness of a brief CBT intervention for caregivers was demonstrated in a study (3) which examined the effectiveness of a two-session caregiver sleep intervention (CASI) (3). The results indicated that compared to controls, the participants who received the CASI treatment showed significantly greater improvements in sleep-onset latency as measured by sleep diaries compared to the baseline period. Additionally, follow-up testing revealed significantly lower sleep-onset latency and higher total sleep time as measured by actigraphy for those receiving the CASI treatment.

Brief Approaches Delivered Using Alternate Formats

The utility of an internet-based brief approach for the treatment of insomnia was evaluated during a five-week period of online treatment that consisted of sleep restriction, stimulus control, sleep hygiene, cognitive restructuring, information about medication withdrawal, and applied relaxation (15). All information was presented via the internet, and two clinical psychologists monitored completion of sleep diaries and responded to participant questions. At posttreatment, the treatment group saw greater improvements in sleep diary variables of total wake time, total sleep time, and sleep efficiency. Additionally, the treatment group had greater improvement of their dysfunctional beliefs about sleep and their medication use compared to the control group. The sleep diary improvements were maintained over the nine-month follow-up period.

Dose-Response Effects of Brief Approaches

A unique approach has been employed to examine the differential effects of increasing the number of treatment sessions using a 'dose-response' study (5). The benefit of this approach is the ability to isolate the effect of treatment length and control for extraneous factors (e.g., therapist qualifications, content of treatment, setting). Treatments consisting of one, two, four, and eight sessions were compared in terms of short and long-term outcomes. All treatment patients received one in-person CBT session lasting 45 to 60 minutes. The session consisted of sleep education, stimulus control, and sleep restriction. Additional treatment for patients receiving more than one session consisted of in-person 15 to 30 minute sessions designed to troubleshoot and modify the time-in-bed prescription as needed. Results indicated that the one and four-session CBT dose resulted in significant pre- to post-treatment improvement in actigraphy total wake time as well as several sleep diary variables, including sleep efficiency, wake time after sleep onset, and total wake time. Additionally, the four-session CBT dose resulted in significant improvement in actigraphy sleep efficiency.

In terms of the durability of outcomes at a six month follow-up period, the participants receiving the one, two, and four session dose of CBT showed significant improvements compared to baseline measures for sleep diary sleep efficiency, total sleep time, and total wake time. Additionally, the four-session CBT dose saw continued improvement in actigraphy sleep efficiency and total wake time. As mentioned above, the sessions subsequent to the first treatment session were primarily 'follow-up' sessions designed to troubleshoot any treatment difficulties.

In summary, while improvements were seen posttreatment with the one and four dose treatments and at follow-up with the one, two, and four dose treatments, it appears that the four dose treatment demonstrated the greatest improvements on both sleep diary and actigraphy measures of sleep. Importantly, the four-session dose consisted of bi-weekly delivery of treatments (compared to a three week intersession interval for the group receiving two sessions and no intersession interval for the group receiving eight sessions). The authors hypothesize that scheduling session bi-weekly may provide sufficient time for the patients to independently develop behavioral changes while still receiving support.

Brief Approaches–Integration of Findings

Overall, the brief treatment approaches reviewed herein exhibited effect sizes ranging primarily from medium to large effects (Table 1). The effect sizes of brief treatments are comparable to the effect sizes for behavioral treatments for insomnia that are of a longer length (40,41) suggesting that treatments of a shorter length can be as effective as traditional behavioral approaches for treating insomnia. Considering that a benefit of briefer approaches is to increase the availability of treatment, it is of interest whether briefer approaches can be effectively delivered by nondoctoral level practitioners. Brief treatments were provided by both doctoral level (4–6,9,15,42) and non-doctoral level practitioners (2,3,8,10,11,14). For the studies utilizing non-doctoral level practitioners, training and supervision was typically provided by doctoral level practitioners.

In terms of treatment length, treatments varying from one to five sessions were found to be efficacious. The one study (5) that compared varying session lengths within the same experiment found that a four-session treatment produced the best outcomes. In the studies that examined one length of treatment (e.g., two sessions) it is possible that although significant improvements were noted for the treatment length, more or fewer sessions may also have resulted in comparable or even greater improvements. Interestingly, Edinger and colleagues (2007) commented that it is not only the *frequency* of treatments that may impact sleep outcomes but also the duration of intervals between sessions that may play a role in treatment effectiveness. Overall, the majority of brief approaches were conducted on a weekly or bi-weekly basis.

The mean ages of participants examined in the brief behavioral treatment studies ranged from 21 to 77 years suggesting that brief treatments are applicable to both adults and older adults. A variety of exclusionary criteria were employed in the studies. Stringent criteria resulted in the inclusion of primarily physically and mentally healthy individuals who were not suffering from a sleep disorder other than insomnia in the majority of studies while a minority of studies included participants with physical and psychiatric complaints. It appears that specialized brief behavioral approaches can be helpful for treating insomnia in specific populations (e.g., those diagnosed with PTSD and caregivers). It is not yet clear how effective brief approaches are with the typical primary care patient diagnosed with medical and psychiatric comorbidities.

Interestingly, the majority of brief approaches were uniform in the content of their CBT sessions. The sessions were multicomponent and typically consisted of sleep education, sleep hygiene, stimulus control, and sleep restriction. Two studies (5,43) also included cognitive restructuring in the treatment regimen.

Brief Approaches – Future Directions

Despite the existence of a body of research examining brief CBT approaches, there are a number of areas that could benefit from future research. First, the majority of studies saw improvement on self-report measures. Few studies employed both objective and subjective measures. It would be interesting to see if the effects of brief behavioral treatments hold over both subjective and objective measures. Second, it would be worthwhile to vary the inter-session time period in future studies in order to examine the impact of duration *between* sessions in addition to examining simply the total number of sessions used. Third, it would be interesting to examine the benefits of additional cognitive approaches (e.g., cognitive restructuring) within a brief model. Fourth, the participants enrolled into the studies were primarily homogenous. It would be helpful to be able to generalize findings regarding brief approaches to individuals with more diverse cultural backgrounds and physical/mental diagnoses. Finally, sessions ranging in number from one to five were found to create significant improvements in sleep. In order to conclusively determine the optimum number of sessions, it would be helpful for more studies to employ a dose-response methodology in order to examine the differential effects of varying numbers of sessions on sleep and sleep-related outcomes.

Conclusions

Examination of the literature investigating brief behavioral approaches to treating insomnia suggests that treatment sessions ranging from one to five can be effective for the treatment of insomnia. While the majority of studies relied on subjective measures of sleep, significant improvements were seen with both subjective and objective measures of sleep (3,5,7,42). In addition to significant posttreatment improvements in sleep, brief behavioral approaches appear to exhibit durability up to six to eight weeks (9,14), three (6,7,10), four (3), six (5,12,42), seven (43), and nine (15) months after treatment. Consequently, it appears that brief approaches are efficacious in the short and longer term (up to nine months) for individuals ranging in age from 21 to 77 years of age.

GROUP INTERVENTION

The ability to simultaneously treat the insomnia symptoms of multiple individuals is an intriguing concept. A growing number of research studies have employed group treatment approaches. Although the majority of these studies appear to have used a group approach due to the cost effectiveness of treating multiple patients at the same time, a few studies have explicitly examined the impact of different aspects of the 'group process' in the treatment of insomnia.

General Overview of the Elements of Group Treatment

One of the most substantial and in-depth accounts of group treatment is found in the classic work by Yalom (1995), The Theory and Practice of Group Psychotherapy. He described eleven therapeutic factors of group therapy that are associated with change in behavior (Table 2).

Table 2 Therapeutic Factors of Group Psychotherapy

1. Installation of hope[a]
2. Universality[a]
3. Imparting information[a]
4. Altruism
5. The corrective recapitulation of the primary family group
6. The development of socializing techniques
7. Imitative behavior[a]
8. Interpersonal learning[a]
9. Cohesiveness
10. Catharsis[a]
11. Existential factors

[a]Factors that could be employed in the group treatment of insomnia.
Source: From Ref. 44.

Table 3 Factors Associated with Group Satisfaction

1. The group meets goals in therapy
2. Satisfaction gained from relationships with other group members
3. Satisfaction gained from participation in the group
4. Satisfaction gained from the group by means of the outside world

Source: Adapted from Ref. 44.

In conjunction with these factors, Yalom (1995) also states that group treatment approaches must be inherently distinct from individual approaches to change. These groups should encompass more than a simple increase in the number of patients present. Group treatment should be based on the group, not on the individualized treatment approach. According to Yalom, in group treatment approaches *"it is the group that is the agent of change"* ((44), p. 109).

In this vein of reasoning, Yalom (1995) has proposed four main factors considered to be essential to patient satisfaction with group treatment (Table 3). These factors generally include the group meeting the patient's needs in alleviating symptoms and the patient's interaction in the group and with group members. While traditional cognitive behavioral treatments of insomnia have proven very efficacious in symptom reduction, the group implementation of such cognitive behavioral treatments seems to be lacking a focus on the group interaction factors. Only a handful of studies employing a group treatment approach have examined aspects of the group interaction.

Group Treatment with a Focus on Group Interaction Factors

Kupych-Woloshyn and colleagues (1993) were the first to describe a group approach to the treatment of insomnia (45). Their approach was based on interpersonal and cognitive-behavioral approaches and integrated group interaction as a mean of therapeutic change with didactic and cognitive-behavioral techniques. Unfortunately, the authors did not present data on the efficacy of their approach. Nonetheless, the theoretical blend of interpersonal and cognitive-behavioral processes makes their model truly unique. They presented seven primary principles that underlie the group treatment of insomnia. These principles are presented in Table 4. However, as described later, the majority of research has opted to focus specifically on the implementation of symptom specific cognitive behavioral techniques.

Only one study was found that examined group therapy process variables in cognitive behavioral treatment for insomnia (46). This intervention, based on interpersonal theory, assessed the impact of patient expectations and perceived therapeutic alliance on sleep outcomes. They found that both early patient expectations and the perceived therapeutic alliance were predictive of sleep outcomes and also differentiated between patients who dropped out of the treatment and those that remained. Patients who had low pretreatment expectations and perceived their therapists as more affiliative had less nightly total wake time; patients who perceived their therapist as more confrontative were less satisfied with treatment and were more likely to drop out of treatment (46). The results suggest the importance of the installation of hope in early sessions and the need for therapists to be nonjudgmental and to strive to form a positive alliance with group members.

Table 4 Principles Proposed Essential to the Group Treatment of Insomnia

1. Normalizing insomnia
2. Flexibility to meet the individual needs and expectation of members
3. Individual differences are recognized and discussed
4. Change is possible following education, and identification and insight within a supportive environment
5. Group validation and acceptance allows individuals to move beyond suffering
6. Individual presentation allows for multiple hypotheses and explanations for sleep disturbances
7. Secure, structured group environments facilitate self-disclosure

Source: Adapted from Ref. 45.

Patient perceived mechanisms of change in the group treatment of insomnia is a difficult variable to assess. However, in comparing the effectiveness of group and individual treatment approaches, it was found that individuals treated in the group format rated their interactions with fellow patients with insomnia as the third most helpful aspect of treatment (47). Only behavioral techniques (sleep restriction and stimulus control) and cognitive restructuring were rated as more helpful. This patient interaction was rated higher than relaxation training. This finding provides support for the stance that the group treatment of insomnia is uniquely different from individualized treatments. However, how to best capitalize on these differences has yet to be answered.

Group Treatment Focusing on Insomnia Symptoms

Community Recruited Volunteers

Traditional individual cognitive behavioral treatment of insomnia has been compared to group cognitive behavioral treatment and telephone consultation (48). In this investigation, all individuals received cognitive behavioral treatment of insomnia that included stimulus control, sleep restriction, cognitive therapy, and sleep hygiene. Treatment arms only differed in the modality of treatment delivery and not in treatment content. Results indicated that from pre- to post-treatment all groups significantly improved their total wake time, sleep efficiency, wake time after sleep onset, sleep efficiency, and sleep quality rating. Total sleep time continued to improve from posttreatment to three-month follow-up. However, no improvements were seen from three-month follow-up to six-month follow-up. Promisingly, 9 out of the 16 group patients (82%) had sleep efficiencies above 80% at six-month follow-up. Importantly, the three treatment groups did not differ significantly in their sleep at any time point, suggesting the comparable nature of the treatment conditions (48).

In patients representing mild cases of insomnia, the effectiveness of relaxation, single-item desensitization, and the combination of relaxation and desensitization, performed in small groups, produced relatively equivocal gains in sleep (49). Pre- to post-treatment improvements in sleep-onset latency and rated difficulty in falling asleep and number of awakenings per night were observed across all groups. A case-by-case examination of the data suggested that the combination therapy may be the most useful group treatment for more severe cases of insomnia (49).

The usefulness of group cognitive behavioral treatment of insomnia as an early intervention for insomnia was examined in subjects who had experienced the onset of insomnia within the previous 3 to 12 months (50). Groups of 6 to 10 patients underwent six weekly sessions of group treatment that included problem solving, relaxation, worry time, distraction, paradoxical intention, observation exercise, sleep hygiene, stimulus control, sleep restriction, cognitive therapy, stress management, sleep beliefs, sleep medications education, coping, and sleep management. Compared to a control group, the group condition demonstrated significant improvements in many self-report sleep variables from baseline to one-year follow-up (i.e., sleep-onset latency, wake time after sleep onset, total sleep time, sleep quality, and sleep efficiency). In addition, the group condition produced more clinically significant gains than the control group at one-year follow-up.

The relationship between group adherence and posttreatment sleep outcomes has been examined in insomnia outpatients (51). Groups of five to six patients underwent seven weekly sessions of cognitive behavioral treatment of insomnia that included sleep hygiene, stimulus control, medication withdrawal, relaxation, sleep restriction, cognitive therapy, stress management, and problem solving. Significant pre- to post-treatment improvements were seen across numerous sleep variables. Interestingly, therapist-rated adherence was the only significant adherence predictor of outcome variables in the group treatment of insomnia. No follow-up data were presented.

Physician/Clinically Referred Patients

Durability of individual CBT-I has been well-established. Similarly, the long-term effectiveness of short-term group cognitive behavioral treatment of insomnia has begun to receive empirical support. For example, 20 physician-referred insomnia patients treated with six weekly sessions of multicomponent group treatment demonstrated significant pre- to post-treatment improvements in total sleep time and sleep efficiency These treatment-induced gains were well maintained at three-year follow-up (52). The immediate and long-term effectiveness of nurse-led group cognitive behavioral treatment of insomnia in general practice patients, as compared to treatment as usual, has also been examined (53). Groups consisted of four to six patients, met for five weekly sessions, and employed stimulus control, sleep restriction, and cognitive therapy. Significant pre- to post-treatment improvements in self-reported sleep for the group condition were observed for sleep onset latency and sleep efficiency. The significant group differences were not maintained at six-month follow-up. However, PSQI measured global sleep disturbance was significantly reduced for the group condition compared to the treatment as usual condition at post-treatment and six-month follow-up (53).

The utility of group cognitive behavioral treatment of insomnia in routine clinical settings has also began to receive empirical support (54). It has been reported that groups of four to eight patients who underwent 11 weekly multicomponent sessions of CBT-I displayed significant improvements in overall sleep quality. Self-reported improvements in sleep at post-treatment included: total sleep time, sleep efficiency, and number of awakenings. No improvements were seen on PSG measures of sleep. Gains in self-reported sleep were maintained at 3- and 12-month follow-up.

Existing data suggest that group and individualized cognitive behavioral treatment of insomnia may produce comparable outcomes. A comparison of group and individual CBT-I found significant improvement in measures of sleep onset, maintenance and efficiency at post-treatment and nine-month follow-up (47). No statistically significant differences were seen as a function of treatment modality. However, when the clinical significance of improvements in sleep was assessed, only 16% of patients receiving group treatment compared to 34% of individually treated patients produced clinically significant gains in sleep, suggesting that individualized CBT-I may produce greater overall gains. It appears the equivalence of treatment modalities in terms of clinical significance needs further investigation.

The above referenced research all suggest the long-term effectiveness of multicomponent CBT-I. However, predictors of patient-perceived improvements following group treatment of insomnia are less well known. To examine potential predictors of patient-perceived improvements following group cognitive behavioral treatment of insomnia, groups of five to six patients met weekly for six sessions and received a multicomponent group CBT-I. Perceived improvement was assessed with the clinical global improvement scale (CGI). Significant improvements from pre- to post-treatment were found for sleep quality, sleep efficiency, sleep duration, and sleep-onset latency. At post-treatment, 41.4% of patients met the criteria for clinically significant improvements. Results indicated that sleep quality and sleep duration were the best predictors of perceived improvements resulting from group treatment of insomnia (55).

Special Populations

The effectiveness of group CBT-I has been assessed in numerous special populations. For example, the utility of group cognitive behavioral treatment of insomnia for improving sleep and preventing recidivism in adolescents with substance abuse problems has been studied (56). Adolescents (between the age of 13 and 19) underwent a multicomponent group treatment and stress reduction administration. Importantly, only 42% of the sample attended at least four treatment sessions. Sleep improvements in individuals that attended at least four treatment sessions were found for sleep efficiency, sleep-onset latency, number of awakenings, total sleep time, and sleep quality. These individuals also strongly endorsed the program at post-treatment. All adolescents increased their substance use during the course of treatment. The authors suggest that the effects of improved sleep on substance abuse in adolescents may manifest over a longer period of time, but group cognitive behavioral treatment of insomnia did produce improved sleep for the adolescents who completed treatment.

The effectiveness of group intervention to treat insomnia secondary to chronic pain has been examined via seven weekly sessions of multicomponent CBT-I. Results indicated significant improvements in sleep (by diary and actigraphy) from pre- to post-treatment for the treated patients compared to controls for sleep onset latency, sleep efficiency, wake time after sleep onset, and PSQI Quality. These reductions were maintained at three-month follow-up. No significant improvements in pain, depression, or medications usage were noted (57).

Cancer patients with insomnia were treated with stimulus control, relaxation, sleep education, worry time, and cognitive restructuring in groups for seven weeks and found to have significant improvements two weeks following treatment for: number of awakenings, wake time after sleep onset, total sleep time, sleep efficiency, sleep quality, and SII (58). Importantly, no participants continued to meet the diagnostic criteria for insomnia at two weeks post-treatment.

Likewise, the effectiveness of group cognitive behavioral treatment of insomnia for individuals with a "serious mental illness" has been investigated. Multicomponent CBT-I was delivered over 10 weekly sessions. From pre- to post-treatment, patients rated their sleep as significantly better (via the SII.). However, no changes in self-reported sleep parameters were noted. This is suspected to be largely due to the small ($n = 10$) sample size (59).

Short-term, group cognitive behavioral treatment of insomnia for "severely mentally ill patients" has been examined (60). Treatment was delivered over two weekly sessions and components used include: sleep education, stimulus control, sleep restriction, and sleep hygiene. From pre- to post-treatment, patients rated their sleep as significantly improved in terms of sleep onset latency and wake time after sleep onset. These improvements were maintained at three-month follow-up.

Group Treatment–Integration of Findings

The growing numbers of empirical research studies that have employed a group-based approach for the treatment of insomnia have varied widely in their approach to the group treatment of insomnia (Table 5 for specific details of each empirical investigation reviewed). In general, the group treatment of insomnia has been successfully employed, based on subjective reports of improved sleep, with a variety of populations, including community recruited volunteers (48–51,61), physician/clinically referred (46,47,52–54), adolescents with substance abuse problems (56), patients with chronic pain (57), patients with cancer (58), and patients with a comorbid mental illness (59,60).

Group sizes have ranged from two (56) to as many as fifteen patients (46). Similarly, treatment length has varied from a minimum of three weekly sessions (49) to a maximum of eleven, 90 minute weekly sessions (54). Patients as young as 13 years (56) and as old as 85 years (46) have been treated in a group format. Typically, group treatment has been conducted by doctoral students in clinical psychology graduate programs (49,56–58). However, treatment has also been successfully implemented by staff psychologists (46,59) and primary care nurses (53). In situations where the individual delivering treatment was not a doctoral-level practitioner, training and supervision was provided by a doctoral-level psychologist.

Although the specific content of the various group treatments have also varied, all the group treatments reported herein have contained one or more components of traditional cognitive behavioral treatment of insomnia as typically employed in individual treatment contexts (i.e., relaxation, sleep hygiene, stimulus control, sleep restriction, cognitive restructuring). Once again, for a complete list of group treatment approaches, please refer to Table 5.

Overall, these group approaches to the implementation of individualized cognitive behavioral treatment of insomnia have shown to be both effective (52–54) and efficacous (48–51,55–61) in improving sleep. All of the studies depicted in Table 5 demonstrated an improvement in subjective sleep characteristics following treatment. The effect sizes of the group treatment approaches reviewed herein ranged from small to large (Table 5) and are comparable to the effect sizes for behavioral treatments for insomnia that are individually administered (40,41). Importantly, many have shown a lasting effect of the treatment many months post-treatment. This has previously been shown in meta-analytic studies of treatment effects on insomnia symptoms. Murtagh and Greenwood (1995) performed a meta-analysis of the effects of psychological treatment on insomnia. They also examined the potential effects of several moderator variables on the treatment effect sizes. These authors found that all psychological treatment approaches produce substantial effect sizes and that the specific type of treatment approach (group vs. individual) did not result in different effect sizes (41). The equality of effects across various modalities of treatment were further demonstrated in direct comparisons of studies (47,48). Overall, the results of these meta-analytic studies as well as the studies reviewed herein suggest

(*text continues on page 338.*)

Table 5 Summary of Research Employing Group Treatment for Insomnia

Source	Patient sample	Exclusionary critieria	Group size	Treatment length	Therapist	Treatment components	Measures	Results	Durability	Effect Size[a]
Backhaus, et al. (52).	20 Physician referred, maen age = 43 yr (SD = 12.2 yr)	Co-morbid psychiatric condition, sleep-relevant somatic disorder	6–8 patients	6 weekly sessions/ 90 min each session	Experienced psychologist	Progressive muscle relaxation, cognitive relaxation, stimulus control (modified), thought stopping, and cognitive restructuring	PSQI, BDI, and STAI	Significant pre to post improvements for SOL (-36.3 min), TST (+53 min), SE (+18%), and BDI (-2.5 points)	3-yr follow-up for TST (+83 min) and SE (+20)	Overall small/medium/large effect sizes PSQI: Pre/post SOL $d = 0.592$, TST $d = 0.620$, SE $d = 1.051$ 3-mo follow-up SOL $d = 0.673$, TST $d = 0.837$, SE $d = 1.222$ 1-yr follow-up SOL $d = 0.529$, TST $d = 0.932$, SE $d = 1.134$ 3-yr followp-up SOL $d = 0.366$, TST $d = 0.826$, SE $d = 0.957$
Bastien, et al. (48).	45 Community-recruited volunteers, mean age = 41.8 yr (SD = 9.9 yr)	Presence of a sleep disorder other than insomnia, presence of an Axis I disorder, sleep disturbance due to substance use, use of hypnotics, current involvement in psychological treatment	4–6 patients	8 weekly sessions/ 90 min each session	Certified clinical psychologists and doctoral students in psychology	Stimulus control, sleep restriction, cognitive therapy, and sleep hygiene	SD, ISI, DBAS, BDI, and BAI	Significant pre to post improvements for TWT (+64 min), SE (+11%), WASO (-31 min), SQR (+6 points), ISI (-11 points), DBAS (-26 points), BDI (-8 points), and BAI (-6 points)	82% had SE above 80% at 6 mo follow-up	Overall medium/large effect sizes Group condition Sleep diary: Pre/post TWT $d = 1.346$, SE $d = 1.193$, WASO $d = .764$, SQR $d = .965$ 3-moh follow-up TWT $d = 1.088$, SE $d = 0.942$, WASO $d = 0.605$, SQR $d = 1.206$ 6-mo follow-up TWT $d = 0.890$, SE $d = 0.477$, WASO $d = 0.662$, SQR $d = 1.033$

(*Continued*)

Table 5 Summary of Research Employing Group Treatment for Insomnia (*Continued*)

Source	Patient sample	Exclusionary critieria	Group size	Treatment length	Therapist	Treatment components	Measures	Results	Durability	Effect Size[a]
Biancosino, et al. (60)	36 Insomnia patients with co-morbid mental illness, mean age = 47.4 yr (SD = 12.6 yr, range = 21–69 yr)	No sleep problem, mental retardation	Not reported	2 weekly sessions/ 60 min each session	Not reported	Sleep educations, stimulus control, sleep hygiene, and sleep restriction	SD, SWAI	Significant pre to post improvements for SOL (-10.3 min) and WASO (-4.5 min)	Improvements maintained at 3 mo	Overall small effect sizes Sleep diary: Pre/post SOL $d = 0.271$, WASO $d = 0.122$ 3-mo follow-up SOL $d = 0.217$, WASO $d = .094$
Bootzin & Stevens (56).	55 Adolescents completed drug abuse counseling, mean age = 16.13 yr (SD = 1.215 yr, range = 13–19 yr)	No complaint of sleep disturbance or daytime impairment, not completing or recently completed substance abuse treatment	2–6 patients	6 weekly sessions with a week break between session 5 and 6/ 90 min each session	Two advanced graduate students	Stimulus control, bright light, sleep hygiene, cognitive therapy, and Mindfulness-Based Stress Reduction	SD, actigraphy, PSWQ, ESS, GMHI, and drug use	SD: SE (+8%), SOL (-19 min), NWAK (-.88 awakenings), TST (+61 min), and SQR (+.76 points). No actigraphy improvements	Decreased drug use at 12-mo follow-up	Overall large effect sizes Sleep diary: Pre/post SE $d = 1.593$, SOL $d = 1.173$, NWAK $d = 1.596$, TST $d = .944$, SQR $d = 1.628$
Borkovec, et al. (49).	24 Community-recruited volunteers, no age information reported	Less than 30 min SOL, use of drugs, current treatment	4 patients	3 weekly sessions	Clinical graduate students	Relaxation alone, desensitization with relaxation, desensitization without relaxation	Daily questionnaires	Posttreatment improvements in SOL (-16 min) and rated difficulty in falling asleep and NWAK	No follow-up	Not enough information provided.
Currie, et al. (57).	60 Patients with co-morbid insomnia and chronic pain, mean age = 45 yr (SD = 8 yr, range = 29–59 yr)	Have fibromyalgia, no sleep complaint, over the age of 60, have major medical and psychiatric conditions, not willing to undergo randomization	5–7 patients	7 weekly sessions/ 2 hours each session	Doctoral students or interns in clinical psychology	Education, sleep restriction, stimulus control, relaxation training, cognitive restructuring, and sleep hygiene	SD and actigraphy, pain, emotional distress, and medication usage	SD: SOL (-27 min), SE (+13%), WASO (-50 min), and PSQI Quality (-5 points)	Maintained at 3-mo follow-up	Overall medium/large effect sizes Group vs wait list Sleep diary: Posttreatment SOL $d = .735$, SE $d = 1.006$, WASO $d = .925$ PSQI: SQR $d = 1.130$ 3-mo follow-up Sleep diary: SOL $d = 0.646$, SE $d = 0.962$, WASO $d = 0.830$ PSQI: SQR $d = 1.534$

Constantino, et al. (46).	86 Physician referred, mean age = 48.95 yr (SD = 15.19 yr, range = 19–85 yr)	None provided	10–15 patients	7 weekly sessions with the final 2 sessions occurring biweekly/ 90 min per session	Licensed clinical psychologists	Sleep education, relaxation, sleep restriction, stimulus control, cognitive restructuring	SD, ISI, Treatment Satisfaction, Patient Expectations, Group Therapy Session Report	↓ TWT, ↓ Daytime interference, patient expectations and therapeutic alliance are important predictors of dropout and satisfaction	No follow-up	Overall large effect sizes Pre/post Sleep diary: TWT $d = .718$
Davidson, et al. (58).	12 Cancer patients with insomnia, mean age = 54.7 yr (SD = 10.4 yr)	Currently receiving cancer treatment (or within 1 mo to baseline), suspicion of a sleep disorder other than insomnia, medical or psychiatric disorder effecting sleep, and medication (hypnotics, prednisone, dexametha-sone, opioids)	4–6 patients	7 weekly sessions with four weeks between session 5 and 6/ 60 – 90 min each session	Doctoral students in clinical psychology	Stimulus control, relaxation training, sleep education, 'worry time', and cognitive restructuring	SD, SII, and HADS	NWAK (-.72 awakenings), WASO (-31 min), TST (+35 min), SE (+16%), SQR (+.9 points), and SII (-11 points)	No follow-up	Overall large effect sizes Pre/post Sleep diary: NWAK $d = 1.041$, WASO $d = 1.557$, TST $d = .559$, SE $d = 1.899$, SQR $d = 1.48$

(*Continued*)

Table 5 Summary of Research Employing Group Treatment for Insomnia (*Continued*)

Source	Patient sample	Exclusionary critieria	Group size	Treatment length	Therapist	Treatment components	Measures	Results	Durability	Effect Size[a]
Dopke, et al. (59).	11 Insomnia patients with comorbid mental illness, mean age = 45.6 yr (SD = 9.85 yr)	None	Unknown	10 weekly sessions/ 50 min each session	Staff clinical psychologist and doctoral student	Sleep education, effects of substances, medical conditions, psychiatric conditions, life circum-stances, and sleep habits on sleep, stimulus control and sleep restriction, and physical, cognitive, and behavioral relaxation	SD and SII	Increased sleep quality via SII. No changes in SD.	No follow-up	Overall small effect sizes Pre/post Sleep diary: SOL $d = .320$, WASO $d = .170$
Espie, et al. (53).	201 General practice patients with insomnia, mean age = 54.2 yr (SD = 14.9 yr)	Deteriorating health or dementia, incapacitating pain or illness, untreated mental health problems, other sleep disorders	4–6 patients	5 weekly sessions/ 60 min per session	Community nurses based in primary care teams	Stimulus control, sleep restriction, and cognitive therapy	SD, actigraphy, and PSQI	SOL (-23.3 min) and SE (+9%) and improved PSQI	SD not maintained at 6-mo follow-up, PSQI maintained	Overall medium effect sizes Group condition Sleep diary: Pre/post SOL $d = .497$, SE $d = .522$ 6-mo follow-up SOL $d = 0.391$, SE $d = 0.417$

Jansson & Linton (50).	136 Community-recruited volunteers, mean age = 49.5 yr (SD = 11 yr)	Not fulfill the diagnostic requirements for insomnia, not of working age (16 – 65 yr old)	6–10 patients	6 weekly sessions with a booster session two mo following session 6/ 2 hours each session	Certified cognitive-behavioral therapists	Problems solving, relaxation, worry time, distraction, paradoxical intention, observation exercise, sleep hygiene, stimulus control, sleep restriction, cognitive therapy, stress management, sleep beliefs, sleep medications, coping, and sleep management	SD, DBAS, and HADS	SOL (-24 min), WASO (-66 min), TST (+60 min), SQR (-1.3 points), and SE (+13%). Improved anxiety HADS	Maintained at 1-yr	Overall small/medium effect sizes Group vs. control Sleep diary: 1-yr follow-up SOL $d = .610$, WASO $d = .386$, TST $d = .272$, SQR $d = .543$, SE $d = .427$
Schramm, et al. (54).	28 Physician referred, mean age = 47.5 yr (SD = 13.5 yr)	Insomnia "secondary" to psychiatric or medical conditions, sleep disorder other than insomnia	4–8 patients	11 weekly sessions/ 90 min each session	Cognitive-behavioral therapist and graduate student in clinical psychology	Behavior analysis, relaxation, sleep education, sleep restriction, stimulus control, cognitive restructuring, stress-management, problem solving, and increasing daytime activities	SD, PSQI, and PSG	Significant improvements in overall sleep quality (PSQI). TST (+28 min), SE (+10%), and NWAK (-.28 awakenings). No PSG improvement.	PSQI maintained at 3- and 12-mo follow-up.	Overall small/medium effect sizes Sleep diary: Pre/post TST $d = .305$, SE $d = .620$, NWAK $d = .282$

(*Continued*)

Table 5 Summary of Research Employing Group Treatment for Insomnia (*Continued*)

Source	Patient sample	Exclusionary critieria	Group size	Treatment length	Therapist	Treatment components	Measures	Results	Durability	Effect Size[a]
Verbeek, et al. (47).	40 Clinically referred patients with chronic insomnia, mean age = 43.68 yr (SD = 10.10 yr)	Psychopathology (depression or anxiety, refusal of group treatment, regular hypnotic use	5–7 patients	6 weekly sessions/ 2 hor and 30 min each session	Unknown	Psychoeducation, stimulus control, sleep hygiene, sleep restriction, cognitive restructuring, and relaxation	SD, DBAS, and SII	Improvements at post-treatment were seen for SOL, WASO, TST, and SE	Maintained at 9-mo follow up	Overall small/medium/large effect sizes Sleep diary: Pre/post SOL $d = .610$, TST $d = .310$, SE $d = 1.136$, WAS0 $d = .513$ 9-mo follow-up SOL $d = 0.567$, TST $d = 0.467$, SE $d = 0.941$, WAS0 $d = 360$
Vincent & Hameed (51).	50 Community-recruited volunteers and respirologist referred patients, mean age = 51.4 yr (SD = 11.4 yr)	Shift work, sleep disorder other than insomnia, brain injury, bipolar disorder, schizophrenia, serious medical condition	5–6 patients	7 weekly sessions/ 90 min each session	Staff psychologist	Sleep hygiene, stimulus control, medication withdrawal, relaxation, sleep restriction, cognitive therapy, stress management, and problem solving	SD, PSQI, DBAS, and ISI	SOL (-20 min), TST (+54 min), SE (+6%), DBAS (-19 points), PSQI (-4.48 points), and ISI (-6.6 points).	No follow-up	Overall large effect sizes Sleep diary: Pre/post TST $d = .833$

Vincent & Lionberg (61).	43 Community-recruited volunteers, mean age = 51.33 yr (SD = 12.37 yr)	Shift work, sleep disorder other than insomnia, brain injury, bipolar disorder, schizophrenia, serious medical condition, concurrent or prior CBTi	5–7 patients	6 weekly sessions	Psychologist and doctoral student	Sleep hygiene, stimulus control, medication withdrawal, relaxation, sleep restriction, and cognitive therapy	SD and SII	No sleep data reported	No follow-up	Not applicable
Vincent, et al. (55).	70 Clinically referred patients, mean age = 49.7 yr (SD = 12.0 yr)	No exclusion criteria	5–6 patients	6 weekly sessions/ 90 min each session	Clinical psychologist	Sleep education, sleep hygiene, relaxation, stimulus control, sleep restriction, medication withdrawal, and cognitive therapy	SD, PSQI, DBAS, and ISI. BDI, PSWQ, and CGI	Improved SQR, SE, Sleep Duration, and SOL as measured by the PSQI. SD: SE (+9%), TST (+42 min), and SOL (-12 min). Improvements for the DBAS, ISI, PSWQ, and BDI	No follow-up	Overall medium/large effect sizes Sleep diary: Pre/post SE $d = .815$, TST $d = .655$, SOL $d = .453$

[a]Effect Size Estimates represent Cohen's *d* and were calculated for pre to post treatment changes for the group condition alone (when no control condition was employed) or represent differences (if adequate control group was used), when sufficient information was available, in subjectively recorded sleep only.

Abbreviations: SD, sleep diary; PSQI, Pittsburg Sleep Quality Index (31); BDI, Beck Depression Inventory (16); BAI, Beck Anxiety Inventory (62); PSG, polysomnography; SOL, sleep-onset latency; WASO, wake time after sleep onset; TWT, total wake time; TST, total sleep time; SE, sleep efficiency; SQR, sleep quality rating; DBAS, Dysfunctional Beliefs and Attitudes About Sleep (19); ISI, Insomnia Severity Index (34); PSWQ, Penn State Worry Questionnaire (63); HADS, Hospital Anxiety and Depression Scale (23); STAI, State-Trait Anxiety Inventory (36); CGI, Clinical Global Improvement Scale; SII, Sleep Impairment Index (34); GMHI, General Mental Health Distress Index (64); SWAI, Sleep-Wake Activity Inventory (65); and ESS, Epworth Sleepiness Scale (20).

that group treatment can be as efficacious and effective as traditional behavioral approaches for treating insomnia.

Future Directions

The research that has previously been conducted on the group treatment of insomnia provides great hope for this modality of implementation. However, many questions are left unanswered. What is the optimal number of patients per group? Are there patients who are better or worse suited for group treatment approaches? What potential patient characteristics might distinguish patients who might most benefit from group treatment? How are these potential patient characteristics best assessed? Are there personal characteristics of group leaders that may lead to improved efficacy of group treatments? Is a purely interpersonal approach to the group treatment of insomnia practical? What is the best way to integrate group processes into the group treatment of insomnia? Which traditional cognitive behavioral treatments of insomnia techniques are best suited for implementation in group contexts?

All of these questions are intriguing. In the age of Health Maintenance Organizations (HMOs), it is critically important to provide empirical evidence of the effectiveness of treatment approaches. The cost-effectiveness of treating multiple patients simultaneously may potentially lead to group-based cognitive behavioral treatment of insomnia as the treatment of choice. While the extant literature suggests that a group approach is an effective treatment for insomnia in many different sub-populations of individuals with insomnia, much work is still needed. Given the high prevalence of insomnia and the preliminary results of group treatment approaches, this line of research warrants continuation and expansion. Furthermore, as presented in Table 5, many of the studies that have employed a group-based treatment approach have included patients with several comorbid conditions. Traditional logic suggests that patients with comorbid conditions are the hardest to successfully treat. Thus far, insomnia comorbid with drug abuse (56), chronic pain (57), cancer (58), and mental illnesses (59) have all been successfully treated within a group approach.

Conclusions

The group treatment of insomnia is a natural extension of individually administered cognitive behavioral treatment of insomnia. While preliminary work suggests these group approaches to be highly efficacious, the majority have apparently not capitalized on the unique therapeutic aspects that group therapy engenders. As Yalom (1995) stated, "groups resting *solely* on other assumptions, such as psycho-educational or cognitive-behavioral principles, fail to reap the full therapeutic harvest of group therapy. Each of these forms of therapy can… be made even more effective by incorporating a focus on interpersonal process" (Yalom, 1995, p. xiv).

Results from the small number of research studies that have employed a group treatment approach are very promising. Given its cost effectiveness, group treatment may prove to be a viable early intervention for insomnia (50) and appears to be suitable for delivery by trained nurses (53). Furthermore, its application to a wide range of clinical populations attests to the durability of this treatment modality. Lastly, patient perceptions of interactions with other individuals with insomnia as therapeutic provide some evidence of the added benefit of group treatment (47).

BRIEF AND GROUP INTERVENTIONS – SUMMARY AND CONCLUSIONS

The traditional approach of individually administering cognitive behavioral treatment of insomnia over the course of 6 to 10 sessions places heavy demands on clinician time and therefore, is not practical for use in 'real world' primary care settings. Briefer intervention protocols and the group administration of cognitive behavioral treatment of insomnia represent attractive alternatives, because they place fewer demands on clinician time. Effect sizes for both brief and group approaches are comparable to cognitive behavioral treatment of insomnia that is longer in duration and individually administered, suggesting that these alternate modes of administration appear to be as efficacious as traditional protocols. Studies of brief and group treatment of insomnia have demonstrated the utility of these approaches across a variety of ages and patient populations. Because the bulk of the research in this area has focused on efficacy trials (with a few notable exceptions) conducted with middle-class participants and delivered in "ideal" settings (academic research), more research on the effectiveness of such approaches is needed in order to fully understand how well such interventions translate to 'real world' primary care settings. To date, the few studies of effectiveness in this area have produced promising results (15,19–21,31,53). More research on the effectiveness of these approaches is needed, because several important questions remain regarding the best approach(es) to administering brief and/or group interventions in applied settings (e.g., Who is best suited to administer such treatment?; What is the ideal length of treatment?; What is the optimal group size for group treatment?).

REFERENCES

1. Morin CM, Bootzin RR, Buysse DJ, et al. Psychological and behavioral treatment of insomnia: Update of the recent evidence (1998–2004). Sleep 2006; 29(11):1398–1414.
2. McCrae CS, McGovern R, Lukefahr R, et al. Research evaluating brief Behavioral sleep treatments for rural elderly (RESTORE): A preliminary examination of effectiveness. Am J Geriatr Psychiatry 2007; 15(11):979–982.
3. Carter PA. A brief behavioral sleep intervention for family caregivers of persons with cancer. Cancer Nurs 2006; 29(2):95–103.
4. Chambers MJ, Alexander SD. Assessment and prediction of outcome for a brief behavioral insomnia treatment program. J Behav Ther Exp Psychiatry 1992; 23(4):289 297.
5. Edinger JD, Wohlgemuth WK, Radtke RA, et al. Dose-response effects of cognitive-behavioral insomnia therapy: A randomized clinical trial. Sleep 2007; 30(2):203–212.
6. Edinger JD, Sampson WS. A primary care "friendly" cognitive behavioral insomnia therapy. Sleep 2003; 26(2):177–182.
7. Friedman L, Benson K, Noda A, et al. An actigraphic comparison of sleep restriction and sleep hygiene treatments for insomnia in older adults. J Geriatr Psychiatry Neurol 2000; 13(1):17–27.
8. Germain A, Moul DE, Franzen PL, et al. Effects of a brief behavioral treatment for late-life insomnia: Preliminary findings. J Clin Sleep Med 2006; 2(4):3.
9. Germain A, Shear MK, Hall M, et al. Effects of a brief behavioral treatment for PTSD-related sleep disturbances: A pilot study. Behav Res Ther 2007; 45(3):627–632.
10. Lichstein KL, Wilson NM, Johnson CT. Psychological treatment of secondary insomnia. Psychol Aging 2000; 15(2):232–240.
11. Means MK, Lichstein KL, Epperson MT, et al. Relaxation therapy for insomnia: Nighttime and day time effects. Behav Res Ther 2000; 38(7):665–678.
12. Pallesen S, Nordhus IH, Kvale G, et al. Behavioral treatment of insomnia in older adults: An open clinical trial comparing two interventions. Behav Res Ther 2003; 41(1):31–48.
13. Bech P, Gudex C, Johansen KS. The WHO (Ten) well-being index: Validation in diabetes. Psychother Psychosom 1996; 65(4):183–190.
14. Riedel BW, Lichstein KL, Peterson BA, et al. A comparison of the efficacy of stimulus control for mediated and nonmedicated insomniacs. Behav Modif 1998; 22(1):3–28.
15. Strom L, Pettersson R, Andersson G. Internet-based treatment for insomnia: A controlled evaluation. J Consult Clin Psychol 2004; 72(1):113–120.
16. Beck AT, Steer RA, Garbin MG. Psychometric properties of the Beck Depression Inventory: Twenty-five years of evaluation. Clin Psychol Rev 1988; 8:77–100.
17. Radloff LS. The CES-D Scale: A self-report depression scale for reseach in the general population. Appl Psychol Meas 1977; 1:385–401.
18. Weitzner MA, McMillan SC. The Caregiver Quality of Life Index-Cancer (CQOLC) scale: Revalidation in a home hospice setting. J Palliat Care 1999; 15(2):13–20.
19. Morin CM, Stone J, Trinkle D, et al. Dysfunctional beliefs and attitudes about sleep among older adults with and without insomnia complaints. Psychol Aging 1993; 8(3):463–467.
20. Johns MW. A new method for measuring daytime sleepiness – The Epworth Sleepiness Scale. Sleep 1991; 14(6):540–545.
21. Krupp LB, Larocca NG, Muirnash J, et al. The Fatigue Severitiy Scale – Appliation to patients with Multiple-Schlerosis and Systematic Lupus-Erythmatosus. Arch Neurol 1989; 46(10):1121–1123.
22. Yesavage JA, Brink TL, Rose TL, et al. Development and validation of a geriatric depression screening scale – A preliminary report. J Psychiatr Res 1983; 17(1):37–49.
23. Zigmond AS, Snaith RP. The Hospital Anxiety and Depression Scale. Acta Psychiatr Scand 1983; 67(6):361–370.
24. Hamilton M. The assessment of anxiety states by rating. British Journal of Medical Psychology 1959.
25. Hamilton M. A rating scale for depression. J Neurol Neurosurg Psychiatry 1960; 23:56–62.

26. Hoelscher TJ, Ware JC, Bond T. Initial validation of the Insomnia Impact Scale. Sleep Res 1993; 22:149.
27. Spielman AJ, Saskin P, Thorpy MJ. Treatment of chronic insomnia by restriction of time in bed. Sleep 1987; 10(1):45–56.
28. Carskadon MA, Dement WC, Mitler MM, et al. Guidelines for the Multiple Sleep Latency Test (MSLT) – A standard measure of sleepiness. Sleep 1986; 9(4):519–524.
29. McNair DM, Lorr M, Droppleman LF. Manual for the Profile of Mood States. San Diego, CA: EDITS, 1971.
30. Meyer TJ, Miller ML, Metzger RL, et al. Development and validation of the Penn State Worry Questionnaire. Behav Res Ther 1990; 28(6):487–495.
31. Buysse DJ, Reynolds CF, Monk TH, et al. The Pittsburgh Sleep Quality Index: A new instrument for psychiatric practice and research. Psychiatry Res 1989 28:193–213.
32. Germain A, Hall M, Krakow B, et al. A brief sleep scale for posttraumatic stress disorder: Pittsburgh Sleep Quality Index Addendum for PTSD. J Anxiety Disord 2005; 19:233–244.
33. Lacks P. Behavioral Treatment for Persistent Insomnia. New York, NY: Pergamon Press, 1987.
34. Morin CM. Insomnia. Psychological Assessment and Management. New York, NY: Guilford Press, 1993.
35. Hoddes E, Zarcone V, Smythe H, et al. Quantification of sleepiness – New approach. Psychophysiology 1973; 10(4):431–436.
36. Spielberger CD, Gorsuch RL, Lushene R, et al. State-Trait Anxiety Inventory, Form Y. Palo Alto, CA: Consulting Psychologists Press, 1983.
37. Miles L. A sleep questionnaire. In: Guilleminault C, ed. Sleeping and Waking Disorders: Indications and Techniques. Stoneham, MA: Butterwork, 1982:Appendix I.:383–413.[CE: Please check highlighted text in this ref.]
38. Perlis ML, Sharpe M, Smith MT, et al. Behavioral treatment of insomnia: Treatment outcome and the relevance of medical and psychiatric morbidity. J Behav Med 2001; 24(3):281–296.
39. Perlis M, Aloia M, Millikan A, et al. Behavioral treatment of insomnia: A clinical case series study. J Behav Med 2000; 23(2):149–161.
40. Irwin MR, Cole JC, Nicassio PM. Comparative meta-analysis of behavioral interventions for insomnia and their efficacy in middle-aged adults and in older adults 55+years of age. Health Psychol 2006; 25(1):3–14.
41. Murtagh DRR, Greenwood KM. Identifying effective psychological treatments for insomnia – A meta-analysis. J Consult Clin Psychol 1995; 63(1):79–89.
42. Edinger JD, Wohlgemuth WK, Radtke RA, et al. Cognitive behavioral therapy for treatment of chronic primary insomnia – A randomized controlled trial. JAMA 2001; 285(14):1856–1864.
43. Chambers MJ, Alexender SD. Assessment and prediction of outcome for a brief behavioral insomnia treatment program. J Abnorm Psychol 1992.
44. Yalom ID. The Theory and Practice of Group Psychotherapy Fourth Edition. New York, NY: BasicBooks, 1995.
45. Kupych-Woloshyn N, MacFarlane J, Shapiro CM. A group-approach for the management of insomnia. J Psychosom Res 1993; 37:39–44.
46. Constantino M, Manber R, Ong J, et al. Patient expectations and therapeutic alliance as predictors of outcome in group cognitive-behavioral therapy for insomnia. Behav Sleep Med 2007; 5(3):210–228.
47. Verbeek I, Konings G, Aldenkamp A, et al. Cognitive behavioral treatment in clinically referred chronic insomniacs: Group versus indivdiual treatment. Behav Sleep Med 2006; 4(3):135–151.
48. Bastien CH, Morin CM, Ouellet MC, et al. Cognitive-behavioral therapy for insomnia: Comparison of individual therapy, group therapy, and telephone consultations. J Consult Clin Psychol 2004; 72(4):653–659.
49. Borkovec TD, Steinmar.Sw, Nau SD. Relaxation training and single-item desensitization in group treatment of insomnia. J Behav Ther Exp Psychiatry 1973; 4(4):401–403.
50. Jansson M, Linton SS. Cognitive-behavioral group therapy as an early intervention for insomnia: A randomized controlled trial. J Occup Rehabil 2005; 15(2):177–190.
51. Vincent N, Hameed H. Relation between adherence and outcome in the group treatment of insomnia. Behav Dleep Med 2003; 1(3):125–139.
52. Backhaus J, Hohagen F, Voderholzer U, et al. Long-term effectiveness of a short-term cognitive-behavioral group treatment for primary insomnia. Eur Arch Psychiatry Clin Neurosci 2001; 251(1): 35–41.
53. Espie CA, MacMahon KMA, Kelly HL, et al. Randomized clinical effectiveness trial of nurse-administered small-group cognitive behavior therapy for persistent insomnia in general practice. Sleep 2007; 30(5):574–584.
54. Schramm E, Hohagen F, Backhaus J, et al. Effectiveness of a multicomponent group treatmetn for insomnia. Behav Cogn Psychother 1995; 23(2):109–127.

55. Vincent N, Penner S, Lewycky S. What predicts patients' perceptions of improvement in insomnia? J Sleep Res 2006; 15(3):301–308.
56. Bootzin RR, Stevens SJ. Adolescents, substance abuse, and the treatment of insomnia and daytime sleepiness. Clin Psychol Rev 2005; 25(5):629–644.
57. Currie SR, Wilson KG, Pontefract AJ, et al. Cognitive-behavioral treatment of insomnia secondary to chronic pain. J Consult Clin Psychol 2000; 68(3):407–416.
58. Davidson JR, Waisberg JL, Brundage MD, et al. Nonpharmacologic group treatment of insomnia: A preliminary study with cancer survivors. *Psychooncology*. 2001; 10(5):389–397.
59. Dopke CA, Lehner RK, Wells AM. Cognitive-behavioral group therapy for insomnia in individuals with serious mental illnesses: A preliminary evaluation. Psychiatr Rehabil J 2004; 27(3):235–242.
60. Biancosino B, Rocchi D, Dona S, et al. Efficacy of short-term psychoeducational intervention for persistent non-organic insomnia in severely mentally ill patients. A pilot study. Eur Psychiatry 2004; 21:460–462.
61. Vincent N, Lionberg C. Treatment preference and patient satisfaction in chronic insomnia. Sleep 2001;24(4):411–417.
62. Beck AT, Epstein N, Brown G, et al. An inventory for measuring clinical anxiety: Psychometric properties. J Consult Clin Psychol 1988; 56:863–897.
63. Carstensen LL, Pasupathi M, Mayr U, et al. Emotional experience in everyday life across the adult life span. J Pers Soc Psychol 2000; 79(4):644–655.
64. Dennis ML. Global Appraisal of Individual Needs – Version 1299. Bloomington, IL: Chestnut Health Systems, 1999.
65. Rosenthal L, Roehrs TA, Roth T. The Sleep-Wake Inventory: A self-report measure of daytime sleepiness. Biol Psychiatry 1993; 34:810–820.

29 Multimodal Cognitive Behavior Therapy

Colleen E. Carney

Department of Psychology, Ryerson University, Toronto, Ontario, Canada

Jack D. Edinger

Psychology Service, VA Medical Center, Department of Psychiatry and Behavioral Sciences, Duke University Medical Center, Durham, North Carolina, U.S.A.

HISTORY AND RATIONALE FOR MULTIMODAL CBT

As described in previous chapters, insomnia is a highly prevalent and often serious health condition that may be precipitated by stress, environmental factors, changes in the sleep–wake cycle, medical or psychiatric illnesses, and/or use of sleep-disrupting substances. Regardless of its initial cause(s), insomnia may assume a chronic course perpetuated by cognitive, emotional, and behavioral factors that persist over time and cause continual sleep disruption (43). Included among the cognitive factors are unhelpful beliefs and attitudes that may contribute to sleep-related performance anxiety and lead to sleep-disruptive bedtime arousal (1). In addition, misconceptions about how one should respond to a poor night's sleep might give way to a variety of compensatory strategies that only further disrupt sleep. For example, daytime napping or spending extra time in bed in pursuit of elusive, unpredictable sleep may interfere with normal homeostatic mechanisms designed to correct for accumulated sleep debt. Alternately, the habit of "sleeping in" beyond the normal rising time following a poor night's sleep may disrupt circadian mechanisms that regulate the normal sleep–wake rhythm. Additionally, engaging in mentally demanding work late into the evening without allotting sufficient wind down time before bed may result in excessive mental arousal that interferes with sleep onset. Over time, these cognitive and behavioral factors may result in the repeated association of the bed and bedroom with unsuccessful sleep attempts and lead to the development of a sleep-disruptive conditioned arousal in response to the home sleeping environment.

Although it seems intuitively obvious that relaxation before bed and practicing good sleep habits (i.e., following a routine sleep–wake schedule; avoiding daytime napping, etc.) facilitates sleep quality, recognition of the effectiveness of these behavioral insomnia remedies did not emerge until the past half century. Between the late 1950s and mid 1980s a number of first generation therapies emerged as viable insomnia treatments. Included among these are such treatments as relaxation training, stimulus control, sleep restriction, and sleep hygiene education, which have been described in detail in the preceding chapters. As outlined in Table 1, each of these therapies is designed to target a fairly-specific subset of the above-mentioned array of cognitive and behavioral factors that can perpetuate insomnia. Consequently, each of these treatments ignores selected cognitive or behavioral that may be more or less important as perpetuating mechanisms across insomnia patients. Therefore, none of these first generation therapies represents a panacea that would be expected to be consistently effective from one insomnia sufferer to the next.

Given this realization, interest in more omnibus, multicomponent behavioral insomnia therapies emerged in the late 1980s and early 1990s. It was during this time-period that the initial trials of what constitutes current-day multimodal cognitive-behavioral insomnia therapy (CBT) were first reported (2–4). These early trials first demonstrated the promise of an insomnia therapy that combines several effective cognitive and behavioral strategies into a comprehensive treatment package. Since that time, various multimodal CBT protocols have been proposed. However, most of these have minimally included stimulus control, sleep restriction, and a cognitively oriented strategy so as to form an insomnia therapy that can be expected to be more broadly and consistently effective across insomnia patients.

Multimodal CBT is appealing for its presumed ability to address the range of insomnia complaints and etiologic factors that can occur in insomnia. For example, it seems unreasonable

Table 1 First Generation Treatment Descriptions and Their Respective Primary Treatment Targets

Type of treatment	Treatment description	Primary treatment target(s)
Relaxation training	• A structured series of mental or muscle-focused exercises designed reduce or eliminate sleep-disruptive physiological (e.g., muscle tension) and/or cognitive (e.g., racing thoughts) arousal. • Examples include progressive muscle relaxation, passive relaxation, autogenic training, biofeedback, imagery training, meditation, and hypnosis.	Sleep-disruptive physiological and/or mental arousal occurring at bedtime or in bed
Stimulus control	• A structured behavioral regimen that instructs the patient to (1) establish a standard rising time; (2) go to bed only when sleepy; (3) get out of bed whenever awake for long periods; (4) avoid reading, watching TV, eating, worrying and other sleep-incompatible behaviors in the bed/bedroom; and (5) refrain from daytime napping. • The goal of this treatment is that of reassociating the bed and bedroom with successful sleep attempts.	Conditioned arousal associated with the bed/bedroom and attempts to sleep Improper sleep–wake scheduling that interferes with circadian control over sleep Daytime napping that reduces homeostatic sleep drive
Sleep restriction	• Sleep restriction therapy reduces nocturnal sleep disturbance primarily by restricting the time allotted for sleep each night so that the time spent in bed closely matches the individual's presumed sleep requirement.	Excessive time spent in bed that reduces homeostatic sleep drive.
Sleep hygiene education	• Patients are educated about normative sleep requirements, healthy sleep behaviors and sleep-conducive environmental conditions. • Typically they are encouraged to exercise daily, eliminate the use of caffeine, alcohol, and nicotine, eat a light snack at bedtime, and ensure that the sleeping environment is quiet, dark, and comfortable.	Patients' misconceptions about sleep. Use of sleep-disruptive substances Lifestyle & environmental factors that disrupt sleep

to expect that a person, who presents with a significant worry component and good sleep habits, should receive the same single component therapy as a patient who presents primarily with an irregular sleep–wake schedule. Since multimodal CBT includes several stand-alone interventions, it presumably casts a wider treatment net, thus providing a more broadly effective therapy across a range of insomnia subtypes (i.e., those with sleep onset insomnia, those with sleep maintenance insomnia, those complaining predominantly of cognitive arousal, etc.).

Given its inclusion of several of the first-generation behavioral treatment strategies, Multimodal CBT is a more complex therapy than are its predecessors. Yet multimodal CBT does not require more time in therapy than do the single component treatments. In fact, CBT is typically administered in one to eight sessions. Given the accumulation of supportive data, CBT arguably has become the nonpharmacologic treatment of choice for insomnia, and most recent RCTs involving psychological interventions for insomnia have focused on various forms of this multicomponent approach.

Multimodal CBT Components

As suggested above, multimodal CBT consists of a number of effective and well-established first generation behavioral insomnia therapies used in combination to form an omnibus and broadly effective insomnia treatment. As its name would imply, this form of therapy includes a number of specific strategies to address both the cognitive factors and sleep disruptive habits that sustain insomnia over time. However, since the time of the earliest descriptions (2–4) of this treatment were published, various versions of multimodal CBT have been proposed. As a result, multimodal CBT currently cannot be characterized as a fixed brand of psychological treatment. In fact, the pertinent empirical and descriptive literature shows that the specific number and nature of treatment components included treatment packages labeled multimodal CBT has varied considerably over the years. Presumably such variability is largely attributable to provide preferences since what constitutes the optimally effect CBT package has yet to be determined. Therefore, a thorough description of CBT treatment components requires discussion of a number of core strategies that are found in most published CBT descriptions as well as a number of add-on strategies, which are commonly included to compliment the core strategies.

Cognitive-behavior therapy, by definition, must include some form of cognitive-focused intervention to merit this descriptive label. In the case of insomnia, a variety of cognitive treatment "targets" may emerge and warrant specific treatment attention. However, the exact nature of the cognitive factors contributing to insomnia may vary considerably across patients so it is often necessary to include an array of specific cognitive therapy techniques in multimodal CBT to meet patients' needs.

Among the common cognitive factors that perpetuate insomnia are a variety of unhelpful beliefs and attitudes about sleep that may heighten sleep-related anxiety and/or promote sleep-interfering habits (5). For example, beliefs that sleep is beyond one's control or that insomnia may have serious negative effects of one's functioning or health can increase anxiety about sleep and, in turn, disrupt the sleep process. Further, insufficient knowledge about how one should respond to a night of poor sleep may promote sleep-disruptive habits (e.g., daytime napping or "sleeping in") that interfere with the next night's sleep. As a result, multimodal CBT typically includes therapeutic strategies designed to alter these unhelpful beliefs. One technique proposed for addressing such beliefs involves providing patients a standardized psychoeducational intervention designed to correct common misconceptions insomnia patients have about their sleep difficulties. Alternately, these unhelpful beliefs may be addressed via formal cognitive restructuring methods. In the latter case, the therapy process may be assisted by use of special questionnaires (4) designed to identify each patient's most problematic sleep-related beliefs or by employing insomnia-focused thought records that modify unhelpful sleep-related beliefs.

For many insomnia patients, cognitive arousal arising from sleep-disruptive practices such as engagement in mentally stimulating activities immediately prior to bedtime or the habit of taking one's worries to bed may confound the sleep process. Encouraging such patients to avoid mentally stimulating activities in the hour or so before bedtime and to schedule an early evening structured problem-solving time to address daily worries (6) are additional cognitive therapy approaches that may be employed to reduce mental arousal during the sleep period. Some CBT packages offer patients systematic instructions for engaging in constructive worry as well as constructive worry worksheets to aid patients in their home application of this technique.

Along with one or more of the mentioned cognitive-focused interventions, multimodal CBT typically includes both stimulus control and sleep restriction instructions as core treatment strategies. As noted earlier, these two interventions are used in combination in most multimodal CBT protocols so as to re-establish normal homeostatic and circadian control over the sleep process and to eliminate conditioned arousal resulting from repeated association of the bed and bedroom with unsuccessful sleep attempts. In some published treatment guides (7), stimulus control and sleep restriction instructions are presented in separate sessions as independent treatment components. However, given the overlapping treatment instructions included in each of these strategies, it is also easy to combine stimulus control and sleep restriction into a single set of instructions that can be presented in a single session. For example, we (2) have employed an instructional set that directs each patient to (1) adhere to a standard rising time; (2) get out of bed whenever awake for > 15 to 20 minutes; (3) avoid reading, watching TV, eating, worrying and other sleep-incompatible behaviors in the bed and bedroom; and (4) refrain from daytime napping; and (5) go to bed when sleepy but not before an individually prescribed bedtime. Consistent with the sleep restriction approach, an average total sleep time (ATST) is determined for each patient using pretherapy sleep logs/diaries and this ATST is used to ascertain a prescribed time in bed (PTIB) for each patient. Once the standard rising time is selected, the PTIB is used to determine the earliest allowable bedtime for each patient and is, thus, incorporated into the modified stimulus control/sleep restriction instructions shown (See Ref. 8 for more details).

As there has been considerable attention devoted to "hyperarousal" as an etiologic factor in insomnia (9), relaxation therapy is often included as a component of multimodal CBT. Relaxation therapy (RT) techniques include strategies such as progressive muscle relaxation, passive relaxation, autogenic training, and imagery (10). Regardless of the specific RT strategy used, treatment entails teaching the insomnia patient formal exercises designed to reduce anxiety and arousal at bedtime so that sleep is facilitated. Most forms of therapy require multiple treatment sessions with additional intersession home practice to achieve optimal results. With this training, the patients are expected to achieve sufficient relaxation skills so as to reduce or eliminate sleep-related performance anxiety and bedtime arousal presumed to perpetuate their insomnia. In addition, RT may have the added, and perhaps unintended, benefit of distracting patients from their usual bedtime worries and intrusive thoughts that interfere with the sleep process (11). As discussed in more detail below, CBT protocols that do not include relaxation have proven highly effective for insomnia management so the value-added of RT as a CBT component remains an open question. Hence, RT may be best classified as a popular add-on rather than a core component of the multimodal CBT package for insomnia.

Inasmuch as one's lifestyle, patterns of consumption, and usual sleeping environment may play a role in sleep difficulties, sleep experts have long recognized the value of addressing these factors in managing insomnia complaints. As such, multimodal CBT protocols often include a set of so-called sleep hygiene (12) education to address such factors. The specifics of sleep hygiene may vary across CBT protocols but typically it includes education about healthy sleep behaviors and sleep-conducive environmental conditions. For example, patients may be encouraged to exercise, reduce caffeine, alcohol, and nicotine use, eat a bedtime snack that includes food items (e.g., milk products, peanut butter) rich in the sleep-promoting amino acid, L-tryptophan, and ensure that the bedroom is quiet, dark, and comfortable. Although sleep hygiene recommendations alone are insufficient for insomnia management, they are often add-on components of CBT protocols to address lifestyle and environmental factors that otherwise may dampen response to the core elements of this therapy.

GENERAL EFFICACY AND EFFECTIVENESS OF CBT

There is substantial evidence supporting the usefulness of multimodal CBT for management of primary insomnia. Both single-case and randomized controlled trials have shown that CBT produces significantly greater sleep improvements for primary insomnia patients than do either no treatment (wait list) control conditions (4,13,14) or such stand-alone therapies as relaxation training (3), sleep hygiene education (15,16) and a credible sham (placebo) psychological treatment. In addition, several randomized trials (17,18) collectively have shown that CBT and pharmacotherapy with common prescription hypnotics (e.g., zolpidem, zolpiclone, temazepam) yield similar sleep improvements during active treatment, but only CBT produces improvements that endure long after active therapy is discontinued. Furthermore, two large clinical effectiveness studies (19,20) have shown multimodal CBT is superior to treatment as usual (most typically pharmacotherapy) for the management of primary insomnia patients who present to medical clinics for care.

Along with these findings, there is growing evidence that multimodal CBT may provide benefits for patients with more complex forms of insomnia. To date, a number of small to moderately sized single-site, randomized clinical trials have suggested that CBT is efficacious for ameliorating sleep problems among patients with chronic peripheral pain syndromes (21), breast cancer survivors, fibromyalgia sufferers (22), older mixed medical patients (14), and those with chronic alcohol abuse. In addition, several case series or clinic-based studies support the efficacy of CBT among patients with mixed mental and medical conditions (23). Moreover, some of these reports have suggested that CBT may also result in improvements in mood status or other disease-specific symptoms. Given these findings along with those derived from studies of primary insomnia patients, multimodal CBT can be regarded as a well-established or frontline therapy for ameliorating sleep disturbance in both simple and complex forms of chronic insomnia.

In addition to improving sleep, one would expect that the multiple components of CBT should address the hypothesized cognitive and behavioral factors that purportedly perpetuate or maintain insomnias. Since multimodal CBT typically has a cognitive component, troublesome thoughts or cognitive arousal should be improved in this modality. Indeed, studies suggest that CBT improves several cognitive factors such as sleep-interfering beliefs (44), sleep-related self-efficacy (e.g., confidence in one's ability to produce sleep) (21), and cognitive arousal (24–26). Likewise, CBT appears to address sleep-interfering behavioral factors such as spending excessive time in bed (27), or varying bedtime and rise times (4,15,17,28). Moreover, although limited in number, the studies that have examined CBT mechanisms have shown that changes in selected, CBT-targeted cognitive and behavioral perpetuating mechanisms appear to mediate improvements in sleep and global insomnia symptoms. Thus, the outcomes achieved with CBT apparently result, at least in part, from the fact that this therapy effectively targets cognitive and behavioral mechanisms critical to sustaining insomnia problems.

MODES OF DELIVERY

Despite the efficacy of multimodal CBT for managing insomnia, access to this treatment can be limited due to the scarcity of providers with CBT expertise. Indeed the number of patients who might benefit from such an intervention currently exceeds the capacity of the number of trained providers of this treatment. This state of affairs has created significant impetus for the development of innovative methods of CBT delivery so as to allow for more facile dissemination of this treatment. Whereas efforts to enhance CBT dissemination is a fairly new effort, there have been a number of innovative CBT delivery methods proposed that might lead to greater public accessibility of this treatment.

Like many other psychological treatments, multimodal CBT is easily adapted to a group therapy format. The obvious advantage of this format is that it allows one trained provider to administer treatment to multiple patients simultaneously. Moreover, a group therapy format can have the added benefit of providing patients peer support as they proceed through the treatment process. Although a previous metaanalytic review (29) suggested a slight superiority of individually administered treatments over group therapy, several controlled evaluations have shown that group CBT models involving six to eight sessions produce notable improvements in subjective/objective sleep patterns, general mood status and unhelpful beliefs about sleep (4,17,19,30). Studies comparing the relative efficacy of individual versus group CBT have been limited, but one recent study did show comparable outcomes for insomnia patients assigned to either group or individualized CBT therapy. Nonetheless, more studies are needed to further explore this issue.

Because most insomnia patients who seek care do so in primary care clinics (31), there has been some interest in developing multimodal CBT protocols suitable for such medication settings. Espie and colleagues (19,20) tested a group CBT protocol administered by office nurses working in outpatient medical clinics and found this approach to be more effective than usual care for managing insomnia patients seen in such settings. However, the treatment effect sizes for this form of intervention appeared to be somewhat smaller than those reported for trials wherein treatment was administered by doctoral-level providers and/or sleep specialists (20,32). As an alternative to this approach, some investigators (15) have proposed abbreviated two-session CBT protocols suitable for delivery by primary care providers. Whereas results from pilot tests of these interventions have been promising, it is yet to be demonstrated that MD-level providers are willing and able to effectively administer such protocols in their busy medical practices. Thus, continued consideration of CBT models suitable for primary care would seem beneficial.

Of course many insomnia sufferers do not seek care from professionals but rather attempt to manage their sleep problems on their own by using over-the-counter sleep aids or other less than optimal "home remedies" such as alcohol (33). With these sorts of individuals in mind, Mimeault and Morin (13) tested a self-help, CBT bibliotherapy with and without supportive phone consultations against a wait list control group. Compared to the control condition, those treated with the bibliotherapy showed substantially greater sleep improvements than control patients, and these improvements were maintained at a three-month follow up. The addition of phone consultations with a therapist conferred some advantage over bibliotherapy alone at posttreatment, but these benefits disappeared by follow up. Oosterhuis and Klip (34) reported promising results from a novel study wherein a multimodal behavioral insomnia therapy was provided via a series of eight, 15-minute educational programs broadcast on radio and television. More than 23,000 people ordered the accompanying course material, and data from a random subset of these showed sleep improvements and reductions in hypnotic use, medical visits, and physical complaints were achieved among those who took part in this educational program. More recently, Strom and colleagues (35) tested a five-week self-help interactive CBT program delivered to insomnia patients via the Internet. Although the treated group did show greater reductions in unhelpful attitudes toward sleep than did untreated patients, the treatment and control groups did not differ on their self-reported sleep improvements. These findings provide a mixed view of self-help protocols but do imply that some guidance from trained therapists (via phone consultation or mass media) may enhance outcomes for these self-help interventions. Hence, the question of how best to optimize the efficacy of these self-help CBT interventions merits research attention.

APPLICATIONS WITH HYPNOTIC USERS

Despite the growing recognition that multimodal CBT is a safe and effective treatment, pharmacotherapy remains the most used first-line intervention provided to those insomnia patients who seek treatment (31,36). Moreover, clinical experience indicates that a sizable proportion of insomnia patients who eventually present seeking nonpharmacological therapy do so while continuing hypnotic medications prescribed for their sleep difficulties. This state of affairs, in turn, leads to a number of important questions in regard to the use of multimodal CBT with such individuals. First, it seems useful to consider whether these patients derive similar benefits from CBT, as do unmedicated patients. Secondly, it seems useful to question if there is an optimal protocol to follow for those patients who wish to combine CBT with pharmacotherapy for insomnia. Finally, it is also useful to determine if CBT and other nonpharmacological approaches might prove useful to hypnotic-dependent patients who ultimately wish to discontinue their sleep medication use.

To date, there have been no studies specifically conducted to compare the CBT responses of patients who do and do not use sleep medications. However, post hoc analyses conducted in a number of published studies suggest a history of hypnotic use does not dampen patients' responses to multimodal CBT interventions. In a large trial (n = 161 CBT-treated patients) that tested a nurse-administered CBT, Espie (19) found that patients who had used hypnotic medications achieved sleep improvements similar to those shown by medication-free patients. Similarly Verbeek et al. (37) conducted a large (n = 127 CBT treated patients) case replication series study and found no differences between the CBT responses of hypnotic users and nonusers. Whereas one single group study (30) showed that unmedicated patients responded better to CBT than did medicated patients, the small sample size (n = 21) of this investigation raises questions about the stability of its results. Thus, the current evidence would suggest that a history of hypnotic medication use should not be considered as a contraindication or limiting factor when screening patients for insomnia treatment with multimodal CBT.

In contrast, the research pertaining to CBT/hypnotic combination therapy has provided somewhat mixed results. Three previous studies (17,18,38) with similar research designs compared treatments consisting of CBT alone, hypnotic medication alone, a CBT + hypnotic treatment combination, and a medication placebo. In each of these studies, patients received treatment for a fix period of time (6–8 weeks) and then entered an extended follow-up period during which they received no addition CBT instruction or medication. In all three of these studies, patients who received CBT alone showed better long-term outcome than did those who received the combined CBT/medication therapy or the other two treatments. One implication of these results is that the presence of medication somehow dampens patients' responses to CBT. However, more recent studies have shown that a sequential treatment protocol in which patients initially receive hypnotic medication with CBT and then are withdrawn from medication and continue with further CBT alone, achieve better short- and long-term outcomes than do patients who receive only CBT intervention. Although more research of this nature is needed, these findings suggest that a time-limited course of hypnotic medication at the outset of CBT therapy may potentiate the treatment effects of this multimodal behavioral intervention.

Of course not all patients are accepting of medications, and some who use hypnotic medications chronically wish to discontinue them and learn to sleep well without sleep aids. For such individuals there is ample evidence that CBT may help some patients achieve this goal. Several studies (13,19,30,37) for example, have shown that a notable proportion of patients who

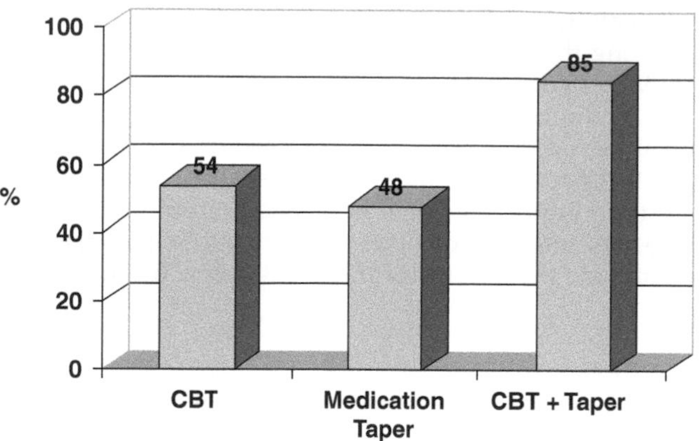

Figure 1 Proportion of patients who were able to stop hypnotic use with treatment

undergo CBT are able to reduce or stop their hypnotic use during the course of this treatment. Perhaps as a result of such observations, some investigators have tested the usefulness of combining multimodal CBT for insomnia with structured medication tapering protocols to aid hypnotic-dependent patients who wish to discontinue sleep medication use. In one such study, Morgan et al. (39) compared a treatment consisting of CBT + medication tapering against a waitlist condition and found the former treatment was superior to the control condition for both improving sleep and producing at least a 50% reduction in sleep medication use by a six-month follow-up. In a subsequent study, Morin compared the relative efficacy of CBT, a guided medication tapering protocol, and a combined CBT + guided taper protocol (40). As shown by Figure 1, the proportion of patients who were able to stop their hypnotic use was substantially higher in the combined treatment condition than in the other two unitary treatment approaches. Patients who received CBT reported greater sleep improvements than those who received only the guided medication tapering protocol. Furthermore, overall hypnotic abstinence rates at a long-term follow-up favored the combined CBT + guided tapering condition over the other two treatments. Given these findings, multimodal CBT appears to be a very useful therapy for helping patients reduces or discontinue their use of hypnotic medications.

SUMMARY AND FUTURE DIRECTIONS

Multimodal CBT is a combination treatment that utilizes effective single-component cognitive and behavioral therapies in a single, easy-to-administer standardized delivery package. This form of therapy has intuitive appeal because it is designed to be a comprehensive intervention strategy suitable for most insomnia subtypes. It also has theoretical appeal as the components of this therapy purportedly address major cognitive and behavioral etiologic factors in insomnia. The inclusion of this therapy in the most recent RCTs suggests it is one of the most commonly used psychological therapies in insomnia treatment. These RCTs have demonstrated that CBT is very effective not only for uncomplicated forms of insomnia but also can be effective for more complicated insomnia sufferers including those with comorbid disorders. Moreover, these studies have shown that CBT is effective for improving sleep and reducing/eliminating sleep medication use even among patients with long-standing histories of hypnotic dependence.

Future research areas for this treatment will likely include dismantling and treatment-matching studies. As noted previously, various versions of multimodal CBT have been proposed. The more streamlined versions tend to include stimulus control, sleep restriction and some form of cognitive therapy. The most complex models include these core components plus additional sleep hygiene education and some form of relaxation therapy. The value-added of the relaxation component is questionable since both CBT with relaxation and CBT without relaxation are currently regarded as well-established insomnia therapies. Head-to-head trial of various CBT models have not yet been conducted so what constitutes the optimal and most cost-effective CBT model remains an open question. Studies to address this question would seem warranted.

Treatment matching relies on a case formulation approach. For example, Patient X and Y complain primarily of cognitive arousal, thus we expect a cognitive approach would be superior to a less cognitively oriented therapy. Patient X is randomly assigned to a cognitively oriented therapy and Patient Y to a predominantly behavioral therapy, and we test whether matching Patient X to a cognitive intervention produces superior treatment outcome to the more behavioral approach. It would be useful to test a matching approach with contemporary treatment approaches and comprehensive outcome measures to determine if tailored approaches are superior to "packaged" treatment approaches.

In this regard, there is also need for research to determine if tailored or augmented CBT protocols need to be developed for complex forms of insomnia. As discussed previously, studies have supported the efficacy of CBT for treating primary insomnia and insomnia with comorbid medical and psychiatric conditions. Nonetheless, to date, no studies have been conducted to evaluate the relative efficacy of CBT delivered in a fixed dose and format to primary and comorbid insomnia patients. Those with comorbid disorders often have symptoms (e.g., pain, lethargy, anxiety, etc.) that can confound sleep and treatment acceptance/adherence. Thus, it is possible that those with comorbid insomnia may respond less well to the CBT dose and format that is optimal for primary insomnia patients. Of course, a corollary of this speculation is that cognitive/behavioral insomnia treatments may benefit from special tailoring or augmentation (41) to better fit the needs of those with various forms of comorbid insomnia. Hopefully, future research will address these questions and speculations.

Lastly, dissemination remains a challenge to this very effective treatment. Given its superior durability to pharmacologic approaches and absence of potentially dangerous side effects, CBT should be a more common first-line approach in primary care and mental health settings (42). This, however, is not the case, so dissemination of the effectiveness of the treatment as well as dissemination of available treatment providers in the community is needed. CBT training facilities are growing but we need more treatment providers to match the prevalence of this disorder. Perhaps a growing number of the recently reported (e.g., self-help, internet, CBT tailored for primary care) (13,15) and yet to be developed alternative delivery modes will increase the treatment accessibility for this very effective intervention.

REFERENCES

1. Morin CM, Stone J, Trinkle D, et al. Dysfunctional beliefs and attitudes about sleep among older adults with and without insomnia complaints. Psychol Aging 1993; 8:463–467.
2. Hoelscher T, Edinger JD. Treatment of sleep-maintenance insomnia in older adults: Sleep period reduction, sleep education and modified stimulus control. Psychol Aging 1988; 3:258–263.
3. Edinger JD, Hoelscher TJ, Marsh GR, et al. A cognitive-behavioral therapy for sleep-maintenance insomnia in older adults. Psychol Aging 1992; 7:282–289.
4. Morin CM, Kowatch RA, Barry T, et al. Cognitive behavior therapy for late-life insomnia. J Consult Clin Psychol 1993; 61:137–147.
5. Edinger JD, Fins AI, Glenn DM, et al. Insomnia and the eye of the beholder: Are there clinical markers of objective sleep disturbances among adults with and without insomnia complaints? J Consult Clin Psychol 2000; 68:586–593.
6. Carney CE, Waters WF. Effects of a Structured Problem-Solving Procedure on Pre-Sleep Cognitive Arousal in College Students with Insomnia. Behav Sleep Med 2006; 4(1):13–28.
7. Morin CM. Insomnia: Psychological Assessment and Management. New York, NY: Guilford Press, 1993.
8. Edinger JD, Carney CE. Overcoming Insomnia: A Cognitive Behavior Therapy Approach Therapist Guide. New York, NY: Oxford University Press, 2008.
9. Bonnet MH, Arand DL. 24-hour metabolic rate in insomniacs and matched normal sleepers. Sleep 1995; 18:581–588.
10. Edinger JD, Wohlgemuth WK. The significance and management of persistent primary insomnia. Sleep Med Rev 1999; 3:101–118.
11. Borkovec T, Hennings BL. The role of physiological attention-focusing in the relaxation treatment of sleep disturbance, general tension, and specific stress reaction. Behav Res Ther 1978; 16: 7–19.
12. Riedel BW. Sleep hygiene. In: Lichstein KL, Morin CM, eds. Treatment of Late Life Insomnia. Thousand Oaks, CA: Sage Publications, Inc, 2000:125–146.

13. Mimeault V, Morin CM. Self-help treatment for insomnia: Bibliotherapy with and without professional guidance. J Consult Clin Psychol 1999; 67(4):511–519.
14. Rybarczyk B, Lopez M, Benson R, et al. Efficacy of two behavioral treatment programs for comorbid geriatric insomnia. Psychol Aging 2002; 17:288–298.
15. Edinger JD, Sampson WS. A primary care "friendly" cognitive behavioral insomnia therapy. Sleep 2003; 26:177–182.
16. Leger D, Guilleminault C, Bader G, et al. Medical and socio-professional impact of insomnia. Sleep 2002; 25:621–625.
17. Morin CM, Colecchi C, Stone J, et al. Behavioral and pharmacological therapies for late-life insomnia: A randomized controlled trial. JAMA 1999; 281:991–999.
18. Jacobs GD, Pace-Schott EF, Stickgold R, et al. Cognitive behavior therapy and pharmacotherapy for insomnia: A randomized controlled trial and direct comparison. Arch Intern Med 2004; 164:1888–1896.
19. Espie CA, Inglis SJ, Tessier S, et al. The clinical effectiveness of cognitive behaviour therapy for chronic insomnia: Implementation and evaluation of a sleep clinic in general medical practice. Behav Res Ther 2001; 39:45–60.
20. Espie CA, MacMahon KMA, Kelly H, et al. Randomized Clinical Effectiveness Trial of Nurse-Administered Small-Group Cognitive Behavior Therapy for Persistent Insomnia in General Practice. Sleep 2007; 30(5):574–584.
21. Currie SR, Wilson KG, Pontefract AJ, et al. Cognitive-behavioral treatment of insomnia secondary to chronic pain. J Consult Clin Psychol 2000; 68:407–416.
22. Edinger JD, Wohlgemuth WK, Krystal AD, et al. Behavioral insomnia therapy for Fibromyalgia patients: A randomized clinical trial. Arch Intern Med 2005; 165:2527–2535.
23. Morin CM, Stone J, McDonald K, et al. Psychological management of insomnia: A clinical replication series with 100 patients. Behav Ther 1994; 25:291–309.
24. Mitchell KR. Behavioral treatment of presleep tension and intrusive cognitions in patients with severe predormital insomnia. J Behav Med 1978; 2:57–69.
25. Mitchell KR, White RG. Self-management of severe predormital insomnia. J Behav Ther Exp Psychiatry 1977; 8:57–63.
26. Sanavio E. Pre-Sleep Cognitive Intrusions and Treatment of Onset-Insomnia. Behav Res Ther 1988; 26(6):451–459.
27. Spielman AJ, Saskin P, Thorpy MJ. Treatment of chronic insomnia by restriction of time in bed. Sleep 1987; 10:45–55.
28. Bootzin RR. Stimulus control treatment for insomnia. Proceedings of the 80th Annual Meeting of the American Psychological Association. 1972;7:395–396.
29. Morin CM, Culbert JP, Schwartz SM. Nonpharmacological interventions for insomnia: A meta-analysis of treatment efficacy. Am J Psychiatry 1994; 151:1172–1180.
30. Backhaus J, Hohagen F, Voderholzer U, et al. Long-term effectiveness of a short-term cognitive-behavioral group treatment for primary insomnia. Eur Arch Psychiatry Clin Neurosci 2001; 251:35–41.
31. Richardson GS. Managing insomnia in the primary care setting: Raising issues. Sleep 2000; 23 (Suppl. 1):S9–S12.
32. Smith MT, Perlis ML, Park A, et al. Comparative Meta-Analysis of pharmacotherapy and behavior therapy for persistent insomnia. Am J Psychiatry 2002; 159:5–11.
33. Mellinger GD, Balter MB, Uhlenhuth EH. Insomnia and its treatment: Prevalence and correlates. Arch Gen Psychiatry 1985; 42:225–232.
34. Oosterhuis A, Klip EC. The treatment of insomnia through mass media: The results of a televised behavioral training programme. Soc Sci Med 1997; 45:1223–1229.
35. Strom L, Pettersson R, Andersson G. Internet-based treatment for insomnia: A controlled evaluation. J Consult Clin Psychol 2004; 72:113–120.
36. Walsh JK, Schweitzer PK. Ten-year trends in the pharmacological treatment of insomnia. Sleep 1998; 22:371–375.
37. Verbeek I, Schreuder K, Declerck G. Evaluation of short-term non-pharmacological treatment of insomnia in a clinical setting. J Psychosom Res 1999; 47:369–383.
38. Wu R, Jinfeng B, Chungai Z, et al. Comparison of sleep condition and sleep-related psychological activity after cognitive behavior and pharmacological therapy for chronic insomnia. Psychother Psychosom 2006; 75:220–228.
39. Morgan K, Dixon S, Mathers S, et al. Psychological treatment for insomnia in the management of long-term hypnotic use: A pragmatic randomised controlled trial. Br J Gen Pract 2003; 53:923–928.
40. Morin CM, Bastien CH, Guay B, et al. Randomized clinical trial of supervised tapering and cognitive behavior therapy to facilitate benzodiazepine discontinuation in older adults with chronic insomnia. Am J Psychiatry 2004; 161:332–342.

41. Smith MT, Huang MI, Manber R. Cognitive Behavior Therapy for chronic insomnia occuring within the context of medical and psychiatric disorders. Clin Psychol Rev 2005; 25:559–592.
42. Stepanski EJ. Hypnotics should not be considered for the initial treatment of chronic insomnia. J Clin Sleep Med 2005; 1(2):125–128.
43. Spielman AJ, Caruso LS, Glovinsky PB. A behavioral perspective on insomnia treatment. Psychiatr Clin North Am 1987; 10:541–553.
44. Morin CM, Blais F, Savard J. Are changes in beliefs and attitudes related to sleep improvements in the treatment of insomnia? Behav Res Ther 2002;40:741–752.

30 Cognitive-Behavior Therapy for Comorbid and Late-Life Insomnia

Kenneth L. Lichstein
Department of Psychology, The University of Alabama, Tuscaloosa, Alabama, U.S.A.

Bruce Rybarczyk
Department of Psychology, Virginia Commonwealth University, Richmond, Virginia, U.S.A.

Haley R. Dillon
Department of Psychology, The University of Alabama, Tuscaloosa, Alabama, U.S.A.

INTRODUCTION

By the mid 1980s, cognitive-behavior therapy for insomnia (CBTi) was a mature science in many respects (1). A substantial literature had accumulated that boasted strong, durable treatment effects with rigorous methodology.

However, the bulk of the research to that point had focused on primary insomnia in young and middle-aged adults. Anticipating possible diminished efficacy and potential safety concerns, individuals with hypnotic-dependent insomnia, individuals with sleep active comorbid conditions, and older adults with insomnia were systematically screened from nearly all of these studies. It was difficult to justify allocating scarce healthcare/scientific resources when confronted by gloomy outcome expectations.

It is now clear that young adult and middle-aged, primary insomnia accounts for a narrow sliver of the insomnia population (see chapter 1 in this volume). Neglecting more complex, severe insomnia also ignores the most needy patients. The literature that has emerged on comorbid and late-life insomnia is now about two decades old and has soundly refuted the apprehensions that denied CBTi treatment to so many in the past.

The present chapter will review the literature in the domains of CBTi for comorbid and late-life insomnia with the intent of estimating clinical efficacy. We will also assess the methodological rigor of these studies to gauge the confidence of their findings. To identify the relevant literature, we searched PsycINFO and MEDLINE for the years 1965 through 2007. We also examined the citations from retrieved studies to identify additional articles.

COMORBID INSOMNIA

General Characteristics

Until recent years chronic insomnia has been classified into two broad categories: as either a 'primary' disorder or one that is 'secondary' to a primary medical or psychiatric disorder (2). The different diagnostic systems for sleep disorders and treatment recommendations for insomnia reflected this basic dichotomy. When a primary medical or psychiatric disorder was present, the standard approach was for treatment to be aimed at the primary disorder, with the expectation that insomnia will improve once the primary disorder remits. A study of specific treatment recommendations made by sleep specialists for patients with insomnia confirmed that this approach was present in actual practice (3).

However, a rapid shift in this clinical logic coincided with the beginning of the 21st century. In a 2000 book chapter, Lichstein (4) outlined the difficulty of determining whether various coexisting medical and psychiatric conditions predate and/or exacerbate the insomnia. Furthermore, beginning in that same year with Lichstein, Wilson and Johnson's (5) study, randomized controlled trials with state-of-the-art behavioral treatments were expanded to populations that were previously overlooked on the grounds that they had secondary insomnia. In the majority of these studies the issue of whether the medical or psychiatric condition predated the insomnia was not addressed in the inclusion criteria (2). Finally, a 2005 State-of-the-Science Conference (6) recommended that *secondary insomnia* be removed from the clinical taxonomy and be replaced with the more descriptive diagnostic term, *comorbid insomnia*. Similarly, treatment guidelines have also shifted such that behavioral methods are recommended as a first-line of treatment for all chronic insomnias, regardless of the presence of a comorbid medical and/or psychiatric condition. The behavioral treatment literature in support of this paradigm shift will be outlined and summarized in the next sections.

Literature Search

We identified 21 published behavioral intervention studies between the years 1989 and 2007. Three additional case studies were published between 1980 and 1990 and four case series studies have been published since 1994. These seven papers were not included in the count of 21 because they were not designed as *a priori* studies. Another paper that focused on caffeine reduction among HIV patients (7) was not included in the count because it employed a single sleep hygiene treatment strategy. Among the 21 studies, 11 were classified as randomized clinical trials (RCT, Table 1), with the remainder being quasi-experimental designs, multiple case studies, or multiple baseline case studies.

Unlike the gradual integration of older adults into the CBTi literature (see below), 15 of the 21 studies have occurred since the year 2000. Consequently, it may not be an exaggeration to say that the comorbid insomnia subset, largely ignored until the 21st century, is now receiving the majority of attention in CBTi research. We will likely to see a wide range of RCT studies applied to different comorbid conditions in the near future and this will be a welcome contribution to the empirical evidence and will hopefully translate into higher levels of behavioral treatment in the clinical setting.

Methodology

Studies of CBTi for comorbid insomnia have employed the full spectrum of methods, including single case studies (e.g., 8–10), multiple case designs (11–15), a large uncontrolled trial (16), a large trial with a convenience sample as a control group (17), RCTs with no-treatment control groups (Table 1), and RCTs with a placebo treatment or other treatment comparisons (Table 1). There have been four additional case-series reports of treatment cases at sleep clinics with a range of comorbidities, usually of a psychiatric nature (18–21).

A variety of types of comorbid conditions have been targeted in the RCTs. In the domain of medical comorbidity, these studies have included mixed chronic illnesses (5,22,23), chronic pain (24), cancer (17,25,26), coronary artery disease (27), osteoarthritis (27), fibromyalgia (28), Alzheimer's disease (29) and pulmonary disease (27). In the domain of psychiatric comorbidity, only two RCT studies have been published and both of those included individuals with or recovering from alcoholism (30,32). Additional, uncontrolled studies included crime victims with posttraumatic stress disorder (16) and individuals with depression and insomnia (15). Accordingly, there is a critical need in CBTi research with comorbid insomnia to address the treatment efficacy of psychiatric comorbidities, including but not limited to anxiety disorders, bipolar disorder, eating disorders and substance abuse disorders.

Most of the RCT studies have been conducted since multicomponent CBTi was established as the "gold standard" for intervention, so all but the two oldest RCTs used this omnibus treatment approach. The specific components within this omnibus approach were fairly uniform, using a combination of stimulus control, sleep restriction, sleep hygiene recommendations, guidelines for discontinuing or reducing hypnotics, and cognitive methods (31). The one exception was relaxation training, which was not included in three of nine multicomponent RCTs (24,25,28). The two earliest RCT studies both employed single modality relaxation training interventions (32,33). The RCT with Alzheimer's patients (29) also employed a necessarily different treatment model, which included caregiver administered changes in activities, sleep windows and light exposure (using a light box). Among the nonRCT studies, multicomponent CBTi was also the norm, but one older study employed only stimulus control and sleep restriction (13). Three studies tested home treatments as comparison groups for in-person multicomponent treatments. These included relaxation training with audiotapes (22), multicomponent CBT delivered via videotape and book instruction (23), and CBT book instruction alone (30).

Table 1 Randomized Clinical Trials of CBT for Comorbid Insomnia

Study	Conditions	Sleep measure	Posttreatment outcome	Follow-up outcome
	Placebo/Treatment comparison control group			
Rybarczyk et al. (27), osteoarthritis, coronary artery disease, and lung disease Rybarczyk (67) report on one yr. f/u data	1 MT (SH, SC, SR, CT, RE) 2 SMW / PL	SD SII PSQI	SD: 1 > 2 (SE, SL, WASO, TTIB) ISI: 1 > 2 PSQI: 1 > 2	SD, TGO, sig. for: SE, SL, WASO, TTIB, ISI & PSQI
Rybarczyk et al., (22), mixed medical illness in older adults	1 MT (SH, SC, SR, CT, RE) 2 HART 3 WLC	SD PSQI ACT	SD: 1 > 3 (SE, WASO, TTIB) 1 = 2 (SE, WASO, TTIB) 2 = 3 (SE, WASO, TTIB) 2 > 1 = 3 (TST) PSQI: 1 = 2 > 3 ACT: ns	SD: 1 = 2 > 3 (SE, WASO) 1 > 3 (TTIB) 1 = 2 (TTIB) 2 = 3 (TTIB) PSQI: 1 = 2 > 3 ACT: ns
Edinger et al. (28), fibromyalgia	1 MT (SH, SC, SR, CT) 2 SH 3 UC	SD ACT	SD: 1 > 3 (SE, WASO, SL) ACT: 1 > 3 (SL)	SD: 1 > 3 (SE, WASO, SL) ACT: 1 > 3 (SL)
Currie et al. (30), recovering alcoholics	1 MT (SH, SC, SR, CT, RE) 2 SHMT 3 WLC	SD PSQI ACT	SD: 1 = 2 > 3 (SE, SL,WASO, SQ) PSQI: 1 = 2 > 3 ACT: ns	SD: 1 = 2 > 3 (SE, SL,WASO, SQ) PSQI: 1 = 2 > 3 ACT: ns
Epstein & Dirksen (25), breast cancer patients	1 MT (SH, SC, SR, CT) 2 SH	SD TER ACT	SD: 1 > 2 (TIB) TER: 1 > 2	N/A
McCurry et al. (29), Alzheimer's Disease	1 MT (ISH, LBE, AI) 2 SH	ACT	ACT: 1 > 2 (TWT, NWAK)	ACT: 1 > 2 (TWT, NWAK)
	No Treatment Control Group			
Cannici et al. (33), cancer	1 RE 2 UC	SD	SD:1 > 2 (SL)	SD:1 > 2 (SL)
Greeff & Conradie (32), alcohol dependency	1 RE 2 WLC	SQ	SQ: 1 > 2	N/A
Currie et al. (24)· chronic pain	1 MT (SH, SC, SR, CT, RE) 2 WLC	SD PSQI ACT	SD: 1 > 2 (SE, SL, WASO) PSQI: 1 > 2 ACT: 1 > 2	SD: 1 > 2 (SE, SL, WASO) PSQI: 1 > 2 ACT: 1 > 2
Lichstein et al. (5), psychiatric and medical illnesses	1 MT (SH, SC, RE) 2 Control	SD	SD: 1 > 2 (SE, WASO, SQ)	SD: 1 > 2 (SE, WASO, SQ)
Savard et al. (26), breast cancer	1 MT (SH, SC, SR, CT, FM) 2 WLC	SD ISI PSG	SD: 1 > 2 (SE, SL, WASO, TWT) ISI: 1 > 2 PSG: n.s.	SD: 1 > 2 (SE, SL, WASO, TWT) ISI: 1 > 2 PSG: n.s.

Note: Posttreatment and follow-up outcomes reflect treatment condition relationships based on the primary or majority of the sleep measures if individual sleep measures are not specified. In reporting outcome, = indicates no statistically significant difference and > indicates a significantly better outcome ($p < 0.05$). This table reports between group comparisons at posttreatment and follow-up, not within group comparisons over time, with the exception of one study's findings at one-year follow up.

Treatment conditions: multicomponent treatment (MT), placebo (PL), stress management and wellness placebo (SMW), home audiotape relaxation treatment (HART), self-help multicomponent treatment (SHMT), relaxation (RE), sleep compression (SCO), sleep hygiene (SH), sleep restriction (SR), stimulus control (SC), cognitive therapy (CT), fatigue management (FM), wait-list control (WLC), usual care (UC), light box exposure (LBE), activity increase (AI), individualized sleep hygiene (ISH), within group analysis for treatment group only (TGO).

Sleep measures: actigraphy (ACT), polysomnography (PSG), sleep diaries (SD), sleep latency (SL), total sleep time (TST), total wake time (TWT), total time in bed (TTIB), number of awakenings (NWAK), sleep efficiency (SE), wake after sleep onset (WASO), Pittsburgh Sleep Quality Inventory (PSQI), sleep questionnaire (SQ), Insomnia Severity Index (ISI), Treatment Effectiveness Rating (TER)

The nine RCT intervention studies employing multicomponent treatment were split relatively evenly between group and individual treatment sessions, with the quantity of treatment ranging between four one-hour individual sessions (5) to as many as eight two-hour group sessions (27). Group treatments are necessarily longer due to the support and interactive content of the classes.

Therapists in the RCTs have ranged from behavioral sleep medicine clinicians (16), psychologists (22,27), masters level mental health professionals (14,25,26) and psychology graduate students (5). All of the group interventions have been led by two clinicians, either two psychologists (22,27) or a psychologist and a graduate student (16). All of the studies delivered treatment in conventional health care settings, with the exception of the self-help interventions (22,23,30) and the innovative caregiver-administered intervention for Alzheimer's patients (29). This intervention included six one-hour in-home sessions delivered by geropsychologists experienced in behavioral interventions for dementia patients and their caregivers.

Outcomes and Meta-Analyses (MA)

As above, the review of outcomes will focus mainly on the RCT findings for multicomponent interventions. Uncontrolled studies are reviewed in a limited way and case studies are not addressed. We were only able to locate a quasi MA for CBTi for comorbid insomnia, published in 2005 (34). Effect sizes were calculated and presented in a table of the literature, along with a systematic review of current and recommended research in this area. Overall, the effect sizes for the RCT studies for self-report variables are in the "moderate" to "strong" range, based on Cohen's (35) criteria, and are generally consistent with those reported in MA for CBTi for primary insomnia (e.g., 36). Thus far, no studies with null findings for most or all sleep variables have been reported in the small body of CBTi literature with comorbid insomnia. One cautionary note is that not all studies employed intent-to-treat analyses, so the effect sizes may be somewhat inflated.

As has been shown with larger MA examining the efficacy of CBTi for primary insomnia (e.g., 36) these effect sizes were strongest with sleep efficiency, wake after sleep onset and sleep quality ratings and absent or smaller for increases in total sleep time. Additionally, as has been the case with primary insomnia (36), these effect sizes were largely maintained at long-term follow-up assessments, ranging from three months to one year in duration. Taken together, these findings suggest that CBTi treatment for comorbid insomnia is both highly effective and robust in its long-term effects on subjective evaluations of sleep.

The findings are much more sparse and inconclusive when it comes to objective measures of sleep. Among the six RCT studies that employed objective outcome measures (i.e., either actigraphy or polysomnography) three found weaker effects compared to self-report (24,28,29) and three found no effects (22,26,30). Only one of the RCT studies employed polysomnography and that study found no significant effects (26). In contrast, two uncontrolled studies (13,14) employed polysomnography measures and both found significant changes on sleep parameters. One of the studies (14) had effect sizes that were 50% smaller compared to sleep diary (though still in the "strong" range) and the other had effect sizes that were comparable to those obtained for self-report for three chronic pain subjects in the study (13). The fact that a number of RCT studies have failed to obtain actigraphy outcomes may be partially due to the limitations of the scoring algorithms for particular populations, as some evidence suggests that it may be suboptimal as a measurement of insomnia in older adults (37) and other specialized populations.

In the comorbid CBTi literature, systematic comparisons of different intervention types are not possible because 9 of 11 of the RCTs employed similar, multicomponent interventions. The two studies employing relaxation interventions (32,33) did obtain strong effects, though outcomes were only measured and analyzed for limited variables. In the three studies which included a self-administered CBTi treatment group, all three found significant effects for self-help treatment, with some additional benefits for professional-led treatment compared to self-help. In the Rybarczyk et al. (22) and Rybarczyk et al. (23) studies, the rate of clinically significant improvement was approximately 50% greater for the in-person treatment compared to self-help treatment. In the Currie et al. (30) study with recovering alcoholics, the outcomes were comparable at posttreatment but professional-led treatment was superior at the six-month follow-up on a measure of clinical significance.

Based on a review of the effect sized calculated in the Smith et al. MA (34), it is apparent that the three case series studies show smaller effect sizes than most of the RCTs. This is most likely due to the fact that relative to carefully screened and incentivized research subjects, "real world" clients often have complicating factors (e.g., lower motivation, lack of treatment adherence) that attenuate treatment efficacy. Also important to note is that in most studies individuals who were using hypnotics were not excluded and this variable was shown to have no impact on the efficacy of the intervention. In fact, several studies determined that hypnotic usage was reduced as a result of the intervention (26,30).

It has been hypothesized that the bi-directional relationship between insomnia and daytime functioning is heightened in comorbid insomnia, for both medical and psychiatric conditions (2). For example, it has been shown that in addition to insomnia being aggravated by increased pain, pain is also increased following nights of insomnia (38). Accordingly, most of the 11 RCT studies hypothesized that secondary daytime medical, mental health and quality of life benefits would follow from improved sleep. In general, secondary findings have been limited to the RCTs addressing insomnia in cancer and Alzheimer's patients. The Quesnel et al. (14) study demonstrated that cancer patients receiving CBTi showed improvements in mood, general and physical fatigue, and global and cognitive dimensions of quality of life. The Savard et al. (26) study showed that cancer patients in the treatment group had lower depression and anxiety as well as greater global quality of life compared to controls. The one study with Alzheimer's patients (29) showed that treatment group participants had reduced symptoms of depression and greater levels of activity compared to controls.

In contrast, in the two studies by Rybarczyk and colleagues (22,27), assessing an array of secondary outcome measures that were relevant to chronic illness, only a single global rating of daytime effects of insomnia produced significant effects in one of the two studies (27). Currie et al. (24) found no secondary benefits among chronic pain patients and Edinger et al. (28) only found pain benefits in his fibromyalgia sample for the sleep hygiene only treatment condition compared to controls. Although the RCTs produced inconsistent findings, all of the seven uncontrolled studies that included daytime functioning measures reported significant findings. However, given the uncontrolled nature of these studies, it is likely that regression to the mean and other threats to internal validity are responsible for a portion of the variance in these findings.

LATE-LIFE INSOMNIA

General Characteristics

Definition

Insomnia is more prevalent, more severe, more chronic, and more impairing in older adults than in any other age group (39–42). Late-life insomnia is simply defined as insomnia occurring in older adults. There is no standard age cut-off for qualifying, but 60 years is commonly used.

It may also be salient to acknowledge that no CBTi study has distinguished between late-life insomnia that initiates in late-life versus chronic middle-aged insomnia that persists into later life. The clinical implications of this distinction are unknown (43).

Literature Search

We identified 41 articles between the years 1974 and 2007 and a frequency distribution of their publication dates are given in Figure 1. The level of interest in CBTi for late-life insomnia is somewhat misleading from this figure. The first six publications either included sleep as a secondary outcome or did not focus on insomnia in older adults, they just did not exclude them and typically included correlations between age and outcome to assess age as a moderating variable. The first study to exclusively focus on CBTi in older adults was published in 1983 (44). The first RCT with an active control group was published in 1999 (45). During the 1990s, interest leveled off to about one article a year and that rate about doubled in the first five years of the 21st century. The prorated rate of publication during the years 2005 to 2007 is greater than two per year.

Five of the 41 studies were on comorbid insomnia in older adults (5,22,23,27,29). These fit equally well in the comorbid section and the late-life section. We arbitrarily chose to include them in the comorbid section above and have omitted them from the reporting of outcomes below to avoid redundant discussion.

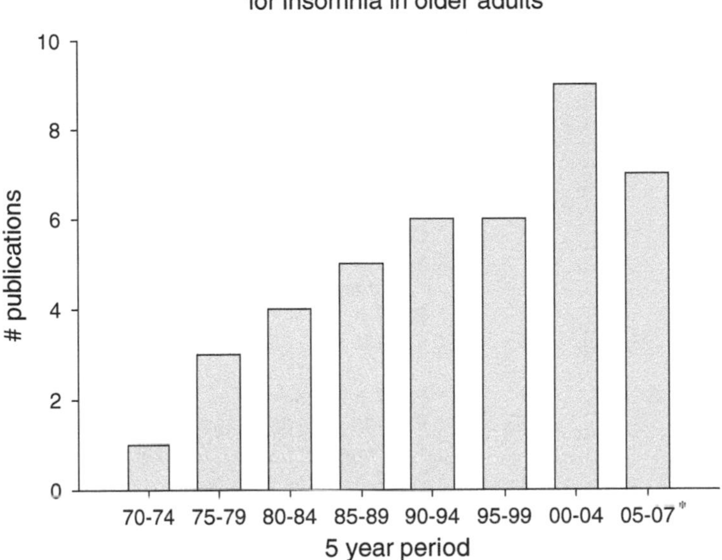

Figure 1 Publication count of the 41 CBT for insomnia studies in five-year periods. *Signifies that the last period, 05–07, is only three years.

Methodology

A variety of methodologies have been used to study late-life insomnia including case studies (e.g., 46,47), single subject experimental designs (e.g., 48,49), RCTs with wait-list control groups (Table 2), and RCTs with placebo or other treatment comparisons (Table 2).

A variety of types of late-life insomnia have been targeted including primary insomnia (e.g., 50,51), comorbid insomnia (e.g., discussed in the above section), hypnotic-dependent insomnia (e.g., 52,53), and insomnia in caregivers (e.g., 54,55).

Therapists have mostly been experienced behavioral sleep medicine clinicians (e.g., 48,50) or psychology graduate students (e.g., 5,56). One study trained nondoctoral counselors and a social worker to present CBTi (57).

Most of the studies delivered treatment in conventional health care settings, but two studies were distinctive. One presented CBTi in primary care (58) and the other in a rural clinic (57).

Outcome Studies

For purposes of efficiency, this discussion will not consider case studies or single-subject design. Excluding the several comorbid insomnia studies reported above, we found six studies that included placebo or treatment comparison controls and 10 studies with a wait list control. A summary of these studies is given in Table 2. This discussion will emphasize the most methodologically rigorous of these studies, those with the placebo or treatment comparison control.

To get a sense of which treatments have received the most attention, we did a frequency distribution among these 16 studies. Stimulus control was the most common (12 studies included a form of this treatment), sleep hygiene, which was usually included as a secondary treatment component, was next (11 studies), and other treatments in decreasing order were sleep restriction/compression (8 studies), relaxation (8 studies), and cognitive therapy (5 studies). Thorough descriptions of these clinical procedures are available elsewhere (59). Every study used sleep diaries as a dependent measure. Actigraphy was also included in one study and polysomnography in six studies.

Of the six placebo/treatment comparison studies, the study by Freidman et al. (60) had the weakest results. The two active treatment groups, sleep restriction fortified with sleep hygiene

Table 2 Randomized Clinical Trials of CBT for Late-Life Insomnia

Study	Conditions	Sleep Measure	Post-treatment Outcome	Follow-up Outcome
	Placebo/Treatment Comparison Control Group			
Friedman et al. (60)	1 SR/SH 2 SR/SH/nap 3 SH	ACT SD	ACT: ns SD: 1 = 2 > 3	ACT: ns SD: ns
Lichstein et al. (62)	1 RE 2 SCO 3 PL	SD PSG CS	SD: 1 = 3 > 2 (TST) 2 > 3 (NWAK) CS: 1 = 2 > 3 No PSG data at post-treatment	SD: ns PSG: ns CS: 2 > 1 = 3
McCrae et al. (57)	1 SH 2 MT (SC, SR, RE)	SD CS	SD: 2 > 1 CS: 2 > 1	No follow-up data
Morin et al. (45)	1 MT (SH, SC, SR, CT) 2 PCT 3 MT/PCT 4 PL	SD PSG SII CS	SD: 1 = 2 = 3 > 4 PSG: 1 = 2 = 3 1 = 2 = 4 3 > 4 SII: 1 = 3 > 2 = 4 CS: 1 = 3 > 4 (SE) 1 = 2 = 3 (SE) 2 = 4 (SE) 1 = 2 = 3 > 4 (SII)	No between group comparisons at follow-up
Morin et al. (63)	1 MW 2 MT (SH, SC, SR, CT) 3 MW/MT	SD PSG MED	SD: 2 = 3 > 1 PSG: ns MED: 3 > 1 = 2	SD: ns PSG: ns MED: ns
Sivertsen et al. (64)	1 MT (SH, SC, SR, CT, RE) 2 PCT 3 PL	SD PSG CS	SD: ns PSG: 1 > 2 = 3 (TWT, SWS) 1 > 3 (SE) 1 = 2 (SE) 2 = 3 (SE) CS: 1 > 2	SD: 1 > 2 (TWT) PSG: 1 > 2 (TWT, SWS, SE) CS: 1 > 2 No follow-up data for group 3
	Wait-List control (WLC) group			
Creti et al. (68)	1 CR 2 RE 3 WLC	SD SQ	SD: ns SQ: ns	SQ: ns No analyses with SD data
Davies et al. (69)	1 CC 2 WLC	SD	SD: 1 > 2	No follow-up data for group 2
Engle-Friedman et al. (70)	1 SH/SU 2 SH/SU/RE 3 SH/SU/SC 4 WLC	SD PSG	SD: 3 > 4 (FR) PSG: ns	SD: 3 > 1 = 2 2 > 1 = 3 (FR) No follow-up data for group 4 No PSG data at follow-up
McCurry et al. (55)	1 MT (SH, SC, SCO, RE) 2 WLC	SD PSQI CS	PSQI: 1 > 2 CS: 1 > 2 No SD data for group 2	PSQI: 1 > 2 No SD data for group 2
Morgan et al. (58)	1 MT (SH, SC, RE, CT) 2 Control	PSQI MED	PSQI: 1 > 2 MED: 1 > 2	PSQI: 1 > 2 MED: 1 > 2
Morin & Azrin (56)	1 SC 2 IT 3 WLC	SD	SD: 1 > 3 (WASO) 1 = 2 (WASO) 2 = 3 (WASO) 1 > 2 = 3 (TST)	SD: ns No follow-up data for group 3

(Continued)

Table 2 Randomized Clinical Trials of CBT for Late-Life Insomnia *(Continued)*

Study	Conditions	Sleep Measure	Post-treatment Outcome	Follow-up Outcome
Morin et al. (71)	1 MT (SH, SC, SR, CT) 2 WLC	SD PSG CS	SD: 1 > 2 PSG: 1 > 2 (TWT) CS: 1 > 2	SD: ns No PSG data at follow-up
Pallesen et al. (72)	1 SH/SC 2 SH/RE 3 WLC	SD	SD: 1 = 2 > 3	SD: 1 = 2 No follow-up data for group 3
Puder et al. (44)	1 SC 2 WLC	SD CS	SD: 1 > 2 CS: 1 > 2	No follow-up data for group 2
Riedel et al. (73)	1 SCO/SH (video plus guidance) 2 SCO/SH (video only) 3 WLC	SD SS	SD: 2 > 1 (TST) SS: 1 > 3 1 = 2 2 = 3	SD: 2 > 3 (TST) SS: 1 > 3 1 = 2 2 = 3

Note: (1) This table excludes several studies on comorbid late-life insomnia reported in the comorbid insomnia section above. (2) Posttreatment and follow-up outcomes reflect treatment condition relationships based on the primary or majority of the sleep measures if individual sleep measures are not specified. (3) In reporting outcome, = indicates no statistically significant difference and > indicates a significantly better outcome ($p < 0.05$). This table reports between group comparisons at post-treatment and follow-up, not within group comparisons over time.

Abbreviations: Treatment conditions: placebo (PL), relaxation (RE), sleep compression (SCO), sleep hygiene (SH), sleep restriction (SR), multicomponent treatment (MT), stimulus control (SC), cognitive therapy (CT), pharmacotherapy (PCT), medication withdrawal/taper (MW), countercontrol (CC), support (SU), imagery training (IT), wait-list control (WLC), cognitive refocusing (CR).

Sleep measures: actigraphy (ACT), polysomnography (PSG), sleep diaries (SD), clinical significance (CS), total sleep time (TST), total wake time (TWT), number of awakenings (NWAK), sleep efficiency (SE), slow-wave sleep (SWS), wake after sleep onset (WASO), feeling refreshed upon awakening (FR), Pittsburgh Sleep Quality Inventory (PSQI), sleep questionnaire (SQ), medication use/reduction (MED), Sleep Impairment Index (SII), sleep satisfaction (SS).

and sleep restriction fortified with sleep hygiene and a daytime nap, demonstrated a stronger effect than sleep hygiene alone at posttreatment and only on self-reported sleep efficiency. All other diary and actigraphy results at posttreatment and follow-up were nonsignificant. Indeed, had a Bonferroni correction been applied to control for testing multiple measures, this one significant effect would have been nullified. These results are particularly discouraging because sleep hygiene is a weak unitary treatment (61).

Lichstein et al. (62) observed modest self-reported sleep gains at posttreatment and follow-up associated with their two active treatments, sleep compression (a method similar to sleep restriction) and relaxation, compared to placebo treatment. No significant PSG effects were demonstrated at follow-up and PSG data were not collected at posttreatment. Clinical significance markers favored sleep compression. As was predicted, differential treatment effects were associated with presence or absence of daytime impairment. Subjects with high daytime fatigue (implying they needed more sleep) responded better to relaxation and patients with low daytime fatigue (implying they did not need more sleep) responded better to sleep compression.

In a recent effectiveness study, McCrae et al. (57) utilized existing providers in rural health clinics to deliver brief multicomponent behavior therapy (stimulus control, sleep restriction, and relaxation) or sleep hygiene education. The group receiving multicomponent therapy fared better at posttreatment on subjective sleep reports (sleep latency and sleep efficiency) and clinical significance markers than participants receiving sleep hygiene education alone. Although no follow-up data were reported, these initial results support the feasibility and value of providing brief behavioral interventions for insomnia in primary care settings.

When compared to a placebo group at posttreatment, Morin et al. (45) observed significant improvements in self-reported sleep for all three active treatment groups, CBT alone, pharmacotherapy alone, and a combination of the two. Only the combined treatment group performed better than the placebo on posttreatment PSGs. While there were no significant differences among the three active treatment conditions, a trend was noted for the combined treatment to result in slightly greater improvements on sleep diary and PSG data than either treatment component alone. However, despite these initial gains, long-term outcomes were highly variable in the combined treatment group and some participants reported significantly worse sleep patterns at follow-up. Participants in the pharmacotherapy only group gradually lost sleep gains over time, while those in the CBT only group maintained improvements in sleep up to 24-months later. Also of note, participants in the combined treatment and CBT only conditions rated themselves as significantly more improved at posttreatment, more satisfied, and having less interference with daytime functioning than participants in the other two conditions.

Another study conducted by Morin et al. (63) tested the efficacy of three interventions for benzodiazepine discontinuation; supervised medication taper alone, CBT alone, and a combination of medication tapering and CBT. In regards to benzodiazepine reduction, the combined treatment group had significantly more medication-free patients at posttreatment than either CBT alone or medication taper alone conditions. The combined treatment group also had more medication-free patients at 3- and 12-month follow-ups, although group differences were no longer statistically significant. PSG data demonstrated sleep gains at posttreatment for all three groups, with no differences between treatment conditions. However, participants receiving insomnia-specific treatments (either CBT alone or CBT combined with medication taper) reported greater improvements in self-reported sleep than the medication taper only condition. Interestingly, all three conditions showed additional gains in self-reported sleep from posttreatment to follow-up, though no significant differences were observed between groups. These results suggest that improvements in sleep may not be noticeable until several months after discontinuing or reducing medication use.

Sivertsen et al. (64) compared CBT with pharmacotherapy and placebo treatment. At six-weeks posttreatment, there were no differences between the three groups on self-reported sleep, although PSG data favored the CBT condition on most sleep variables. The CBT group demonstrated greater increases in PSG-recorded slow wave sleep compared to pharmacotherapy or placebo conditions, while the pharmacotherapy condition actually showed decreases in slow wave sleep at posttreatment. Six-month follow-up data for the two active treatments indicated that the pharmacotherapy group maintained sleep gains, but the CBT group produced significantly better results on all self-reported and PSG outcome variables except for total sleep time. Clinical significance markers also favored CBT at both posttreatment and follow-up.

Daytime functioning is plausibly expected to profit from sleep improvement but it is not always measured before and after treatment. Only three of the active controlled studies assessed changes in daytime functioning. One study reported substantial daytime functioning gains accruing to CBTi (45) and two others did not (60,62).

Most of the studies reviewed above included a multicomponent treatment condition that consisted of several behavioral and cognitive techniques for addressing insomnia. Of the studies comparing specific interventions, two trials found that behavioral treatments were more effective than sleep hygiene alone, although neither study included a placebo or additional control group for comparison (57,60). Lichstein et al. (62) also reported sleep gains for two different behavioral treatments, with stronger effects for sleep compression. The two trials that compared psychological treatments with pharmacotherapy found conflicting results for pharmacotherapy conditions, but both found positive treatment effects for CBT (45,65). In particular, the study by Morin et al. (45) raises question as to the lasting benefits of combining CBT with pharmacotherapy and whether the addition of pharmacotherapy might undermine the long-term effectiveness of CBT. A trial focused on chronic users of benzodiazepine medication found that supervised medication tapering is safe and effective with older adults and suggested that combining CBT with a medication taper may facilitate benzodiazepine discontinuation by targeting insomnia and withdrawal symptoms (63). Taken together, the most consistent finding across these controlled studies is that including components of CBTi when treating late-life insomnia generally produces statistically and clinically significant improvements in subjective sleep that are well maintained over time. More research is needed to determine the individual components of CBTi that are responsible for these treatment effects and to clarify the risks and benefits of using pharmacotherapy by itself or in conjunction with other treatments for late-life insomnia.

Meta-Analyses

Meta-Analyses (MA) have the ability to digest large numbers of articles efficiently and provide a broad perspective of the field from a quantitative perspective. The three MA presented below are all based on self-reported sleep data.

One of the first MA on CBT for insomnia found that treatment effects did not significantly vary with age (36). Two MA focused on CBT for older adults with insomnia. The first reported results for 13 studies (65). Effect sizes based on therapeutic increment above control group changes found the largest effect for WASO, d = 0.61, the smallest effect for TST, d = 0.15, with NWAK and SOL intermediate. More recently, a MA compared CBT effects on insomnia in middle-aged and older individuals (66). There was no significant difference in treatment effects in these two age groups for sleep quality ratings, SOL, or WASO. The younger group exhibited stronger treatment effects for TST and SE.

To summarize the MA findings, CBTi for late-life insomnia is often as effective as with younger adults. Differential effectiveness has been observed indicating greater treatment effects are sometimes obtained in younger adults. Interestingly, sleep maintenance insomnia (characterized by WASO), which may be the most common form of insomnia in older adults, does not exhibit diminished responsiveness in older samples.

CONCLUSIONS

CBTi for comorbid and late-life insomnia is effective, and the pattern of characteristics in these two literatures is very similar. The following conclusions apply equally well to both domains.

- Strong insomnia efficacy is consistently demonstrated.
- There exists good methodological rigor in many of these studies including well- controlled RCTs.
- There is good long-term maintenance of sleep effects.
- Self-reported sleep improvement is often stronger than objective findings. This may be disquieting to researchers but is good news for patients.
- There is inconsistent improvement in daytime functioning associated with sleep improvement.

Overall, we strongly conclude that earlier reluctance to apply CBT to comorbid and late-life insomnia was not justified and deprived patients of effective treatment.

ACKNOWLEDGEMENT

Preparation of this chapter was supported in part by National Institute on Drug Abuse grant DA13574 awarded to the first author and National Institute of Aging grant AG017491 awarded to the second author.

REFERENCES

1. Lichstein KL, Fischer SM. Insomnia. In: Hersen M, Bellack AS, eds. Handbook of clinical behavior therapy with adults. New York, NY: Plenum Press, 1985:319–352.
2. Stepanski E, Rybarczyk B. Emerging research on the treatment and etiology of secondary or comorbid insomnia. Sleep Med Rev 2006; 10:7–18.
3. Buysse D, Reynolds C, Kupfer D, et al. Effects of diagnosis on treatment recommendations in chronic insomnia—a report from the APA/NIMH DSM-IV field trial. Sleep 1997; 20;542–552.
4. Lichstein KL. Secondary insomnia. In: Lichstein KL, Morin CM eds. Treatment of Late-life Insomnia. Thousand Oaks, CA: Sage Publications Inc., 2000.
5. Lichstein KL, Wilson NM, Johnson CT. Psychological treatment of secondary insomnia. Psychol Aging 2000; 15:232–240.
6. State-of-the-Science Panel. National Institutes of Health State of the Science Conference Statement: Manifestations and management of chronic insomnia in adults, June 13–15, 2005. Sleep 2005; 28:1049–1057.
7. Dreher HM. The effect of caffeine reduction on sleep quality and well being in persons with HIV. J Psychosom Res 2003; 54:191–198.
8. Morin CM, Kowatch RA, O'Shanick G. Sleep restriction for the inpatient treatment of insomnia. Sleep 1990; 13:183–186.

9. Stam HJ, Bultz BD. The treatment of severe insomnia in a cancer patient. J Behav Ther Exp Res 1986; 17:33–37.
10. Varni JW. Behavioral treatment of disease-related chronic insomnia in a hemophiliac. J Behav Ther Exp Psychiatry 1980; 11:143–145.
11. Davidson JR, Waisberg JL, Brundage MD, et al. Nonpharmacologic group treatment of insomnia: A preliminary study with cancer survivors. Psychooncology 2001; 10:389–397.
12. DeViva JC, Zayfert C, Pigeon WR, et al. Treatment of residual insomnia after CBT for PTSD: Case studies. J Trauma Stress 2005; 18:155–159.
13. Morin CM, Kowatch RA, Wade JB. Behavioral management of sleep disturbances secondary to chronic pain. J Behav Ther Exp Psychiatry 1989; 20:295–302.
14. Quesnel C, Savard J, Simard S, et al. Efficacy of cognitive-behavioral therapy for insomnia in women treated for nonmetastatic breast cancer. J Consult Clin Psychol 2003; 71:189–200.
15. Taylor DJ, Lichstein KL, Weinstock J, et al. A pilot study of cognitive-behavioral therapy of insomnia in people with mild depression. Behav Ther 2007; 38(1):49–57.
16. Krakow B, Johnston L, Melendrez D. An open-label trial of evidence-based cognitive behavior therapy for nightmares and insomnia in crime victims with PTSD. Am J Psychiatry 2001; 158(12):2043–2047.
17. Simiet R, Deck R, Conta-Marx B. Sleep management training for cancer patients with insomnia. Supportive Care Cancer 2004; 12:176–183.
18. Dashevsky BA, Kramer M. Behavioral treatment of chronic insomnia in psychiatrically ill patients. J Consult Clin Psychol 1998; 59:693–699.
19. Morawetz, D. Depression and insomnia: Which comes first? Aus J Counsel Psychol 2001; 3(1):19–24.
20. Morin CM, Stone J, McDonald K, et al. Psychological management of insomnia: A clinical replication series with 100 patients. Behav Ther 1994; 25:291–309.
21. Perlis ML, Sharpe M, Smith MT, et al. Behavioral treatment of insomnia: Treatment outcome and the relevance of medical and psychiatric morbidity. J Behav Med 2001; 24:281–296.
22. Rybarczyk B, Lopez M, Benson R, et al. Efficacy of two behavioral treatment programs for comorbid geriatric insomnia. Psychol Aging 2002; 17:288–298.
23. Rybarczyk B, Lopez M, Schelble K, et al. Home-based video CBT for comorbid geriatric insomnia: A pilot study using secondary data analyses. Behav Sleep Med 2005; 3:158–175.
24. Currie SR, Wilson KG, Pontefract AJ, et al. Cognitive-behavioral treatment of insomnia secondary to chronic pain. J Consult Clin Psychol 2000; 69:50–57.
25. Epstein DR, Dirksen SR. Randomized trial of a cognitive-behavioral intervention for insomnia in breast cancer survivors. Oncol Nurs Forum 2007; 34(5):E51–E59.
26. Savard J, Simard S, Ivers H, et al. Randomized study on the efficacy of cognitive-behavioral therapy for insomnia secondary to breast cancer, part I: Sleep and psychological effects. J Clin Oncol 2005; 23(25):6083–6096.
27. Rybarczyk B, Stepanski E, Fogg L, et al. A placebo-controlled test of cognitive-behavioral therapy for comorbid insomnia in older adults. J Consult Clin Psychol 2005; 73:1164–1174.
28. Edinger JD, Wohlgemuth WK, Krystal AD, et al. Behavioral insomnia therapy for fibromyalgia patients: A randomized clinical trial. Arch Intern Med 2005; 165(21):2527–2535.
29. McCurry SM, Gibbons LE, Logsdon RG, et al. Nighttime insomnia treatment and education for Alzheimer's disease: A randomized, controlled trial. J Am Geriatr Soc 2005; 53:793–802.
30. Currie SR, Clark S, Hodgins DC, et al. Randomized controlled trial of brief cognitive-behavioral interventions for insomnia in recovering alcoholics. Addiction 2004; 9:1121–1132.
31. Morin CM. Insomnia: Psychological assessment and management. New York: Guilford, 1993.
32. Greeff AP, Conradie WS. Use of progressive relaxation training for chronic alcoholics with insomnia. Psychol Rep 1998; 82:407–412.
33. Cannici J, Malcolm R, & Peek LA. Treatment of insomnia in cancer patients using muscle relaxation training. J Behav Ther Exp Psychiatry 1983; 14:251–256.
34. Smith MT, Huang MI, Manber R. Cognitive behavior therapy for chronic insomnia occurring within the context of medical and psychiatric disorders. Clin Psychol Rev 2005; 25(5):559–592.
35. Cohen J. Statistical Power Analysis for the Behavioral Sciences. New York, NY: Academic Press, 1977:274–281.
36. Morin CM, Culbert JP, Schwartz SM. Nonpharmacological interventions for insomnia: A meta-analysis of treatment efficacy. Am J Psychiatry 1994; 151:1172–1180.
37. Sivertsen B, Omvik S, Havik OE, et al. A comparison of actigraphy and polysomnography in older adults treated for chronic primary insomnia. Sleep 2006; 29:1353–1358
38. Roizenblatt S, Moldofsky H, Benedito-Silva A, et al. Alpha sleep characteristics in fibromyalgia. Arthritis Rheum 2001; 44:222–230.
39. Lichstein KL, Durrence HH, Riedel BW, et al. Epidemiology of sleep: Age, gender, and ethnicity. Mahwah, NJ: Erlbaum, 2004.

40. Morgan K. Sleep and aging. In: Lichstein KL, Morin CM, eds. Treatment of late-life insomnia. Thousand Oaks, CA: Sage, 2000:3–36.
41. Morphy H, Dunn KM, Lewis M, et al. Epidemiology of insomnia: a longitudinal study in a UK population. Sleep 2007; 30:274–280.
42. Stewart R, Besset A, Bebbington P, et al. Insomnia comorbidity and impact and hypnotic use by age group in a national survey population aged 16 to 74 years. Sleep 2006; 29:1391–1397.
43. Morgan K, Clarke D. Longitudinal trends in late-life insomnia: Implications for prescribing. Age Ageing 1997; 26:179–184.
44. Puder R, Lacks P, Bertelson AD, et al. Short-term stimulus control treatment of insomnia in older adults. Behav Ther 1983; 14:424–429.
45. Morin CM, Colecchi C, Stone J, et al. Behavioral and pharmacological therapies for late-life insomnia: A randomized controlled trial. J Am Med Assoc 1999; 281:991–999.
46. Lichstein KL. Sleep compression treatment of an insomnoid. Behav Ther 1988; 19:625–632.
47. McCurry SM, Logsdon RG, Teri L. Behavioral treatment of sleep disturbance in elderly dementia caregivers. Clin Gerontol 1996; 17(2):35–50.
48. Edinger JD, Hoelscher TJ, Marsh GR, et al. A cognitive-behavioral therapy for sleep-maintenance insomnia in older adults. Psychol Aging 1992; 7:282–289.
49. Morin CM, Colecchi CA, Ling WD, et al. Cognitive behavior therapy to facilitate benzodiazepine discontinuation among hypnotic-dependent patients with insomnia. Behav Ther 1995; 26:733–745.
50. Friedman L, Bliwise DL, Yesavage JA, et al. A preliminary study comparing sleep restriction and relaxation treatments for insomnia in older adults. J Gerontol 1991; 46:P1–P8.
51. Lichstein KL, Johnson RS. Relaxation for insomnia and hypnotic medication use in older women. Psychol Aging 1993; 8:103–111.
52. Baillargeon L, Landreville P, Verreault R, et al. Discontinuation of benzodiazepines among older insomniac adults treated with cognitive-behavioural therapy combined with gradual tapering: A randomized trial. Can Med Assoc J 2003; 169:1015–1020.
53. Cooper TV, Lichstein KL, Aguillard RN. Hypnotic dependent insomnia in an older adult with addiction-prone personality. Clin Case Studies 2003; 2:247–258.
54. McCrae CS, Tierney CG, McNamara JPH. Behavioral intervention for insomnia: Future directions for nontraditional caregivers at various stages of care. Clin Gerontol 2005; 29(2):95–114.
55. McCurry SM, Logsdon RG, Vitiello MV, et al. Successful behavioral treatment for reported sleep problems in elderly caregivers of dementia patients: A controlled study. J Gerontol Psychol Soc Sci 1998; 53B:P122–P129.
56. Morin CM, Azrin NH. Behavioral and cognitive treatments of geriatric insomnia. J Consult Clin Psychol 1988; 56:748–753.
57. McCrae CS, McGovern R, Lukefahr R, et al. Research evaluating brief behavioral sleep treatments for rural elderly (RESTORE): A preliminary examination of effectiveness. Am J Geriatr Psychiatry 2007; 15:979–982.
58. Morgan K, Dixon S, Mathers N, et al. Psychological treatment for insomnia in the management of long-term hypnotic drug use: A pragmatic randomised controlled trial. Br J Gen Pract 2003; 53:923–928.
59. Lichstein KL, Morin CM, eds. Treatment of late-life insomnia. Thousand Oaks, CA: Sage, 2000.
60. Friedman L, Benson K, Noda A, et al. An actigraphic comparison of sleep restriction and sleep hygiene treatments for insomnia in older adults. J Geriatr Psychiatry Neurol 2000; 13:17–27.
61. Stepanski EJ, Wyatt JK. Use of sleep hygiene in the treatment of insomnia. Sleep Med Rev 2003; 7:215–225.
62. Lichstein KL, Riedel BW, Wilson NM, et al. Relaxation and sleep compression for late-life insomnia: A placebo-controlled trial. J Consult Clin Psychol 2001; 69:227–239.
63. Morin CM, Bastien C, Guay B, et al. Randomized clinical trial of supervised tapering and cognitive behavior therapy to facilitate benzodiazepine discontinuation in older adults with chronic insomnia. Am J Psychiatry 2004; 161:332–342.
64. Sivertsen B, Omvik S, Pallesen S, et al. Cognitive behavioral therapy vs zopiclone for treatment of chronic primary insomnia in older adults: A randomized controlled trial. J Am Med Assoc 2006; 295:2851–2858.
65. Pallesen S, Nordhus IH, Kvale G. Nonpharmacological interventions for insomnia in older adults: A meta-analysis of treatment efficacy. Psychotherapy 1998; 35:472–482.
66. Irwin MR, Cole JC, Nicassio PM. Comparative meta-analysis of behavioral interventions for insomnia and their efficacy in middle-aged adults and in older adults 55 + years of age. Health Psychol 2006; 25:3–14.
67. Rybarczyk BD, Stepanski E, Alsten C, et al. Applying cognitive-behavioral treatment to comorbid insomnia: Successes and challenges. Paper presented at: The Annual Meeting of the American Psychological Association; 2007; San Francisco, CA.

68. Creti L, Libman E, Bailes S, et al. Effectiveness of cognitive-behavioral insomnia treatment in a community sample of older individuals: More questions than conclusions. J Clin Psychol Med Settings 2005; 12:153–164.
69. Davies R, Lacks P, Storandt M, et al. Countercontrol treatment of sleep-maintenance insomnia in relation to age. Psychol Aging 1986; 1:233–238.
70. Engle-Friedman M, Bootzin RR, Hazlewood L, et al. An evaluation of behavioral treatments for insomnia in the older adult. J Clin Psychol 1992; 48:77–90.
71. Morin CM, Kowatch RA, Barry T, et al. Cognitive-behavior therapy for late-life insomnia. J Consult Clin Psychol 1993; 61:137–146.
72. Pallesen S, Nordhus IH, Kvale G, et al. Behavioral treatment of insomnia in older adults: An open clinical trial comparing two interventions. Behav Res Ther 2003; 41:31–48.
73. Riedel BW, Lichstein KL, Dwyer WO. Sleep compression and sleep education for older insomniacs: Self-help versus therapist guidance. Psychol Aging 1995; 10:54–63.

31 Pharmacology of the $GABA_A$ Receptor Complex

Alan N. Bateson
Institute for Membrane and Systems Biology, Faculty of Biological Sciences, University of Leeds, Leeds, U.K.

INTRODUCTION

Gamma-aminobutyric acid (GABA) is an amino acid neurotransmitter, first discovered more than 50 years ago (1). Approximately 30% of synapses in the vertebrate central nervous system have been show to contain GABA, making it the most abundant inhibitory neurotransmitter. Consequently it is not surprising that GABAergic neurotransmission plays a key role in the normal physiological function of the brain, including sleep regulation (2–5), as well as various pathophysiological sequelae (6). GABA receptors have traditionally been classified according to pharmacological criteria into three groups, $GABA_A$, $GABA_B$ and $GABA_C$ receptors. $GABA_A$ and $GABA_C$ receptors are ligand-gated ion channels whereas $GABA_B$ receptors are G protein-coupled receptors (7). Molecular cloning studies have revealed the structural basis for this classification, a heterogeneity hitherto unrealized (particularly in the case of $GABA_A$ receptors) and that $GABA_C$ receptors should be considered part of the $GABA_A$ receptor family (7,8).

$GABA_A$ receptors posses a rich pharmacology with a number of distinct binding sites for a variety of molecular entities that are separate to that of the agonist GABA. These binding sites are often, though not exclusively, modulatory such that their occupation leads to an allosteric modulation of the action of GABA or other agonists. Benzodiazepines, barbiturates, alcohol and certain anesthetics all bind to $GABA_A$ receptors and modulate their activity. From the perspective of sleep medicine it is clearly the benzodiazepine binding site that has attracted the most interest. Elucidation of the molecular composition of $GABA_A$ receptors has revealed that compounds that interact with the benzodiazepine site can modulate GABA-induced receptor activity in a positive or negative fashion.

Members of the $GABA_A$ receptor family are the targets for both the traditional benzodiazepine hypnotics and as well as the newer non-benzodiazepine "Z" drugs (zaleplon, zolpidem, zopiclone and eszopiclone) (9). The realization from basic science studies that the $GABA_A$ receptor is not a single entity but a family of related receptors has opened the door to the possible targeting of specific $GABA_A$ receptor subtypes in the pursuit of novel therapeutic interventions for sleep and other disorders. This chapter provides an overview of $GABA_A$ receptor pharmacology, with particular reference to classic and newer hypnotics. It also discusses the ongoing elucidation of $GABA_A$ receptor heterogeneity and how this might be relevant to the understanding of the physiology sleep, its disorders and their treatment. The rich pharmacology of this receptor family and the specific distribution patterns and physiological functions of its members means that there is significant potential for the further development of novel hypnotics that act at members of this important receptor family.

$GABA_A$ RECEPTOR HETEROGENEITY

$GABA_A$ receptors are members of the cys-cys loop ligand-gated ion channel superfamily (7) that includes the nicotinic acetylcholine, glycine and serotonin type 3 ($5HT_3$) receptors. That is to say, all these receptor families share a degree of primary amino acid sequence identity to such an extent that they display three-dimensional structural similarities. Indeed, the nicotinic acetylcholine receptor is considered the archetypal member of the cys-cys loop receptor superfamily and has provided the lead in studies examining receptor structure (10). All receptors in this family are pseudosymmetric pentamers with an integral ion channel pore (11,12). Evolutionary studies indicate that members of this superfamily are highly conserved even down to invertebrates (13). Within a single receptor family there is a greater degree of sequence identity than between families (14).

The $GABA_A$ receptor family comprises of at least 19 genes each encoding a single subunit. Comparisons of sequence identity between individual $GABA_A$ receptor subunits have led to their classification into seven isoform groups (α, β, γ, δ, ε, θ, π, ρ; 1,7,9,16). In mammals there are six α, three β, three δ, one each of ε, θ and π, and three ρ subunit genes, the latter being previously classified as $GABA_C$ receptors (7,8). Alternate splice forms have been described for a number of $GABA_A$ receptor gene transcripts, thereby potentially increasing diversity. Combinatorial association of these subunits into pentameric receptors results in the production of a large number of $GABA_A$ receptor subtypes. The actual number of $GABA_A$ receptor subtypes in mammalian brain is not currently known, but although the theoretical number of combinations is immense, evidence exists for a few dozen rather than thousands of different $GABA_A$ receptor subtypes (8,15). α and β subunits commonly occur together with γ subunits, although δ subunits do occur in place of a γ subunit. The most abundant receptor subtype comprises of two α1, two β2 and one γ2 subunit (7,9,16).

$GABA_A$ RECEPTOR DISTRIBUTION

Prior to the molecular cloning of $GABA_A$ receptor subunit genes, pharmacological analysis of $GABA_A$ receptor subtypes suggested at least two subtypes (BZ1 and BZ2) existed that could be differentiated by their affinity for CL218872, a nonbenzodiazepine triazolopyridazine ligand that binds to the benzodiazepine site. BZ1 binding sites showed high affinity for CL218872 and distribution primarily in the cerebellum, whereas BZ2 binding sites exhibited lower affinity for CL218872 and were found in hippocampal and cortical structures (17,18). It is now clear that each $GABA_A$ receptor subunit gene exhibits a specific spatial (and temporal) expression pattern, with the distribution of some subunits being wide and others more limited (18).

That specific neuronal populations express a subset of $GABA_A$ receptor genes has been known for some time (19,20). What has become apparent in recent years is that the subcellular localization of $GABA_A$ receptor subtypes is also subject to control. The mechanisms governing the distribution of specific $GABA_A$ receptor subtypes are beginning to be understood. For example, analysis of intracellular proteins that interact with certain $GABA_A$ receptor subunits has revealed that one of these, gephyrin, is necessary, along with the γ2 subunit, for the correct postsynaptic clustering of $GABA_A$ receptors (21–23). Further, immunohistochemical studies have revealed that certain GABA receptor subtypes are concentrated in specific regions of hippocampal pyramidal neurons, with α1 subunit-containing receptors being detected on the cell soma while α2 subunit-containing receptors localize to the axon initial segment. These postsynaptic localizations correspond to neuron-specific innervation. Thus parvalbumin-positive basket cells form GABAergic terminals on the cell soma of hippocampal pyramidal neurons and parvalbumin-positive chandelier cells innervate axon initial segment (21).

Finally, perhaps the most exciting development in recent years in this area has been the realization that $GABA_A$ receptors are present outside of the traditional synaptic structure as extrasynaptic receptors (16,24). These have been shown to be present on a number of different neuronal types, each possessing a specific extrasynaptic $GABA_A$ receptor subtype (16,21,25,26).

POSTSYNAPTIC AND EXTRASYNAPTIC $GABA_A$ RECEPTORS MEDIATE PHASIC AND TONIC INHIBITION

Postsynaptic $GABA_A$ receptors are responsible for phasic inhibition. In response to an action potential, GABA is released from the presynaptic membrane and diffuses into the synaptic cleft at a high concentration. It binds to and activates the postsynaptic receptors causing the postsynaptic membrane to hyperpolarise by opening the integral chloride ion channel of the $GABA_A$ receptor. Two processes terminate the action of this phasic release of GABA. One is a general mechanism involving the rapid removal of the neurotransmitter GABA from the synaptic cleft by GABA transporters (16,27). A second, $GABA_A$ receptor subtype-specific mechanism, leads to the termination of GABA activation and is governed by the specific kinetic properties of the receptor. $GABA_A$ receptor subtypes exhibit varying rates of desensitization with many of the synaptic subtypes showing quite rapid rates. Before released GABA can be removed from the synaptic cleft, $GABA_A$ receptors that have been activated can move into a desensitized closed configuration. Thus phasic GABAergic neurotransmission is determined by a combination of the structure of the synaptic cleft, the uptake mechanisms for removal of neurotransmitter from the synaptic cleft, and the kinetic properties of the postsynaptic $GABA_A$ receptor subtypes (16).

Many postsynaptic GABA$_A$ receptors contain γ2 subunits, which given the linked role of these subunits with that of gephyrin in postsynaptic localization is perhaps not surprising (21). This is not a simple one-to-one correlation, however, as γ2 subunit-containing GABA$_A$ receptors have been shown to be located beyond the immediate postsynaptic area (18) and different neuronal types exhibit differing GABA$_A$ receptor subtypes at postsynaptic sites (15).

In contrast to postsynaptic GABA$_A$ receptors, some of the best characterized extrasynaptic GABA$_A$ receptor subtypes possess kinetic properties that allow them to function effectively in the absence of the high concentrations of GABA seen in the synaptic cleft immediately following phasic release. Low millimolar concentrations of "ambient" GABA are found extrasynaptically which arise from spillover or leakage from GABAergic synapses and are not likely to exhibit the rapid changes in concentration seen within a GABAergic synaptic cleft (16,22). Thus, the combination of α6, β2 or β3, and δ subunits, which is found in cerebellar granule cells, and the α4β2/3δ combination, which is found in dentate gyrus granule neurones and thalamocortical neurons of the ventro-basal complex, are located extrasynaptically (16,15,24,26,28). These subunit combinations result in receptors with high affinity for GABA and slow desensitization properties. Their high affinity for GABA means that they bind the neurotransmitter even when it is present at the low concentrations found outside of the synapse. Further, the slow desensitization properties of some extrasynaptic GABA$_A$ receptors means that once they are activated they produce a longer lasting (tonic) inhibition. These properties are particular to those receptor subtypes that contain α4 or α6 subunits in combination with a δ subunit (16,22). It has been estimated that under these particular conditions a greater charge transfer occurs via such extrasynaptic GABA$_A$ receptor-mediated tonic inhibition than that which occurs via phasic inhibition by postsynaptic GABA$_A$ receptors (29). Extrasynaptic GABA$_A$ receptors have been identified that comprise of other subunit combinations, and which exhibit different kinetic properties; the consequences of this are currently under investigation (18,28).

GABA$_A$ RECEPTOR SUBTYPES EXHIBIT SPECIFIC PHARMACOLOGICAL PROFILES

The functional consequences of the cell and subcellular localization of specific GABA$_A$ receptor subtypes are not fully understood, but are clearly dependent upon the specific properties of these different GABA$_A$ receptor subtypes. The cloning of GABA$_A$ receptor subunit cDNAs in the late 1980s and early 1990s revealed the existence of the GABA$_A$ receptor gene family. Determination of the contribution that individual subunits make to the physiological and pharmacological properties of GABA$_A$ receptors became the goal of numerous research laboratories in the following years and relating these to *in vivo* receptor properties is ongoing. What has emerged is a picture in which related subunits confer specific physiological features to the receptor, which include GABA affinity and kinetic properties such as desensitization rates, as well as pharmacological characteristics such as benzodiazepine binding site affinity and efficacy of benzodiazepine action. Thus, the combinatorial association of different GABA$_A$ receptor subunits exquisitely determines the functional characteristics of GABA$_A$ receptor subtypes as well playing a role in their localization (9,15).

The earliest indication that subunit heterogeneity determined the pharmacological profile of GABA receptors came a year after publication of the first GABA$_A$ receptor cDNA clones (30,31). Although the 1987 study had indicated that the full pharmacological profile of GABA$_A$ receptors was recapitulated in heterologous expression systems using only the α and β subunits (31), it became apparent that the benzodiazepine response was not robust and a third subunit class, the γ subunits, needed to be co-expressed with an α and a β subunit in order to achieve potentiation of GABA$_A$ receptor activity with classical benzodiazepines (30).

A molecular explanation of BZ1 and BZ2 binding profile soon followed with α1 subunits conferring the BZ1 binding phenotype and α2, α3 and α5 the BZ2 binding phenotype (30,32,33). Further, specific amino acids in the N-terminal domains of these α subunits were identified as being responsible for these different pharmacological profiles (34). In contrast, receptors incorporating α4 or α6 subunits with β and γ subunits could not bind classical benzodiazepine agonists, although they did bind antagonists and inverse agonists (see below) (35,36). Thus α subunits play a key role in the benzodiazepine recognition properties of GABA receptor subtypes.

What of the γ subunits? While it was known that they were necessary for benzodiazepine recognition (30), it soon became apparent that different γ subunit isoforms contribute to benzodiazepine recognition and functional properties in combination with α subunits (37). For example, in contrast to those containing γ2 or γ3 subunits, γ1-containing receptors show little affinity for the antagonist flumazenil (Ro15–1788). Further, methyl β-carboline-3-carboxylate (βCCM), which binds to $GABA_A$ receptors at the benzodiazepine site, is a positive modulator at some receptor subunit compositions and a negative modulator at others (37). Thus both α and γ subunits determine the recognition and functional properties of the benzodiazepine binding site of the $GABA_A$ receptor.

The δ subunit has a discrete expression profile and is found in combination with a variety of α and β subunits in place of a γ subunit. δ subunit-containing receptor subtypes exhibit an interesting pharmacology in that they do not bind classical benzodiazepine agonists but play an important role in the mechanism of action of the natural modulators neurosteroids (25).

Recent studies combining DNA mutagenesis, transgenic technology and psychopharmacology have shed light on the role played by specific $GABA_A$ receptor subtypes in the pharmacological profile of drugs that act at $GABA_A$ receptors (18,38,39). For example, the sedative properties of the classical benzodiazepine diazepam are mediated via α1 subunit-containing receptors while its anxiolytic properties are mediated by α2 subunit-containing receptors at low receptor occupancy and both α2 and α3 subunit-containing receptors at high receptor occupancy (28,38). Thus the principle of targeting a single $GABA_A$ receptor subtype (or a limited number) in order to achieve a specific pharmacological outcome has been established.

It is clear therefore that the subunit combination, as well as the site(s) of expression, both with respect to cell compartment and cell type, should be taken into account when considering $GABA_A$ receptors as therapeutic targets.

THE BENZODIAZEPINE SITE AS TARGET FOR SLEEP MEDICINES

Classical benzodiazepine agonists have long been used as therapeutics for the treatment of anxiety and sleep disorders but, as indicated above, it is only in recent years that the identities of their molecular targets have become apparent. A salient lesson from these studies is that the pharmacology of benzodiazepines, or other compounds that act at the benzodiazepine binding site of the $GABA_A$ receptor, can only be defined when both the compound and the precise $GABA_A$ receptor subtype is specified. While this is currently possible for a number of $GABA_A$ receptor subtypes, particularly the most abundant (α1,β2,γ2), our lack of a full appreciation of $GABA_A$ receptor heterogeneity *in vivo* means that this is still a goal rather than a reality.

Progress has been made, however, in defining the molecular site of interaction between certain benzodiazepines and their binding site on the $GABA_A$ receptor protein. Specific amino acids have been identified on both the α and γ subunits that play roles in determining both the affinity and the efficacy of benzodiazepine interactions. These studies have demonstrated that the benzodiazepine-binding pocket lies at the interface of the α and γ subunit, thereby explaining why both α and γ subunit isoforms play a role in determining benzodiazepine pharmacological properties (40).

Compounds that act at the benzodiazepine site which are sedative-hypnotics can be divided into two broad classes; classical benzodiazepine agonists and newer nonbenzodiazepine agonists. Although chemically distinct, they all bind to the same site on the $GABA_A$ receptor and are believed to produce their actions by similar molecular mechanisms that result in the potentiation of the actions of GABA leading to an increase in $GABA_A$ receptor-meditated inhibition. The pharmacological differences between these therapeutic agents, both within a class and between the classes, lie in their specificity of action with respect to $GABA_A$ receptor subtypes and their pharmacokinetics. With respect to the latter, it is obvious that the pharmacokinetic properties of an ideal hypnotic would include rapid onset of action (to promote sleep induction) and an appropriate half-life (to limit drug-mediated daytime effects) of both the parent drug and any active metabolites (2,41).

CLASSICAL BENZODIAZEPINE HYPNOTICS

The classical 1,4-benzodiazepines are hypnotics that also display sedative, anxiolytic, anticonvulsant, muscle relaxant and amnesic activities. Those indicated for treatment of insomnia include estazolam (U.S.A.), flurazepam (U.S.A., U.K.), quazepam (U.S.A.), temazepam (U.S.A., U.K.) nitrazepam (U.K.), loprazolam (U.K.), lormetazepam (U.K.) and triazolam (USA) (42,43).

Most classical benzodiazepine hypnotics appear not to differentiate between different GABA$_A$ receptor subtypes, although there are a few studies, which indicate that quazepam and lormetazepam show a 10- and 3-fold, respectively, selectivity for receptors containing α1 subunits (30,44).

Significant advances in our understanding of the mechanisms of action of classical benzodiazepines have occurred more than the past 10 years, largely due to use of transgenic animal studies. Therefore we now have a much clearer, though by no means complete, understanding of which GABA$_A$ receptor subtypes mediate specific aspects of the complex pharmacological profile of classical benzodiazepine agonists. Unfortunately, these studies have largely used diazepam as an exemplar and hence we can only draw conclusions based upon the very similar pharmacodynamic profile that diazepam shares with the currently prescribed classical benzodiazepine hypnotics indicated above.

Two sorts of transgenic studies have shed light on this area: gene knock-out mice, where the expression of a specific GABA$_A$ receptor subunit gene is ablated; and knock-in mice, where a specific amino acid is altered in one subunit to alter its pharmacology (e.g., to change its recognition properties from diazepam sensitive to diazepam insensitive) (39). These allow the analysis of the sedative-hypnotic properties of benzodiazepine-site compounds when combined with such behavioral tests as locomotor activity and loss of righting reflex (39). However, such studies are not without problems, particularly in knock-out animals where compensation for the loss of expression of one GABA$_A$ receptor gene has been seen in the form of up regulation of the expression of other GABA$_A$ receptor genes (e.g., 45) making interpretation difficult. Thus in α1-subunit knock-out mice diazepam's hypnotic action was increased, which was opposite to the effects of the α1 subunit-specific hypnotic zolpidem (39,45). In contrast, using α1-subunit knock-in mice it was clearly demonstrated that the sedative effects of diazepam were mediated via the α1 subunit (46,47). Changes in EEG patterns caused by diazepam during sleep are well known but experiments with knock-in mice suggested that the α1 (48) and α3 (49) subunits do not mediate these particular effects, but there is an involvement of α2 subunit-containing receptors in the diazepam-mediated modulation of delta-wave activity (50).

NON-BENZODIAZEPINE HYPNOTICS

There are a number of nonbenzodiazepine compounds of various structural classes that bind to the benzodiazepine site of the GABA$_A$ receptor and which are very effective hypnotics. These include the so-called "z-drugs" zaleplon (pyrazolopyrimidine), zopiclone and eszopiclone (cyclopyrrolones), and zolpidem (imidazopyridine), as well as others such as indiplon (pyrazolopyrimidine). Some of these are licensed in the USA (43) but, somewhat controversially, while the "z-drugs" are licensed in the UK, they are not recommended by the National Institute for Health and Clinical Excellence (42,51,52).

In general these hypnotics all show selectivity for α1-subunit containing GABA$_A$ receptors, although to varying degrees. Data from published studies indicate a range of values for affinity and potency at defined GABA$_A$ receptors subtypes, dependent to an extent on the methodology used by different laboratories.

Zaleplon shows a ~10 fold higher affinity for α1 subunit-containing receptors over those containing α2 or α3 subunits, and a ~30 fold higher affinity over those containing the α5 subunit (53). The difference in zopiclone's affinity for α1 versus α2, α3 or α5 subunit-containing receptors is less (2–6 fold: 53,54,55). Zolpidem shows the greatest selective affinity for α1 subunit-containing receptors compared to those containing α2 (5–24 fold), α3 (14–19 fold), or α5 (>1000 fold) subunits (32,54). One study reported similar values for zolpidem for α1 and α3 but not α2 subunit-containing receptors where they were unable to detect binding of zolpidem (53). Although not tested on defined receptor subtypes, the *S*(+)-enantiomer of zopiclone (eszopiclone) displays approximately 50- and 25-fold higher affinities for GABA$_A$ receptor benzodiazepine binding sites in mouse brain than the racemate zolpidem or the *R*(+)-enantiomer, respectively (56).

Studies on the relative potency of these drugs at different receptor subtypes further demonstrates their selectivity for α1 subunit-containing receptors, although the actual values vary markedly from study to study. Overall, it is clear however, that zaleplon, zopiclone, eszopiclone, zolpidem and indiplon are more potent at α1 compared to α2 (2–9 fold) and $\alpha3$ (3–29 fold) subunit-containing receptors (2,57,58). At $\alpha5$ subunit-containing receptors, however, a different picture emerges which serves to differentiate these compounds further. Zopiclone shows similar potency to that exhibited at $\alpha1$ subunit-containing receptors (57), zaleplon and indiplon demonstrate a 3 to 30 fold (study dependent) selective potency for receptors with $\alpha1$ subunits (2,57–59) and two studies report that zolpidem does not potentiate $\alpha5$ subunit-containing receptors at all (57,58).

These findings using defined receptor subtypes concur with those produced using less reductionist approaches such as isolated neurons, brain membranes or whole animals, which indicate that all of these compounds act primarily through $\alpha1$-subunit containing receptors (BZ1 type receptors) to produce their pharmacological effects (e.g., 60–63). Only zolpidem, however, has been investigated using transgenic animals, demonstrating that its sedative effects are produced exclusively via $\alpha1$ subunit-containing receptors (64).

Another important aspect of the non-benzodiazepine hypnotics' pharmacology is their pharmacokinetic profile, in particular their half-lives. The very nature of the use of hypnotics for the treatment of insomnia dictates that a short half-life is desirable to limit or obviate day-time effects. The half-lives of these hypnotics are: zaleplon, 1 hour; zopiclone, 4.4 hour; zolpidem 1.9 (52); and indiplon 1.5 to 2 hour (65). This fits the ideal better than the "short-acting" benzodiazepines such as temazepam, for example, which has a half life of 9 h (52).

The pharmacodynamic and pharmacokinetic profiles of these nonbenzodiazepine hypnotics are markedly suited for the treatment of insomnia. Their selectivity for $\alpha1$ subunit-containing $GABA_A$ receptors predicts a more limited side-effect profile compared to classical benzodiazepines. Studies using transgenic mice demonstrate that tolerance to the sedative effects of diazepam require the presence of receptors containing the $\alpha5$ subunit (66). Given that zolpidem does not act at $\alpha5$ subunit containing receptors, it might be expected that zolpidem would exhibit reduced tolerance and while there is data to support this notion, not all studies agree (see 67 for discussion). The abuse liability of benzodiazepines is widely recognized and a number of studies have indicated that nonbenzodiazepine hypnotics present a lower, albeit non-zero, potential for abuse (52,68,69). Thus the selectivity of nonbenzodiazepine hypnotics coupled with their short half lives comprise advantages over classical benzodiazepines.

THE GABA-AGONIST SITE AS TARGET FOR SLEEP MEDICINES

Given the utility of modulating $GABA_A$ receptor activity in order to induce or maintain sleep, it is perhaps surprising that direct activation of $GABA_A$ receptors has not been utilized for the same end more extensively. Indeed, although ~60%of $GABA_A$ receptors comprise $\alpha1\beta2\gamma2$ and there a number of other γ subunit-containing receptor subtypes, there are also $GABA_A$ receptors which do not comprise of the appropriate subunit complement for modulation by benzodiazepines (28). Ligands that act at the GABA-agonist site therefore have the potential to promote inhibition of neurons that are not modulated by benzodiazepines. Despite this, few such ligands have been successfully developed as sleep medications. The most promising of these in recent years was a rigid analogue of GABA, 4,5,6,7-tetrahydroisoxazolo(5,4-c)pyridin-3-ol (THIP) developed under the name gaboxadol, which although reaching phase 3 trials was withdrawn from further development in 2007 by Lundbeck and Merck due to some safety and efficacy concerns. Nevertheless, the proof-of-principle was established by the data from preclinical experimentation and clinical trails that gaboxadol is an effective sleep medication that works via $GABA_A$ receptors but by mechanisms distinct from that of the benzodiazepine-site agonists (2,22,27,70).

Gaboxadol has an interesting pharmacological profile that suggests new possibilities for targeting the $GABA_A$ receptor to promote sleep. It has high potency at $\alpha4\beta3\delta$ $GABA_A$ receptors with a greater maximum response than GABA, while at receptors containing γ subunit instead of a δ subunit gaboxadol is a low potency partial agonist (71). This receptor subtype has been shown to be present extrasynaptically in thalamocortical neurons of the ventrobasal complex where they regulate oscillatory activity that is associated with sleep (25,26). Examination of other GABA-site agonists, particularly with respect to their subtype specificity, has the potential to develop new hypnotics that target this site (2,22,24).

OTHER GABA$_A$ RECEPTOR SITES AS TARGET FOR SLEEP MEDICINES

GABA$_A$ receptors display a rich pharmacology with a multitude of distinct modulatory sites for ligands from a variety of chemical classes. Our lack of a complete understanding of the mechanisms by which compounds that act at these various sites produce their modulatory activity and whether (and how) they are receptor-subtype selective, indicates that there is even further potential for targeting the GABA$_A$ receptor beyond that of the benzodiazepine and GABA-agonist sites. The sleep-promoting effects of barbiturates and alcohol are well established, but problems of abuse and overdose limit their usefulness.

The general anesthetics halothane and enflurane have been shown to produce a loss of righting reflex in mice that is mediated in part by the β3 subunit of the GABA$_A$ receptor (28). Further, GABA$_A$ receptors that contain the ε subunit appear to be less sensitive to the actions of the general anesthetic propofol (72), demonstrating GABA$_A$ receptor subtype specificity. The loss of consciousness produced by general anesthetics has EEG features that are similar to those seen in various stages of sleep and it has been proposed that normal sleep and anesthetic-induced loss of consciousness may share some neuronal pathways in common, particularly those that involve the thalamus (3). Hence it is possible that a greater understanding of the molecular and neurobiological mechanisms by which general anesthetics operate via GABA$_A$ receptors may yield novel ways of modulating sleep.

One the most exciting, yet underdeveloped sites on the GABA$_A$ receptor, is the target of a class of natural modulators of GABA$_A$ receptor function the neurosteroids (73). It has long been known that neurosteroids can modulate sleep in both rats (74) and man (75). The recent finding that activation and modulation of GABA$_A$ receptor activity occurs at separate sites on the receptor (76) coupled with the observation of subunit-selectivity and brain region-specific action of neurosteroids (73), further indicates that the capacity of the GABA receptor as a target for novel hypnotics is only likely to increase in the future.

CONCLUSION

The benzodiazepine site of the GABA$_A$ receptor has proven to be a most effective site for the pharmacological manipulation of sleep. Our growing understanding of this receptor family, in particular: the pharmacological distinctiveness of GABA$_A$ receptor subtypes; the diverse expression patterns of individual GABA$_A$ receptor subtypes; and the emerging physiological roles of specific GABA$_A$ receptors subtypes; all indicate that this receptor family is likely to provide a rich vein for the development of GABA$_A$ receptor-mediated hypnotics in the future.

REFERENCES

1. Owens DF, Kriegstein AR. Is there more to GABA than synaptic inhibition? Nat Rev Neurosci 2002; 3:715–727.
2. Ebert B, Wafford KA, Deacon S. Treating insomnia: Current and investigational pharmacological approaches. Pharmacol Ther 2006;112:612–629.
3. Franks NP. General anaesthesia: From molecular targets to neuronal pathways of sleep and arousal. Nat Rev Neuro 2008; 9:370–386.
4. Saper CB, Scammell TE, Lu J. Hypothalamic regulation of sleep and circadian rhythms. Nature 2005; 437:1257–1263.
5. Watson CJ, Soto-Calderon S, Lydic R, et al. Pontine reticular formation (PnO) administration of hypocretin-1 increases PnO GABA levels and wakefulness. Sleep 2008; 31:453–464.
6. Mohler H. GABA$_A$ receptors in central nervous system disease: Anxiety, epilepsy, and insomnia. J Recept Signal Transduct Res 2006a; 26:731–740.
7. Barnard EA, Skolnick P, Olsen RW, et al. International Union of Pharmacology. XV. Subtypes of γ-aminobutyric acid A receptors: Classification on the basis of subunit structure and receptor function. Pharmacol Rev 1998; 50:291–313.
8. Olsen RW, Sieghart W. International Union of Pharmacology. LXX. Subtypes of γ-aminobutyric acid(A) receptors: Classification on the basis of subunit composition, pharmacology, and function. Update. Pharmacol Rev 2008; 60:243–260.
9. Bateson AN. The benzodiazepine site of the GABA$_A$ receptor: An old target with new potential? Sleep Med 2004; 5(suppl 1):S9–S15.
10. Unwin N. Refined structure of the nicotinic acetylcholine receptor at 4 A resolution J Mol Biol 2005; 346:967–989.

11. Barrera NP, Betts J, You H, et al. Atomic force microscopy reveals the stoichiometry and subunit arrangement of the α4β3δ $GABA_A$ receptor. Mol Pharmacol 2008; 73:960–967.
12. Nayeem N, Green TP, Martin IL, et al. Quaternary structure of the native $GABA_A$ receptor determined by electron microscopic image analysis. J Neurochem 1994; 62:815–818.
13. Tsang SY, Ng SK, Xu Z, et al. The evolution of $GABA_A$ receptor-like genes. Mol Biol Evol 2007; 24:599–610.
14. Cockcroft VB, Osguthorpe DJ, Barnard EA, et al. Ligand-gated ion channels. Homology and diversity. Mol Neurobiol 1990; 4:129–169.
15. Mohler H. GABA(A) receptor diversity and pharmacology. Cell Tissue Res 2006b; 326:505–516.
16. Farrant M, Nusser Z. Variations on an inhibitory theme: Phasic and tonic activation of $GABA_A$ receptors. Nat Rev Neurosci 2005; 6:215–229.
17. Doble A, Martin IL. Multiple benzodiazepine receptors: No reason for anxiety. Trends Pharmacol Sci 1992; 13:76–81.
18. Mohler H, Fritschy JM, Rudolph U. A new benzodiazepine pharmacology. J Pharmacol Exp Ther 2002; 300:2–8.
19. Laurie DJ, Seeburg PH, Wisden W. The distribution of 13 $GABA_A$ receptor subunit mRNAs in the rat brain. II. Olfactory bulb and cerebellum. J Neurosci 1992; 12:1063–1076.
20. Wisden W, Laurie DJ, Monyer H, et al. The distribution of 13 $GABA_A$ receptor subunit mRNAs in the rat brain. I. Telencephalon, diencephalon, mesencephalon. J Neurosci 1992; 12:1040–1062.
21. Luscher B, Keller CA. Regulation of $GABA_A$ receptor trafficking, channel activity, and functional plasticity of inhibitory synapses. Pharmacol Ther 2004; 102(3):195–221.
22. Wafford K, Ebert, B. Gaboxadol – a new awakening in sleep. Curr Opin Pharmacol 2006; 6:30–36.
23. Yu W, Jiang M, Miralles CP, et al. Gephyrin clustering is required for the stability of GABAergic synapses. Mol Cell Neurosci 2007; 36:484–500.
24. Bateson AN. Further potential of the $GABA_A$ receptor in the treatment of insomnia. Sleep Med 2006; 7(suppl 1):S3–S9.
25. Belelli D, Peden DR, Rosahl TW, et al. Extrasynaptic $GABA_A$ receptors of thalamocortical neurons: A molecular target for hypnotics. J Neurosci 2005; 25:11513–11520.
26. Jia F, Pignataro L, Schofield CM, et al. An extrasynaptic $GABA_A$ receptor mediates tonic inhibition in thalamic VB neurons. J Neurophysiol 2005; 94:4491–4501.
27. Borden LA. GABA transporter heterogeneity: Pharmacology and cellular localization. Neurochem Int. 1996; 29:335–356.
28. Rudolph U, Mohler H. GABA-based therapeutic approaches: $GABA_A$ receptor function. Curr Op Pharmacol 2006; 6:18–23.
29. Brickley SG, Cull-Candy SG, Farrant M. Development of a tonic form of synaptic inhibition in rat cerebellar granule cells resulting from persistent activation of $GABA_A$ receptors. J Physiol 1996; 497:753–759.
30. Pritchett DB, Sontheimer H, Shivers BD, et al. Importance of a novel $GABA_A$ receptor subunit for benzodiazepine pharmacology. Nature 1989; 338:582–585.
31. Schofield PR, Darlison MG, Fujita N, et al. Sequence and functional expression of the $GABA_A$ receptor shows a ligand-gated receptor super-family. Nature 1987; 328:221–227.
32. Pritchett DB, Seeburg PH. γ-aminobutyric $acid_A$ receptor alpha 5-subunit creates novel type II benzodiazepine receptor pharmacology. J Neurochem 1990; 54:1802–1804.
33. Pritchett DB, Lüddens H, Seeburg PH. Type I and type II $GABA_A$-benzodiazepine receptors produced in transfected cells. Science 1989; 245:1389–1392.
34. Pritchett DB, Seeburg PH. γ-Aminobutyric acid type A receptor point mutation increases the affinity of compounds for the benzodiazepine site. Proc Natl Acad Sci U S A 1991;88:1421–1425.
35. Lüddens H, Pritchett DB, Köhler M, et al. Cerebellar $GABA_A$ receptor selective for a behavioural alcohol antagonist. Nature 1990; 346:648–651.
36. Wisden W, Herb A, Wieland H, et al. Cloning, pharmacological characteristics and expression pattern of the rat $GABA_A$ receptor a4 subunit. FEBS Lett 1991; 289:227–230.
37. Bateson AN. Basic pharmacological mechanisms involved in benzodiazepine tolerance and withdrawal. Curr Pharm Des 2002; 8:5–21.
38. Reynolds DS. The value of genetic and pharmacological approaches to understanding the complexities of $GABA_A$ receptor subtype functions: The anxiolytic effects of benzodiazepines. Pharm Biochem Behav 2008; 90:37–42.
39. Rudolph U, Mohler H. Analysis of $GABA_A$ receptor function and dissection of the pharmacology of benzodiazepines and general anesthetics through mouse. Ann Rev Pharmacol Toxicol 2004; 44: 475–498.
40. Sigel E, Buhr A. The benzodiazepine binding site of $GABA_A$ receptors. Trends Pharmacol Sci 1997; 18:425–429.

41. Mendelson WB, Roth T, Cassella J, et al. The treatment of chronic insomnia: Drug indications, chronic use and abuse liability. Sleep Med Rev 2004; 8:7–17.
42. British National Formulary 58. 2010. http://www.bnf.org/
43. Passarella S, Duong MT. Diagnosis and treatment of insomnia. Am J Health Syst Pharm 2008; 65: 27–34.
44. Ozawa M, Nakada Y, Sugimachi K, et al. Interaction of the hypnotic lormetazepam with central benzodiazepine receptor subtypes omega-1, omega-2 and omega-3. Nippon Yakurigaku Zasshi (Folia Pharmacol Jap) 1991; 98:399–408
45. Kralic JE, O'Buckley TK, Khisti RT, et al. $GABA_A$ receptor α1 subunit deletion alters receptor subtype assembly, pharmacological and behavioral responses to benzodiazepines and zolpidem. Neuropharm 2002; 43:685–694.
46. McKernan RM, Rosahl TW, Reynolds DS, et al. Sedative but not anxiolytic properties of benzodiazepines are mediated by the $GABA_A$ receptor α1 subtype. Nat Neurosci 2000; 3:587–592.
47. Rudolph U, Crestani F, Benke D, et al. Benzodiazepine actions mediated by specific gamma-aminobutyric acid(A) receptor subtypes. Nature 1999; 401:796–800.
48. Tobler I, Kopp C, Deboer T, et al. Diazepam-induced changes in sleep: Role of the α1 $GABA_A$ receptor subtype. Proc Natl Acad Sci USA 2001; 98:6464–6469.
49. Kopp C, Rudolph U, Keist R, et al. Diazepam-induced changes on sleep and the EEG spectrum in mice: Role of the α3-$GABA_A$ receptor subtype. Eur J Neurosci 2003; 17:2226–2230.
50. Kopp C, Rudolph U, Löw K, et al. Modulation of rhythmic brain activity by diazepam: $GABA_A$ receptor subtype and state specificity. Proc Natl Acad Sci U S A 2004; 101:3674–3679.
51. NICE. Guidance on the use of zaleplon, zolpidem and zopiclone for the short-term management of insomnia. 2005; http://www.nice.org.uk/TA077guidance.
52. Nutt DJ. NICE: The National Institute of Clinical Excellence – or Eccentricity? Reflections on the Z-drugs as hypnotics. J Psychopharmacol 2005; 19:125–127.
53. Damgen K, Luddens H. Zaleplon displays a selectivity to recombinant $GABA_A$ receptors different from zolpidem, zopiclone and benzodiazepines. Neurosci Res Comm 1999; 25:139–148.
54. Smith A, Alder L, Silk J, et al. Effect of a subunit on allosteric modulation of ion channel function in stably expressed human recombinant γ-aminobutyric acidA receptors determined using 36 Cl ion flux. Mol Pharmacol 2001; 59:1108–1118.
55. Davies M, Newell JG, Derry JM, et al. Characterization of the interaction of zopiclone with γ-aminobutyric acid type A receptors. Mol Pharmacol 2000; 58:756–762.
56. Blaschke G, Hempel G, Muller W. Preparative and analytical separation of the zopiclone enantiomers and determination of their affinity to the benzodiazepine receptor binding site. Chirality 1993; 5: 419–421
57. Petroski RE, Pomeroy JE, Das R, et al. Indiplon is a high-affinity positive allosteric modulator with selectivity for α1 subunit-containing $GABA_A$ receptors. J Pharmacol Exp Ther 2006; 317:369–377.
58. Sanna E, Busonero F, Talani G, et al. Comparison of the effects of zaleplon, zolpidem, and triazolam at various $GABA_A$ receptor subtypes. Eur J Pharmacol 2002; 451:103–110.
59. Fleck MW. Molecular actions of (S)-desmethylzopiclone (SEP-174559), an anxiolytic metabolite of zopiclone. J Pharmacol Exp Ther 2002; 302:612–618.
60. Foster AC, Pelleymounter MA, Cullen MJ, et al. In vivo pharmacological characterization of indiplon, a novel pyrazolopyrimidine sedative-hypnotic. J Pharmacol Exp Ther 2004; 311:547–559.
61. Noguchi H, Kitazumi K, Mori M, et al. Binding and neuropharmacological profile of zaleplon, a novel nonbenzodiazepine sedative/hypnotic. Eur J Pharmacol 2002; 434:21–28.
62. Sanger DJ, Morel E, Perrault G. Comparison of the pharmacological profiles of the hypnotic drugs, zaleplon and zolpidem. Eur J Pharmacol 1996; 313:35–42.
63. Sullivan SK, Petroski RE, Verge G, et al. Characterization of the interaction of indiplon, a novel pyrazolopyrimidine sedative-hypnotic, with the $GABA_A$ receptor. J Pharmacol Ther 2004; 311; 537–546.
64. Crestani F, Martin JR, Möhler H, et al. Mechanism of action of the hypnotic zolpidem in vivo. Br J Pharmacol 2000; 131:1251–1254.
65. Rosenberg R, Roth T, Scharf MB, et al. Efficacy and tolerability of indiplon in transient insomnia. J Clin Sleep Med 2007: 3:374–379.
66. van Rijnsoever C, Tauber M, Choulli MK, et al. Requirement of α5-$GABA_A$ receptors for the development of tolerance to the sedative action of diazepam in mice. J Neurosci 2005; 24:6785–6790.
67. Wafford KA. $GABA_A$ receptor subtypes: Any clues to the mechanism of benzodiazepine dependence? Curr Opin Pharmacol 2005; 5:47–52.
68. Evans SM, Funderburk FR, Griffiths RR. Zolpidem and triazolam in humans: Behavioral and subjective effects and abuse liability. J Pharmacol Exp Ther 1990; 255:1246–1255.

69. Hajak G, Muller WE, Wittchen HU, et al. Abuse and dependence potential for the non-benzodiazepine hypnotics zolpidem and zopiclone: A review of case reports and epidemiological data. Addiction 2003; 98:1371–1378.
70. Roth T. A physiological basis for the evolution of pharmacotherapy for insomnia. J Clin Psychiatry 2007; 68(suppl 5):13–18.
71. Brown N, Kerby J, Bonnert TP, et al. Pharmacological characterization of a novel cell line expressing human $\alpha 4\beta 3\delta$ $GABA_A$ receptors. Br J Pharmacol 2002; 136:965–974.
72. Davies PA, Hanna MC, Hales TG, et al. Insensitivity to anaesthetic agents conferred by a class of $GABA_A$ receptor subunit. Nature 1997; 385:820–823.
73. Belelli D, Lambert JJ. Neurosteroids: Endogenous regulators of the $GABA_A$ receptor. Nat Rev Neuro 2005; 6:565–575.
74. Damianisch K, Rupprecht R, Lancel M. The influence of subchronic administration of the neurosteroid allopregnanolone on sleep in the rat. Neuropsychopharm 2001; 25:576–584.
75. Steiger A, Trachsel L, Guldner J, et al. Neurosteroid pregnenolone induces sleep-EEG changes in man compatible with inverse agonistic $GABA_A$-receptor modulation. Brain Res 1993; 615:267–274.
76. Hosie AM, Wilkins ME, da Silva HM, et al. Endogenous neurosteroids regulate $GABA_A$ receptors through two discrete transmembrane sites. Nature 2006; 444:486–449.

32 Benzodiazepine Receptor Agonists: Indications, Efficacy, and Outcome

Andrew D. Krystal

Insomnia and Sleep Research Laboratory, Department of Psychiatry and Behavioral Sciences, Duke University School of Medicine, Durham, North Carolina, U.S.A.

INTRODUCTION

Many different agents are prescribed to treat insomnia. These agents represent at least 12 different medication classes. Among these classes are agents which mediate their therapeutic effect by binding to sites on the gamma-aminobutyric acid (GABA) type A receptor complex, thereby enhancing the inhibition that occurs when GABA binds to this receptor (1,2). These agents represent a set of chemically related compounds referred to as benzodiazepines and include triazolam, temazepam, flurazepam, diazepam, alprazolam, lorazepam, and oxazepam (2) (Table 1). The benzodiazepines can have a diverse set of effects via their modulation of $GABA_A$ receptors. These effects include sedation, anxiolysis, myorelaxation, antiseizure effects, and psychomotor impairment (2). There appears to be variation among the benzodiazepines in their profile of relative potency for these effects; however, all of them have some degree of sleep enhancement. However, only five of these agents are indicated for insomnia treatment by the U.S. Food and Drug Administration (FDA): triazolam, temazepam, flurazepam, estazolam, and quazepam (Table 1) (3).Agents that modulate $GABA_A$ receptors at the same binding sites as the benzodiazepines but that are unrelated chemically to these medications have been referred to as "nonbenzodiazepines" (3). Nonbenzodiazepines indicated for the treatment of insomnia in the United States include zolpidem, zolpidem CR, zaleplon, and eszopiclone. Together the benzodiazepines and nonbenzodiazepines have been referred to as "benzodiazepine receptor agonists" (BzRAs). While these agents are actually allosteric modulators and not agonists, because this is the most commonly used term for these medications, it will be adopted here as well (1). The BzRAs have dominated the pharmacologic management of insomnia for the last 50 years. They represent nearly all of the medications that have been approved by the FDA for the treatment of insomnia during this period. There is a substantial body of literature documenting their therapeutic effects in the treatment of insomnia. This chapter reviews this literature with the goal of providing an overview of their indications, the evidence for efficacy, and the data related to treatment outcome.

INDICATIONS

The first step in determining whether a BzRA might be indicated in a given patient is determining whether there is an indication to implement treatment for insomnia. This decision should involve weighing the risks/costs associated with not treating a patient for insomnia (the adverse effects of the untreated insomnia) against the anticipated benefits and risks of the available insomnia therapies (3). Factors that should be taken into account when assessing risks include medical and psychiatric conditions the patient may have such as obstructive sleep apnea, chronic obstructive pulmonary disease, pregnancy, etc., which may alter the risks of administering particular treatments. Treatment should be administered if at least one insomnia therapy is expected to deliver improvements in quality of life and/or function that outweigh the associated side effects and costs. The greater the impairment an individual experiences because of insomnia, the greater is the cost of not implementing treatment and the greater the possible benefit with treatment and therefore, the greater the motivation to institute treatment (35).

Once a decision has been made to implement treatment for insomnia, it is then necessary to decide which treatment to administer. In addition to the BzRAs, available options primarily include nonpharmacologic therapies such as cognitive behavioral therapy (CBT)

Table 1 Properties of BzRAs

Agent[c]	FDA indication	T_{max} (hr)	$t_{1/2}$ (hr)	Metabolism	Sleep-onset efficacy[a]	Sleep-maintenance efficacy[a]
Flurazepam[b]	Insomnia	0.5–1.5	40–250	CYP2C19 CYP3A4	+	+
Quazepam[b]	Insomnia	2	20–120	CYP3A4, CYP2C19	+	+
Estazolam[b]	Insomnia	1.5–2	10–24	CYP3A4	+	+
Temazepam[b]	Insomnia	1–3	8–20	Glucuronide conjugation	+	+
Triazolam[b]	Insomnia	1–3	2–5.5	CYP3A4 Glucuronide conjugation	+	+
Clonazepam[b]	Seizures Anxiety	1–2	35–40	CYP2B CYP3A4 Acetylation		
Lorazepam[b]	Anxiety	1–3	12–15	Glucuronide conjugation		
Alprazolam[b]	Anxiety	1–3	12–14	CYP3A4/5 CYP2C19		
Diazepam[b]	Anxiety Muscle Spasm Seizures	0.5–2	20–50	CYP2B, CYP2C19 CYP3A4 Glucuronide conjugation		
Chlordiazepoxide[b]	Anxiety ETOH Withdrawal	0.5–4	5–100	CYP2B, CYP2C19 CYP3A4 Glucuronide conjugation		
Zolpidem (CR)[c]	Insomnia	1.7–2.5	2.0–5.5	CYP3A4 CYP1A2 CYP2C9	+	+ (CR only)
Zaleplon[c]	Insomnia	1.1	0.9–1.1	Aldehyde Oxidase; CYP3A4	+	
Eszopiclone[c]	Insomnia	1.3–1.6	6–7	CYP3A1 CYP2E1	+	+

[a]Efficacy in at least one double-blind, placebo-controlled trial employing either self-report or polysomnographic endpoints.
[b]Benzodiazepine.
[c]Nonbenzodiazepine; $t_{1/2}$ includes the half-lives of the parent compound and major active metabolites.
Abbreviations: CYP, Cytochrome P450.
Information in the table is from Refs. 4–34.

for insomnia, antidepressants, antipsychotics, anticonvulsants, melatonin receptor agonists, and antihistamines (3). In determining which therapy to recommend, the anticipated risks and benefits of all of the treatment options should be weighed and discussed with the patient in the context of their personal preferences. The treatment which has the overall most favorable risks-to-benefits ratio taking all of these factors into account should be recommended (3).

In order for clinicians to effectively carry out this decision-making process, they must have access to data from placebo-controlled trials delineating the therapeutic and adverse effects of the insomnia treatment options in the population of the patient in question (same age range, comorbid condition, etc.). The BzRAs and the melatonin agonist ramelteon are the medications currently in common use that have by far the strongest empirical support and have an indication for insomnia treatment from the FDA (3). CBT also has a strong empirical basis (36). It is noteworthy that some of the most commonly administered insomnia medications, including antidepressants, antipsychotics, and anticonvulsants, have yet to be studied in controlled trials in insomnia patients and are prescribed "off label" (3,37). Without controlled trials of these agents, it is not possible to determine on empirical grounds whether they might be indicated for use over BzRAs in a given patient. However, there are some factors relevant to deciding whether treatment with a BzRA is indicated that do not derive from placebo-controlled clinical trials.

One such consideration is abuse potential. Some degree of abuse potential exists for all BzRAs; therefore, another therapy should be considered when abuse is a concern (3). However, it is important to note that the population of insomnia patients that is at risk for abuse of BzRAs is actually relatively small (38). The available evidence suggests that insomnia patients, by and large, take their medications for therapeutic purposes and do not abuse insomnia agents (39). Abuse of BzRAs appears to be limited to a relatively small subgroup of polysubstance abuse-prone individuals (38,39). As a result, when treating a patient known not to have a history of substance abuse, the risk of abuse is extremely small and should not be a significant factor in considering treatment options. However, in many cases, it remains uncertain whether the patient in question may be abuse prone and in these circumstances some risk of abuse should be assumed in making treatment decisions. It is important to note that abuse potential is not related to duration of medication therapy. It is as likely on the first day of treatment as the 1000th. Dependence [seeking medication because of loss of benefit over time (tolerance), withdrawal, or drug inaccessibility], however, is a phenomenon that increases in likelihood the longer the duration of treatment. The tendency for this to occur can only be determined from placebo-controlled trials of treatment (discussed in the following section).

Another important consideration in deciding whether a particular BzRA might be indicated in a patient is the route of metabolism. This factor becomes particularly important when treating individuals with significant hepatic or renal disease. Those agents, which are primarily metabolized via a hepatic cytochrome P450 pathway, will be relatively more affected by hepatic disease than those metabolized via glucuronide conjugation or other mechanisms (40). This would suggest that, among the BzRAs, the use of temazepam and lorazepam would be relatively preferred in this setting (Table 1) (41–44). In those with significant renal disease, agents eliminated by glucuronide conjugation are relatively contraindicated. Among BzRAs this includes temazepam, lorazepam, chlordiazepoxide, diazepam, and triazolam (41–44).

A final treatment-related consideration related to the choice of BzRAs versus other therapies is the relative availability, feasibility, and likelihood of efficacy of nonpharmacologic therapy. CBT for insomnia is a highly effective form of treatment, which is primarily limited by the lack of availability of trained practitioners in clinical settings (45). As a result, despite a substantial literature supporting the use of this treatment, many practitioners turn to pharmacotherapy such as BzRAs (45). In some individuals, medications are preferable due to unwillingness or inability to undergo CBT or a lack of maladaptive behaviors/cognitions that are targeted by CBT (46).

These considerations should complement the evidence base as a means to optimize therapy rather than serve as a basis for making decisions that are not supported by the available data. As we will review in the next section, a substantial body of data from placebo-controlled trials has been collected on the effects of BzRAs in insomnia patients. The available studies far outnumber those of any other insomnia medications and provide data on the efficacy and safety of BzRAs that can be used as a basis for clinical decision making.

EFFICACY

This section reviews the available double-blind, placebo-controlled trials of the treatment of insomnia with BzRAs. Efficacy has been assessed via continuous measures of self-reported or polysomnographic sleep-onset latency or sleep maintenance (either wake time after sleep onset or number of awakenings) as has long been the standard in insomnia research. The results are organized for presentation into the following subsections: (1) efficacy in adults with primary insomnia, (2) efficacy in older adults with primary insomnia, (3) efficacy in children, (4) efficacy in comorbid insomnia, (5) efficacy as a function of treatment duration, (6) efficacy in intermittent dosing, and (7) comparative efficacy studies.

Table 2 BzRA Dosages with Efficacy in ≥1 Double-Blind, Placebo-Controlled Trials

Agent	Onset in adults (mg)	Onset in elderly (mg)	Maintenance in adults (mg)	Maintenance in elderly (mg)	Efficacy in comorbid insomnia
Flurazepam		15 30	30	30	
Quazepam	30		30		
Estazolam	1 2		1 2		
Triazolam	0.25 0.5	0.125 0.25 0.4 0.5 0.8	0.5	0.125 0.25 0.4 0.8	RA: 0.125–0.25 mg COPD: 0.125–0.25 mg
Temazepam	30		30	7.5–30	
Zolpidem	10	5	10		Menopause: 10 mg COPD: 10 mg
Zolpidem CR	12.5		12.5		MDD: 12.5 mg; GAD: 12.5 mg
Zaleplon	10 20	5 10			
Eszopiclone	2 3	2	2 3	2	MDD: 3 mg; GAD: 3 mg; RA: 3 mg; Menopause: 3 mg

Abbreviations: MDD, major depressive disorder; GAD, generalized anxiety disorder, RA, rheumatoid arthritis.
Information in the table is from Refs. 4–34 and 47–59.

Efficacy in Adults with Primary Insomnia

Up to this point in time, there have been 22 double-blind, placebo-controlled studies of the treatment of primary insomnia patients with BzRAs in adults where a significant difference compared with placebo was reported on at least one sleep-onset or sleep-maintenance measure (Table 2) (5,7,9–12,14,17,18,20,22,24,25,27–31,34,75). One challenge in applying this body of literature to clinical practice is uncertainty about how to best account for the variation among agents in the number of positive studies. The tendency, particularly in the past, not to publish negative studies makes it difficult to assume efficacy when there has only been one positive study, as is the case for several BzRAs.

The available studies provide evidence of sleep-onset efficacy in adults for triazolam (three studies), flurazepam (two studies), estazolam (two studies), quazepam (one study), temazepam (one study), zolpidem (five studies), zolpidem CR (two studies), zaleplon (three studies), and eszopiclone (three studies). On this basis, triazolam, flurazepam, estazolam, zolpidem, zolpidem CR, zaleplon, and eszopiclone could be considered for the treatment of sleep-onset problems in adults with relative confidence. There is also evidence for sleep-maintenance efficacy in adults for triazolam (one study), flurazepam (one study), estazolam (three studies), quazepam (one study), temazepam (one study), zolpidem (one study), zolpidem CR (two studies), and eszopiclone (3 studies). The strongest support for sleep-maintenance efficacy exists for estazolam, zolpidem CR, and eszopiclone. These same agents have the strongest base of support for use in patients with both onset and maintenance problems.

Efficacy in Older Adults with Primary Insomnia

In the elderly, 11 double-blind, placebo-controlled trials of the treatment of primary insomnia have been carried out (6,8,13,15,16,19,21,23,26,32,33). Sleep-onset efficacy has been reported for triazolam (five studies), flurazepam (two studies), zolpidem (one study), zaleplon (two studies), and eszopiclone (two studies). Evidence for sleep-maintenance efficacy in this population exists for triazolam (three studies), flurazepam (one study), temazepam (one study), and eszopiclone (two studies). The available data provide relative support for the efficacy of triazolam, flurazepam, zaleplon, and eszopiclone in addressing sleep-onset problems in older adults, and triazolam and eszopiclone for treating sleep-maintenance problems in this population.

Efficacy in Children with Insomnia

The most glaring deficiency in the literature on the treatment of insomnia with BzRAs is the absence of any placebo-controlled trials in children (3).

In fact, there has yet to be a placebo-controlled trial of any insomnia agent in this population. Given the fact that pharmacotherapy of insomnia in children is common in clinical practice, such studies are greatly needed (60).

Efficacy in Comorbid Insomnia

Twelve studies of the treatment of insomnia comorbid with medical and psychiatric conditions have been carried out with BzRAs (Table 2) (47–59). Agents with a significant effect versus placebo on sleep in patients with comorbid major depressive disorder (MDD) are lormetazepam, clonazepam, eszopiclone, and zolpidem CR (48–52). Each was the subject of one published trial in this population. Eszopiclone and zolpidem CR have also been noted to have efficacy in a study of the treatment of insomnia occurring with generalized anxiety disorder (GAD) (53,59). In patients with insomnia occurring with rheumatoid arthritis, both eszopiclone and triazolam were reported to improve sleep versus placebo in a single study (57,58). Triazolam has been reported to have efficacy in the treatment of insomnia occurring with chronic obstructive pulmonary disease in two studies, while the efficacy of zolpidem in this population has been noted in one study (55,56). Lastly, single studies demonstrate the efficacy of zolpidem and eszopiclone in the treatment of menopausal insomnia (47,54).

Efficacy as a Function of Treatment Duration

The duration of treatment for which efficacy has been demonstrated may also be relevant to clinical decision making. Because it is not possible to predict how long any individual will experience insomnia, it is not possible to plan in advance how long pharmacotherapy will be needed (3). As a result, periodic trial discontinuations may be helpful to determine the ongoing need for medication via carrying out risk–benefit analyses of continued therapy following each trial tapering of medication (3). At the same time, it is important to know how long efficacy can be expected with a given agent to plan such trial discontinuations.

Despite the high prevalence of long-lasting insomnia, large-scale pharmacologic trials of treatment beyond four to five weeks have only recently been carried out (14,16,61,62). These studies contradict the long-held view that the pharmacologic treatment of insomnia with BzRAs for longer periods of time is inevitably associated with tolerance (loss of benefit over time) and/or withdrawal symptoms (63). The available data do not rule out the possibility that such dependence phenomena occur in some individuals (the risk depends on the agent and dosage and may vary among individuals); however, it has now been established that dependence phenomena are not characteristic of nightly treatment for up to one year with some agents. Among the BzRAs, eszopiclone has been the subject of two placebo-controlled trials demonstrating efficacy over six months of nightly treatment (14,62). In one of these studies, subjects were switched to single-blind placebo therapy for an additional six months during which there was evidence for continued efficacy out to one year (76). An open-label study of zaleplon employing nightly treatment for up to one year provided evidence for minimal adverse effects occurring as a function of treatment duration (61). For other agents commonly in use, the longest durations of efficacy that have been demonstrated in controlled trials are eight weeks for temazepam (in the elderly) and five weeks for zolpidem and zaleplon (9,16,25,30). All of the other BzRAs have been studied for maximal periods of four weeks or less.

Efficacy in Intermittent Dosing

It is important to note that the studies discussed so far have employed nightly dosing of medication. Intermittent dosing, prescribed to approximately 41% of insomnia patients, is a potential means to lower costs and lessen exposure to medication's side effects, particularly over longer periods of treatment (3,64). Three placebo-controlled studies of the intermittent dosing of BzRAs have been carried out in primary insomnia patients (18,28,34). Two of these demonstrated the efficacy of zolpidem when dosed three to five nights per week for periods of two and three months (18,28). One additional study reported the efficacy of zolpidem CR when dosed three to seven nights per week over a six-month period (34). These studies, which set minimum and maximum requirements for pill-taking each week, provide the best available indicators of the properties of "as needed" dosing of insomnia medication. Studies of true "as needed" dosing will be needed to determine if the required pill-taking frequencies in these studies affected the results. In terms of the clinical application of these findings, we currently lack data to indicate which patients with insomnia are best treated with this regimen. From a practical viewpoint, the effective implementation of intermittent dosing requires that an individual must be able to predict prior to going to bed that they are likely to have sleep difficulty (3). While there may be some individuals who can effectively implement dosing following unsuccessful attempts to sleep, there is a concern that this practice might be problematic from a behavioral viewpoint. Such a practice may increase the focus on sleep and contribute to the perpetuation of conditioned insomnia through allowing patients to experience ongoing sleep difficulty (3).

Comparative Efficacy Studies

Eleven studies have been carried out, which compared the efficacy of BzRAs to the efficacy of (1) other BzRAs or (2) other treatments (7,8,16,19,24,26,27,65,66,67). The following comparisons of medication therapies have been carried out: estazolam 2 mg versus flurazepam 30 mg, zaleplon 10 to 20 mg versus triazolam 0.25 mg, zolpidem 10 mg versus trazodone 50 mg, triazolam 0.25 mg versus flurazepam 15 mg, triazolam 0.4 to 0.8 mg versus flurazepam 15 to 30 mg, triazolam 0.25 to 0.5 mg versus 250 to 500 mg chloral hydrate, and eszopiclone 3 mg versus zolpidem 10 mg (7,8,12,19,24,26,27,65,66). Generally, these studies were not powered to detect differences between the active treatments. Their primary aim was focused on documenting differences between the active treatments and placebo. It is not surprising, therefore, that significant differences in sleep effects between medication therapies were only reported for two studies. In one of these studies, triazolam 0.5 mg led to shorter sleep-onset latency and fewer awakenings than 250 to 500 mg of chloral hydrate, while triazolam 0.25 mg was associated with longer total sleep time than both dosages of chloral hydrate (66). The other study, carried out in elderly insomnia patients, reported that triazolam 0.25 mg led to significantly longer total sleep time and higher ratings of sleep quality and restedness in the morning compared with flurazepam 15 mg (19). When interpreting these data, it is important to bear in mind that the results apply only to the dosages assessed, which may not have been optimal in some cases.

Two studies have been carried out comparing BzRAs (zolpidem 10 mg and temazepam 7.5 to 30 mg) with CBT (16,67). A limitation of these studies is that they employed a control for pill-taking but did not employ a control for the behavioral therapy administered. These studies did not find significant differences between the treatments during acute therapy; however, in follow-up assessment, advantages for CBT over temazepam 7.5 to 30 mg and zolpidem 10 mg were observed (16,67). It is important to note that the follow-up assessments were carried out following BzRA discontinuation. As a result, they speak more to the degree of insomnia present after a period of BzRA therapy rather than to the acute therapeutic effects of these agents. The findings suggest that greater persistence of benefit occurs after a course of CBT than occurs following discontinuation of a period of treatment with temazepam or zolpidem in primary insomnia patients.

OUTCOME

The studies of the efficacy of BzRAs reviewed in the prior section provide an important basis for making treatment decisions. However, they reflect only one aspect of outcome. In clinical practice it is necessary to take other considerations into account, such as treatment-emergent adverse effects and the degree of improvement in function occurring with treatment. Here, we have reviewed the available literature on the effects of BzRAs on nonsleep aspects of outcome as well as global outcome measures. The following five types of outcomes are reviewed in the subsequent sections: (1) syndromal insomnia measures, (2) patient and clinician global impressions, (3) measures of daytime function, (4) the severity of comorbid conditions, and (5) adverse effects of treatment.

Syndromal Insomnia Measures

Measures that assess the entire constellation of features that constitute the syndrome of insomnia have only recently been employed as outcome measures in placebo-controlled trials of BzRAs. A syndromal insomnia measure that has been used in several BzRA trials is the Insomnia Severity Index (ISI) (68). The ISI consists of seven items, each of which is a 5-point Likert scale rating of a *DSM-IV* defined insomnia symptom. Several thresholds for defining levels of insomnia severity have been established—ISI 0 to 7: not clinically significant; ISI 8 to 14: subthreshold insomnia; ISI 15 to 21: moderate insomnia; ISI 22 to 28: severe insomnia (62,68,69). Significantly greater improvement versus placebo in the ISI total score has been reported in a number of recent controlled trials of eszopiclone in adults and elderly with primary insomnia, insomnia comorbid with MDD, and in menopausal insomnia (15,49,54,58,62). In three of these studies, active treatment led to a significantly greater percentage of the subjects meeting ISI criteria for subthreshold and not clinically significant insomnia and a lower percentage meeting criteria for moderate and severe insomnia compared with placebo (49,54,62). These studies provide evidence that treatment leads to improvement in the overall severity of the insomnia syndrome and significantly increases the percentage of individuals who are not substantively affected by the disorder. These studies illustrate how a syndromal measure could have relevance to clinical practice and speak to the need to adopt consensus response and remission criteria and employ them in controlled trials of BzRA treatment.

Patient and Clinician Global Impressions

While not a specific measure of the insomnia syndrome, global impression data can also provide valuable, highly clinically relevant outcome data. These data have also been used to generate categorical response criteria analogous to the analyses carried out with ISI data discussed in the previous section. Several recent studies have employed global impression assessments completed by patients (PGI) and/or clinicians (CGI) (18,34,53). In a three-month study in primary insomnia patients, zolpidem 10 mg dosed three to five nights per week led to significantly greater improvement in CGI score than placebo treatment (18). Zolpidem CR taken three to seven nights per week for six months by primary insomnia patients led to a greater percentage of responders (rating of much improved or very much improved with treatment) on both CGI and PGI compared with placebo (34). In a study of the treatment of insomnia comorbid with GAD, subjects treated with eszopiclone 3 mg and escitalopram had greater CGI improvement ratings than subjects treated with placebo and escitalopram (53).

Measures of Daytime Function

Syndromal and global measures of insomnia take into account daytime function; however, they do not provide a specific indicator of the degree of functional impairment. While impairment in daytime function is required in order to make a diagnosis of insomnia according to the established criteria, measures of daytime function have generally not been included in insomnia outcome assessment and have never been among the primary outcome measures in an insomnia treatment trial (35,70). No studies have been powered to detect effects on a measure of daytime function and no studies have required that subjects have daytime impairment on any instrument as a requirement for study entry (35). These factors decrease the likelihood of finding a significant effect of treatment on daytime function. For this reason, we review the studies of BzRAs that had a significant effect versus placebo on at least one measure of daytime function but do not cite the studies where no effect was found. Seven studies of eszopiclone dosed at 3 mg in adults and 2 mg in older adults reported significant effects on at least one measure of daytime function which included (1) Likert ratings of "daytime alertness," "ability to concentrate or think clearly," "ability to function," or "sense of physical well-being" (14,49,53,54,58,62,71); (2) a decrease in napping among those who napped (15,71); (3) morning sleepiness ratings (71); (4) the Epworth Sleepiness Scale (62); (5) the Fatigue Severity Scale (62); (6) the Quality of Life Enjoyment and Satisfaction Questionnaire (QLESQ) (71); (7) the Work Limitations Questionnaire (62); (8) either the "vitality," "physical functioning," or "social functioning" subscales of the SF-36; (15,62) and (9) at least one subscale of the Sheehan Disability Scale (54,62). Zolpidem 10 mg was reported to have a significant effect versus placebo on the SF-36 "vitality" subscale in patients with MDD in remission who had residual insomnia (72). In a study of intermittent dosing with zolpidem CR 12.5 mg in primary insomnia patients, significant effects were observed on Likert ratings of "morning sleepiness" and "ability to concentrate," as well as the Epworth Sleepiness Scale (34). These findings indicate the potential for BzRAs to improve daytime function and suggest the need for better integration of measures of daytime function into insomnia research and clinical practice.

Severity of Comorbid Conditions

The majority of chronic insomnia occurs in association with medical and psychiatric disorders (73). For many years, chronic insomnia was viewed as a symptom of these medical and psychiatric conditions (63). As such, guidelines recommended treating the causative underlying condition and discouraged administering insomnia-specific treatment (63). However, recent studies have provided convincing evidence that this view is incorrect and suggest that the relationship between insomnia and comorbid conditions is complex and, in some cases, the causality may be bidirectional (3). This emerging view legitimizes the use of measures of the severity of the comorbid medical and psychiatric conditions associated with insomnia in assessing the outcome of insomnia treatment. Six studies have reported statistically significant improvement in measures related to the severity of associated medical or psychiatric conditions with BzRA therapy compared with placebo (49,51,53,54,57,58). One of these was a study of the treatment of insomnia comorbid with MDD where greater improvement in the Hamilton Depression Rating Scale (HAM-D) occurred with clonazepam compared with placebo (51). Greater improvement in the HAM-D with and without the sleep items as well as a greater depression remission and response rate were also noted with eszopiclone 3 mg compared with placebo (49). Eszopiclone 3 mg also improved the HAM-D as well as the Hamilton Anxiety Scale (HAM-A) to a significantly greater extent than placebo in patients with insomnia comorbid with GAD (53). Two studies have demonstrated improvement in pain in patients with insomnia occurring in association with rheumatoid arthritis (57,58). In the first such study, triazolam 0.125 to 0.25 mg significantly improved morning stiffness ratings compared with placebo (57). The second study reported that eszopiclone 3 mg led to significantly lower Arthritis Efficacy Scale score, lower pain severity ratings, and fewer tender joints than placebo (58). Lastly, in a study of the treatment of menopausal insomnia, eszopiclone 3 mg led to significant improvement in the Menopause Specific Quality of Life Scale, the Greene Climacteric Scale Score, and the Montgomery–Asberg Depression Rating Scale score, and also decreased awakenings due to hot flashes compared with placebo (54). These studies provide clear evidence that the treatment of insomnia with at least some BzRAs can improve the severity of comorbid medical and psychiatric conditions. Whether this is a byproduct of improving insomnia or is a specific effect of these agents remains unresolved. However, recent studies of insomnia comorbid with GAD and MDD treated with zolpidem CR 12.5 mg reported significant improvement in sleep compared with placebo but did not note corresponding improvement in depression or anxiety severity (48,59). These findings may suggest that some of the effects of BzRA treatment on the severity of comorbid conditions may be medication specific, though other factors such as differences in study design may confound interpretation.

Adverse Effects of Treatment

In making treatment decisions and assessing the outcome of therapies, the beneficial effects of treatment must be weighed against the associated adverse effects. The available studies are relatively limited in their capacity to detect between-treatment differences in adverse effects. Studies have generally not been powered to detect differences from placebo in adverse effects. Further, adverse effects data are derived from spontaneous symptoms reported and not from a systematic or standardized assessment of symptoms. As a result, instead of including studies where significant differences were found between BzRAs and placebo, we report the relative rates of adverse effects in these groups. This overview is focused on data from studies in the elderly as this population is relatively vulnerable to a number of potential BzRA adverse effects. We, therefore, expect that studies in older adults provide a more sensitive indicator of potential adverse effects than studies in younger adults. The results are broken down into two groups: (1) daytime sedation and (2) other adverse effects.

Daytime sedation: One study reported a statistically significantly greater rate of incidence of somnolence as an adverse event with flurazepam compared with placebo and temazepam (74). Relative frequencies of somnolence in BzRA therapies and placebo that have been reported are zolpidem 5 mg 10% versus zaleplon 10 mg 4% versus placebo 2% (6) and eszopiclone 2 mg 6.6% versus placebo 5.5% (15).

Other adverse effects: Temazepam dosed at 7.5 to 30 mg was associated with an 8% overall incidence of adverse effects compared with 11% for placebo treatment (16). Zolpidem 5 mg was noted to have a rate of CNS adverse effects of 25% versus 14% with placebo and zaleplon 10 mg (6). Eszopiclone 2 mg led to unpleasant taste in 12% compared with 0% in placebo, dizziness in 6% versus 2% in placebo, and dry mouth in 7% compared with 2% in the placebo group (15).

In summary, the available data would suggest a relatively low rate of adverse effects for the BzRAs compared with placebo. However, adverse effects data were available for a limited number of the BzRAs.

CONCLUSIONS

BzRAs consist of the benzodiazepines and a chemically unrelated set of medications (zolpidem, zaleplon, eszopiclone), which affect sleep via a related mechanism. These agents have dominated the pharmacologic treatment of insomnia for the last 50 years. Nine BzRAs are indicated for insomnia treatment by the FDA. A risk–benefit analysis should be used to decide whether to administer treatment for insomnia in an individual, whether to use a BzRA, and which BzRA to use. This analysis should be based on the published placebo-controlled trials of insomnia therapies. More studies have been carried out documenting the efficacy and adverse effects of BzRAs than any other agents. A number of BzRAs have been documented to have efficacy in the treatment of sleep onset and/or maintenance difficulties with relatively minimal risk of adverse effects. The available literature has some significant limitations, most notably the complete absence of any controlled trials of insomnia pharmacotherapy in children. Another gap in the literature is limited availability of studies of some of the most commonly prescribed insomnia agents in key comorbid conditions. In addition to data from placebo-controlled trials, there are some other factors that should be considered when deciding whether a BzRA is indicated for a given patient, including abuse potential, route of metabolism, and the availability and feasibility of other treatments. There is also a small amount of evidence that BzRAs have therapeutic effects on syndromal measures of insomnia, global outcome, and daytime function. Further studies employing such outcomes are needed to better characterize the treatment effects of BzRAs.

REFERENCES

1. Downing SS, Lee YT, Farb DH, et al. Benzodiazepine modulation of partial agonist efficacy and spontaneously active GABA(A) receptors supports an allosteric model of modulation. Br J Pharmacol 2005; 145(7):894–906.
2. Katzung BG, ed. Basic & Clinical Pharmacology, 8th ed. New York: Lange Medical Books/McGraw-Hill, 2001.
3. Krystal AD. A compendium of placebo-controlled trials of the risks/benefits of pharmacologic treatments for insomnia: The empirical basis for U.S. clinical practice. Sleep Med Rev. 2009; 13(4):265–274.
4. Krystal AD, Erman M, Zammit GK, et al. Long-term efficacy and safety of zolpidem extended-release 12.5 mg, administered 3 to 7 nights per week for 24 weeks, in patients with chronic primary insomnia: A 6-month, randomized, double-blind, placebo-controlled, parallel-group, multicenter study. Sleep. 2008; 31(1):79–90.
5. Aden GC, Thatcher C. Quazepam in the short-term treatment of insomnia in outpatients. J Clin Psychiatry 1983; 44(12):454–456.
6. Ancoli-Israel S, Walsh JK, Mangano RM, et al. A novel nonbenzodiazepine hypnotic, effectively treats insomnia in elderly patients without causing rebound effects. Prim Care Companion J Clin Psychiatry 1999; 1(4):114–120.
7. Drake CL, Roehrs TA, Mangano RM, et al. Dose-response effects of zaleplon as compared with triazolam (0.25 mg) and placebo in chronic primary insomnia. Hum Psychopharmacol 2000; 15(8):595–604.
8. Elie R, Frenay M, Le Morvan P, et al. Efficacy and safety of zopiclone and triazolam in the treatment of geriatric insomniacs. Int Clin Psychopharmacol 1990; 5(suppl 2):39–46.
9. Elie R, Ruther E, Farr I, et al. Sleep latency is shortened during 4 weeks of treatment with zaleplon, a novel nonbenzodiazepine hypnotic. Zaleplon Clinical Study Group. J Clin Psychiatry 1999; 60(8):536–44.

10. Fabre LF Jr, Brachfeld J, Meyer LR, et al. Multi-clinic double-blind comparison of triazolam (Halcion) and placebo administered for 14 consecutive nights in outpatients with insomnia. J Clin Psychiatry 1978; 39(8):679–682.
11. Fillingim JM. Double-blind evaluation of the efficacy and safety of temazepam in outpatients with insomnia. Br J Clin Pharmacol 1979; 8(1):73S–77S.
12. Hajak G, Clarenbach P, Fischer W, et al. Zopiclone improves sleep quality and daytime well-being in insomniac patients: Comparison with triazolam, flunitrazepam and placebo. Int Clin Psychopharmacol 1994; 9:251–261.
13. Hedner J, Yaeche R, Emilien G, et al. Zaleplon shortens subjective sleep latency and improves subjective sleep quality in elderly patients with insomnia. The Zaleplon Clinical Investigator Study Group. Int J Geriatr Psychiatry 2000; 15(8):704–712.
14. Krystal AD, Walsh JK, Laska E, et al. Sustained efficacy of eszopiclone over six months of nightly treatment: Results of a randomized, double-blind, placebo controlled study in adults with chronic insomnia. Sleep 2003; 26:793–799.
15. McCall WV, Erman, M, Krystal AD, et al. A polysomnography study of eszopiclone in elderly patients with insomnia. Curr Med Res Opin 2006; 22:1633–1642.
16. Morin CM, Colecchi C, Stone J, et al. Behavioral and pharmacological therapies for late-life insomnia: A randomized controlled trial. JAMA 1999; 281(11):991–999.
17. Nair NP, Schwartz G, Dimitri R, et al. A dose-range finding study of zopiclone in insomniac patients. Int Clin Psychopharmacol 1990; 5(suppl 2):1–10.
18. Perlis ML, McCall WV, Krystal AD, et al. Long-term, non-nightly administration of zolpidem in the treatment of patients with primary insomnia. J Clin Psychiatry 2004; 65(8):1128–1137.
19. Reeves RL. Comparison of triazolam, flurazepam, and placebo as hypnotics in geriatric patients with insomnia. J Clin Pharmacol 1977; 17(5–6):319–323.
20. Roehrs T, Zorick F, Lord N, et al. Dose-related effects of estazolam on sleep of patients with insomnia. J Clin Psychopharmacol 1983; 3(3):152–156.
21. Roehrs T, Zorick F, Wittig R, et al. Efficacy of a reduced triazolam dose in elderly insomniacs. Neurobiol Aging 1985 Winter; 6(4):293–296.
22. Roth T, Seiden D, Sainati S, et al. Effects of ramelteon on patient-reported sleep latency in older adults with chronic insomnia. Sleep Med 2006; 7(4):312–318.
23. Scharf M, Erman M, Rosenberg R, et al. A 2-week efficacy and safety study of eszopiclone in elderly patients with primary insomnia. Sleep 2005; 28(6):720–727.
24. Scharf MB, Roth PB, Dominguez RA, et al. Estazolam and flurazepam: A multicenter, placebo-controlled comparative study in outpatients with insomnia. J Clin Pharmacol 1990; 30(5):461–467.
25. Scharf MB, Roth T, Vogel GW, et al. A multicenter, placebo-controlled study evaluating zolpidem in the treatment of chronic insomnia. J Clin Psychiatry 1994; 55(5):192–199.
26. Sunshine A. Comparison of the hypnotic activity of triazolam, flurazepam hydrochloride, and placebo. Clin Pharmacol Ther 1975; 17(5):573–577.
27. Walsh JK, Erman M, Erwin CW, et al. Subjective hypnotic efficacy of trazodone and zolpidem in DSM-III-R primary insomnia. Hum Psychopharmacol 1998; 13:191–198.
28. Walsh JK, Roth T, Randazzo A, et al. Eight weeks of non-nightly use of zolpidem for primary insomnia. Sleep 2000; 23(8):1087–1096.
29. Walsh JK, Targum SD, Pegram V. A multi-center clinical investigation of estazolam: Short-term efficacy. Curr Ther Res 1984; 36:866–874.
30. Walsh JK, Vogel GW, Scharf M, et al. A five week, polysomnographic assessment of zaleplon 10 mg for the treatment of primary insomnia. Sleep Med 2000; 1(1):41–49.
31. Zammit GK, McNabb LJ, Caron J, et al. Efficacy and safety of eszopiclone across 6-weeks of treatment for primary insomnia. Curr Med Res Opin 2004; 20:1979–1991.
32. Piccione P, Zorick F, Lutz T, et al. The efficacy of triazolam and chloral hydrate in geriatric insomniacs. J Int Med Res 1980; 8(5):361–367.
33. Scharf M, Erman M, Rosenberg R, et al. A 2-week efficacy and safety study of eszopiclone in elderly patients with primary insomnia. Sleep 2005; 28(6):720–727.
34. Krystal AD, Erman M, Zammit GK, et al. Long-term efficacy and safety of zolpidem extended-release 12.5 mg, administered 3 to 7 nights per week for 24 weeks, in patients with chronic primary insomnia: A 6-month, randomized, double-blind, placebo-controlled, parallel-group, multicenter study. Sleep. 2008; 31(1):79–90.
35. Krystal AD. Treating the health, quality of life, and functional impairments in insomnia. J Clin Sleep Med 2007; 3(1):63–72.
36. Morin CM, Bootzin RR, Buysse DJ, et al. Psychological and behavioral treatment of insomnia: Update of the recent evidence (1998–2004). Sleep 2006; 29(11):1398–1414.

37. Walsh JK. Drugs used to treat insomnia in 2002: Regulatory-based rather than evidence-based medicine. Sleep 2004; 27(8):14441–14442.
38. Hajak G. A comparative assessment of the risks and benefits of zopiclone: A review of 15 years' clinical experience. Drug Saf 1999; 21:457–469.
39. Roehrs T, Pedrosi B, Rosenthal L, et al. Hypnotic self administration and dose escalation. Psychopharmacology (Berl) 1996; 127:150–154.
40. Crone CC, Gabriel GM. Treatment of anxiety and depression in transplant patients: Pharmacokinetic considerations. Clin Pharmacokinet 2004; 43(6):361–394.
41. Friedman H, Redmond DE Jr, Greenblatt DJ. Comparative pharmacokinetics of alprazolam and lorazepam in humans and in African Green Monkeys. Psychopharmacology (Berl) 1991; 104(1):103–105.
42. Fukasawa T, Suzuki A, Otani K. Effects of genetic polymorphism of cytochrome P450 enzymes on the pharmacokinetics of benzodiazepines. J Clin Pharm Ther 2007; 32(4):333–341.
43. Greenblatt DJ, Harmatz JS, Engelhardt N, et al. Pharmacokinetic determinants of dynamic differences among three benzodiazepine hypnotics. Flurazepam, temazepam, and triazolam. Arch Gen Psychiatry 1989; 46(4):326–332.
44. Locniskar A. Greenblatt DJ. Oxidative versus conjugative biotransformation of temazepam. Biopharm Drug Dispos 1990; 11:499–506.
45. Edinger JD, Sampson WS. A primary care "friendly" cognitive behavioral insomnia therapy. Sleep 2003; 26(2):177–182.
46. Wohlgemuth WK, Krystal AD. Hypnotics should be considered for the initial treatment of chronic insomnia. Pro. J Clin Sleep Med 2005; 1(2):120–124.
47. Dorsey CM, Lee KA, Scharf MB. Effect of zolpidem on sleep in women with perimenopausal and postmenopausal insomnia: A 4-week, randomized, multicenter, double-blind, placebo-controlled study. Clin Ther 2004; 26(10):1578–1586.
48. Fava M, Asnis GM, Shrivastava R, et al. Zolpidem extended-release improves sleep and next-day symptoms in comorbid insomnia and generalized anxiety disorder. J Clin Psychopharmacol 2009; 29(3):222–230.
49. Fava M, McCall WV, Krystal A, et al. Eszopiclone co-administered with fluoxetine in patients with insomnia co-existing with major depressive disorder. Biol Psychiatry 2006; 59:1052–1060.
50. Krystal AD, Fava M, Rubens R, et al. Evaluation of eszopiclone discontinuation after co-therapy with fluoxetine for insomnia with co-existing depression. J Clin Sleep Med 2007; 3:48–55.
51. Londborg PD, Smith WT, Glaudin V, et al. Short-term cotherapy with clonazepam and fluoxetine: Anxiety, sleep disturbance and core symptoms of depression. J Affect Disord 2000; 61:73–79.
52. Nolen WA, Haffmans PM, Bouvy PF, et al. Hypnotics as concurrent medication in depression. A placebo-controlled, double-blind comparison of flunitrazepam and lormetazepam in patients with major depression, treated with a (tri)cyclic antidepressant. J Affect Disord 1993; 28(3):179–188.
53. Pollack M, Kinrys G, Krystal A, et al. Eszopiclone coadministered with escitalopram in patients with insomnia and comorbid generalized anxiety disorder. Arch Gen Psychiatry 2008; 65(5):551–562.
54. Soares CN, Joffe H, Rubens R, et al. Eszopiclone in patients with insomnia during perimenopause and early postmenopause: A randomized controlled trial. Obstet Gynecol 2006; 108(6):1402–1410.
55. Steens RD, Pouliot Z, Millar TW, et al. Effects of zolpidem and triazolam on sleep and respiration in mild to moderate chronic obstructive pulmonary disease. Sleep 1993; 16(4):318–326.
56. Timms RM, Dawson A, Hajdukovic RM, et al. Effect of triazolam on sleep and arterial oxygen saturation in patients with chronic obstructive pulmonary disease. Arch Intern Med 1988; 148(10):2159–2163.
57. Walsh JK, Muehlbach MJ, Lauter SA, et al. Effects of triazolam on sleep, daytime sleepiness, and morning stiffness in patients with rheumatoid arthritis. J Rheumatol 1996; 23(2):245–252.
58. Roth T, Price JM, Amato DA, et al. The effect of eszopiclone in patients with insomnia and coexisting rheumatoid arthritis: a pilot study. Prim Care Companion J Clin Psychiatry 2009; 11(6):292–301.
59. Fava M, Asnis GM, Shrivastava R, et al. Zolpidem extended-release improves sleep and next-day symptoms in comorbid insomnia and generalized anxiety disorder. J Clin Psychopharmacol 2009; 29(3):222–230.
60. Mindell JA, Emslie G, Blumer J, et al. Pharmacologic management of insomnia in children and adolescents: Consensus statement. Pediatrics 2006; 117(6):e1223–e1232.
61. Ancoli-Israel S, Richardson GS, Mangano RM, et al. Long-term use of sedative hypnotics in older patients with insomnia. Sleep Med 2005; 6(2):107–113.
62. Walsh JK, Krystal, AD, Amata DA, et al. Nightly treatment of primary insomnia with eszopiclone for six months: Effect on sleep, quality of life, and work limitations. Sleep 2007; 30(8):959–968.
63. National Institutes of Health. Consensus conference. Drugs and Insomnia. The use of medications to promote sleep. JAMA 1984; 251(18):2410–2414.

64. Estivill E. Behavior of insomniacs and implication for their management. Sleep Med Rev 2002; 6 (suppl 1):S3–S6.
65. Erman MK, Zammit G, Rubens R, et al. A polysomnographic placebo-controlled evaluation of the efficacy and safety of eszopiclone relative to placebo and zolpidem in the treatment of primary insomnia. J Clin Sleep Med 2008; 4(3):229–234.
66. Piccione P, Zorick F, Lutz T, et al. The efficacy of triazolam and chloral hydrate in geriatric insomniacs. J Int Med Res 1980; 8(5):361–367.
67. Jacobs GD, Pace-Schott EF, Stickgold R, et al. Cognitive behavior therapy and pharmacotherapy for insomnia: a randomized controlled trial and direct comparison. Arch Intern Med 2004; 164(17):1888–1896.
68. Morin CM. Insomnia: Psychological Assessment and Management. New York: Guilford Press; 1993.
69. Smith S, Trinder J. Detecting insomnia: Comparison of four self-report measures of sleep in a young adult population. J Sleep Res 2001; 10:229–235.
70. Edinger JD, Bonnet MH, Bootzin RR, et al. American Academy of Sleep Medicine Work Group. Derivation of research diagnostic criteria for insomnia: report of an American Academy of Sleep Medicine Work Group. Sleep 2004; 27(8):1567–1596.
71. Scharf M, Erman M, Rosenberg R, et al. A 2-week efficacy and safety study of eszopiclone in elderly patients with primary insomnia. Sleep 2005; 28(6):720–727.
72. Asnis GM, Chakraburtty A, DuBoff EA, et al. Zolpidem for persistent insomnia in SSRI-treated depressed patients. J Clin Psychiatry 1999; 60:668–676.
73. Ford DE, Kamerow DB. Epidemiologic study of sleep disturbances and psychiatric disorders. An opportunity for prevention? JAMA 1989; 262:1479–1484.
74. Sunshine, 1979.
75. Roth T, Soubrane C, Titeux L; Zoladult Study Group. Efficacy and safety of zolpidem-MR: A double-blind, placebo-controlled study in adults with primary insomnia. Sleep Med 2006; 7(5):397–406.
76. Roth T, Walsh JK, Krystal A, et al. An evaluation of the efficacy and safety of eszopiclone over 12 months in patients with chronic primary insomnia. Sleep Med 2005; 6(6):487–495.

33 Benzodiazepine Receptor Agonist Safety

Timothy Roehrs and Thomas Roth

Sleep Disorders and Research Center, Henry Ford Hospital, and Department of Psychiatry and Behavioral Neuroscience, School of Medicine, Wayne State University, Detroit, Michigan, U.S.A.

INTRODUCTION

The major side effect and safety issues associated with benzodiazepine receptor agonist (BzRA) hypnotic use include psychomotor and cognitive (i.e., anterograde amnesia) impairment, parasomnia-like episodes, discontinuation effects, and dependence liability. Some of these side effects are mediated by the primary pharmacodynamic activity, sedation, of BzRAs and directly relate to the pharmacokinetic properties of specific BzRAs. Other side effects can be attributed to both pharmacokinetics and receptor selectivity of the drug. Finally, drug dose, duration of use, and concomitant medications, comorbid medical, or sleep disorders may determine side effects.

The side effect–safety profile of the BzRAs has to be weighed against the various alternatives to treating insomnia, including no treatment, self-treatment, and alternative nonhypnotic medications (i.e., drugs used as hypnotics that have sedative effects but are indicated for another disorder). Unfortunately, comparisons to alternative nonhypnotics are limited by the fact that there is little systematic information regarding the safety of the various alternative medications being used as hypnotics. This includes an absence of data at the lower doses frequently used for sleep and for the effects on sleep-related activity (e.g., rebound insomnia, effects on sleep-related breathing disorders). Importantly, the risks associated with nontreatment and self-treatment also have to be compared with those of the BzRAs. The risks of nontreatment and self-treatment are known.

This chapter will review the evidence and discuss the determinants of the side effects of BzRA hypnotics. It will compare these risks to the risks associated with alternative drugs used as hypnotics and self-treatment, as well as those risks associated with no treatment. Finally, we will discuss ways by which the clinician can minimize the various side effect–safety risks associated with BzRAs.

Benzodiazepine Receptor Agonist Risks

Psychomotor Impairment

Psychomotor impairment with BzRAs has been shown on various measures (i.e., as slowed reaction times, response errors, tracking errors, lapses of attention, and driving deviations) in laboratory performance testing and on actual roadway driving assessments. At their peak plasma concentrations BzRA-associated impairments relate directly to the level of plasma concentration, which is a function of dose. To illustrate, a study compared the daytime administration effects of 0.125, 0.25, and 0.50 mg triazolam; 5, 10, and 20 mg zolpidem; and 15, 30, and 60 mg temazepam (1). These BzRAs were compared on the basis of their differing pharmacokinetics and receptor selectivity. Temazepam is known to be longer acting than zolpidem and triazolam, and zolpidem is considered to be more receptor selective than triazolam and temazepam. Each drug—zolpidem, triazolam, and temazepam—produced orderly dose-related impairment in learning and recall and psychomotor performance at their peak concentrations (1).

The duration of the impairment relates to the duration of action mediated by both the half-life and dose of a specific BzRA. In the study cited earlier, the functions relating impairment to time since ingestion for the three drugs revealed a six-hour duration impairment relative to placebo with 60 mg temazepam and a three-hour duration impairment with 20 mg zolpidem, although these two drugs and doses had comparable impairing effects at their peak (1). Although zolpidem is considered more $GABA_A$ α_1-receptor selective than triazolam and temazepam, it did not produce a differential pattern of impairment.

When the BzRA impairment extends to the morning following a nighttime administration, this impairment is referred to as "residual effects." Residual effects are merely the prolongation of the therapeutic effect of the drug into next-day wakefulness. BzRAs with longer durations of action, as determined by the half-life of the drug and secondarily by the dose of the drug (e.g., higher doses and longer half-lives extend duration of action), are more likely to produce residual effects. Using performance and driving assessments and the Multiple Sleep Latency Test (MSLT), studies have found differences in residual effects between short- and long-acting drugs and between doses of the same drug. For example, an early study in healthy elderly compared the daytime residual effects of triazolam 0.25 mg and flurazepam 15 mg administered before sleep (2). Both drugs produced a comparable one hour increase in total sleep time, but flurazepam, a long-acting drug, produced increased daytime sleepiness on the MSLT the following day, while triazolam, a short-acting drug, reduced sleepiness on the MSLT. In the same study, next-day vigilance performance was impaired with flurazepam, but not with triazolam.

Given a desired sleep period of eight hours, middle-of-the-night administration of a short half-life drug (i.e., three to five hours) is likely to produce residual effects. In other words, the likelihood of residual effects is determined by the time of administration relative to the desired time of arising and the pharmacokinetics of the given drug. A study comparing the residual effects of the short half-life drug (2.5–4.5 hours), zolpidem (10 mg), with the ultra short half-life drug (1 hour), zaleplon (10 mg), illustrates this point (3). The drugs were administered in the middle of the night at either 3, 4, 5, or 6 AM before a desired 8 AM awakening, translating to an awakening that occurred—two to five hours postadministration. Zolpidem produced residual effects on digit symbol substitution and immediate and delayed memory recall after all middle-of-the-night administrations, but zaleplon administration had no effects at 8 AM, even after the 6 AM (two hours postadministration). The FDA label for recently approved hypnotics, given their distinct pharmacokinetics, now includes the caution that "x" hours be devoted to sleep when using the medication. For example, the zaleplon label cautions four or more hours, while the zolpidem-CR formulation cautions eight hours.

Falls in the elderly are often cited as a special case of psychomotor impairment associated with BzRAs, either due to elevated peak plasma concentrations or residual effects. Several questions arise, including whether the reported association is unique to BzRAs, whether that risk is greater than the untreated condition, and if truly associated, how it can be minimized, which will be discussed later. Falls in the elderly are not unique to BzRAs, which are not independent predictors of falls when controlling for comorbid diseases. A case–control study of community-living persons aged 66 years and older who visited emergency departments for injurious falls during one year in a Canadian health district identified seven medication classes, including sedatives, that were associated with falls (4). After controlling for comorbid conditions, narcotics, anticonvulsants, and antidepressants were independent predictors, but not hypnotics. In a prospective study of elderly women and fractures, narcotics and antidepressants were associated with increased risk for fractures, while benzodiazepines and anticonvulsants were not independent predictors (5).

There are data to suggest that sleep problems and daytime sleepiness in elderly are independent factors increasing risk of accidental injury and falls. A representative sample of elderly adults from northern California was surveyed by telephone (6). Nighttime sleep problems were a risk for fractures and remained so after controlling for demographic variables and concurrent medical diseases. A more recent study assessing the risk of BzRA-associated falls in elderly controlled for insomnia (7). This large study of nursing home residents in Southeastern Michigan found that insomnia represents a significant risk for falls but BzRAs do not. Thus, the risk of falls associated with BzRAs was actually less than untreated insomnia.

Cognitive Impairment

Another major side effect of BzRAs is cognitive impairment, most typically anterograde amnesia. Anterograde, in contrast to retrograde, amnesia is failure to recall information presented after consumption of the drug. The degree of amnesia is determined by the level of plasma concentration at the time of information input. It can be because of attentional and/or consolidation failures in the memory process. At peak plasma concentration, very orderly dose-dependent amnesic effects have been demonstrated for BzRAs (1). The amnesia is, in part, related to the sedative effects of the BzRAs, as the degree of the amnesia parallels the sedative effects of the drug as measured by the MSLT (8). Failure to consolidate the newly acquired material is one cause of the amnesia. This explanation is supported by a study in which the drug-induced rapid return to sleep was delayed for 15 minutes (i.e., wakefulness was maintained for 15 minutes) and memory was preserved (9). The extent to which the sedative effects mediate the amnesic effects has been debated extensively. Several studies have attempted to dissociate these two effects. The amnestic effects of drugs with differing sedative effects were compared, or the antagonist, flumazenil, was used to dissociate sedative and amnestic effects, but the studies had equivocal results (10,11). The problem in these studies was that sedation was self-reported rather than objectively assessed. Another important complication is that sleep, even brief sleep periods, produce retrograde amnesia.

Amnesia is associated with the receptor selectivity of the BzRAs. These act as allosteric modulators of $GABA_A$ receptors and gene knockin studies have identified and characterized various $GABA_A$ receptor subunits for their pharmacological profiles (12). The animal data indicate that the α_1-receptor subtype mediates both the sleep and amnesic effects of the BzRAs (12). When zolpidem, a nonbenzodiazepine hypnotic, was introduced, it was hypothesized that because of the receptor selectivity of zolpidem, amnesia could be avoided. But, as noted above, the α_1-receptor–selective agent zolpidem did not differ from nonselective benzodiazepines in its amnesic effects (1). Zopiclone and its *S*-isomer, eszopiclone, are less selective for α_1-receptors than zopidem and more selective for α_3-receptors, but we are unaware of studies that have compared their amnestic effects, although adverse events characterized as amnesia have been reported. It must be concluded that all BzRAs that act extensively at the α_1-receptor produce dose-dependent anterograde amnesia with as yet no studies demonstrating differences between the various drugs when sedative potency is controlled.

Finally, long-term BzRA use is purportedly associated with cognitive impairment, particularly in elderly. One has to distinguish time-limited impairment (i.e., the time over which drug is present in plasma) in acute use from long-term impairment in chronic use. There have been reports of "global amnesia" associated with BzRAs (13). The reported total amnesia lasted for several hours after consuming triazolam, 0.5 mg, but the triazolam use was also accompanied by variable amounts of reported alcohol consumption.

These reports of acute global amnesia contrast with the suggestion that chronic BzRA use is associated with cognitive impairment. The results of studies assessing cognitive function in elderly chronic BzRA users are equivocal, with some studies reporting impairment and others finding minimal or no impairment (14–16). It is difficult to reach definitive conclusions because these reports are cross-sectional and retrospective in nature with a number of confounds. Further, determining the appropriate controls for these studies is problematic. Most of the information on BzRA cognitive impairment is from patients with anxiety disorders, who are using long-acting benzodiazepines. The relevance of these data to current best clinical practice for insomnia pharmacotherapy (i.e., use of short-acting nonbenzodiazepine hypnotics) is questionable.

Discontinuation Effects

The most frequently reported discontinuation effect of the BzRAs in clinical use is rebound insomnia (17). Rebound insomnia is defined as worsened sleep for one or two nights relative to baseline. It can occur after even one to two nights of previous BzRA use (17). The rebound insomnia does not appear to increase in severity with the duration of nightly use, at least in the short term. Rebound insomnia was reported with the 0.5-mg dose, but not the 0.25-mg dose, of the short-acting drug, triazolam (17). Proper multiple-dose studies that explore the threshold dose for rebound with other BzRA hypnotics have not been done. Many studies report an absence of rebound, but do not include a positive control that demonstrates that the study design is robust enough to detect rebound. Rebound is likely to occur after high doses (i.e., beyond minimally effective doses) of all short- and intermediate-acting BzRAs. This prediction is made based on the multiple-dose studies of daytime performance impairment that have compared various BzRAs to triazolam and find comparable impairment at triazolam doses that produce rebound (1). Rebound is unlikely to occur with a long-acting drug because of the gradual decline in plasma concentrations inherent to its pharmacology.

Rebound insomnia is an exacerbation of the original symptom (i.e., difficulty falling and or staying asleep), and thus, differs from recrudescence, which is the return of the original symptom at its original severity. It is not a withdrawal syndrome (i.e., expression of new symptoms), at least in the available short-term studies (i.e., two weeks and less), which induced rebound but no other new symptoms (17). Its time course differs from that of a withdrawal syndrome, lasting for one or two nights only. Finally, there is no evidence to suggest that the benzodiazepine and nonbenzodiazepine BzRAs differ in the likelihood of producing rebound (17,18).

The extent to which duration of use and dose might combine to increase the likelihood of rebound, even at clinical doses, when used in the long-term is unknown. A recent study assessed rebound after six months of the nightly use of eszopiclone 3 mg, its clinical dose (19). Over the 14 days studied after discontinuation of eszopiclone, no increase in self-reported sleep latency or wake after sleep onset relative to baseline was observed. These data need to be considered cautiously as no positive control was used in this study. It also has been suggested that the experience of rebound insomnia leads to continued chronic use of the hypnotic. Importantly, a study, which directly tested that notion, showed that the experience of rebound insomnia does not alter the subsequent likelihood of self-administering triazolam 0.25 mg (20). In summary, while rebound insomnia is a reliable effect associated with BzRAs, its clinical significance, if any, is yet to be identified.

Abuse Liability

There has long been concern that behavioral or physical dependence develops with chronic use of BzRAs. The concern is based on reports of physical and behavioral dependence with long-term daytime anxiolytic use of therapeutic doses of BzRAs (21). Systematic information regarding the dependence liability of long-term therapeutic use of BzRA hypnotics at clinical doses is very limited. A majority of persons in population-based studies report using hypnotics for two weeks or less (22,23). Two recent placebo-controlled, double-blind studies of eszopiclone 3 mg reported no evidence of physical or behavioral dependence after six months of nightly use (19,24). But, neither of these studies directly tested for physical and behavioral dependence liability.

Short-term studies directly testing the behavioral dependence liability of BzRA hypnotics suggest that they have a low behavioral dependence liability (25). Behavioral dependence liability can be directly tested by assessing the self-administration of active drug versus placebo administered as color-coded capsules. After sampling each color-coded capsule over 7 to 14 subsequent nights' patients choose the desired capsule based on its color. Hypnotic self-administration by insomniacs is not associated with dose escalation with repeated use when provided opportunity to self-administer multiple capsules (26), does not increase with rebound insomnia (20), does not generalize to daytime use (27), and varies as a function of the nature and severity of the patients' sleep disturbance (25). These short-term studies lead to the conclusion that insomnia patients' hypnotic self-administration is a therapy-seeking behavior and not drug seeking or abuse. It should be noted that these conclusions are true for insomniacs and normal controls, but not for individuals with a drug abuse history.

One important question is the extent to which receptor subtype selectivity may influence the abuse liability of the BzRAs. One assessment of the relative abuse liability of hypnotic drugs failed to find differential receptor subtype selectivity in abuse liability among drugs used as hypnotics (28). For example, the α_1 selective drug, zolpidem, did not differ from various nonselective BzRAs. However, there are very few studies comparing multiple doses of multiple drugs and thus the rating had to be made across a variety of methodologies and data sources. In addition, the rating also included drug toxicities and thus was not specific to what is more narrowly defined as drug abuse liability.

Amnestic Parasomnia Episodes

Reports of parasomnia-like side effects associated with BzRA hypnotics have appeared in the public print and video media. These reports of "global amnesia", somnambulism, sleep driving, and sleep-related eating disorder are problematic; they are not peer-reviewed, generally not independently documented, are subject to confirmation bias, and likely overrepresent the real risk. Further, they do not provide information that can lead to a scientific medical understanding of the phenomena, and they raise unnecessary concern among patients and their physicians.

In the scientific medical literature peer-reviewed case reports of parasomnia-like BzRA-associated side effects have also appeared. But, again one must be cautious. Case reports do provide some information about contributing factors, but it is not placebo-controlled information. Most importantly, the real risk of BzRA-associated parasomnia is unknown because the rate of exposure is not known. The number of prescriptions written and doses consumed at the time of the event is unknown and consequently, the incidence of the events cannot be determined. Finally, there have been several publications that suggest that the appearance of media reports and medical articles distort the true prevalence of adverse events.

As noted earlier, transient global amnesia has been reported in association with the use of triazolam by otherwise healthy individuals experiencing sleep disturbance (13,29). The memory loss was for all autobiographical events transpiring over an 8- to 12-hour period. In some of these cases in which clinical doses were used, prior stress, sleep deprivation, and a virus may have contributed to produce the amnesia. In other cases, supraclinical doses and alcohol ingestion are likely contributory factors. It is unlikely that this phenomenon is unique to triazolam as similar kinds of amnesia are produced by the intravenous administration of other benzodiazepines.

Somnambulism has been reported with zolpidem and zaleplon (30,31). These episodes of somnambulism have occurred with two to three times the clinical doses of the drug, in individuals with a prior history of somnambulism and in individuals with prior traumatic head injury. Zolpidem-associated somnambulism also has been reported in combination with antidepressant treatment (32). Somnambulism is believed to be associated with partial arousals from sleep, which alcohol and sleep deprivation also exacerbate. Not surprisingly, both alcohol and sleep deprivation also exacerbate somnambulism.

Finally, there are case reports of sleep-related eating disorder associated with psychotropic medications, including BzRAs (33–35). There is a dispute as to whether sleep-related eating disorder is a disorder of partial arousal from sleep with altered levels of consciousness or is the psychiatric disorder of nocturnal eating with awareness and recall (36,37). Sleep related eating disorder is hypothesized to share a common pathophysiology with somnambulism. Zolpidem was reported to exacerbate sleep-related eating disorder and in several cases induce it de novo (37). In some of these cases greater than 10 mg of zolpidem doses were being used and in other cases there was use of sedating antidepressants. Sleep-related eating disorder has also been reported with triazolam (38,39).

These case reports have a common thread running through them—excessive hypnotic activity or sleep drive. The excessive hypnotic activity is produced by high doses, clinical doses in vulnerable individuals (i.e., those with a past history of sleep disorders or brain injury), the combination of clinical or high doses with prior sleep deprivation due to stress or illness, or the combination of clinical or high doses with the prior consumption of alcohol or other CNS drugs. The types of behaviors described in these case reports also share a commonality. They all are symptoms of excessive hypnotic activity or excessive sleepiness. Amnesia and memory difficulties are reported by patients with excessive daytime sleepiness. Sleep deprivation produces intense slow wave sleep and abrupt arousals from slow wave sleep after prior sleep deprivation is known to be associated with sleep inertia–behaving individuals with little consciousness and memory. Patients with excessive sleepiness are known to engage in automatic behavior, and sleep deprivation is known to induce somnambulism in individuals with a previous history of somnambulism. Taken together the data suggest that parasomnia reports associated with BzRAs are the result of excessive hypnotic/sedative activity in vulnerable individuals.

Risks Associated with Alternatives

Good clinical practice requires that the risk of BzRA insomnia treatment be weighed against the risks associated with the alternatives. The common alternatives include no treatment, self-treatment, and treatment with nonhypnotic medications, most typically low-dose sedative antidepressants and antipsychotics. Epidemiological data indicate that a very small percentage of people reporting insomnia are treated medically for their insomnia (40). In the population, approximately one-third of those reporting insomnia self-medicate with either over-the-counter (OTC) medications or alcohol (23). Finally, most patients receiving medical treatment for insomnia are prescribed off-label medications (41).

Nontreatment

Untreated insomnia has well-documented morbidity. Insomniacs report reduced quality of life on the Short-Form-16 Quality of Life Questionnaire across all of its domains, and they rate their quality-of-life akin to that of patients with other chronic disorders such as congestive heart failure and clinical depression (42,43). Compared to individuals without insomnia, insomniacs self-report increased days of restricted activity due to illness and increased days spent in bed as a result of illness (44). Higher rates of absenteeism are reported by those with insomnia compared with controls, and rates of work-related accidents and traffic accidents are higher (42,45). Among nursing home residents, the risk of falls and fractures was higher in the untreated insomniacs than those treated with hypnotics (7). This finding contradicts the general perception based on earlier studies that hypnotic treatment in elderly is associated with greater risk of falls and the risk reversal likely relates to a wider current use of short-acting rather than long-acting hypnotics as in the earlier studies. Importantly, those earlier studies did not control for insomnia, which itself is a risk factor for falls.

Untreated insomnia is associated with increased risk of incident cases and relapse of psychiatric disorders and with an exacerbation of medical diseases. A number of studies have now demonstrated a heightened risk of future depression in persons reporting insomnia without a current or previous history of depression, and a study has shown insomnia precedes incident depression as well as relapse (46–48). In addition, there is an increased risk of anxiety disorders and drug and alcohol abuse associated with insomnia (46). Whether treating insomnia would reduce these risks is yet to be determined. However, one recent study did find that adjunctive pharmacological treatment of insomnia coexisting with primary depression not only improved the insomnia, but also improved depressive symptoms beyond that found with standard antidepressant monotherapy (49).

Insomnia is comorbid with various medical diseases and evidence indicates that disturbed sleep exacerbates medical disease, specifically diseases with pain as a prominent symptom. In a prospective study, self-ratings of sleep and pain in patients with fibromyalgia showed that nights with poor sleep were followed by days with greater pain (50). Also, patients with rheumatological disorders frequently report insomnia and disturbed sleep. In two small studies, treatment of insomnia associated with rheumatoid arthritis with either triazolam or zopiclone failed to show concurrent improvement in both sleep and pain (51,52). However, in a recent large study of patients with rheumatoid arthritis and coexisting insomnia, eszopiclone 3 mg improved both nighttime sleep and daytime joint pain (53). Studies in healthy normals have suggested that poor sleep may exacerbate pain. Studies have found that total sleep deprivation is hyperalgesic and a recent study in healthy normals has shown that only a four-hour reduction of sleep time for a single night is hyperalgesic to a radiant heat stimulus (54).

Self-Medication

The pursuit of ineffective and potentially dangerous self-treatments is not fully appreciated as a risk of not treating the patient with insomnia. In a population-based study in Southeastern Michigan, respondents with insomnia reported poorer sleep hygiene practices than noninsomniacs (55). Among the compensatory self-help behaviors reported by insomniacs is napping and sleeping on weekends, behaviors that can potentially exacerbate and perpetuate the insomnia.

Insomniacs use nonprescription substances to self-treat their insomnia, including OTC medications, herbals, and alcohol (23). The active component of all OTC sleep aids is H_1 antihistamine, typically diphenhydramine 25 to 50 mg. Beyond there being no clear placebo-controlled studies that show diphenhydramine has *hypnotic* efficacy, rapid tolerance development to its *sedative* effects has been shown (56). Low-dose alcohol as a sleep aid is potentially dangerous for two reasons. Low-dose alcohol initially improves the sleep of insomniacs, which is why they self-administer it as a sleep aid (57). However, within six nights tolerance develops, sleep is worsened beyond that of baseline, and larger alcohol doses are self-administered to achieve the sleep effect (57–59). Insomniacs who reported using alcohol as a sleep aid also reported greater levels of daytime sleepiness than those who used prescription or OTC drugs for sleep (23).

Nonhypnotic Medications

The most commonly used drugs to treat insomnia according to the *Physician Drug and Diagnosis Audit* (PDDA) database in 2002 (the most recently available published data) were sedating antidepressants (60). They were 1.53 times more likely to be prescribed for insomnia than BzRAs and the three most common were trazodone, amitriptyline, and mirtazapine. These prescribing data may not represent current practice given the very recent introduction of a number of new FDA-approved BzRA hypnotics. Nevertheless, the safety of sedating antidepressants used to promote sleep, as opposed to treating depression, merits discussion.

Information on antidepressant safety is primarily derived from use in depressed patients and the data are for higher doses (e.g., antidepressant doses) than typically used for insomnia. As an example, the doses reported in the PDDA for trazodone were 50 mg in 53% of those mentioned, 100 mg in 31% and 150 mg in 14% (60). The 150-mg dose is the usual daily antidepressant dose. However, on the basis of recent studies of low-dose doxepin as a hypnotic, antidepressants at low doses are likely safer than the higher antidepressant doses (61).

Trazodone: Sedation is a widely reported side effect with trazodone use, which possibly relates to its approximate 12-hour half-life in elderly patients, although in younger patients the half-life is 6 hours (62). On an average across studies, 29% of depressed patients reported daytime drowsiness at antidepressant doses. Even at the lower 50-mg dose, the only placebo-controlled trial of its use as treatment for primary insomnia reported 23% of patients over the two-week treatment had problems with daytime somnolence compared to 8% with placebo and 16% with zolpidem (63). Trazodone has significant cardiovascular risks including hypotension, orthostatic hypotension, ventricular arrhythmias, conduction disturbances, and exacerbation of ischemic attacks. Finally, trazodone is associated with priapism in many case reports and an analysis found that most cases occurred with 50 to 150 mg daily doses, which are the doses more typically used for insomnia (64). However, this case report information on priapism may suggest a higher incidence than the estimated incidence of 1/5000.

Amitriptyline: It is known for its anticholinergic side effects, including blurred vision, dry mouth, urinary retention, orthostatic hypotension, flushing, tachycardia, and confusion (65). Cardiac toxicity in overdoses has been reported, and at clinical doses in patients with known cardiovascular disease, there are increased cardiac risks. But it should be emphasized that this information may not be relevant to the lower doses often used to treat insomnia.

Mirtazapine: The major side effects associated with mirtazapine are weight gain and increased appetite. Increased daytime sleepiness and dizziness have also been reported (65).

Quetiapine and olanzapine: In the PDDA data for 2002, the antipsychotics quetiapine and olanzapine and the antihistamines hydroxyzine and diphenhydramine were also frequently used as hypnotics. As is true of the sedating antidepressants, there is no safety information for these drugs at the doses used for hypnotic effects. These drugs are chosen for their reported sedating effects, generally produced by their H_1 antagonism. To the extent that a given drug has a long half-life (i.e., olanzapine's half-life is 20–50 hours), its duration of action will be extended to the following day, producing residual impairment of function. But they also affect other neurotransmitter systems, which produce other side effects such as dizziness and hypotension.

Minimizing the BzRA Risks

The risk of next-day psychomotor impairment can be minimized by choosing drugs that have a duration of action that is limited to the desired sleep period. Drugs with half-lives greater than 5 hours will likely result in residual sedation. The lowest effective dose should be utilized. Low doses also will reduce the likelihood of impairment during nighttime bathroom visits and as discussed earlier, will reduce the likelihood of amnestic parasomnia episodes and decrease the chances of experiencing rebound insomnia.

With regard to amnestic parasomnia episodes, two points should be emphasized. Firstly, excessive sleep drive and hypnotic activity produced by high doses above the approved clinical doses, a combination of sedating drugs, or a combination of prior sleep deprivation and a sedating drug in vulnerable individuals should be avoided. Thus, dose, concurrent use of other sedating drugs, and time-in-bed after drug ingestion should be carefully monitored. Secondly, by most indications these are very rare side effects when the medications are used appropriately.

As with psychomotor impairment, the risk of cognitive impairment is reduced by attention to duration of action and dose. Special caution should be taken for patients who are elderly. Both duration of action and peak plasma concentration can be enhanced in elderly with the result being a greater likelihood of psychomotor and cognitive impairment. The same is true for patients with renal or hepatic problems. In addition, elderly patients are more likely to be using multiple drugs, many of which have sedating effects, further enhancing risks of cognitive impairment.

Rebound insomnia can be minimized with short- and intermediate-acting drugs by gradually tapering the dose over several nights. Its impact can be reduced with patient instructions that include the caution that rebound can occur, but that rebound endures for one to two nights, when it does occur.

Finally, identifying patients with an enhanced liability of dependence development, whether physical or behavioral, is quite difficult. The most reliable predictor is a previous history of drug or alcohol abuse. While treating patients, possible dose escalation should be closely monitored and the use of the medication outside of the therapeutic context noted. Thus, any daytime use of a hypnotic, except for night workers who are day sleepers, should be discouraged and when observed should be a sign of concern.

REFERENCES

1. Rush CR, Griffiths RR. Zolpidem, triazolam, and temazepam: Behavioral and subject-rated effects in normal volunteers. J Clin Psychopharmacol 1996; 16:146–157.
2. Carskadon MA, Seidel WF, Greenblatt DJ, et al. Daytime carryover of triazolam and flurazepam in elderly insomniacs. Sleep 1982; 5:361–371.
3. Danjou P, Fruncillo PR, Worthington P, et al. A comparison of the residual effects of zaleplon and zolpidem following administration 5 to 2 h before awakening. Br J Clin Pharmacol 1999; 48:367–374.
4. Kelly KD, Pickett W, Yiannakaoulias N, et al. Medication use and falls in community-dwelling older persons. Age Ageing 2003; 32:503–509.
5. Ensrud KE, Blackwell T, Mangione CM, et al. Central nervous system active medications and risk for fractures in older women. Arch Intern Med 2003; 163:949–957.
6. Brassington GS, King AC, Bliwise DL. Sleep problems as a risk factor for falls in a sample of community-dwelling adults aged 64–99 years. J Am Geriatr Soc 2000; 48:1234–1240.
7. Avidan AY, Fries BE, James ML, et al. Insomnia and hypnotic use recorded in the minimum data set as predictors of fall and hip fractures in Michigan nursing homes. J Am Geriatr Soc 2005; 53:955–962.
8. Roehrs T, Merlotti L, Zorick F, et al. Sedative, memory and performance effects of hypnotics. Psychopharmacology 1994; 116:130–134.
9. Roehrs T, Zorick F, Sicklesteel J, et al. Effects of hypnotics on memory. J Clin Psychopharmacol 1983; 3:310–313.
10. Green JF, McElholm A, King DJ. A comparison of the sedative and amnestic effects of chlorpromazine and lorazepam. Psychopharmacology 1996; 128:67–73.
11. Curran HV, Birch B. Differentiating the sedative, psychomotor and amnesic effects of benzodiazepines: A study with midazolam and the benzodiazepine antagonist, flumazenil. Psychopharmacology 1991; 103:519–523.
12. Mohler H, Crestani F, Rudolph. GABA-A receptor subtypes: A new pharmacology. Curr Opin Pharmacol 2001; 1:22–25.
13. Shader RI, Greenblatt DJ. Triazolam and anterograde amnesia: All is not well in the z-zone. J Clin Psychopharmacol 1983; 3:273.
14. Paterniti S, Dufouil C, Alperovitch A. Long-term benzodiazepine use and cognitive decline in the elderly: The Epidemiology of Vascular Aging Study. J Clin Psychopharmacol 2002; 22:285–293.
15. Allard J, Artero S, Ritchie K. Consumption of psychotropic medication in the elderly: A re-evaluation of its effect on cognitive performance. Int J Geriatr Psychiatry 2003; 18:874–878.
16. McAndrews MP, Weiss RT, Sandor P, et al. Cognitive effects of long-term benzodiazepine use in older adults. Hum Psychopharmacol Clin Exp 2003; 18:51–57.
17. Roehrs TA, Vogel G, Roth T. Rebound insomnia: Its determinants and significance. Am J Med 1990; 88:43S–46S.
18. Roth T, Soubrane C, Titeux L, et al. Efficacy and safety of zolpidem-MR: A double-blind, placebo-controlled study in adults with primary insomnia. Sleep Med 2006;7:397–406.

19. Walsh J, Krystal A, Amato DA, et al. Nightly treatment of primary insomnia with eszopiclone for six months: Effect on sleep quality of life, and work limitations. Sleep 2007; 30:959–968.
20. Roehrs T, Merlotti L, Zorick F, et al. Rebound insomnia and hypnotic self administration. Psychopharmacology 1992; 107:480–484.
21. Woods JH, Winger G. Current benzodiazepine issues. Psychopharmacology 1995; 118:107–103.
22. Mellinger GD, Balter MB, Uhlenhuth EH. Insomnia and its treatment. Arch Gen Psychiatry 1985; 42:225–232.
23. Roehrs T, Hollebeek E, Drake C, et al. Substance use for insomnia in Metropolitan Detroit. J Psychosom Res 2002; 53:571–576.
24. Krystal AD, Walsh JK, Laska E, et al. Sustained efficacy of eszopiclone over 6 months of nightly treatment: Results of a randomized, double-blind, placebo-controlled study in adults with chronic insomnia. Sleep 2003; 26:793–799.
25. Roehrs T, Bonahoom A, Pedrosi B, et al. Disturbed sleep predicts hypnotic self administration. Sleep Med 2002; 3:61–66.
26. Roehrs T, Pedrosi B, Rosenthal L, et al. Hypnotic self administration and dose escalation. Psychopharmacology 1996; 127:150–154.
27. Roehrs T, Bonahoom A, Pedrosi B, et al. Nighttime versus daytime hypnotic self-administration. Psychopharmacology 2002; 161:137–142.
28. Griffiths RR, Johnson MW. Relative abuse liability of hypnotic drugs: A conceptual framework and algorithm for differentiating among compounds. J Clin Psychiatry 2005; 66(suppl 9): 31–41.
29. Morris HH, Estes ML. Traveler's amnesia. Transient global amnesia secondary to triazolam. JAMA 1987; 258:945–946.
30. Yang W, Dollear M, Muthukrishnan SR. One rare side effect of zolpidem—sleepwalking: A case report. Arch Phys Med Rehabil 2005; 86:1265–1266.
31. Liskow B, Pikalov A. Zaleplon overdose associated with sleepwalking and complex behavior. J Am Acad Child Adoles Psychiatry. 2004; 43:927–928.
32. Lange CL. Medication-associated somnambulism. J Am Acad Child Adoles Psychiatry 2005; 44: 211–212.
33. Paquet V, Strul J, Servais L, et al. Sleep-related eating disorder induced by olanzapine. J Clin Psychiatry 2002; 63:7.
34. Lu ML, Shen WW. Sleep-related eating disorder induced by risperidone. J Clin Psychiatry 2004; 65:273–274.
35. Morgenthaler TI, Silber MH. Amnestic sleep-related eating disorder associated with zolpidem. Sleep Med 2002; 3:323–327.
36. Schenk CH, Mahowald MW. Review of nocturnal sleep-related eating disorders. Int J Eat Disord 1994; 15:343–356.
37. Vetrugno R, Manconi M, Strembi LF, et al. Nocturnal eating: Sleep related eating disorder or nocturnal eating syndrome? A videopolysomnographic study. Sleep 2006; 29:876–877.
38. Menkes DB. Triazolam-induced nocturnal bingeing with amnesia. Aust N Z J Psychaitry 1992; 26: 320–321.
39. Lauerma H. Nocturnal wandering caused by restless legs and short-acting benzodiazepines. Acta Psychiatr Scand 1991; 83:492–493.
40. Ancoli-Israel S, Roth T. Characteristics of insomnia in the United States: Results of the 1991 National Sleep Foundation Survey. Sleep 1999; 22:S347–S353.
41. Johnson EO, Roehrs T, Roth T, et al. Epidemiology of alcohol and medication as aids to sleep in early adulthood. Sleep 1998; 21:178–186.
42. Zammit GK, Weiner J, Damato N, et al. Quality of life in people with insomnia. Sleep 1999; 22 (suppl 2):S379–S385.
43. Katz DA, McHorney CA. The relationship between insomnia and health-related quality of life in patients with chronic illness. J Fam Pract 2002; 51:229–235.
44. Simon GE, Von Korff M. Prevalence, burden, and treatment of insomnia in primary care. Am J Psychiatry 1997; 154:1417–1423.
45. Leger D, Guilleminault C, Bader G, et al. Medical and socio-professional impact of insomnia. Sleep 2002; 25:625–629.
46. Breslau N, Roth T, Rosenthal L, et al. Sleep disturbance and psychiatric disorders: A longitudinal epidemiological study of young adults. Biol Psychiatry 1996; 39:411–418.
47. Chang PP, Ford DE, Mead LA, et al. Insomnia in young men and subsequent depression. The Hohns Hopkins Precursor Study. Am J Epidemiol 1997; 146:105–114.
48. Perlis ML, Giles DE, Buysse DJ. Self-reported sleep disturbance as a prodromal symptom in recurrent depression. J Affect Disord 1997; 42:209–212.

49. Fava M, McCall WV, Krystal A, et al. Eszopiclone co-administered with fluoxetine in patients with insomnia coexisting with major depressive disorder. Bio Psychiatry 2006.
50. Affleck G, Urrows S, Tennen H, et al. Sequential daily relations of sleep, pain intensity, and attention to pain among women with fibromyalgia. Pain 1996; 68:363–368.
51. Walsh JK, Muehlbach MJ, Lauter SA, et al. Effect of triazolam on sleep, daytime sleepiness and morning stiffness in patients with rheumatoid arthritis. J Rheumatol 1996; 23:245–252.
52. Drewes AM, Bjerregard K, Jorgensen T, et al. Zopiclone as night medication in rheumatoid arthritis. Scand J Rheumatol 1998; 27:180–187.
53. Schnitzer T, Rubens R, Price J, et al. The effect of eszopiclone 3 mg compared with placebo in patients with rheumatoid arthritis and co-existing insomnia. Poster presented at: Sleep; 2006; Salt Lake City, UT. Abstract.
54. Roehrs T, Hyde M, Blaisdell B, et al. Sleep loss and REM sleep loss are hyperalgesic. Sleep 2006; 29:145–151.
55. Jefferson CD, Drake Cl, Scofield HM, et al. Sleep hygiene practices in a population-based sample of insomniacs. Sleep 2005; 28:611–615.
56. Richardson G, Roehrs T, Rosenthal L, et al. Tolerance to daytime sedative effects of H1 antihistamines. J Clin Psychopharmacol 2002; 22:511–515.
57. Roehrs T, Papineau K, Rosenthal L, et al. Ethanol as a hypnotic in insomniacs: Self administration and effects of sleep and mood. Neuropsychopharmacology 1999; 20:279–286.
58. Roehrs, Blaisdell B, Cruz N, et al. Tolerance to hypnotic effects of ethanol in insomnias. Sleep 2004; 27(abstract suppl):A52.
59. Roehrs TA, Blaisdell B, Richardson GS, et al. Insomnia as a path to alcoholism: Dose escalation. Sleep 2003; 26(abstract suppl):A307.
60. Compton-McBride S, Schweitzer, Walsh JK. Most commonly used drugs to treat insomnia in 2002. Sleep 2004; 27(abstract suppl):A255.
61. Roth T, Durrence H, Gotfried M, et al. Efficacy and safety of doxepin 1 and 3 mg in a 3-month trial of elderly adults with chronic primary insomnia. Sleep 2008; 31(abstract suppl):A230.
62. Mendelson WB. A review of the evidence for the efficacy and safety of trazodone in insomnia. J Clin Psychiatry 2005; 66:469–476.
63. Walsh JK, Erman M, Erwin CW, et al. Subjective hypnotic efficacy of trazodone and zolpidem in DSM-III-R primary insomnia. Hum Psychopharmacol 1998;13:191–198.
64. Thompson JW, Ware MR, Blashfield RK. Psychotropic medication and priapism: A comprehensive review. J Clin Psychiatry 1990; 51:430–433.
65. Flores BH, Schatzberg AF. Mirtazepine. In: Schatzberg A, Nemeroff C, eds. The American Psychiatric Publishing Textbook of Psychopharmacology. Washington, DC: American Psychiatric Publishing, Inc., 2004:341–347.

ACKNOWLEDGEMENT

Supported in part by NIDA grant # ROI DA17355 awarded to Dr Roehrs

34 Off-label Use of Prescription Medications for Insomnia: Sedating Antidepressants, Antipsychotics, Anxiolytics, and Anticonvulsants

W. Vaughn McCall

Department of Psychiatry and Behavioral Medicine, Wake Forest University School of Medicine, Winston-Salem, North Carolina, U.S.A.

The inclusion of a separate chapter regarding the off-label use of prescription medications for insomnia in this book is a reflection of the peculiarities of the treatment of insomnia in the United States. The idiosyncratic nature of off-label prescribing in the field of insomnia is underlined by the absence of similar chapters devoted to off-label prescribing in standard textbooks on cardiac pharmacology, pulmonary pharmacology, etc. The need for such a chapter in a textbook on insomnia treatment is derived from statistics on physician prescribing that, until recently, revealed that off-label medications were prescribed preferentially for insomnia, in lieu of medications that are FDA approved for insomnia. As recently as 2002, the most-prescribed medication for insomnia in the United States was trazodone, which is approved by the FDA as an antidepressant, not as a hypnotic (1) (Table 1). It had not always been this way, as in 1986 the FDA-approved hypnotics triazolam, flurazepam, and temazepam were the leading choices among physicians (2). Somehow during the late 1980s and early 1990s, FDA-approved hypnotics were surpassed by trazodone. It is not entirely clear how and why this happened, but we can hypothesize the action of several factors including

- a belief among prescribers that trazodone, other antidepressants, and later, some antipsychotics were reliably effective for treating insomnia;
- a belief among prescribers that trazodone, other antidepressants, and later, some antipsychotics may be safer for patients than FDA-approved hypnotics;
- a belief among prescribers that FDA-approved hypnotics would be needed or asked for by patients for a duration of time that outstripped their FDA-approved indication of use, thus exposing the prescriber to potential liability if there was an untoward event.

The beliefs contained in the three hypotheses are for the most part unsubstantiated, as there are few placebo-controlled trials to show that any non-FDA approved sleep aid is effective in insomnia, or has fewer side effects than approved medications. However, it is true that until recently, the use of FDA-approved hypnotics in the United States appeared to be constrained by package labeling that recommended that schedule IV hypnotics not be given for more than two consecutive weeks, unless the patient was reevaluated. FDA-approved treatments for insomnia generally require (1) two randomized, placebo-controlled clinical trials in insomnia patients showing a superior induction/maintenance of sleep for the investigational medication as compared with placebo and (2) evidence of superiority in both patient report and an objective measurement of sleep [i.e., polysomnography (PSG)]. The data supporting trazodone and other non–FDA-approved medicines prescribed for sleep generally lack one or more of these elements. The importance of each of these elements is defined below:

1. *The importance of a placebo comparison*
   Many investigations of the sleep properties of non-FDA sleep aids have omitted a placebo comparator and instead, have looked at improvement in insomnia symptoms over time that came with administration of the investigational drug, as compared with a pretreatment baseline. This flaw in this approach is revealed in the studies that show a strong placebo effect in insomnia clinical trials. Reductions in sleep latency

Table 1 Drug "Occurrences" for Insomnia 2002: The Verispan Data Base (In Millions)

Antidepressants	
Amitriptyline	0.8
Doxepin	0.2
Mirtazapine	0.7
Trazodone	2.7
FDA-approved hypnotics	
Flurazepam	0.2
Temazepam	0.6
Zaleplon	0.4
Zolpidem	2.0
Sedatives	
Alprazolam	0.3
Clonazepam	0.4
Lorazepam	0.3
Antipsychotics	
Olanzapine	0.2
Quetiapine	0.5
Antihistamines/sedative	
Hydoxyzine	0.3

(SL) and increases in total sleep time (TST) are routinely seen with administration of placebo alone, making it impossible to assume improvement in insomnia seen with an investigational drug and is attributable to the drug and not the placebo effect, in the absence of a placebo comparator (3,4).

2. *The importance of testing in insomnia patients*
   Needless to say, medications may have different effects in persons who are ill than in persons who are well. A classic example in insomnia research is the contrast of the effect of the beta-blocker propranolol in good sleepers versus anxious sleepers. Placebo-controlled comparisons of propranolol in good sleepers have shown a deterioration of sleep (5,6), while a study in sleepers who were anticipating surgery the next day showed better sleep with propranolol than with placebo (7). The take-home message is "in the absence of testing done directly in the population of interest, it is hazardous to predict how a medication might work in an ill-population"
3. *The importance of measuring both patient-report as well as objective testing*

Many non-FDA approaches to insomnia treatment have relied upon patient-report of improvement without confirmation with an independent objective method (i.e., PSG), or occasionally have relied upon PSG improvement, absent patient-reported improvement. The hazards of both approaches are illustrated in the following two studies. The first study examined the serotonin reuptake inhibitor (SSRI) fluoxetine in depressed insomniacs, showing a perception of benefit, but concurrent PSG testing showed some worsening of EEG-defined sleep in the same patients (8). In the second study, the anticonvulsant tiagabine was found to enhance slow wave sleep (SWS), which is generally believed to connote a benefit, but the same insomniac patients did not appreciate a meaningful subjective improvement in their sleep (9). These two studies show that patient's impressions and PSG data may dissociate in the direction of their effect. At the present time, it is impossible to discern the meaning of patient benefit in the absence of PSG-benefit, or PSG-benefit in the absence of patient-reported benefit. So, the present standard for showing anti-insomnia efficacy is the demonstration of both patient-reported and PSG benefit.

The preferential use of non-FDA-approved approaches for insomnia entails its own unique set of problems, over and above the risks inherent in the particular off-label medication prescribed. In general, the FDA does not prohibit the use of approved medications for off-label indications, as the FDA recognizes the judgment of the prescriber to best understand the needs of the patient (10). However, the preferential avoidance of approved approaches and embrace

Table 2 Drug "Occurrences" for Insomnia 2007: The Verispan Data Base

Antidepressants	
Amitriptyline	0.5
Mirtazapine	0.7
Trazodone	2.1
FDA-approved hypnotics	
Eszopiclone	1.4
Ramelteon	0.9
Temazepam	0.6
Zaleplon	0.2
Zolpidem	3.6
Sedatives	
Alprazolam	0.3
Clonazepam	0.5
Lorazepam	0.5
Antipsychotics	
Quetiapine	0.9
Others	
Clonidine	0.2
Cyclobenzaprine	0.2
Tizanidine	0.2

of nonapproved approaches require, at a minimum, some discussion between the prescriber and the patient on how the prescriber arrived at the choice of treatment. Further, this discussion should be documented in the patient's medical record (11).

Recently, there is evidence that the tide is turning back in favor of FDA-approved hypnotics as the preferred treatment for insomnia (James Walsh, personal communication, 2009) (Table 2). Zolpidem has bested trazodone for first place in the list of approaches to insomnia, with trazodone falling to second place. This dynamic may be explained by (1) the availability of generic, less-expensive zolpidem in 2007; (2) the more liberal package labeling of newer anti-insomnia agents, which have no specific comments against prescription for longer than two weeks; (3) vigorous direct-to-consumer advertising that has raised consumer awareness of FDA-approved hypnotics. Still, despite the relative decline in trazodone usage within the last five years, antidepressants, antipsychotics, and other medications not approved for insomnia continue to play a large role in insomnia treatment. We have reviewed the literature regarding the sleep effects of some of the most commonly used off-label prescribed medications for insomnia, focusing on the best evidence available for each medication.

ANTIDEPRESSANTS

Trazodone

Pharmacology

Trazodone is a triazolopyridine antidepressant that was introduced in the United States in 1982 under the brand name Desyrel. It has relatively weak SSRI properties, and is a blocker of postsynaptic serotonin receptors 5-HT_{1A}, 5-HT_{1C}, and 5-HT_2, as well as postsynaptic α_1-adrenergic receptors. It has an elimination half-life of about five to nine hours. When prescribed as an antidepressant, the usual doses of trazodone are $\geq$ 150 mg daily.

Sleep Efficacy

Although the sleep effects of trazodone have been poorly documented in persons who do not have psychiatric disorders, it is widely believed to have beneficial effects on sleep, as reflected in its favored status in the rank order of prescribing rates (Tables 1 and 3). Furthermore, a recent survey revealed that trazodone was the first-line choice of 78% of psychiatrists when prescribing for SSRI-related insomnia (12). This favoritism is baffling given the sparse evidence

Table 3 Trends in Pharmacological Treatment of Insomnia 1987–1996 (Number of Drugs Mentioned in Thousands) (1)

	1987	1996
Antidepressants		
Amitriptyline	421	748
Doxepin	263	269
Trazodone	222	1328
FDA-approved hypnotics		
Flurazepam	1677	373
Temazepam	1201	904
Triazolam	3199	209
Zolpidem	—	1218
Sedatives		
Alprazolam	397	250
Clonazepam	28	330
Lorazepam	346	398

of sleep effect in psychiatric patients. In 17 patients with insomnia associated with fluoxetine or bupropion, the Pittsburgh Sleep Quality Index improved after one week of trazodone 50 mg, compared with placebo (13). In seven patients with insomnia associated with the monoamine oxidase inhibitor brofaromine, SWS increased and the number of polysomnographic awakenings decreased after one week of trazodone 50 mg administration, compared with placebo (14).

The best evidence for a beneficial sleep effect comes from a single, large study in primary insomniacs, albeit the period of study was for only two weeks. Walsh et al. conducted a three-armed randomized comparison of bedtime doses of trazodone 50 mg, versus zolpidem 10 mg and versus placebo in 278 primary insomniacs. Trazodone and zolpidem were both superior to placebo in patient-reported reduction in SL for week 1, but trazodone did not separate from placebo by week 2, while zolpidem maintained its efficacy in week 2. TST effects were mixed, with both trazodone and zolpidem showing an advantage over placebo at week 1, but not week 2 (15).

In normal sleepers, trazodone 50 to 200 mg increases SWS over short periods of time ($\leq$2 weeks) compared to placebo in 9, 8, and 6 subjects, respectively (16–18). As stated above, the clinical significance of an increase in SWS is not always clear, although it is usually inferred to be a sign of potential benefit.

Side Effects

The most common side effects of small bedtime doses of trazodone may be residual morning sedation. Daytime doses of trazodone (TRZ) 100 mg impairs critical flicker fusion and choice reaction time one to four hours later (19,20). Bedtime doses of TRZ 100 mg lowers BP and impairs critical flicker fusion the next morning (21). Less common side effects include orthostatic hypotension (from peripheral adrenergic blockade) and priapism (22). Priapism has an incidence of about 1/6000 persons and can occur at low doses, early in treatment.

Amitriptyline

Pharmacology

Prior to the introduction of fluoxetine in the United States in 1987, tricyclic antidepressants (TCAs) were first-line somatic treatment of major depressive episode (MDE), and TCA therapy could be counted upon to produce reliable, early improvement in the sleep of persons with insomnia and MDE, as compared to the relative lack of effect of psychotherapy on insomnia (23). Amitriptyline is a TCA with a half-life of 20 to 30 hours. Its synaptic effects include reuptake blockade of 5-HT, as well as anticholinergic, antihistaminergic, and α_1-blockade. Typical antidepressant dosages are $\geq$ 75 mg.

Sleep Efficacy

There are no data on the effect of amitriptyline on sleep in primary insomnia. However, in depressed inpatients (many of whom are presumed to have had insomnia) a four-week course of amitriptyline, escalated from 50 mg at bedtime (qhs) to 50 mg four times per day (qid), was associated with an increase in PSG-determined TST, and a reduction in SL, early morning awakening, and a general suppression of Rapid Eye Movement Sleep (REM) as compared to baseline (24). This study did not have a placebo comparison and did not provide patient-reports.

Doxepin

Pharmacology

Doxepin is a TCA with a half-life of 10 to 25 hours. Like amitriptyline, at standard antidepressant doses, doxepin has 5-HT and noradrenergic (NE) reuptake blockade properties, as well as blockade of cholinergic, histaminergic, and α-adrenergic activity. Typical antidepressant doses of doxepin are ≥ 75 mg daily. Smaller doses have been tested for hypnotic potential in primary insomniacs. It is likely that at very low doses (<10 mg) doxepin's meaningful pharmacologic activity is almost exclusively antihistaminergic, with little or no significant effect in serotonergic or adrenergic systems. Theoretically, this low-dose profile would facilitate sleep without other side effects.

Sleep Efficacy

Doxepin 25 to 50 mg was superior over 4 weeks in 47 primary insomniacs in improving PSG total sleep time, sleep efficiency and sleep quality, and daytime ability to work (25). These effects were confirmed in a study of 67 young adults with primary insomnia who underwent a four-period crossover design comparison of placebo versus doxepin 1, 3, and 6 mg (26). Each treatment period lasted for two days. All three doses of doxepin in increased PSG-defined TST and reduced Wake Time after Sleep Onset (WASO), while only the 6-mg dose reduced SL compared with placebo. REM% decreased with the 3- and 6-mg dose with no change in SWS. Patient-report showed superiority for doxepin in reducing SL and increasing TST only for the 6-mg dose.

Side Effects

The side effects of low-dose doxepin in primary insomniacs were infrequent and numerically similar to placebo with the two-day exposure, four-way crossover design (26).

Nortriptyline

Pharmacology

Nortriptyline is a TCA with a half-life of 22 to 39 hours, potent reuptake blockade of NE, and weaker reuptake of 5-HT. It also has anticholinergic effects as well as weak α_1-adrenergic and histaminergic blockade.

Sleep Efficacy

There is no data regarding the efficacy of nortriptyline in primary insomnia, but in a sample of 20 depressed insomniacs, acute exposure to nortriptyline reduced PSG-determined SL and suppressed most measures of REM sleep. Patient-report was not described in this study (27). In a somewhat different design, a comparison was made in the sleep profiles of previously depressed, now-remitted elderly patients who had received one year of maintenance treatment for depression with either nortriptyline versus placebo. Interestingly, the nortriptyline patients had longer PSG-determined SL and no advantages in sleep maintenance, but the nortriptyline patients did exhibit more intense SWS (28).

Side Effects

The most frequent side effect is dry mouth (29).

Mirtazapine

Pharmacology

Mirtazapine is a tetracyclic piperazinoazepine with a half-life of 22 to 40 hours. It has minimal effect on monoamine uptake, but is a potent inhibitor of 5-HT_2 and 5-HT_3 receptors, as well as central α_2-adrenergic receptors (30). Typical antidepressant doses are $\geq$15 mg daily.

Sleep Efficacy

There are no placebo-RCT in primary insomniacs. However, mirtazapine 30 mg reduced PSG sleep latency and increased SWS in six good sleepers on the first night in the sleep lab compare to placebo in a crossover design (31). Mirtazapine 30 mg increased PSG sleep efficiency and SWS compared to placebo on the third night in the laboratory in 20 good sleepers in parallel-arm clinical trial (32). In 22 depressed insomniacs randomized to either mirtazapine 45 mg or fluoxetine 40 mg, the conclusion of 8 weeks of treatment saw greater reductions in PSG-determined SL and increases in TST for mirtazapine as compared with fluoxetine. Patient-report was not described (33).

Side Effects

Bedtime doses of Mirtazapine were associated with prolonged motor reaction times the next day (34) and impaired actual driving performance at 30 mg, compared with placebo with acute, but not chronic dosing (30).

ANTIPSYCHOTICS

Quetiapine

Pharmacology

Quetiapine is an atypical antipsychotic with a half-life of two to three hours. It has high affinity for 5-HT_{2A} receptors and weak affinity for dopamine, muscarinic, and adrenergic receptors. Typical antipsychotic doses are 150 to 800 mg daily.

Sleep Efficacy

There are no randomized controlled trials in primary insomnia. Quetiapine 25 or 100 mg at bedtime was superior to placebo for one night in increasing PSG total sleep time and subjective sleep quality in 14 good sleepers under noisy conditions. The authors speculate that the beneficial sleep effect was mediated through blockade of histaminergic, dopaminergic, and adrenergic receptors. Of note, the 100-mg dose induced periodic limb movements (PLMs) (35). Quetiapine has been tested in an open study of doses of 25 to 75 mg at bedtime for 6 weeks in 18 patients with primary insomnia, finding there were PSG-determined and patient-report improvements in TST, but not SL, compared to baseline (36). Quetiapine has been tested against placebo in demented patients with associated sleep disturbance. Doses of quetiapine started at 25 mg and could be increased to 125 mg by the fifth week. Quetiapine was associated with increases in actigraphically determined TST as early as the first week, and this advantage was still seen at the end of the fifth week (37).

Side Effects

Quetiapine is associated with weight gain, with the potential for glucose intolerance. Similar to other atypical antipsychotics, the FDA has required a black box warning for quetiapine noting increased risk of cerebrovascular accident in elderly patients.

Olanzapine

Pharmacology

Olanzapine is an atypical antipsychotic and a derivative of thienobenzodiazepines. It has potent antagonist properties for 5-HT_{2A} and 5-HT_{2C} receptors, with weak affinity for dopamine receptors. Olanzapine also is active at muscarinic, α_1-adrenergic, and histaminergic receptors (38). Olanzapine has a half-life of 36 hours. Typical antipsychotic dosages are $\geq$5 mg daily.

Sleep Efficacy

There are no studies of Olanzapine in primary insomnia. The only placebo-controlled study of Olanzapine was conducted in nine good sleepers, using a three-way crossover comparison of three-nights exposure to placebo versus Olanzapine 5 or 10 mg. Both doses of Olanzapine were associated with PSG-determined reductions in SL and WASO, increases in TST and SWS, and suppression of REM. These volunteers also reported better sleep quality with olanzapine than placebo (38). The same authors later examined the addition of a three-week course of olanzapine 2.5 to 10 mg to ongoing SSRI therapy in 12 depressed patients with an inadequate response to SSRI monotherapy. There was no placebo control. The findings were similar to the earlier study, with reductions in SL and WASO, and gains in TST and SWS. Unexpectedly, patients reported difficulty getting up in the morning, with an approximate one-hour increase in time in bed at home (39). Similar small, uncontrolled studies of olanzapine have been undertaken in persons with schizophrenia, using doses up to 20 mg for up to four weeks, and again reported PSG-determined increases in TST and SWS, and reductions in WASO (40,41).

Side Effects

Olanzapine is associated with weight gain, with the potential for glucose intolerance. Similar to other atypical antipsychotics, the FDA has required a black box warning for olanzapine noting increased risk of cerebrovascular accident in elderly patients.

Other Antipsychotics

Although the atypical antipsychotics risperidone and ziprasidone and the conventional antipsychotics haloperidol and thiothixene are not among the most common medications prescribed for insomnia (Tables 1–3), it is noteworthy that in general their sleep effects mirror to a greater or lesser degree what is reported for quetiapine and olanzapine, namely increases in TST and SWS (42–44).

Anxiolytics

Pharmacology

Lorazepam, clonazepam and alprazolam are all classic benzodiazepines with rapid absorption and respective half-lives of 10 to 20, 24 to 56, and 10 to 15 hours. All three are indicated for treatment of anxiety states, and clonazepam is also indicated for epilepsy. There are no fundamental differences between those benzodiazepine approved for insomnia and those not approved for insomnia, other than pharmacokinetics and route of administration.

Lorazepam

Sleep Efficacy

Lorazepam 2.5 mg was compared in a parallel design against midazolam 15 mg and placebo in 60 adults who were dosed the night before surgery. Outcomes were recorded by direct nursing observation and found that while midazolam was superior for sleep induction, lorazepam was significantly superior to placebo for sleep maintenance and patient-reported quality of sleep (45). A similar study of sleep on the night before surgery was conducted in 60 adults allocated in a randomized, balanced, parallel design to either lorazepam 2 mg, lorazepam 4 mg, nitrazepam 10 mg, lormetazepam 1 mg, lormetazepam 2 mg, or placebo. Both doses of lorazepam were associated with longer sleep on the preoperative night as compared to placebo (46). A crossover study of six good sleepers compared on night dosing of lorazepam 1 mg versus zolpidem 10 mg, zopiclone 7.5 mg, triazolam 0.25 mg, and placebo under noisy conditions found that lorazepam reduced SL and increased TST (47).

Lorazepam 0.5 mg tid and then 1.5 mg at bedtime were examined in a two-stage crossover comparison with placebo in 12 adults with primary insomnia. Each treatment phase lasted for four days. Both dosing strategies of lorazepam were superior to placebo in both subjective and PSG sleep (48). A single-blind examination of lorazepam 3 mg was conducted for 7 nights in 6 adults with primary insomnia without the benefit of a placebo comparison. By both patient-report and PSG, lorazepam was associated with decreased SL and increased TST (49).

Lorazepam 2 mg showed improvement compared to baseline in 30 patients over 4 nights in subjective sleep, with no placebo comparator (50).

Side Effects

In six adults with primary insomniacs, lorazepam 3 mg was associated with poorer performance on the digit symbol substitution task (DSST) and timed card-sorting task as compared with performance at baseline (49). In 30 adults with primary insomnia, lorazepam 2 mg was associated with greater reported problems with dizziness, drowsiness, and poor coordination than placebo (50). A single dose of lorazepam 4 mg at bedtime was associated with more complaints of sleepiness, confusion, slurred speech, clumsiness, and blurred vision than placebo presurgical patients (46). Morning alertness was reduced in a different study of presurgical patients after a single bedtime dose of lorazepam 2.5 mg. A one-week exposure to lorazepam 1 mg at bedtime was compared against bedtime doses of alprazolam 0.25 mg and placebo in six good sleepers using a blinded, randomized crossover design. Lorazepam, but not alprazolam, was associated with slower reaction time the morning following the final dose in each treatment phase (51). Lorazepam has also been associated with drug-withdrawal insomnia after as little as seven nights of continuous use of either 2 mg (52) or 4 mg (53).

Clonazepam

There are no double-blind randomized placebo-controlled trials of clonazepam in primary insomnia. However, a single-blind study found that clonazepam 0.5 mg reduced PSG-determined total wake time over seven nights of dosing as compared with the pretreatment baseline (54). However, clonazepam has been tested using double-blind randomized placebo-controlled trials in patients with PLMs and depression associated with insomnia.

In 80 depressed patients receiving fluoxetine, the coadministration of clonazepam 0.5 to 1.0 at bedtime for 21 days was superior to placebo in improving scores on the Hamilton Rating Scale for Depression (HRSD) sleep items over the entire three weeks (55). The success of this study led the authors to repeat the study using a longer period of drug administration: 50 depressed patients received fluoxetine and the coadministration of clonazepam 0.5 to 1.0 versus placebo at bedtime for 18 weeks. Again, clonazepam was superior to placebo in Hamilton Rating Scale for Depression sleep items for the first three weeks, but clonazepam did not separate from placebo after three weeks (56). Neither study reported an advantage for clonazepam for any clinical parameter other than sleep.

In a mixed sample of 10 restless leg syndrome patients and 16 PLM patients, a single bedtime dose of clonazepam 1 mg reduced PSG-determined SL and increased TST compared with baseline, without impacting the rate of PLMs (57). In a sample of 20 PLM patients, including 8 with insomnia, one month of clonazepam 0.5–2.0 mg was superior to placebo in a parallel-design comparison (58). In this study, clonazepam was associated with PSG-determined reductions in SL, PLM frequency, PLM arousals, and increases in TST.

Alprazolam

There are no randomized, placebo-controlled trials of alprazolam for insomnia. Using a single-blind design, alprazolam 1 mg was administered for one week at bedtime in six adults with primary insomnia. Compared with baseline, alprazolam was associated with PSG-determined reduction in SL and WASO, and increases in TST. However, a worsening compared with baseline was seen during the first week of single-blind discontinuation of alprazolam (59).

ANTICONVULSANTS

Although no anticonvulsants appear on the list of most common medications prescribed for sleep, several studies have shown potential clinical promise of anticonvulsants in selected populations.

Gabapentin and Pregabalin

Many alcoholics experience persistent insomnia during abstinence from alcohol and those that do experience insomnia are at a greater risk of relapse. Treatment of insomnia during abstinence would seem to be a potential pathway to prevent relapse, but other than ramelteon,

FDA-approved treatments for insomnia are controlled substances and convey some risk for abuse in alcoholics. Gabapentin, 1-(aminomethyl) cyclohexane acetic acid, is a GABA analogue excreted unchanged through the kidneys. Gabapentin is not a controlled substance, is not thought to have potential for abuse, and can be used in alcoholics with reduced hepatic function. It has also been shown to increase SWS in normals (60).

Gabapentin may also be helpful in treating insomnia during alcoholic abstinence. Fifty alcohol-dependent outpatients with persisting insomnia were treated with either gabapentin or trazodone for four to six weeks, according to the prescriber's preference. Thirty-four were treated with gabapentin (mean dose 888 mg) at bedtime and 16 were treated with trazodone (105 mg) at bedtime. The gabapentin group improved significantly more than the trazodone group in insomnia severity (61).

Finally, gabapentin has been shown to reduce alcohol use and cravings, as compared with placebo (62).

Gabapentin has also been shown to reduce pain-related sleep disturbance in a variety of pain syndromes, including fibromyalgia (63), peripheral neuropathy (64–66), and traumatic nerve injury pain (67). Dosing of gabapentin for neuropathic pain is higher than what is used for alcohol abstinence insomnia; doses of 2400 to 3600 mg/day would be common.

Pregabalin is closely related to gabapentin, and like gabapentin, it interferes with influx of calcium into nerve terminals. Pregabalin's half-life is five to six hours and it is exclusively eliminated by the kidney. It is FDA approved for the treatment of fibromyalgia, neuropathic pain, postherpetic neuralgia, and epilepsy. It has a robust literature showing that treatment of these pain syndromes with pregabalin results in less patient-reported, pain-related sleep disturbance at doses of 150 to 600 mg/day (68–71). Like gabapentin, pregabalin enhances SWS in normal volunteers (72).

Valproic Acid

Sleep loss has been described as a risk factor for the precipitation or perpetuation of acute mania. Therefore, it is likely that treatments for acute mania should have effects that support sleep induction or sleep maintenance. Valproic acid in the form of divalproex was tested in 377 patients with acute mania, with patients randomly assigned in a 1:1 ratio to 21 days of double-blind treatment with divalproex ER ($N = 192$) or placebo ($N = 185$). Daily dosage was increased to 500 mg daily by day 3. Treatment with divalproex was associated with improvement on a mania rating scale, but specifically with reported improvement in sleep (73).

Tiagabine

Tiagabine is a GABA uptake inhibitor with a half-life of seven to nine hours. Two hundred and thirty-two men and women with primary insomnia were randomly assigned to receive tiagabine 4, 6, 8, 10 mg or placebo in a randomized, double-blind, parallel-group study. Efficacy was assessed using PSG and self-report measures. No significant differences were observed between tiagabine and placebo in wake after sleep onset, latency to persistent sleep, or TST. This study is important for testing the concept of whether induction of SWS is pathognomonic for an effective insomnia agent, showing that SWS induction and anti-insomnia efficacy are dissociable (9). Tiagabine is no longer under commercial development as a hypnotic.

CONCLUSIONS

Doxepin is the only medication with frequent off-label use for insomnia that is supported by double-blind, placebo-controlled studies in primary insomnia, confirming superior activity confirmed by both patient-report and PSG. Doxepin may receive FDA approval by the time this chapter is published. Although none of the other medications described in this chapter meet this same standard, there is still a suggestion of sleep efficacy for most of them. Intriguingly, many of these medications enhance SWS, a feature not seen in the most recent FDA-approved hypnotics (74–76). Although the lessons learned from tiagabine have shown that enhancement of SWS can be divorced from the usual signs of sleep efficacy, enhancement of SWS seems to be a near-universal feature of the off-label approaches to insomnia treatment.

If the use of off-label medications is driven in part by the belief that these medications are in some way safer than FDA-approved hypnotics, then it is surprising how little safety information is there about use of these off-label approaches in insomniacs. What data does exist typically shows some degree of next-day impairment, bringing into question whether these off-label approaches are really any safer than FDA-approved insomnia treatments.

RECOMMENDATIONS

None of the off-label approaches to treating insomnia can be recommended as first-line treatment for primary insomnia, perhaps with the exception of low-dose doxepin. However, off-label medications may be justified as monotherapy or as add-on therapy if FDA-approved treatments fail, or if the patient has a strong preference for avoiding controlled substances. Also, off-label approaches may be indicated in specific clinical circumstances, such as given in the following:

- Trazodone, tricyclic antidepressants, or mirtazapine for insomnia associated with depression
- Quetiapine or olanzapine for insomnia associated with psychosis
- Lorazepam, clonazepam, or alprazolam for insomnia associated with anxiety
- Clonazepam for insomnia associated with PLMs
- Valproic acid for insomnia associated with bipolar disorder
- Gabapentin or pregabalin for insomnia associated with alcohol abstinence or pain

REFERENCES

1. Walsh JK. Drugs used to treat insomnia in 2002: Regulatory-based rather than evidence-based medicine. Sleep 2004; 27:1441–1442.
2. Walsh JK, Schweitzer PK. Ten-year trends in the pharmacological treatment of insomnia. Sleep 1999; 22:371–375.
3. McCall V, D'Agostino RB Jr, Dunn A. A meta-analysis of sleep changes associated with placebo in hypnotic clinical trials. Sleep Med 2003; 4:57–62.
4. McCall V, Perlis M, Tu X, et al. A comparison of placebo and no-treatment during a hypnotic clinical trial. Int J Clin Pharmacol Ther 2005; 43:355–359.
5. Betts TA, Alford C. Beta-blockers and sleep: A controlled trial. Eur J Clin Pharmacol 1985; 28:65–68.
6. Kostis JB, Rosen RC. Central nervous system effects of beta-adrenergic-blocking drugs: The role of ancillary properties. Circulation 1987; 75:204–212.
7. Chierichetti SM, Moise G, Galeone M, et al. Beta-blockers and psychic stress: A double-blind, placebo-controlled study of bopindolol vs lorazepam and butalbital in surgical patients. Int J Clin Pharmacol Ther Toxicol 1985; 23:510–514.
8. Gillin JC, Rapaport M, Erman MK, et al. A comparison of nefazodone and fluoxetine on mood and on objective, subjective, and clinician-rated measures of sleep in depressed patients: A double-blind, 8-week clinical trial. J Clin Psychiatry 1997; 58:185–192.
9. Walsh J, Perlis M, Rosenthal M, et al. Tiagabine increases slow-wave sleep in a dose-dependent fashion without affecting traditional efficacy measures in adults with primary insomnia. J Clin Sleep Med 2006; 2:35–41.
10. Kuntz R. Off-label prescribing of antidepressants and anxiolytics: An attorney's guide to psychoactive drugs. J Psychiatry and the Law 1998; 26:519–532.
11. Kramer S, McCall V. Off-label prescribing: 7 steps for safer, more effective treatment. Curr Psychiatr 2006; 5:15–28.
12. Dording C, Mischoulon D, Petersen T, et al. The pharmacologic management of SSRI-induced side effects: A survey of psychiatrists. Ann Clin Psychiatry 2002; 14:143–147.
13. Nierenberg A, Adler LA, Peselow E, et al. Trazodone for antidepressant-associated insomnia. Am J Psychiatry 1994; 151:1069–1072.
14. Haffmans PMJ. The effects of trazodone on sleep disturbances included by brofaromine. Eur Psychiatry 1999; 14:167–171.
15. Walsh JK, Erman M, Erwin CW, et al. Subjective hypnotic efficacy of trazodone and zolpidem in DSMIII-R primary insomnia. Hum Psychopharmacol 1998; 13:191–198.
16. Montgomery I, Oswald I, Morgan K, et al. Trazodone enhances sleep in subjective quality but not in objective duration. Br J Clin Pharmacol 1983; 16:139–144.
17. Yamadera H, Nakamura S, Suzuki H, et al. Effects of trazodone hydrochloride and imipramine on polysomnography in healthy subjects. Psychiatry Clin Neurosci 1998; 52:439–443.
18. Ware JC, Pittard JT. Increased deep sleep after trazodone use: A double-blind placebo-controlled study in healthy young adults. J Clin Psychiatry 1990; 51:18–22.

19. Burns M, Hoskowitz H, Jaffe J. A comparison of the effects of trazodone and amitriptyline on skills performance by geriatric subjects. J Clin Psychiatry 1986; 47:252–254.
20. Warrington SJ, Ankier SI, Turner P. An evaluation of possible interactions between ethanol and trazodone or amitriptyline. Br J Clin Pharmacol 1984; 18:549–557.
21. Saletu-Zyhlarz G, Abu-Bakr M, Anderer P, et al. Insomnia related to dysthymia: Polysomnographic and psychometric comparison with normal controls and acute therapeutic trials with trazodone. Neuropsychobiology 2001; 44:139–149.
22. James S, Mendelson W. The use of trazodone as a hypnotic: A critical review. J Clin Psychiatry 2004; 65:752–755.
23. DiMascio A, Weissman MM, Prusoff BA, et al. Differential symptom reduction by drugs and psychotherapy in acute depression. Arch Gen Psychiatry 1979; 36:1450–1456.
24. Kupfer DJ, Spiker DG, Coble P, et al. Amitriptyline and EEG sleep in depressed patients: I. Drug effect. Sleep 1978; 1:149–159.
25. Hajak G, Rodenbeck A, Voderholzer U, et al. Doxepin in the treatment of primary insomnia: A placebo-controlled, double-blind, polysomnographic study. J Clin Psychiatry 2001; 62:453–463.
26. Roth T, Rogowski R, Hull S, et al. Efficacy and safety of doxepin 1 mg, 3 mg, and 6 mg in adults with primary insomnia. Sleep 2007; 30:1555–1561.
27. Kupfer DJ, Spiker DG, Rossi A, et al. Nortriptyline and EEG sleep in depressed patients. Biol Psychiatry 1982; 17:535–546.
28. Reynolds CF III, Buysse D, Brunner D, et al. Maintenance nortriptyline effects on electroencephalographic sleep in elderly patients with recurrent major depression: Double-blind, placebo- and plasma-level-controlled evaluation. Biol Psychiatry 1997; 42:560–567.
29. Haggstram FM, Chatkin JM, Sussenbach-Vaz E, et al. A controlled trial of nortriptyline, sustained-release bupropion and placebo for smoking cessation: Preliminary results. Pulm Pharmacol Ther 2006; 19:205–209.
30. Wingen M, Bothmer J, Langer S, et al. Actual driving performance and psychomotor function in healthy subjects after acute and subchronic treatment with escitalopram, mirtazapine, and placebo: A crossover trial. J Clin Psychiatry 2005; 66:436–443.
31. Ruigt GSF, Kemp B, Groenhout CM, et al. Effect of the antidepressant Org 3770 on human sleep. Eur J Clin Pharmacol 1990; 38:551–554.
32. Aslan S, Isik E, Cosar B. The effects of mirtazapine on sleep: A placebo controlled, double-blind study in young healthy volunteers. Sleep 2002; 25:677–679.
33. Winokur A, DeMartinis NA III, McNally DP, et al. Comparative effects of mirtazapine and fluoxetine on sleep physiology measures in patients with major depression and insomnia. J Clin Psychiatry 2003; 64:1224–1229.
34. Ridout F, Meadows R, Johnsen S, et al. A placebo controlled investigation into the effects of paroxetine and mirtazapine on measures related to car driving performance. Hum Psychopharmacol 2003; 18:261–269.
35. Cohrs S, Rodenbeck A, Guan Z, et al. Sleep-promoting properties of quetiapine in healthy subjects. Psychopharmacology 2004; 174:421–429.
36. Wiegand M, Landry F, Bruckner T, et al. Quetiapine in primary insomnia: A pilot study. Psychopharmacology 2008; 196:337–338.
37. Nanda F, Singer C. Placebo-controlled trial of quetiapine for sleep disturbance in dementia and MCI [abstract]. Am J Geriatr Psychiatry 2008; 16(3)(suppl I):A126.
38. Sharpley AlL, Vassallo CM, Cowen PJ. Olanzapine increases slow-wave sleep: Evidence for blockade of central 5-HT2 C receptors in vivo. Soc Biol Psychiatry 2000; 47:468–470.
39. Sharpley AL, Attenburrow EJ, Hafizi S, et al. Olanzapine increases slow wave sleep and sleep continuity in SSRI-resistant depressed patients. J Clin Psychiatry 2005; 66:450–454.
40. Salin-Pascual RJ, Herrera-Estrella M, Galicia-Polo L, et al. Olanzapine acute administration in schizophrenic patients increases delta sleep and sleep efficiency. Biol Psychiatry 1999; 46: 141–143.
41. Muller MJ, Rossbach WMK, Roschke J, et al. Subchronic effects of olanzapine on sleep EEG in schizophrenic patients with predominantly negative symptoms. Pharmacopsychiatry 2004; 37: 157–162.
42. Maixner S, Tandon R, Eiser A, et al. Effects of antipsychotic treatment on ploysomnographic measures in schizophrenia: A replication and extension. Am J Psychiatry 1998; 155:1600–1602.
43. Cohrs S, Meier A, Neumann A, et al. Improved sleep continuity and increased slow wave sleep and REM latency during ziprasidone treatment: A randomized, controlled, crossover trial of 12 healthy male subjects. J Clin Psychiatry 2005; 66:989–996.
44. Sharpley AL, Bhagwager Z, Hafizi S, et al. Risperidone augmentation decreases rapid eye movement sleep and decreases wake in treatment-resistant depressed patients. J Clin Psychiatry 2003; 64:192–196.

45. Mattila MAK, Salmela J, Vaananen A, et al. Midazolam vs lorazepam and placebo as hypnotic premedication before surgery. A controlled, double-blind study. Drugs Exp Clin Res 1985; 12:841–844.
46. Sanders LD, Yeomans WA, Rees J, et al. A double-blind comparison between nitrazepam, lorazepam, lormetazepam and placebo as preoperative night sedatives. Eur J Anaesthesiol 1988; 5:377–383.
47. Parrino L, Boselli M, Spaggiari MC, et al. Multidrug comparison (lorazepam, triazolam, zolpidem, and zopiclone) in situational insomnia: Polysomnographic analysis by means of the cyclic alternating pattern. Clin Neuropharmacol 1997; 20:253–263.
48. Bonnet MH, Arand DL. The use of lorazepam TID for chronic insomnia. Int Clin Psychopharmacol 1999; 14:81–89.
49. Walsh JK, Schweitzer PK, Parwatikar S. Effects of lorazepam and its withdrawal on sleep, performance, and subjective state. Clin Pharmacol Ther 1983; 34:496–500.
50. Cohn JB. Double-blind crossover comparison of triazolam and lorazepam in the posthypnotic state. J Clin Psychiatry 1984; 45:104–107.
51. Jurado JL, Fernandez-Mas R, Gernandez-Guardiola A. Effects of 1 week administration of two benzodiazepines on the sleep and early daytime performance of normal subjects. Psychopharmacology 1989; 99:91–93.
52. Kales A, Bixler EO, Soldatos C, et al. Lorazepam: Effects on sleep and withdrawal phenomena. Pharmacology 1986; 32:121–130.
53. Scharf MB, Kales A, Bixler EO, et al. Lorazepam—efficacy, side effects, and rebound phenomena. Clin Pharmacol Ther 1982; 31:175–179.
54. Kales A, Manfredi RL, Vgontzas AN, et al. Clonazepam: Sleep laboratory study of efficacy and withdrawal. J Clin Psychopharmacol 1991; 11:189–193.
55. Londborg PD, Smith WT, Glaudin V, et al. Short-term cotherapy with clonazepam and fluoxetine: Anxiety, sleep disturbance and core symptoms of depression. J Affect Disord 2000; 61:73–79.
56. Smith WT, Londborg PD, Glaudin V, et al. Is extended clonazepam cotherapy of fluoxetine effective for outpatients with major depression? J Affect Disord 2002; 70:251–259.
57. Saletu M, Anderer P, Saletu-Zyhlarz G, et al. Restless legs syndrome (RLS) and periodic limb movement disorder (PLMD). Acute placebo-controlled sleep laboratory studies with clonazepam. Eur Neuropsychopharmacol 2001; 11:153–161.
58. Peled R, Lavie P. Double-blind evaluation of clonazepam on periodic leg movements in sleep. J Neurol Neurosurg Psychiatry 1987; 50:1679–1681.
59. Kales A, Bixler EO, Vela-Bueno A, et al. Alprazolam: Effects on sleep and withdrawal phenomena. J Clin Pharmacol 1987; 27:508–515.
60. Foldvary-Schaefer N, De Leon Sanchez I, Karafa M, et al. Gabapentin increases slow-wave sleep in normal adults. Epilepsia 2002; 43:1493–1497.
61. Karam-Hage M, Brower K. Open pilot study of gabapentin versus trazodone to treat insomnia in alcoholic outpatients. Psychiatry Clin Neurosci 2003; 57:542–544.
62. Furieri F, Nakamura-Placios E. Gabapentin reduces alcohol consumption and craving: A randomized, double-blind, placebo-controlled trial. J Clin Psychiatry 2007; 68:1691–1700.
63. Arnold LM, Goldenberg D, Stanford S, et al. Gabapentin in the treatment of fibromyalgia: A randomized, double-blind, placebo-controlled, multicenter trial. Arthritis Rheum 2007; 56:1336–1344.
64. Hahn K, Arendt G, Braun J, et al. A placebo-controlled trial of gabapentin for painful HIV-associated sensory neuropathies. J Neurol 2004; 251:1260–1266.
65. Rice A, Maton S; Postherpetic Neuralgia Study Group. Gabapentin in postherpetic neuralgia: A randomised, double blind, placebo controlled study. Pain 2001; 94:215–224.
66. Backonja M. Gabapentin monotherapy for the symptomatic treatment of painful neuropathy: A multicenter, double-blind, placebo-controlled trial in patients with diabetes mellitus. Epilepsia 1990;40(suppl):S57–S59.
67. Gordh T, Stubhaug A, Jenson T, et al. Gabapentin in traumatic nerve injury pain: A randomized, double-blind, placebo-controlled, cross-over, multi-center study. Pain 2008; 138:255–266.
68. Arnold LM, Russell I, Diri E, et al. A 14-week, randomized, double-blinded, placebo-controlled monotherapy trial of pregabalin in pateints with fibromyalgia. J Pain 2008; 9:792–805.
69. Freeman R, Durso-Decruz E, Emir B. Efficacy, safety, and tolerability of pregabalin treatment for painful diabetic peripheral neuropathy: Findings from seven randomized, controlled trials across a range of doses. Diabetes Care 2008; 31:1448–1454.
70. Mease P, Russell I, Arnold LM, et al. A randomized, double-blind, placebo-controlled, phase III trial of pregabalin in the treatment of patients with fibromyalgia. J Rheumatol 2008; 35:502–514.
71. Siddall P, Cousins M, Otte A, et al. Pregabalin in central neuropathic pain associated with spinal cord injury: A placebo-controlled trial. Neurology 2006; 67:1792–1800.
72. Hindmarch I, Dawson J, Stanley N. A double-blind study in healthy volunteers to assess the effects on sleep of pregabalin compared with alprazolam and placebo. Sleep 2005; 28:187–193.

73. Bowden CL, Swann A, Calabrese J, et al. A randomized, placebo-controlled, multicenter study of divalproex sodium extended release in the treatment of acute mania. J Clin Pyshciatry 2006; 67: 1501–1510.
74. Zammit GK, McNabb LJ, Caron J, et al. Efficacy and safety of eszopiclone across 6-weeks of treatment for primary insomnia. Curr Med Res Opin 2004; 20:1979–1991.
75. Roth T, Soubrane C, Titeux L, et al. Eficacy and safety of zolpidem-MR: A double-blind, placebo-controlled study in adults with primary insomnia. Sleep Med 2006; 7:397–406.
76. Zammit GK, Erman M, Wang-Weigand S, et al. Evaluation of the efficacy and safety of ramelteon in subjects with chronic insomnia. J Clin Sleep Med 2007; 3:495–504.

35 Melatonin in Sleep-Wake Regulation

Phyllis C. Zee and Kathryn J. Reid

Department of Neurology, Feinberg School of Medicine, Northwestern University, Chicago, Illinois, U.S.A.

INTRODUCTION

The circadian system plays an essential role in regulating the daily cycles of physiological and behavioral functions, such as core body temperature, hormonal rhythms of cortisol and melatonin secretion, and levels of sleepiness, alertness, and performance (1). Circadian rhythms are endogenously generated cellular, physiologic or behavioral cycles with a genetically encoded period of approximately 24 hours. In mammals, circadian rhythms are regulated by a central circadian clock located in the suprachiasmatic nucleus (SCN) of the anterior hypothalamus (2–4). The endogenous circadian period in humans has been shown to be approximately 24.2 hours (5). Because under normal conditions, the circadian system is synchronized or entrained to the 24-hour rotation of the earth, individuals with an endogenous period longer or shorter than 24 hours require a daily net advance or delay of the SCN-driven rhythm (6). Light, melatonin, and high-intensity physical activity have been shown to act as synchronizing agents for the circadian clock. However, light is the primary circadian synchronizing agent in humans (7).

In humans, the most apparent function of the circadian system is the regulation of the sleep–wake cycle (8). Circadian propensity for sleep and wakefulness is regulated by multisynaptic pathways from the SCN to wake and sleep promoting areas of the brain (9–12). Circadian synchronizing agents such as light and melatonin not only reset the timing of circadian rhythms but also can influence the firing rate of SCN neurons and thus modulate levels of alertness and sleepiness. Thus, both light and melatonin have been studied for the treatment of sleep disorders, including insomnia. In this chapter, we will discuss the evidence for a role of endogenous melatonin in sleep regulation and the use of exogenous melatonin and melatonin receptor agonists as treatments for insomnia.

ROLE OF MELATONIN IN SLEEP–WAKE REGULATION

Melatonin, an indoleamine hormone secreted by the pineal gland, was originally described in 1958 (13). Since its initial description, researchers have made significant gains in further understanding this hormone's role in the organization of circadian rhythms and sleep. The circadian rhythm of melatonin production is regulated by a multisynaptic pathway that originates from the SCN via the paraventricular nucleus (PVN) to the sympathetic preganglionic thoracic spinal cord neurons, which in turn project to the superior cervical ganglia (SCG) (Fig. 1). The superior cervical ganglia releases norepinephrine to stimulate the β-adrenergic receptors of the pineal gland to produce melatonin (14). This multistep process of melatonin production occurs at night, when the firing rate of SCN neurons slow (15).

There is a distinct circadian rhythm of melatonin production, with high levels at night and low levels in the daytime. In humans, the high nocturnal levels of melatonin reflect the biological night, a time when sleep occurs. In an entrained individual with a conventional sleep–wake time between 11 PM and 7 AM, the onset of melatonin secretion begins at about 9 PM or about 2 hours before typical sleep onset (16). Melatonin secretion reaches its peak between 2 and 4 AM, and then declines to almost undetectable levels by about 9 AM (17).

The primary site of action of melatonin is on melatonin receptors (MT_1, MT_2, MT_3) in the SCN. Melatonin acts on its receptors to inhibit SCN neuronal firing, leading to further melatonin production (14). In contrast, exposure to bright light in the evening or night (at a time when melatonin is being produced) will increase the firing rate of SCN neurons (18) and suppress melatonin production. Melatonin binding to MT_1 receptors produces inhibition of SCN neuron firing, which has been linked to the sleep promoting effects of melatonin (19,20).

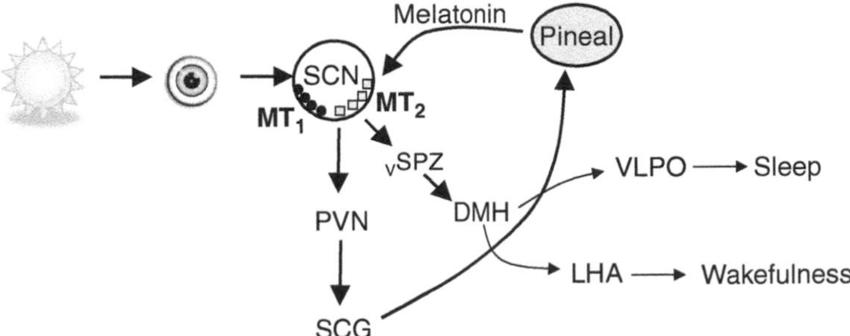

Figure 1 This is a schematic representation of the role of the circadian system and pineal melatonin in the regulation of sleep and wakefulness. Light–dark information is received by the retina (retinal ganglion cells that are most responsive to short wavelength (blue) light) and travels via the retinohypothalamic tract to the SCN. Information travels from the SCN via the paraventricular nucleus (PVN) to the sympathetic preganglionic thoracic spinal cord neurons, which in turn project to the superior cervical ganglia (SCG) to signal the pineal to produce melatonin. Melatonin binding to the MT_1 receptors primarily produces inhibition of SCN neuron firing, and melatonin binding primarily to MT_2 receptors phase shift neural firing rhythms in the SCN. The SCN influences sleep and wakefulness via efferent projections to other brain sleep [ventrolateral preoptic nucleus (VLPO)] and arousal [lateral hypothalamus (LHA)] centers. The SCN sends projections to the ventral subparaventricular zone (vSPZ) which in turn sends projections to the dorsomedial nucleus of the hypothalamus (DMH) and finally to the VLPO and LHA.

It is thought that exogenous melatonin promotes sleep by its ability to inhibit electrical activity or wake promoting signal from the SCN. Activation of MT_1 and MT_2 SCN receptors (primarily MT2) can also reset the timing of circadian rhythms (21–23). Although the function of the MT_3 receptor is not well understood, it is not likely to play an important role in sleep regulation (24). Under normally entrained conditions, the activity of the MT_1 and MT_2 receptors promotes sleep and also synchronizes the regular timing of the sleep–wake cycle. These distinct roles for the different melatonin receptors offer opportunities for receptor-specific drug therapies of circadian-based sleep disorders and insomnia.

EXOGENOUS MELATONIN

Exogenous melatonin has been shown to be efficacious for the treatment of sleep disturbances associated with circadian rhythm sleep disorders. Substantial evidence shows that when timed appropriately, melatonin is able to realign and synchronize circadian rhythms. On the basis of its phase–response curve, melatonin, when given in the late afternoon/evening (prior to the nadir of the core body temperature rhythm), produces phase advances, whereas, in the late night/early morning (after the nadir of the core body temperature rhythm), it produces phase delays in physiological and behavioral rhythms, including that of the sleep–wake cycle (25,26). Because melatonin possesses both chronobiotic as well as soporific effects, it has been studied and indicated for the treatment of circadian rhythm sleep disorders, such as delayed sleep phase disorder, free-running disorder in blind people, jet lag disorder, and shiftwork sleep disorder (27–30). However, in this section, we will focus on the use of exogenous melatonin for the treatment of insomnia.

When Dr. Aaron Lerner first identified the pineal hormone melatonin, he connected it to previously described lightening effects of pineal extracts on amphibian skin. He gave melatonin to patients with vitiligo, hoping to treat the skin condition, but instead noted that his patients became sleepy (13,31). Since then, several other studies have shown that administration of exogenous melatonin during the biological day (when endogenous melatonin levels are low) can promote sleep (32,33). These findings, together with findings of an association between decreased level of nocturnal melatonin and pineal calcification (34,35) with insomnia provide further rationale for using melatonin to improve sleep quality in insomniacs. However, clinical studies on the efficacy of melatonin for the treatment of insomnia have yielded inconsistent results. Such inconsistencies may be due to differences in pharmacokinetic properties of the melatonin preparation, purity of the formulations, doses, and timing of administration that were used in the various studies (36). Furthermore, clinical studies have not used well-defined inclusion and exclusion criteria, and outcome measures to evaluate melatonin's efficacy have been inconsistent across studies.

This latter point is highlighted in recent meta-analyses and systematic reviews that evaluated the efficacy and safety of exogenous melatonin in the treatment of primary and secondary sleep disorders (37,38). One meta-analysis of 14 randomized controlled trials concluded that with short-term use, melatonin was ineffective in treating most primary sleep disorders, including insomnia. Although the authors did note that melatonin may be useful for the treatment of sleep-onset insomnia associated with delayed sleep phase disorder (38). However, a meta-analysis of 17 studies that included mixed populations of healthy volunteers, insomnia patients, and individuals with psychiatric conditions concluded that melatonin is both effective in improving sleep efficiency and decreasing sleep-onset latency (37).

Some of the more positive effects of melatonin treatment for insomnia have come from studies in older adults (39–43), in particular those with low melatonin levels (34,39,41,44). Of the various formulations of melatonin used, the prolonged-release (PR) formulations appear to produce more consistent improvements in sleep maintenance (41), latency to persistent sleep (LPS) (42), and subjective sleep quality (43). The effects of three-week prolonged-release melatonin 2 mg was evaluated in a multicenter, randomized placebo-controlled study in 170 patients, aged 55 years and older with primary insomnia (43). In this large study, prolonged-release melatonin improved measures of subjective sleep quality and morning alertness. There were no withdrawal or rebound symptoms upon discontinuation and the adverse effects were generally mild and not significantly different from placebo. Yet, it is important to note that there are also studies in which melatonin did not improve sleep quality in older adults with insomnia (45,46).

Melatonin has also been studied for the treatment of sleep disturbances in older adults with dementia. Similar to the studies in general adults, studies in patients with dementia have yielded inconsistent results (47,48). The largest multicenter randomized placebo-controlled study of patients with Alzheimer Disease failed to show significant improvements in actigraphy derived sleep measures with melatonin 5 mg, but there was a trend for improvement in the group that received 10 mg (47,48). A recent randomized controlled trial in older adults with dementia showed that melatonin 2.5 mg taken in the evening shortened sleep-onset latency and increased average sleep duration by 27 minutes (47,48). However, melatonin had negative effects on affect and also increased withdrawn behavior. Interestingly, these adverse effects were not seen if melatonin was given in combination with daytime bright light, suggesting that in this patient population, although low-dose melatonin can improve sleep, it is more effective when combined with bright light exposure during the day (49).

While melatonin has been shown to be effective in treating insomnia in some studies, the lack of large-scale, double-blind, placebo-controlled clinical trials in the general adult population with insomnia, the variety of available preparations, differences in doses used, and concerns about long-term effects have led the NIH State-of-the Science Consensus Statement on Chronic Insomnia panel to conclude that "While melatonin appears to be effective for the treatment of circadian rhythm disorders, little evidence exists for efficacy in the treatment of insomnia or its appropriate dosage. In short-term use, melatonin is thought to be safe, but there is no information about the safety of long-term use" (50).

MELATONIN RECEPTOR AGONISTS

Ramelteon, a selective MT_1 and MT_2 receptor agonist is the first melatonin receptor agonist to be approved by the FDA for the treatment of insomnia, characterized by sleep-onset difficulty [for a review (51)]. In comparison with melatonin, ramelteon had longer half-life (1–2.6 hours), greater affinity and selectivity for the MT_1 and MT_2 receptor binding sites, and low affinity for the MT_3 binding site (52). Ramelteon is metabolized via cytochrome P450 (CYP isoenzymes), predominantly CYP1A2 to several metabolites. One of these metabolites, M-II, is a much less potent MT_1 and MT_2 receptor agonist, with a half-life of 2 to 4 hours.

Randomized multicenter clinical trials have shown that ramelteon reduces sleep-onset latency in those with transient (53,54) and chronic insomnia (55–59). In a model of transient insomnia in healthy adults, administration of ramelteon significantly decreased the time to fall asleep when compared to placebo (53,54). In patients with chronic primary insomnia, ramelteon 8 mg taken 30 minutes before bedtime improved LPS in the first week and for the duration of five-week (55,60) and six-month studies (61). Subjective sleep latency improved in some, but not in all studies, and was not maintained at all time points throughout the six-month period. Improvements in other objective and self-reported sleep parameters, including total sleep time were inconsistent among various studies.

Ramelteon has also been studied in special populations, such as older adults. Older adults are particularly interesting because melatonin levels may decline with aging (62,63). In a large study of older adults, 65 to 93 years with chronic insomnia ramelteon administration over a five-week period significantly decreased self-reported sleep latency (56,57,64). However, there were no significant differences between ramelteon and placebo on sleep quality and number of awakenings.

In the clinical studies, ramelteon was generally well tolerated and was not associated with withdrawal, abuse or rebound insomnia (55,57,65). The most common adverse events were headache, somnolence, dizziness, and fatigue (55,56). Furthermore, ramelteon had no significant effect on cognitive or psychomotor function compared to placebo (58,65) and no impact on balance in the middle-of-the-night testing (61,66). Studies of long-term use (six months) on endocrine function showed increases in prolactin in women, without measurable effects on reproductive function (67). Other safety studies have included patients with mild to moderate (68) and severe (69) chronic obstructive pulmonary disease (COPD) or obstructive sleep apnea (70) in which administration of 8 mg of ramelteon showed no significant reductions in oxygen saturation (68,69).

Melatonin Receptor Agonists in Development

Since the introduction of ramelteon in 2005, there has been an interest to develop other melatonin receptor agonist for the treatment of circadian rhythm sleep disorders and insomnia. Of these, clinical data is available for agomelatine, tasimelteon, and TIK-301.

There is limited clinical trial data on the efficacy and tolerability of TIK-301 (β-methyl-6-chloromelatonin). This compound is a melatonin analogue with high affinity for the MT_1 and MT_2 receptors. In a double-blind placebo-controlled phase II trial in patients with moderate to severe primary insomnia, TIK-301 was shown to produce a dose dependent (5–100 mg) reduction in sleep latency (71).

Agomelatine (S20098) is a high-affinity MT_1 and MT_2 receptor agonist (72) and a 5-HT_{2C} and 5-HT_{2B} receptor antagonist (73). Agomelatine has been shown to have effects on both the circadian system and in mood regulation. Its circadian effects include promotion of sleep via its action on melatonin receptors in the SCN (74) and resetting of the timing of circadian rhythms (56). Although agomelatine is being developed primarily for the treatment of anxiety (75) and depression (76–78). [for a review (79)] It has also been shown to improve sleep quality in studies of major depressive disorder (43) and generalized anxiety disorder (75).

Tasimelteon (VEC-162) is an MT_1 and MT_2 agonist that has been studied in phase II and phase III trials in healthy adults in a model of transient insomnia induced by a 5-hour phase advance of the sleep–wake cycle (80). In both the phase II and phase III trials, tasimelteon was given 30 minutes prior to bedtime at doses of 10 mg, 20 mg, 50 mg, and 100 mg. In the phase II trial, only tasimelteon 100 mg significantly advanced dim light melatonin onset compared to the placebo group. In the phase III trial, tasimelteon increased sleep efficiency and total sleep time and decreased LPS (80). The most consistent improvements in objective and subjective sleep quality measures were seen with tasimelteon 50 mg. Tasimelteon was generally well tolerated.

SUMMARY

Endogenous melatonin produced by the pineal gland plays an important role in sleep–wake regulation. While exogenous melatonin has been shown to possess sleep-promoting properties, studies on its effectiveness in the treatment of adults with chronic insomnia have yielded inconsistent results. Some of these inconsistencies may be related to the differences in the study populations, type of formulation, dose, and outcome measures of efficacy between studies. Within the area of insomnia, the most promising results for melatonin come from studies in late-middle age and older adults. Although melatonin has been shown to be effective in some short-term studies of insomnia and found to be generally safe in low doses of 1 to 5 mg, more short-term and long-term multicenter randomized clinical trials are needed before evidence-based clinical guidelines can be established for its use in the treatment of insomnia.

The development of melatonin receptor agonists with more specific and stronger affinities for particular receptor subtypes within the SCN will likely lead to improved understanding of the role of endogenous melatonin in sleep regulation and help develop more targeted therapies for insomnia.

ACKNOWLEDGMENTS

Funding for this work was provided by a National Institutes of Health grant R01HL069988.

REFERENCES

1. Zee PC, Manthena P. The brain's master circadian clock: Implications and opportunities for therapy of sleep disorders. Sleep Med Rev 2007; 11(1):59–70.
2. Inouye ST. Ventromedial hypothalamic lesions eliminate anticipatory activities of restricted daily feeding schedules in the rat. Brain Res 1982; 250(1):183–187.
3. Meijer JH, Rietveld WJ. Neurophysiology of the suprachiasmatic circadian pacemaker in rodents. Physiol Rev 1989; 69(3):671–707.
4. van den Pol, The hypothalamic suprachiasmatic nucleus of rat: Intrinsic anatomy. J Comp Neurol 1980; 191(4):661–702.
5. Czeisler CA, et al. Stability, precision, and near-24-hour period of the human circadian pacemaker. Science 1999; 284(5423):2177–2181.
6. Moore-Ede MC, Czeisler CA, Richardson GS. Circadian timekeeping in health and disease. Part 1. Basic properties of circadian pacemakers. N Engl J Med 1983; 309(8):469–476.
7. Czeisler CA, Wright KPJ. Influence of light on circadian rhythmicity in humans. In: FW Turck, PC Zee, eds. Neurobiology of Sleep and Circadian Rhythms. New York: Marcel Dekker, 1999:149–180.
8. Dijk DJ, Lockley SW. Integration of human sleep-wake regulation and circadian rhythmicity. J Appl Physiol 2002; 92(2):852–862.
9. Aston-Jones G. Brain structures and receptors involved in alertness. Sleep Med 2005; 6(suppl 1):S3–S7.
10. Chou TC et al. Afferents to the ventrolateral preoptic nucleus. J Neurosci 2002; 22(3):977–990.
11. Deurveilher S, Semba K. Indirect projections from the suprachiasmatic nucleus to major arousal-promoting cell groups in rat: Implications for the circadian control of behavioural state. Neuroscience 2005; 130(1):165–183.
12. Zhang S et al. Lesions of the suprachiasmatic nucleus eliminate the daily rhythm of hypocretin-1 release. Sleep 2004; 27(4):619–627.
13. Lerner AB et al. Isolation of melatonin, the pineal gland factor that lightens melanocytes. J Am Chem Soc 1958; 80:2587.
14. Moore RY. Suprachiasmatic nucleus in sleep-wake regulation. Sleep Med 2007; 8(suppl 3):27–33.
15. Moore RY. Neural control of the pineal gland. Behav Brain Res 1996; 73(1–2):125–130.
16. Burgess HJ et al. The relationship between the dim light melatonin onset and sleep on a regular schedule in young healthy adults. Behav Sleep Med 2003; 1(2):102–114.
17. Monk TH et al. Circadian rhythms in human performance and mood under constant conditions. J Sleep Res 1997; 6(1):9–18.
18. Nakamura TJ et al. Light response of the neuronal firing activity in the suprachiasmatic nucleus of mice. Neurosci Lett 2004; 371(2–3):244–248.
19. Jin X et al. Targeted disruption of the mouse Mel(1b) melatonin receptor. Mol Cell Biol 2003; 23(3):1054–1060.
20. Liu C et al. Molecular dissection of two distinct actions of melatonin on the suprachiasmatic circadian clock. Neuron 1997; 19(1):91–102.
21. Dubocovich ML. Melatonin receptors: Role on sleep and circadian rhythm regulation. Sleep Med 2007; 8(suppl 3):34–42.
22. Hunt AE et al. Activation of MT(2) melatonin receptors in rat suprachiasmatic nucleus phase advances the circadian clock. Am J Physiol Cell Physiol 2001; 280(1):C110–C118.
23. Dubocovich ML et al. Molecular pharmacology, regulation and function of mammalian melatonin receptors. Front Biosci 2003; 8:d1093–d1108.
24. Nosjean O et al. Identification of the melatonin-binding site MT3 as the quinone reductase 2. J Biol Chem 2000; 275(40):31311–31317.
25. Burgess HJ, Revell VL, Eastman CI. A three pulse phase response curve to three milligrams of melatonin in humans. J Physiol 2008; 586(2):639–647.

26. Lewy AJ et al. The human phase response curve (PRC) to melatonin is about 12 hours out of phase with the PRC to light. Chronobiol Int 1998; 15(1):71–83.
27. Mundey K et al. Phase-dependent treatment of delayed sleep phase syndrome with melatonin. Sleep 2005; 28(10):1271–1278.
28. Nagtegaal JE et al. Delayed sleep phase syndrome: A placebo-controlled cross-over study on the effects of melatonin administered five hours before the individual dim light melatonin onset. J Sleep Res 1998; 7(2):135–143.
29. Lewy AJ et al. Capturing the circadian rhythms of free-running blind people with 0.5 mg melatonin. Brain Res 2001; 918(1–2):96–100.
30. Sack RL et al. Entrainment of free-running circadian rhythms by melatonin in blind people. N Engl J Med 2000; 343(15):1070–1077.
31. Nordlund JJ, Lerner AB. The effects of oral melatonin on skin color and on the release of pituitary hormones. J Clin Endocrinol Metab 1977; 45(4):768–774.
32. Reid K, van den Heuvel C, Dawson D. Day-time melatonin administration: Effects on core temperature and sleep onset latency. J Sleep Res 1996; 5(3):150–154.
33. Wyatt JK et al. Sleep-facilitating effect of exogenous melatonin in healthy young men and women is circadian-phase dependent. Sleep 2006; 29(5):609–618.
34. Leger D, Laudon M, Zisapel N. Nocturnal 6-sulfatoxymelatonin excretion in insomnia and its relation to the response to melatonin replacement therapy. Am J Med 2004; 116(2):91–95.
35. Mahlberg R et al. Degree of pineal calcification (DOC) is associated with polysomnographic sleep measures in primary insomnia patients. Sleep Med 2008; 10(4):439–445.
36. Doghramji K. Melatonin and its receptors: A new class of sleep-promoting agents. J Clin Sleep Med 2007; 3(5)(suppl):S17–S23.
37. Brzezinski A et al. Effects of exogenous melatonin on sleep: A meta-analysis. Sleep Med Rev 2005; 9(1):41–50.
38. Buscemi N et al. The efficacy and safety of exogenous melatonin for primary sleep disorders. A meta-analysis. J Gen Intern Med 2005; 20(12):1151–1158.
39. Garfinkel D et al. Improvement of sleep quality in elderly people by controlled-release melatonin. Lancet 1995; 346(8974):541–544.
40. Wurtman RJ, Zhdanova I. Improvement of sleep quality by melatonin. Lancet 1995; 346(8988):1491.
41. Haimov I et al. Melatonin replacement therapy of elderly insomniacs. Sleep 1995; 18(7): 598–603.
42. Hughes RJ, Sack RL, Lewy AJ. The role of melatonin and circadian phase in age-related sleep-maintenance insomnia: Assessment in a clinical trial of melatonin replacement. Sleep 1998; 21(1): 52–68.
43. Lemoine P et al. Prolonged-release melatonin improves sleep quality and morning alertness in insomnia patients aged 55 years and older and has no withdrawal effects. J Sleep Res 2007; 16(4): 372–380.
44. Zhdanova IV et al. Melatonin treatment for age-related insomnia. J Clin Endocrinol Metab 2001; 86(10):4727–4230.
45. Dawson D et al. Effect of sustained nocturnal transbuccal melatonin administration on sleep and temperature in elderly insomniacs. J Biol Rhythms 1998; 13(6):532–538.
46. Baskett JJ et al. Does melatonin improve sleep in older people? A randomised crossover trial. Age Ageing 2003; 32(2):164–170.
47. Asayama K et al. Double blind study of melatonin effects on the sleep-wake rhythm, cognitive and non-cognitive functions in Alzheimer type dementia. J Nippon Med Sch 2003; 70(4):334–341.
48. Singer C et al. A multicenter, placebo-controlled trial of melatonin for sleep disturbance in Alzheimer's disease. Sleep 2003; 26(7):893–901.
49. Riemersma-van der Lek RF et al. Effect of bright light and melatonin on cognitive and noncognitive function in elderly residents of group care facilities: A randomized controlled trial. JAMA 2008; 299(22):2642–2655.
50. National Institutes of Health. NIH State-of-the-Science Conference Statement: Manifestations and Management of Chronic Insomnia in Adults. NIH Consensus and State-of-the-Science Statements. Bethesda: National Institutes of Health 2005; 22(2): 1–30.
51. Simpson D, Curran MP. Ramelteon: A review of its use in insomnia. Drugs 2008; 68(13):1901–1919.
52. Kato K et al. Neurochemical properties of ramelteon (TAK-375), a selective MT1/MT2 receptor agonist. Neuropharmacology 2005; 48(2):301–310.
53. Roth T, Stubbs C, Walsh JK. Ramelteon (TAK-375), a selective MT1/MT2-receptor agonist, reduces latency to persistent sleep in a model of transient insomnia related to a novel sleep environment. Sleep 2005; 28(3):303–307.
54. Zammit G et al. The effects of ramelteon in a first-night model of transient insomnia. Sleep Med 2009; 10(1):55–59.

55. Mini L, Wang-Weigand S, Zhang J. Ramelteon 8 mg/d versus placebo in patients with chronic insomnia: Post hoc analysis of a 5-week trial using 50% or greater reduction in latency to persistent sleep as a measure of treatment effect. Clin Ther 2008; 30(7):1316–1323.
56. Mini LJ, Wang-Weigand S, Zhang J. Self-reported efficacy and tolerability of ramelteon 8 mg in older adults experiencing severe sleep-onset difficulty. Am J Geriatr Pharmacother 2007; 5(3):177–184.
57. Roth T et al. Effects of ramelteon on patient-reported sleep latency in older adults with chronic insomnia. Sleep Med 2006; 7(4):312–318.
58. Roth T et al. A 2-night, 3-period, crossover study of ramelteon's efficacy and safety in older adults with chronic insomnia. Curr Med Res Opin 2007; 23(5):1005–1014.
59. Stigler KA, Posey DJ, McDougle CJ. Ramelteon for insomnia in two youths with autistic disorder. J Child Adolesc Psychopharmacol 2006; 16(5):631–636.
60. Zammit G et al. Evaluation of the efficacy and safety of ramelteon in subjects with chronic insomnia. J Clin Sleep Med 2007; 3(5):495–504.
61. Wang-Weigand S, Mayer G, Roth-Schechter B. Long Term Efficacy and Safety of Ramelteon 8 mg Treatment in Adults with Chronic Insomnia: Results of a Six Month, Double Blind, Placebo Controlled, Polysomnography Trial in World Congress of the World Federation of Sleep Research and Medicine Societies. Cairns, Queensland, Australia; 2007: A525.
62. Iguchi H. Age dependent changes in the serum melatonin concentrations in healthy human subjects and in patients with endocrine and hepatic disorders and renal failure (author's transl). Fukuoka Igaku Zasshi 1981; 72(7):423–430.
63. Sack RL et al. Human melatonin production decreases with age. J Pineal Res 1986; 3(4):379–388.
64. Turek FW, Gillette MU. Melatonin, sleep, and circadian rhythms: Rationale for development of specific melatonin agonists. Sleep Med 2004; 5(6):523–532.
65. Johnson MW, Suess PE, Griffiths RR. Ramelteon: A novel hypnotic lacking abuse liability and sedative adverse effects. Arch Gen Psychiatry 2006; 63(10):1149–1157.
66. Hajak G, Ebrahim I, M H. Effect of ramelteon and zopiclone on body sway at peak plasma levels in chronic insomnia [abstract NR611]. In: Conference Proceedings of the160thAnnual Meeting of the American Psychiatric Association; 2007; San Diego, CA.
67. Richardson G, Wang-Weigand S. Effects of long-term exposure to ramelteon, a melatonin receptor agonist, on endocrine function in adults with chronic insomnia. Hum Psychopharmacol 2008; 24(2):103–111.
68. Kryger M et al. Effect of ramelteon, a selective MT(1)/MT (2)-receptor agonist, on respiration during sleep in mild to moderate COPD. Sleep Breath 2008; 12(3):243–250.
69. Kryger M et al. The effects of ramelteon on respiration during sleep in subjects with moderate to severe chronic obstructive pulmonary disease. Sleep Breath 2009; 13(1):79–84.
70. Kryger M, Wang-Weigand S, Roth T. Safety of ramelteon in individuals with mild to moderate obstructive sleep apnea. Sleep Breath 2007; 11(3):159–164.
71. Zemlan FP et al. The efficacy and safety of the melatonin agonist beta-methyl-6-chloromelatonin in primary insomnia: A randomized, placebo-controlled, crossover clinical trial. J Clin Psychiatry 2005; 66(3):384–390.
72. Yous S et al. Novel naphthalenic ligands with high affinity for the melatonin receptor. J Med Chem 1992; 35(8):1484–1486.
73. Millan MJ et al. The novel melatonin agonist agomelatine (S20098) is an antagonist at 5-hydroxytryptamine2 C receptors, blockade of which enhances the activity of frontocortical dopaminergic and adrenergic pathways. J Pharmacol Exp Ther 2003; 306(3):954–964.
74. Ying SW et al. Melatonin analogues as agonists and antagonists in the circadian system and other brain areas. Eur J Pharmacol 1996; 296(1):33–42.
75. Stein DJ, Ahokas AA, de Bodinat C. Efficacy of agomelatine in generalized anxiety disorder: A randomized, double-blind, placebo-controlled study. J Clin Psychopharmacol 2008; 28(5):561–566.
76. Bourin M, Mocaer E, Porsolt R. Antidepressant-like activity of S 20098 (agomelatine) in the forced swimming test in rodents: Involvement of melatonin and serotonin receptors. J Psychiatry Neurosci 2004; 29(2):126–133.
77. Montgomery SA, Kasper S. Severe depression and antidepressants: Focus on a pooled analysis of placebo-controlled studies on agomelatine. Int Clin Psychopharmacol 2007; 22(5):283–291.
78. Loo H, Hale A, D'Haenen H. Determination of the dose of agomelatine, a melatoninergic agonist and selective 5-HT(2C) antagonist, in the treatment of major depressive disorder: A placebo-controlled dose range study. Int Clin Psychopharmacol 2002; 17(5):239–247.
79. Dolder CR, Nelson M, Snider M. Agomelatine treatment of major depressive disorder. Ann Pharmacother 2008; 42(12):1822–1831.
80. Rajaratnam SM et al. Melatonin agonist tasimelteon (VEC-162) for transient insomnia after sleep-time shift: Two randomised controlled multicentre trials. Lancet 2008; 373(9662):482–491.

36 Nonprescription Pharmacotherapies: Alcohol, Over-the-Counter, and Complementary and Alternative Medicines

David N. Neubauer

Department of Psychiatry, Johns Hopkins Bayview Medical Center, Johns Hopkins University School of Medicine, Baltimore, Maryland, U.S.A.

Kelleen N. Flaherty

Department of Biomedical Writing, University of the Sciences in Philadelphia, Philadelphia, Pennsylvania, U.S.A.

INTRODUCTION

A large percentage of individuals with insomnia self-medicate with alcohol, over-the-counter (OTC) antihistamines, or complementary and alternative preparations (1,2). In the United States, the formulation and manufacture of OTC products are regulated by the U.S. Food and Drug Administration (FDA). Other products not requiring a prescription, such as dietary supplements, are unregulated. The National Center for Complementary Health and Alternative Medicine (NCCAM) at the National Institutes of Health (NIH) defines "complementary and alternative medicine (CAM)" as "practices that are unproven by science and not presently considered an integral part of conventional medicine" (3). CAM encompasses a variety of dietary supplements, herbal compounds, or formulations containing a mixture of these (4,5). Individuals seeking relief from insomnia may also combine two or more of *any* agents for insomnia (including prescription medications, OTC agents, alcohol, and CAM preparations) (6). Alcohol is the substance most commonly used to self-medicate for insomnia. Some 1.6 million noninstitutionalized adults with insomnia are estimated to use CAM to treat their insomnia or difficulties in sleeping (7); 20% of the population using herbals alone (8). The popularity of CAM in general is increasing; a 2007 national survey of adults and children found that 38.3% of U.S. adults using any CAM increased from 36% in 2002. Of those individuals using CAM in 2007, 1.4% of adults and 1.8% of children were doing so for insomnia. Nonvitamin, nonmineral products accounted for most (17%) CAM use (9).

Despite the perceived efficacy of these agents by the individuals who use them, there are several concerns associated with their use. There have been very few controlled studies conducted on most of these substances, and the available evidence has demonstrated little or no clinical efficacy. Safety data are similarly scant or lacking (10,11). Since CAM preparations are not regulated by the FDA, the consistent potency and product purity are not assured (10,12–14). Compounding this, many herbal products are mixtures of more than one type of herb. The FDA may intervene to remove a product from the market or issue advisories or warnings only when significant safety concerns are evident, as was the case with tryptophan in 1990 (10,13,15,16) and kava kava in 2002 (17). Although generally regarded as benign, the use of CAM substances may be associated with clinically important and sometimes lethal adverse effects, such as the liver toxicity reported for kava kava, as well as the myriad problems associated with excessive alcohol use (10,12,18). CAM tends to be used more by individuals experiencing insomnia comorbid with other chronic conditions, particularly psychiatric illness (e.g., anxiety and mood disorders), congestive heart failure, hypertension, and obesity (7,19). Apart from the fact that comorbid conditions themselves may lower the risk threshold associated with use of certain OTC and CAM products (such as CNS and GI effects with antihistamine use (20) or hepatotoxicity with kava kava) (8,10,18), the potential for pharmacologic interactions is also significant (10,13). St. John's wort, for example, is an inducer of cytochrome P450 isoenzymes (8,10) and has the potential to interfere with protease inhibitors, chemotherapeutic agents, and oral contraceptives (21). Kava kava, valerian, and St. John's wort may interact with anesthetics (22), and tryptophan may have toxic effects when used concomitantly with certain psychiatric medications (11). Further complicating these issues, most of the OTC and CAM products are perceived by patients to be safe, as they often are touted to be "natural" (8), or are not considered dangerous since they do not require a prescription. Frequently patients do not report their use of these agents to their physicians when listing their "real" medications and physicians are not necessarily aware that they should inquire about them (12,19).

ALCOHOL

Large-scale studies have estimated that 13% to 28% of individuals with insomnia use alcohol specifically to induce sleep (6,23). One Japanese study reported the use of alcohol as a sleep-promoting agent in 48% of male survey respondents (24). A National Sleep Foundation (NSF) survey conducted in 1991 found that some 30% of their respondents with chronic insomnia used alcohol as a sleep aid, and that 67% of them found it to be effective in reducing sleep latency (25). Alcohol is a CNS depressant; its hypnotic properties may be a consequence of multiple pharmacologic effects, including its interaction with gamma-aminobutyric acid (GABA) and glutamate (26,27). Its effects on sleep have been investigated for decades, often in controlled trials, but frequently with conflicting results. Some studies have shown that alcohol does, in fact, decrease sleep latency (28–31), while others have shown that it does not (23,32,33). The effects of alcohol on sleep typically are dose dependent (10,23) and may also depend upon the chronicity of the insomnia as compared with individuals without insomnia (23). While total sleep time (TST) is not usually affected by alcohol intake, a dose-dependent redistribution of REM sleep and NREM sleep stages is common, although this has not been demonstrated consistently. A common finding is REM suppression during the first half of the night, followed by REM rebound (or "mini withdrawal") during the latter half of the night as the alcohol is metabolized and the serum level decreases (23,26,30,31). An increase in NREM stages 3 and 4 sleep during the first half of the night may be associated with alcohol ingestion (31), as may an increase in NREM stage 1 and waking in the latter half of the night (30). Low doses of alcohol have been shown to increase TST and therefore, may result in mildly beneficial effects (23,32). Development of tolerance to alcohol develops quickly, often within three nights in healthy volunteers (31), and is associated with a concomitant return to normal sleep architecture (26). Use of alcohol as a sleep aid has also been shown to impair secretion of growth hormone (GH), independent of slow wave sleep (SWS) alterations (26,34); exacerbate snoring and sleep apnea (23,35); and worsen restless legs syndrome (RLS) (2). Nightly use of alcohol can cause or worsen insomnia or exacerbate other psychiatric conditions such as depression or anxiety (36). Chronic use of alcohol for insomnia may lead to the development of alcohol dependence (36,37). Finally, it has been argued that an improved mood associated with the use of alcohol may be contributing to beneficial effects on sleep (23). Given the potentially significant problems associated with the regular use of alcohol as a sleep-inducing agent, its use should be discouraged.

ANTIHISTAMINES

First-generation antihistamines, such as diphenhydramine, doxylamine, chlorpheniramine (as well as the prescription drugs hydroxyzine and doxepin), are pharmacodynamic antagonists at central histamine H_1 receptors. The first-generation antihistamines are liposoluble and readily cross the blood-brain barrier, and may be associated with significant anticholinergic and sedative effects, hence their popularity as OTC sleep aids (38–40). Diphenhydramine is by far the most common antihistamine encountered in OTC sleep aids, either by itself (e.g., Nytol®, Sominex®) or in combination with pain relievers in "nighttime" or "PM" formulations (e.g., Tylenol PM®). Diphenhydramine has a t_{max} of 1.7 (±1) hours, a $t_{1/2}$ of 9.2 (±2.5) hours, and a duration of action of approximately 12 hours (39). Subjective improvement of sleep onset and sleep quality are common in subjects taking diphenhydramine (typically at a dose of 25–50 mg) (2,10,41–45), but few randomized, placebo-controlled studies assessing the safety and efficacy of diphenhydramine in the treatment of insomnia have been conducted. Efficacy in at least one sleep parameter has been demonstrated in populations of adults (41), geriatric subjects (including those in long-term care) (44,45), pediatric subjects (42), and psychiatric patients (43). A 1983 double-blind, placebo-controlled, crossover study evaluated the use of diphenhydramine 50 mg in adult subjects complaining of difficulty with sleep onset. On the basis of subjective assessments (daily sleep logs), diphenhydramine was significantly more effective than placebo at decreasing sleep latency, decreasing frequency of awakenings, decreasing wake time after sleep onset (WASO), increasing sleep duration, and increasing quality of sleep. Subjective physician assessment of efficacy was similar (41).

While diphenhydramine has been shown to be associated with sedation and improvement in sleep parameters such as sleep onset, duration, and quality, it also is associated with significant safety concerns regarding its relatively long half-life and its anticholinergic properties resulting from postsynaptic muscarinic receptor antagonism. Complaints of residual sedation, drowsiness, or grogginess during the morning or daytime following bedtime use are common (11,38,41). The anticholinergic activity has the potential to cause other side effects, such as diminished cognitive function and delirium, dry mouth, blurred vision, urinary retention, constipation, and risk of increased intraocular pressure in individuals with narrow-angle glaucoma (11). Undesired sedation, delirium, and anticholinergic effects are of particular concern in geriatric patients (11,46). Additionally, there are potential pharmacokinetic and pharmacodynamic interactions with concomitant medications, CAM substances, and alcohol. Caution is advised when patients are taking other medications with anticholinergic effects. Diphenhydramine also exacerbates the adverse effects of ethanol upon oculomotor coordination, cognitive function, and driving ability (40). An additional concern with the use of diphenhydramine as a sleep aid is the possible development of tolerance to its sedating effects. In one study in healthy volunteers, diphenhydramine was administered 50 mg twice daily and sleepiness was assessed both objectively and subjectively throughout the day. Development of tolerance to the sedating effects of diphenhydramine was observed after administration of the medication for four consecutive days (47). The development of tolerance results in reduced efficacy and may contribute to the development of dependence or abuse. Tolerance to the antihistamine sedating effects may lead to dose escalation and other possible reinforcing effects, such as euphoria. Antihistamine abuse has been documented; case reports exist for doses of diphenhydramine as high as 3000 mg per day (48). The position of the American Academy of Sleep Medicine (AASM) on diphenhydramine is as follows: "Sufficient evidence does not exist to support over-the-counter (OTC) sleep aids . . . OTC sleep aids that contain antihistamine may provide modest, short-term benefits for adults with mild cases of insomnia. It is important to be aware, however, that the use of antihistamines may produce a variety of side effects" (49).

MELATONIN

Melatonin is a pineal hormone involved in the regulation of circadian rhythms. Although it has sleep-promoting effects on healthy volunteers and has been assessed in a small number of controlled clinical trials, its efficacy in the treatment of insomnia has not been well established (50,51), and some controlled studies have shown it to be indistinguishable from placebo (52). Melatonin generally is considered to be safe, but its safety in long-term use has not been demonstrated (11,50). Melatonin is a very popular dietary supplement. The 2002 Alternative Health/Complementary and Alternative Medicine Supplement to the National Health Interview Survey (NHIS) interviewed an age and socioeconomically representative population of 31,044 individuals about use of 25 pharmacologic and nonpharmacologic CAM therapies, including melatonin. The use of melatonin was reported by 5.2% of the respondents and of those individuals, 27.5% identified insomnia as at least one reason for its use. Most melatonin use occurred without physician consultation (52). A retrospective meta-analytic study was conducted in 2005 by Buscemi and colleagues evaluating the safety and efficacy of melatonin in the treatment of primary insomnia. Initially, 1884 melatonin studies were identified; however, only 14 met the randomized-controlled trial criteria for assessment of efficacy and only 10 met the criteria for safety assessment (50). Mean improvement of sleep latency was 11.7 minutes. Two studies in the insomnia meta-analysis also investigated the efficacy of melatonin in shortening sleep onset in subjects with delayed sleep phase syndrome (DSPS). Subjects with DSPS taking melatonin experienced an average improvement in sleep latency of 38.8 minutes, as compared with 7.2 minutes in subjects with insomnia. The meta-analysis also assessed secondary outcome measures such as sleep efficiency, sleep quality, wakefulness after sleep onset (WASO), TST, and percentage of time spent in REM sleep. None of these secondary measures reached statistical significance. Safety assessment (headache, nausea, dizziness, drowsiness) showed no significant difference in adverse events between melatonin and placebo. The study group for the meta-analysis concluded that there was little evidence supporting the use of melatonin as an exogenous sleep aid, although it might be useful for treating DSPS. The researchers also concluded that melatonin appears to be safe, at least for short-term use (up to three months) (50).

A second meta-analysis by Brzezinski and colleagues evaluated the effects of exogenous melatonin on sleep in 17 randomized, double-blind, placebo-controlled trials using objective measures of sleep evaluation and including at least six adult subjects with no severe disabling systemic disease (53). Crossover and parallel group designs were included, but case studies were not. This meta-analysis was a review of the trials investigating the effects of melatonin on sleep and not on insomnia per se. However, nine of the trials in this meta-analysis involved participants with insomnia (five of the insomnia studies were also included in the Buscemi meta-analysis). In a subanalysis of healthy subjects with no relevant medical condition other than insomnia, subjects administered exogenous melatonin had shorter sleep onset by an average of 3.9 minutes, higher sleep efficiency by an average of 3.1%, and a longer TST by an average of 13.7 minutes. The authors concluded that there was statistically significant evidence demonstrating that the use of exogenous melatonin improves sleep latency, sleep efficiency, and TST (53). However, it remains unclear whether these modest changes represent clinically significant improvements. The meta-analysis authors also concluded that melatonin generally is safe, at least for short-term use in adults.

The role of melatonin in sleep-wake regulation and the use of exogenous melatonin and melatonin agonists as sleep aids is discussed further in chapter 35.

L-TRYPTOPHAN

L-tryptophan is an essential amino acid and dietary precursor of serotonin. The role it plays in the biochemistry of sleep and its impact on sleep architecture have not been fully elucidated, although it has been regarded as a "natural" sleep aid. Its purported positive effects on sleep onset and maintenance are based on very few and mostly uncontrolled clinical studies that often included noninsomniac subjects (10,19,54–57). L-tryptophan may be most beneficial in subjects with mild insomnia or in normal subjects with situational insomnia accompanied by longer-than-average sleep onset (58,59). Tryptophan generally is considered to be safe and reportedly is not associated with visuomotor, cognitive, or memory impairment. However, L-tryptophan as a supplement was removed from the market in 1989 because of the development of an often serious and sometimes fatal (37 attributed deaths) eosinophilia myalgia syndrome (EMS) in some individuals who had taken one of several tryptophan-containing products. The cause of the eosinophilia myalgia syndrome was ultimately traced to a contaminant from a single manufacturer, and L-tryptophan is once again available (2,15,16). Nevertheless, the NIH chronic insomnia State-of-the-Science summary report cautions against the use L-tryptophan due to possible adverse effects, particularly if used in conjunction with psychiatric medications (11). When concern about L-tryptophan developed and its availability became limited, 5-hydroxy-L-tryptophan (5-HTP, the immediate precursor to serotonin, or 5-HT) grew in popularity as a "natural hypnotic." After the L-tryptophan recall, scrutiny of 5-HTP for serious adverse events was high, but no definitive toxicity with use of the agent has been confirmed (15). 5-HTP is commercially produced by extraction from the seeds of *Griffonia simplicifolia,* a woody African shrub. Effects of 5-HTP on insomnia are inconclusive (10,19).

HERBAL PREPARATIONS AND DIETARY SUPPLMENTS

Herbal products used as CAM are prepared from roots, stems, flowers, buds, or leaves of plants. These plant products can be used whole, dried, crushed, and steeped as tea; other preparations contain extracts. While some herbal preparations have shown some efficacy in improving some sleep parameters in a few studies, most studies are small and uncontrolled or anecdotal in nature. As production of these compounds is not overseen by the FDA, purity and consistency are not assured. Significant adverse events may be associated with the use of some of these herbal products. Individuals perceive these agents to be safe because they're "natural" and frequently do not report use of these supplements to their physicians.

Valerian (Valerian Root, All Heal, Garden Heliotrope, Vandal Root)

Valeriana officinalis is a perennial herb used in a variety of herbal supplements either by itself or in combination with other agents. Among its major ingredients are valerenic acid, valepotriates, sesquiterpenes, and hydroxypinoresinol; aqueous extracts contain significant concentrations of gamma aminobutyric acid (GABA). The sedative and anxiolytic effects of valerian have been attributed to the valepotriates and sesquiterpenes in the volatile oils (19). Studies have also shown that valerian extract and valerenic acid are partial agonists of the 5-HT_{5A} receptor (60). Valerian-containing preparations have been assessed in many studies, including some randomized, placebo-controlled trials, subjective assessments, and polysomnographic studies. However, given the multiple pharmacologically active components of the herb and the lack of consistency in manufacturing, the elucidation of its effects is difficult (2,10). Significant improvements in both objective and subjective measures of sleep onset, wakefulness after sleep onset, and sleep quality have been reported, but many studies also have shown no statistical improvement in these measures. Valerian has not been shown to affect sleep architecture. Response to valerian is typically dose dependent (10,22). Although generally considered to be safe, some concerns exist about its potential for interaction with alcohol (61), anesthetics (22), the CYP3A4 metabolic pathway, as well as for potential interactions with sedatives, such as benzodiazepines or barbiturates (2,61). Hallucinations, hepatotoxicity, and withdrawal effects also have been reported (2,19,62), but case reports are rare. In the Alternative Health/Complementary and Alternative Medicine Supplement to the NHIS, 5.9% of individuals surveyed reported using valerian, 29.9% of whom identified insomnia as at least one reason for doing so. As with melatonin use in this study, less than half of the individuals using valerian did so without consultation with a health care provider (52). The 2005 NIH chronic insomnia State-of-the-Science summary report concluded that the limited evidence shows no benefit compared with placebo (11).

Kava Kava (Awa, Kawa, Intoxicating Pepper)

Kava kava, which is derived from a pepper plant, *Piper methysticum,* is reported to have sedative and anxiolytic properties (22). Its CNS pharmacologic effects are thought to include blockade of voltage-gated sodium and calcium ion channels, enhanced ligand binding to $GABA_A$ receptors (although there is also evidence for lack of binding to GABA or benzodiazepine receptors), diminished excitatory neurotransmitter release, and reduced neuronal reuptake of norepinephrine. Several of these pharmacodynamic actions may contribute to the purported hypnotic properties (18,19). Sleep-promoting effects of kava kava have been reported, although mostly in anecdotal or uncontrolled studies, and not necessarily in populations of insomnia subjects (63). Most research on the safety and efficacy of kava kava has been with anxiety outcomes. One internet-based, randomized, placebo-controlled trial showed no statistical difference in improvement of sleep scores (Insomnia Severity Index, sleep latency, and frequency of nocturnal awakening) with the use of kava kava as compared with placebo (64). Another nonblinded trial assessing the efficacy of treating stress-related insomnia did, however, show significant improvement of symptoms with use of kava kava as compared with placebo (63). While there are concerns about the interaction of kava kava with other medications such as CNS depressants and dopamine antagonists (22,65), the major concern associated with its use is hepatotoxicity. Seventy-eight cases of hepatotoxity (via diffuse hepatocellular necrosis, cholestatic hepatitis, or isolated gamma-GTP increase) were recognized after 1998, including 11 cases requiring liver transplantation (4 resulting in death). The supplement was banned in the European Union and Canada, and the U.S. FDA issued a consumer advisory in 2002 (17,18). Its use should be strongly discouraged for this reason, particularly in any individual with hepatic impairment.

St. John's Wort (Amber Touch and Heal, Goat Weed, Hardhay, Hypericum, SJW, Klamath Weed, Millepertuis, Rosin Rose, Tipton Weed)

Hypericum perforatum is a perennial herb indigenous to Europe, but found across the United States. It has been used for medicinal purposes for millennia. The above-ground portion of the plant is dried and a red liquid is extracted to create the dietary supplements. There are several pharmacologically active compounds in St. John's wort, but those most likely to be responsible for sleep-promoting effects are hypericin and hyperforin. *Hypericum* may exert its effects through impact on catecholamine neurotransmission, via inhibition of neurotransmitter metabolism, modulation of neurotransmitter receptor density and sensitivity, and synaptic reuptake inhibition (14). Although the exact mechanism of action of *Hypericum* remains unknown, hyperforin has been demonstrated to inhibit the reuptake of serotonin, norepinephrine, dopamine, GABA, and L-glutamate (10). Almost all of the safety and efficacy studies of St. John's wort have been for its utility in managing depression; none have been conducted for insomnia. However, the effects of St. John's wort on sleep architecture have been assessed in healthy volunteers with varying results, including inconsistent reports of increased latency to REM sleep and increased percentage of slow wave sleep (10,14). Adverse events associated with the use of St. John's wort include fatigue, gastrointestinal upset, dizziness, anxiety, headache, photosensitivity, and phototoxicity. The significant concern associated with the use of St. John's wort, however, is its potential interactions with other drugs. Of all the popular herbal supplements, St. John's wort is the most problematic as far as pharmacokinetic interactions are concerned. St. John's wort is an inducer of several CYP450 isoenzymes, including CYP3A4. Studies have shown that St. John's wort decreases cyclosporine levels; may be associated with breakthrough bleeding in women on oral contraceptives; lowers concentration levels of statins, midazolam, nifedepine, protease inhibitors, theophylline, and tricyclic antidepressants; decreases the effects of warfarin; can have significant interactions with SSRI antidepressants, anesthetics, digoxin, loperamide, chemotherapeutic agents, and thyroid medications; and may contribute to the development of the serotonin syndrome (14,21). Individuals taking any medications that are metabolized by the CYP450 system should be cautioned against using St. John's wort.

Miscellaneous Herbs Used as Sleep Aids

Passionflower (*Passiflora incarnata*), Skullcap (*Scutellaria laterifolia*), Jamaica dogwood (*Piscidia erythrina* or *Piscidia piscipula*), chamomile (*Anthemis nobilis*), hops (*Humulus lupulus*), lavender (*Lavandula officinalis*), wild lettuce (*Lactuca virosa*), California poppy (*Escholtzschia californica*), lemon balm (*Melissa officinalis*) and other herbs (and combinations of herbs) are commonly marketed as natural remedies for insomnia. Little or no safety and efficacy studies have been performed on these botanicals. Apart from Jamaica dogwood, which can be toxic if used in large amounts (it is used as a fish poison and is the source of rotenone), no reports of toxicities to any of these plant products has been made.

The position of the AASM on herbal supplements as a remedy for insomnia is as follows: "There is only limited scientific evidence to show that herbal supplements are effective sleep aids. Because these products may be marketed and sold without FDA approval and may involve dangerous side effects or adverse drug interactions, they should be taken only if approved by a physician" (66).

Vitamin and Mineral Supplements

Minimal information (often case reports) is available on the use of vitamins to treat sleep disturbances. There are no randomized controlled clinical trials, and conclusions from studies that have been performed are preliminary and provide the caveat that more studies are needed. Some vitamins and minerals are hypothesized to have an impact on sleep based on evidence that subjects who have taken high doses of certain vitamins and minerals experience disturbed sleep or grogginess as a side effect (vitamin A and calcium are examples) (10,67). Two small, uncontrolled trials evaluating nicotinamide have reported improved sleep (increased REM sleep in one, and increased sleep efficiency in another) (68). Magnesium has been reported to enhance the secretion of melatonin and therefore, may help promote sleep, but no studies on its use with insomnia have been published (69). Vitamin B_{12} has been shown to have a significant effect on circadian rhythm disorder in some case reports, but also has not been investigated for the treatment of insomnia (10). In one large study of 519 subjects assessing the relationship between vitamin use and sleep, significantly impaired sleep was seen in subjects taking multivitamins or multiple single vitamins as compared with those not taking vitamins. Concomitant use of herbal medicines, however, was not taken into account for this study. The authors concluded that these results may be explained by the possibility that vitamins cause poor sleep, poor sleepers seek vitamins, or unidentified factors promote both poor sleep and vitamin use, and that more controlled studies are needed (67).

Table 1 Nonprescription Pharmacotherapeutic Agents used as Sleep Aids

Nonprescription agent	Reported effects on sleep in ≥ 1 study	Safety concerns
Alcohol		
Alcohol	Decreases sleep latency (28–31) Does *not* decrease sleep latency (23,32,33) ↑ TST by low doses (23,32) ↓ REM first half of night ↑ REM latter half of night ↑ NREM 3/4 first half of night (23,26,30,31) ↑ NREM 1, ↑ waking in second half of night (30)	Tolerance (31) ↓ Secretion GH (26,34) ↑ Snoring, sleep apnea (23,35) Worsens RLS (2) Cause or worsen insomnia (36) Exacerbate comorbid psychiatric conditions (36) Dependence (36,37)
Antihistamines		
Diphenhydramine	Subjective (physician and subject) improvement of sleep onset and quality, ↓ awakenings, ↑ TST (2,10, 41–45) Efficacy in at least one sleep parameter seen in adults, geriatric subjects, pediatric subjects, and psychiatric patients (41–45)	Anticholinergic effects, particularly in older individuals (11,38–40,46) Residual sedation, grogginess; long half-life (11,38,41) Interaction with concomitant medications, CAM agents, alcohol Tolerance (47) Abuse (48)
Dietary Supplements		
Melatonin	↓ Onset in some studies (50) Effective in DSPS (50)	Essentially not different from placebo; safe in short-term (≤ 3 months) (53)
L-tryptophan	Might be beneficial in mild or situational insomnia (58,59)	Removed from market in 1989 due to fatality-related impurities; has since been restored with caveats (2,15,16) Possible interactions if used with psychiatric medicines (11)
Valerian	Significant improvements in both objective and subjective measures of sleep onset, WASO, and sleep quality have been reported (10,22) Not been shown to affect sleep architecture (10,22)	Potential interaction with alcohol, (61) anesthetics, (22) the CYP3A4 metabolic pathway, and sedatives (2, 61) Hallucinations, hepatotoxicity, and withdrawal effects have been reported (2,19,62)
Kava kava	Sleep-promoting effects have been observed in anecdotal/uncontrolled studies (63) Improvement in stress-related insomnia symptoms in 1 trial (63)	Interaction with CNS depressants and dopamine antagonists (22,65) Significant hepatotoxicity that can lead to liver transplantation and death (17,18) Warning: *do not take with hepatic impairment*
St. John's wort	Inconsistent results of ↑ latency to REM sleep, ↑ % SWS (10,14)	Fatigue, GI upset, dizziness, anxiety, headache, photosensitivity, phototoxicity (14,21) Significant concern with drug interactions; induces several CYP450 enzymes, especially CYP3A4 Studies: may cause decreased concentrations of or have significant interactions with certain prescription medications Warning: *do not take concomitantly with medications that are metabolized by the CYP 450 system*
Nicotinamide	↑ REM sleep (68; small, uncontrolled trial) ↑ Sleep efficiency (68; small, uncontrolled trial)	

Abbreviations: CAM, complementary and alternative medicine; DSPS, delayed sleep phase syndrome; GH, growth hormone; GI, gastrointestinal; NREM, non rapid-eye movement (sleep); REM, rapid-eye movement (sleep); RLS, restless leg syndrome; SWS, slow wave sleep; TST, total sleep time; WASO, wakefulness after sleep onset.

SUMMARY

A variety of nonprescription pharmacologic agents are widely used as sleep aids (Table 1). Although the most frequently used substance to induce sleep, alcohol has not been determined to be safe or efficacious as a sleep aid or in the treatment of insomnia. OTC antihistamine sleep aids may be popular because they are readily accessible, do not require a prescription, and are perceived to be safe. Herbal and dietary supplements, such as melatonin and valerian, may be appealing to consumers because they are viewed as "natural" products. Accordingly, it are not surprising that the use of OTC and CAM compounds is widespread. However, data are scant or lacking on the safety and efficacy of most of these agents, some can have serious side effects or cause significant drug interactions, and consistent purity and concentration of the unregulated marketed agents are not assured. Increased awareness of the potential safety issues associated with OTC and CAM agents is required by both consumers and health care professionals alike.

REFERENCES

1. Roehrs T, Hollebeek E, Drake C, et al. Substance use for insomnia in Metropolitan Detroit. J Psychosom Res 2002; 53 (1):571–576.
2. Curry DT, Eisenstein RD, Walsh JK. Pharmacologic management of insomnia: Past, present, and future. Psychiatr Clin North Am 2006; 29 (4):871–893.
3. Expanding Horizons of Health Care: NCCAM Strategic Plan, 2005–2009. National Center for Complementary Health and Alternative Medicine, National Institutes of Health; 2004.
4. Cvetanovic I, Golbin D. Polysomnographic evaluations of the effect of Nytex (natural supplements) in insomniac patients. Sleep 2007; 30(abstract Suppl):A230–A231.
5. Morin CM, Koetter U, Bastien C, et al. Valerian-hops combination and diphenhydramine for treating insomnia: A randomized placebo-controlled clinical trial. Sleep 2005; 28(11):1465–1471.
6. Johnson EO, Roehrs T, Roth T, et al. Epidemiology of alcohol and medication as aids to sleep in early adulthood. Sleep 1998; 21(2):178–186.
7. Pearson NJ, Johnson LL, Nahin RL. Insomnia, trouble sleeping, and complementary and alternative medicine: Analysis of the 2002 National Health Interview Survey data. Arch Intern Med 2006; 166(16):1775–1782.
8. Bent S. Herbal medicine in the United States: Review of efficacy, safety, and regulation: Grand rounds at University of California, San Francisco Medical Center. J Gen Intern Med 2008; 23(6):854–859.
9. Barnes PM, Bloom B, Nahin RL. Complementary and Alternative Medicine use Among Adults and Children: United States, 2007. National Health Statistics Reports, No. 12. Hyattsville, MD: National Center for Health Statistics, 2008.
10. Meoli AL, Rosen C, Kristo D, et al. Oral nonprescription treatment for insomnia: An evaluation of products with limited evidence. J Clin Sleep Med 2005; 1(2):173–187.
11. National Institutes of Health. National Institutes of Health State of the Science Conference Statement on Manifestations and Management of Chronic Insomnia in Adults, June 13–15, 2005. Sleep 2005; 28(9):1049–1057.
12. Huntley A. Over-the-counter herbals and drug interactions: Getting the (right) message across. Expert Opin Drug Saf 2006; 5(1):5–6.
13. Cobert BL. Herbal remedies and drug interactions: An issue overlooked by health authorities. Expert Opin Drug Saf 2006; 5(1):7.
14. Greeson JM, Sanford B, Monti DA. St. John's wort *(Hypericum perforatum):* A review of the current pharmacological, toxicological, and clinical literature. Psychopharmacology (Berl) 2001; 153(4): 402–414.
15. Das YT, Bagchi M, Bagchi D, et al. Safety of 5-hydroxy-L-tryptophan. Toxicol Lett 2004; 150(1): 111–122.
16. Criswell LA, Sack KE. Tryptophan-induced eosinophilia-myalgia syndrome. West J Med 1990; 153(3):269–274.
17. U.S. Food and Drug Administration Center for Food Safety and Applied Nutrition. Kava-containing Dietary Supplements May Be Associated with Severe Liver Injury. http://www.fda.gov/Food/ResourcesForYou/Consumers/ucm085482.htm. Published March 25, 2002. Updated May 4, 2009. Accessed June 1, 2009.
18. Clouatre DL. Kava kava: Examining new reports of toxicity. Toxicol Lett 2004; 150(1):85–96.
19. Fugh-Berman A, Cott JM. Dietary supplements and natural products as psychotherapeutic agents. Psychosom Med 1999; 61(5):712–728.
20. Cirillo V, Tempero K. Pharmacology and therapeutic use of antihistamines. Am J Hosp Pharm 1976; 33(1200):1207.
21. Hammerness P, Basch E, Ulbricht C, et al. St John's wort: A systematic review of adverse effects and drug interactions for the consultation psychiatrist. Psychosomatics 2003; 44(4):271–282.

22. Ang-Lee MK, Moss J, Yuan CS. Herbal medicines and perioperative care. JAMA 2001; 286(2):208–216.
23. Roehrs T, Papineau K, Rosenthal L, et al. Ethanol as a hypnotic in insomniacs: Self administration and effects on sleep and mood. Neuropsychopharmacology 1999; 20(3):279–286.
24. Kaneita Y, Uchiyama M, Takemura S, et al. Use of alcohol and hypnotic medication as aids to sleep among the Japanese general population. Sleep Med 2007; 8(7–8):723–732.
25. Ancoli-Israel S, Roth T. Characteristics of insomnia in the United States: Results of the 1991 National Sleep Foundation Survey. I. Sleep 1999; 22(suppl 2):S347–S353.
26. Roehrs T, Roth T. Sleep, sleepiness, and alcohol use. Alcohol Res Health 2001; 25(2):101–109.
27. Koob GF. The neuropharmacology of ethanol's behavioral action: New data, new paradigms, new hope. In: Dietrick RA, Erwin VG, eds. Pharmacological Effects of Ethanol on the Nervous System. New York: CRC Press, 1996:1–12.
28. Rundell OH, Lester BK, Griffiths WJ, et al. Alcohol and sleep in young adults. Psychopharmacologia 1972; 26(3):201–218.
29. MacLean AW, Cairns J. Dose-response effects of ethanol on the sleep of young men. J Stud Alcohol 1982; 43(5):434–444.
30. Williams DL, MacLean AW, Cairns J. Dose-response effects of ethanol on the sleep of young women. J Stud Alcohol 1983; 44(3):515–523.
31. Williams H, Salamy A. Alcohol and sleep. In: Kissin B, Begleiter H, eds. The Biology of Alcoholism. New York: Plenum Press, 1972:435–483.
32. Stone BM. Sleep and low doses of alcohol. Electroencephalogr Clin Neurophysiol 1980; 48(6):706–709.
33. Dijk DJ, Brunner DP, Aeschbach D, et al. The effects of ethanol on human sleep EEG power spectra differ from those of benzodiazepine receptor agonists. Neuropsychopharmacology 1992; 7(3):225–232.
34. Ekman AC, Vakkuri O, Ekman M, et al. Ethanol decreases nocturnal plasma levels of thyrotropin and growth hormone but not those of thyroid hormones or prolactin in man. J Clin Endocrinol Metab 1996; 81(7):2627–2632.
35. Dawson A, Bigby BG, Poceta JS, et al. Effect of bedtime alcohol on inspiratory resistance and respiratory drive in snoring and nonsnoring men. Alcohol Clin Exp Res 1997; 21(2):183–190.
36. Weissman MM, Greenwald S, Nino-Murcia G, et al. The morbidity of insomnia uncomplicated by psychiatric disorders. Gen Hosp Psychiatry 1997; 19(4):245–250.
37. Janson C, Lindberg E, Gislason T, et al. Insomnia in men—A 10-year prospective population based study. Sleep 2001; 24(4):425–430.
38. Roth T, Roehrs T, Koshorek G, et al. Sedative effects of antihistamines. J Allergy Clin Immunol 1987; 80(1):94–98.
39. del Cuvillo A, Mullol J, Bartra J, et al. Comparative pharmacology of the H1 antihistamines. J Investig Allergol Clin Immunol 2006; 16(suppl 1):3–12.
40. Montoro J, Sastre J, Bartra J, et al. Effect of H1 antihistamines upon the central nervous system. J Investig Allergol Clin Immunol 2006; 16(suppl 1):24–28.
41. Rickels K, Morris RJ, Newman H, et al. Diphenhydramine in insomniac family practice patients: A double-blind study. J Clin Pharmacol 1983; 23(5–6):234–242.
42. Russo RM, Gururaj VJ, Allen JE. The effectiveness of diphenhydramine HCl in pediatric sleep disorders. J Clin Pharmacol 1976; 16(5–6):284–288.
43. Kudo Y, Kurihara M. Clinical evaluation of diphenhydramine hydrochloride for the treatment of insomnia in psychiatric patients: A double-blind study. J Clin Pharmacol 1990; 30(11):1041–1048.
44. Meuleman JR, Nelson RC, Clark RL Jr. Evaluation of temazepam and diphenhydramine as hypnotics in a nursing-home population. Drug Intell Clin Pharm 1987; 21(9):716–720.
45. Glass JR, Sproule BA, Herrmann N, et al. Effects of 2-week treatment with temazepam and diphenhydramine in elderly insomniacs: A randomized, placebo-controlled trial. J Clin Psychopharmacol 2008; 28(2):182–188.
46. Conn DK, Madan R. Use of sleep-promoting medications in nursing home residents: Risks versus benefits. Drugs Aging 2006; 23(4):271–287.
47. Richardson GS, Roehrs TA, Rosenthal L, et al. Tolerance to daytime sedative effects of H1 antihistamines. J Clin Psychopharmacol 2002; 22(5):511–515.
48. Thomas A, Nallur DG, Jones N, et al. Diphenhydramine abuse and detoxification: A brief review and case report. J Psychopharmacol 2009; 23(1):101–105.
49. American Academy of Sleep Medicine. AASM Position Statement: Treating Insomnia with Over-the-Counter Sleep Aids. Westchester, IL: American Academy of Sleep Medicine, 2006.
50. Buscemi N, Vandermeer B, Hooton N, et al. The efficacy and safety of exogenous melatonin for primary sleep disorders. A meta-analysis. J Gen Intern Med 2005; 20(12):1151–1158.
51. Reiter RJ. Melatonin: Clinical relevance. Best Pract Res Clin Endocrinol Metab 2003; 17(2):273–285.
52. Bliwise DL, Ansari FP. Insomnia associated with valerian and melatonin usage in the 2002 National Health Interview Survey. Sleep 2007; 30(7):881–884.

53. Brzezinski A, Vangel MG, Wurtman RJ, et al. Effects of exogenous melatonin on sleep: A meta-analysis. Sleep Med Rev 2005; 9(1):41–50.
54. Lindsley JG, Hartmann EL, Mitchell W. Selectivity in response to L-tryptophan among insomniac subjects: A preliminary report. Sleep 1983; 6(3):247–256.
55. Boman B. L-tryptophan: A rational anti-depressant and a natural hypnotic? Aust N Z J Psychiatry 1988; 22(1):83–97.
56. Hartmann E. L-tryptophan: A possible natural hypnotic substance [editorial]. JAMA 1974; 230(12): 1680–1681.
57. Hartmann E. L-tryptophan: A rational hypnotic with clinical potential. Am J Psychiatry 1977; 134(4): 366–370.
58. Hartmann E. Effects of L-tryptophan on sleepiness and on sleep. J Psychiatr Res 1982; 17(2):107–113.
59. Schneider-Helmert D, Spinweber CL. Evaluation of L-tryptophan for treatment of insomnia: A review. Psychopharmacology (Berl) 1986; 89(1):1–7.
60. Dietz BM, Mahady GB, Pauli GF, et al. Valerian extract and valerenic acid are partial agonists of the 5-HT5a receptor in vitro. Brain Res Mol Brain Res 2005; 138(2):191–197.
61. Miller LG. Herbal medicinals: Selected clinical considerations focusing on known or potential drug-herb interactions. Arch Intern Med 1998; 158(20):2200–2211.
62. Winslow LC, Kroll DJ. Herbs as medicines. Arch Intern Med 1998; 158(20):2192–2199.
63. Wheatley D. Medicinal plants for insomnia: a review of their pharmacology, efficacy and tolerability. J Psychopharmacol 2005; 19(4):414–421.
64. Jacobs BP, Bent S, Tice JA, et al. An internet-based randomized, placebo-controlled trial of kava and valerian for anxiety and insomnia. Medicine (Baltimore) 2005; 84(4):197–207.
65. Bressler R. Herb-drug interactions: Interactions between kava and prescription medications. Geriatrics 2005; 60(9):24–25.
66. American Academy of Sleep Medicine. AASM Position Statement: Treating Insomnia with Herbal Supplements. Westchester, IL: American Academy of Sleep Medicine, 2006.
67. Lichstein KL, Payne KL, Soeffing JP, et al. Vitamins and sleep: An exploratory study. Sleep Med 2008; 9(1):27–32.
68. Robinson CR, Pegram GV, Hyde PR, et al. The effects of nicotinamide upon sleep in humans. Biol Psychiatry 1977; 12(1):139–143.
69. Durlach J, Pages N, Bac P, Bara M, Gviet-Bara A. Biorhythms and possible central regulation of magnesium status, phototherapy, darkness therapy, and chronopathologic forms of magnesium depletion. Magnes Res 2002; 15(1–2):49–66.

37 Current Advances in the Pharmacotherapy of Insomnia: Pipeline Agents

Michael J. Sateia

Department of Psychiatry, Dartmouth Medical School, Lebanon, New Hampshire, U.S.A.

Medications used for the treatment of insomnia during the past century have largely employed two basic mechanisms for sleep promotion. Prescription sleeping pills such as barbiturates, benzodiazepines (BZDs), and other BZD receptor agonistic modulators (BzRAs) act at the $GABA_A$ receptor complex to enhance GABA inhibitory activity and promote sleep. Over-the-counter sleep medications have been and continue to be formulations of nonselective histamine antagonists such as diphenhydramine or doxylamine. Advances in the understanding of neurochemical control of sleep–wake, coupled with identification of previously unknown transmitters, such as hypocretin/orexin, have created new horizons in the pharmacotherapy of insomnia. While some pipeline development continues to target activation of sleep-promoting GABAergic mechanisms, many of the current pharmaceutical efforts are directed at the identification of safe and efficacious medications that antagonize wake-active transmitter systems such as orexin, $5\text{-}HT_{2A}$, and histamine. Other agents are targeted at the melatonin system, potentially expanding the choice of such agents beyond ramelteon. Certain pipeline drugs offer multiple potential mechanisms of sleep-promoting action.

The following chapter attempts to capture the cross section of compounds in development as of 2009. However, a review of this literature underscores the unpredictability of pharmacological research and development. Failures to replicate initially promising efficacy data, emergence of unforeseen adverse reactions, shifts in the competitive environment, and numerous other factors create an ever-changing field. In recent years, numerous promising drugs have been derailed, sometimes in late stages of development. Therefore, in considering compounds discussed in this chapter, one should keep in mind that, in all likelihood, many, if not most, of the drugs discussed will never achieve FDA approval. Despite that, the research engendered in discovery and development of these agents often serves to advance our knowledge of not only pharmacotherapy but also sleep–wake biology itself.

GABA AGONISTIC MODULATORS

GABA is the major inhibitory neurotransmitter in the brain, and GABAergic neurons of the ventrolateral preoptic (VLPO) region of the hypothalamus demonstrate maximum firing rates during sleep. For most of the past century, prescription agents for the treatment of insomnia have exerted their primary mechanism of action on the GABA receptor complex. This is true for the barbiturate compounds, widely used in the first half of the 20th century, as well as the benzodiazepine agents, the dominant prescription medications since the late 1960s. The BZDs and their more recently developed cousins (imidazopyridines, pyrazolopyrimidines, and cyclopyrrolones), collectively referred to as benzodiazepine receptor agonists (BzRA), bind at various subunits of the BZD receptor, located on the $GABA_A$ receptor complex, and exert a modulating action that, in the presence of GABA, enhances chloride flux across the membrane and hyperpolarizes the cell. BZDs themselves show little selectivity in receptor subtype binding, while newer agents demonstrate greater selectivity primarily for the α_1-receptor subunit. The pharmacology and clinical application of these agents is discussed extensively in preceding chapters.

One newer BzRA agent, indiplon, has been in the pipeline for some time and undergone full phase III trials (1–5). Indiplon, in both immediate and modified-release formulations, was submitted for FDA approval that was denied in 2006. Particular concerns focused on the higher dose, extended-release formulation, which was deemed not approvable. To date, the future of this agent remains uncertain.

EVT 201 (Evotec AG), a partial positive allosteric GABA receptor modulator in pre-clinical studies, has undergone initial assessments for the treatment of primary insomnia. Sleep was evaluated in 75 subjects who received placebo, EVT 201 (1.5 or 2.5 mg), in a cross-over design (6). Two nights of polysomnography (PSG) and subjective sleep ratings indicated significantly shorter latency to persistent sleep, greater total sleep time (TST), fewer awakenings, and reduced wake after sleep onset. Sleep maintenance improvements were observed into the third and fourth quarters of the night. Quality ratings were improved and no major adverse events were reported, although mild effects on morning digit symbol substitution test were noted. A phase II, randomized, placebo-controlled study (7) of EVT 201 in 149 elderly primary insomnia subjects demonstrated increased TST, reduced latency to persistent sleep (LPS) and wakefulness after sleep onset (WASO), and objective improvements in daytime alertness by multiple sleep latency test (MSLT).

Adipiplon (NG2-73; Neurogen) has also been demonstrated to have partial GABA agonist activity selective for the BZD α_3-subunit in pre-clinical studies. The unique selectivity profile would theoretically promote both hypnotic and antianxiety effect. Phase I/II trials have been conducted. These demonstrated significant reductions in sleep latency, reduction in WASO, and improvements in TST and sleep efficiency (8,9). However, in a more recent phase II/III trial, with an Ambien CR comparison, an unexpectedly high rate of adverse effects was reported (10). As a result, Neurogen announced in 2008 that they had no further plans to advance adipiplon at that time.

Further modifications to existing BzRA agents are also in various stages of development. A longer-acting preparation (SKP-1041) of zaleplon, a short-acting agent with an elimination half-life of only about one hour, is currently being evaluated. Somnus Therapeutics, Inc., has allied with SkyePharma (SKP) to develop a longer-acting preparation using SKP's GeoLock controlled release technology. To date, only phase I assessment data of pharmacodynamics, using varied formulations, have been published (11,12). Results show differing time courses of sleep promotion using the MSLT as a primary evaluation tool, suggesting potential efficacy for sleep-maintenance problems. Further clinical studies are currently underway. Intec Pharma has also reported on development of a gastro-retentive formulation of zaleplon (zaleplon GR), which provides a sustained duodenal infusion of the drug through the night.

An oral spray form of zolpidem (ZolpiMist®; NovaDel Pharma, Inc.) was approved in late 2008 for short-term treatment of sleep-onset insomnia. At dosages of 5 and 10 mg, the spray formulation produced therapeutic levels more rapidly than standard zolpidem tablets (13). Commercialization efforts for the product are in progress.

A sublingual preparation of zolpidem (Edluar®, formerly Sublinox®) was approved for short-term treatment of sleep initiation difficulty in March, 2009, and is now marketed in the U.S. Recent studies (14) have demonstrated that sleep latency with this formulation is significantly more rapid compared to standard, orally administered zolpidem. Another zolpidem sublingual preparation (Intermezzo®; Transcept Pharmaceuticals, Inc.), in low-dose formulation (1.75 mg and 3.5 mg) is being evaluated for treatment of middle-of-the-night (MOTN) awakening (15). Eighty-two patients with primary sleep maintenance problems were administered sublingual zolpidem (1.75 mg or 3.5 mg) or placebo following awakening. Latency to persistent sleep after middle-of-the-night awakenings were significantly lower and TST increased compared to placebo. Subjective ratings of sleep quality were improved at the higher dose. There was no evidence of morning impairment by Digit Symbol Substitution or subjective assessment of sleepiness. As of this writing, the FDA has requested additional safety data for MOTN dosing.

Other, novel agents targeted at the GABA receptor have also been explored. Gaboxadol, a GABA analogue and select agonist, unlike BzRAs enhances slow wave activity and has been shown to reduce sleep latency and improve efficiency in healthy subjects and insomniacs (16–21). However, efforts to obtain FDA approval for gaboxadol for the treatment of insomnia have been abandoned at the present time.

OREXIN ANTAGONISTS

The orexin (hypocretin) system was independently described by two groups in the late 1990s (22,23). This system consists of a relatively small number of neurons located in the lateral hypothalamus, with extensive projections to brain regions involved in the regulation of sleep–wake, among others. Subsequent determinations that disruptions of this system play a key role in the pathogenesis of narcolepsy with cataplexy fueled further interest in the role of orexin neurons in sleep–wake regulation (24,25). It has since been demonstrated that orexin neurons serve a controller function for other wake–active systems of the brain, including other hypothalamic regions [histaminergic neurons of the tubero-mamillary nucleus (TMN)], cholinergic basal forebrain and lateral dorsal / pedunculopontine nuclei, noradrenergic locus coeruleus, and serotonergic dorsal raphe neurons (26). Orexin receptors are widely distributed in the brain. Activation of orexin neurons and their downstream targets promotes wakefulness.

Orexins are neuropeptides derived from a larger neuropeptide, prepro-orexin. Orexin A (hypocretin-1) and orexin B (hypocretin-2) act on two receptors, OX_1 and OX_2 (27). OX_1 receptors are most heavily distributed in locus coeruleus while OX_2 receptors are expressed particularly in histaminergic hypothalamic regions (TMN). Current evidence suggests that these receptors play a critical role in induction/maintenance of wakefulness. Thus, it is not surprising that there is significant ongoing investigation of orexin antagonists as potential sleep-promoting medications.

Although there are a number of orexin antagonists in various stages of evaluation, the most extensively studied to date is almorexant (Actelion-078573), a dual, selective and competitive antagonist at both OX_1 and OX_2 receptors. Almorexant has an elimination half-life that varies from 6 to 19 hours. Its effects on sleep have been evaluated in rats, dogs and humans. Brisbare-Roch et al. (28). reported that almorexant, administered during the active period in rats, increased indices of both NREM and REM sleep. Increases in NREM efficiency were comparable to those observed with zolpidem and significantly greater than placebo. The increased proclivity to sleep was accompanied by reduced locomotor activity as well. Similar effects were observed with repeated dosing.

In humans, doses from 1 to 1000 mg were administered during morning hours. Brief (25 minutes) quantitative electroencephalographic (EEG) recordings were conducted 90 minutes following administration and showed dose-dependent reduction in latency to persistent sleep. Increases in theta and delta power were observed in the almorexant group but not in the zolpidem group. Sedating effects resolved in dose-dependent fashion with effects no longer evident for all but the maximal (1000 mg) dosage by 6.5 hours.

In these studies, the agent was apparently well tolerated; the most common adverse events included somnolence, fatigue, reduced attention, dizziness, and diplopia. Of note, no evidence of cataplectic-type events was observed in any species.

Initial proof-of-concept trials (29) in humans involved a randomized, placebo-controlled crossover study of 161 primary insomnia subjects who underwent two nights polysomnography. Dose-dependent improvement of sleep efficiency (by PSG) was observed at 50, 100, 200, and 400 mg. A dose-dependent trend to decrease in latency to persistent sleep and WASO was also reported. A reduction in REM latency was noted but there was overall maintenance or increase of REM%. No evidence of waking REM-intrusion symptoms was seen. Subjective ratings of sleep were improved and the drug was apparently well tolerated with an absence of significant daytime impairments.

Currently, almorexant is in phase III trials (RESTORA), which began in 2008 with expected enrollment of 670 primary insomnia patients (30). Primary endpoints of the randomized, placebo-controlled study will include measures of sleep onset and maintenance. A zolpidem reference arm is also included.

GSK 649868 (GlaxoSmithKline Pharmaceuticals Ltd.) is a second orexin antagonist currently in phase II trials. Preliminary data (31) in healthy subjects and 52 patients with primary insomnia show dose-dependent improvement versus placebo of sleep latency, wake after sleep time, and TST at doses of 30 and 60 mg. REM sleep was also increased at the higher dose.

Other orexin antagonists are also being investigated but are in earlier phases of development. The OX_2 antagonist, JNJ-10397049, is highly selective, with little evidence of binding at OX_1 receptors (32). Comparison studies between almorexant and JNJ-10397049 have been performed in rats. This preliminary work demonstrates that both agents reduce latency to persistent NREM sleep, although the selective OX_2 demonstrated this effect at dosages 10 times lower than the dual antagonist (almorexant). MK-4305 (Merck & Co., Inc.) is also currently in phase II development (33).

5-HT_{2A} ANTAGONISTS

Serotonergic neurons of the dorsal raphe play an important role in regulation of sleep and wakefulness. An understanding of the function of serotonin (5-HT) in control of sleep–wake has continued to evolve and is complicated by the heterogeneity of numerous receptor subtypes. Serotonin activity of the dorsal raphe is at its highest firing rate during wake. Firing rate of these neurons decreases with onset of NREM sleep and becomes negligible during REM sleep. A great deal of research in this area has focused on the 5-HT_2 family of receptors. It has been shown that activation of 5-HT_{2A} receptors is associated with tonic inhibition of NREM sleep (34). Correspondingly, antagonism at the 5-HT_{2A} receptor results in promotion of increased slow wave activity in sleep (35).

These observations have led to significant interest in 5-HT_2 antagonists as potential therapies in the management of insomnia. Ritanserin, a potent 5-HT_2 antagonist, has been studied with respect to its effects on sleep in animals and humans. Early work demonstrated that administration of ritanserin to young, poor sleepers resulted in a doubling of slow wave activity, with a corresponding decrease in N2 (stage 2 sleep) (36). Subsequent work has revealed comparable increases in slow wave sleep in healthy volunteers (37), middle-aged poor sleepers (38), and dysthymic patients (39). Some of these data have also suggested a reduction in frequency of awakening (38) and improvement in subjective sleep quality (36). Ritanserin has also been evaluated as a treatment for patients with schizophrenia (40). However, its patent has expired without the drug ever becoming FDA-approved. In recent years, atypical antipsychotic medications with potent 5-HT_{2A} and H_1 antagonistic properties such as quetiapine and olanzapine have been utilized off-label as sleep aids, particularly in psychiatric populations.

Eplivanserin (Ciltyri; Sanofi-aventis) is a 5-HT_{2A} antagonist currently in phase III trials for treatment of insomnia. A randomized, double-blind study (41) of 351 adults with chronic insomnia treated to 4 weeks with either 1 mg or 5 mg of eplivanserin or placebo in the evening found that the 5-mg dose resulted in a mean 39-minute reduction in the baseline 84-minute wake time after sleep onset. This was significantly greater than the mean 26-minute reduction with placebo. Eplivanserin 5 mg/day resulted in a 64% reduction in the number of nocturnal awakenings, compared with a 36% decrease with placebo. More eplivanserin-treated patients reported a significant improvement in the refreshing quality of sleep.

In two phase III, 12-week randomized controlled trial (RCTs) of eplivanserin (42,43) with open-label extension, sleep maintenance insomnia subjects were treated with eplivanserin 5 mg or placebo. Significantly greater reductions in WASO (least square means (LSM) difference = 11.5 min and 13.5 min, respectively) and number of awakenings was observed at 12 weeks with eplivanserin with associated reported improvement in subjective sleep quality and morning concentration. Other studies have demonstrated very significant increase in N3 sleep (44) and delta frequency power on quantitative electroencephalographic analysis (45). In September, 2009, the FDA requested further information from Sanofi-aventis concerning risk–benefit ratio for eplivanserin.

Sanofi-aventis has a second 5-HT_{2A} antagonist, volinanserin, in development, although this agent has not progressed as far in the pipeline as eplivanserin.

Pruvanserin (LY2422347; Eli Lilly and Company) was originally developed by Hypnion, Inc., and obtained by Eli Lilly and Company in 2007. A phase II trial of this drug, which examined its efficacy in the management of sleep-maintenance insomnia, was reportedly commenced in 2006. Published results for this trial were not identified. Eli Lilly and Company does not currently (as of July 1, 2009) list pruvanserin among its pipeline agents (46) and appears to be focused primarily on LY2624803, which has both 5-HT_{2A} antagonist and antihistaminergic properties (discussed in the following section).

Pimavanserin (ACP-103) is a selective 5-HT_{2A} inverse agonist being developed by Acadia Pharmaceuticals, Inc. Although the primary indication in development is for treatment of Parkinson disease (PD) psychosis, a secondary evaluation of its effects on sleep maintenance has also been pursued. In trials with older PD patients, pimavanserin improved psychosis and also resulted in significant increase in slow wave sleep (47).

Another 5-HT_{2A} inverse agonist, ADP-125 (Arena) showed promise in initial smaller trials for treatment of insomnia. However, in late 2008 it was announced that the compound had failed to meet primary or secondary endpoints in a larger phase II study. Indications at that time were that the company no longer planned to pursue development.

In summary, these agents have theoretical promise as a treatment for sleep maintenance insomnia and largely unexplored potential for improving sleep quality in other conditions by virtue of their enhancement of slow wave sleep activity. However, development has been fraught with setbacks and it appears that several of the drugs are no longer in the active pipeline. Eplivanserin is closest to market and its future currently rests on its developer's ability to respond adequately to FDA concerns.

MELATONIN AGONISTS

Melatonin is an endogenous peptide that is synthesized and released by the pineal gland. It represents the key "darkness" signal in mammalian CNS. Exogenously administered melatonin, available as an over-the-counter nutritional supplement, has been used by millions in the treatment of insomnia, particularly over the past two decades. Distinct from its usage as an effective chronobiological agent, its efficacy for chronic insomnia is not especially well established. Meta-analyses (48,49) show mixed results with pooled data suggesting very modest improvement in sleep parameters of uncertain clinical significance. Against this background, the only currently approved melatonin agonist, ramelteon, was launched in 2005. This agent produces modest reductions of sleep latency in patients with chronic insomnia, but its very short half-life limits its application primarily to sleep-onset difficulties.

Other melatonin agonists are presently in testing. Tasimelteon (VEC-162; Vanda Pharmaceuticals, Inc.), a potent MT1/MT2 receptor agonist has been studied in phase II and III trials. The phase II trial (50) involved 39 healthy subjects who were studied at baseline for 3 nights, for 3 treatment nights with tasimelteon (at dosages of 20 mg, 50 mg, or 100 mg) or placebo, with a 5-hour phase advance of schedule, and for one night following treatment. Reductions of PSG sleep latency and improved sleep efficiency were observed, along with a dose-dependent advance in melatonin rhythm. In the phase III trial (50) of 411 healthy subjects using the same 5-hour phase advance model of transient insomnia, latency to persistent sleep was significantly reduced and sleep efficiency increased. Wake after sleep onset was reduced at the two lower (20 and 50 mg) dosages. The subjects appeared to tolerate the drug well and there were no indications of adverse events in excess of those seen with placebo.

A subsequent phase III trial (51) of 322 subjects with chronic insomnia characterized by sleep initiation difficulty showed significant reductions of latency to persistent sleep, which persisted throughout the five-week study period. No significant improvements were observed in standard measures for wake after sleep onset. Subjects did not show evidence of daytime impairment following use of tasimelteon. Submission of a marketing application for tasimelteon is expected by mid-2011.

Preliminary phase II results of another melatonin agonist, PD-6735, were announced in 2004 (52). Significant reductions in sleep latency were seen in 40 insomnia subjects. However, further development data has not been released on this compound.

TRICYCLIC, COMBINED ACTION, AND OTHER COMPOUNDS

Since the advent of tricyclic medications, the sedative action of many of these drugs has been recognized. Agents such as amitriptyline have been and continue to be employed in low dosages as sleep aids in a variety of conditions. In the past 20 years, the heterocyclic compound, trazodone, has come to occupy an important role in the pharmacological management of insomnia, despite a paucity of data supporting its efficacy. The mechanism of sedation of these medications varies. Doxepin, developed as an antidepressant in 1968, is a tricyclic medication with proven antidepressant efficacy. Its sedative properties have long been recognized. In recent years, doxepin, in dosages far lower than typical antidepressant dosages, has been developed as a sleep-inducing agent. It appears likely that much of its sedative action is derived from potent antihistaminergic properties, although other actions such as anticholinergic effect may also contribute to sedation. One of the initial investigations of doxepin's hypnotic action was conducted in 2001 (53). This RCT of primary insomnia patients demonstrated significant improvements in sleep efficiency and TST on night 1 and night 28 on doxepin dosages of 25 to 50 mg, while WASO was significantly reduced only on night 1. Sleep latencies were not altered since this population was predominantly sleep-maintenance insomniacs with relatively normal baseline sleep latencies. Subjective sleep and daytime performance ratings were likewise significantly improved. Subsequently, smaller dosages (1, 3, and 6 mg, Silenor®; Somaxon Pharmaceuticals) have been evaluated in phase III trials involving adult (54) and elderly adult (55) primary insomnia subjects. Each subject underwent two nights of PSG during each of five trials separated by 5 to 12 days in a multiple crossover design. An initial single-blind placebo assessment was followed by randomized assignment to one of four sequences with every subject receiving all three doses of doxepin plus placebo. The primary endpoint of wake during sleep showed significant reductions at the 3- and 6-mg dosage. TST, sleep efficiency, and WASO were improved at all three doses. The 6-mg dose produced reduction of subjective time to fall asleep. The efficacy assessment in elderly insomniacs was conducted with identical design and demonstrated comparable results. All dosages were generally well tolerated without indication of significant anticholinergic or other side effects. There did not appear to be significant daytime residual effects. In late 2009 Somaxon received an FDA response to its second submission for approval which indicated continued efficacy concerns and denied approval of the drug in its current form.

Several current pipeline agents demonstrate dual or multiple mechanisms of action, which may prove effective in management of insomnia. One of the most widely studied agents, agomelatine (Servier; as Valdoxan in the European Union), is in development primarily as an antidepressant drug and has already received approval in the European Union. It is in phase III trials in the United States, licensed to Novartis International AG, which expects submission of FDA application no sooner than 2012. The agent has a combined action of 5-HT_{2C} antagonism, coupled with potent melatonin agonistic properties. In addition to its proven antidepressant properties, it demonstrates significant sedative properties.

Lemoine et al. (56) reported significantly greater subjective improvement in "getting to sleep" and sleep quality in 332 patients with major depressive disorder treated with agomelatine 25 to 50 mg qd compared to venlafaxine. Other studies have demonstrated increased TST and sleep efficiency and reduced WASO without significant change in REM% or latency in patients with major depressive disorder (MDD) (57). Support for the contention that agomelatine stabilized NREM sleep is derived from studies indicating that NREM cyclic alternating pattern (CAP) is reduced by this agent (58). Additional reports (59) have found significant improvement in subjective sleep latency in generalized anxiety disorder patients treated with agomelatine. In addition to its direct effects on sleep continuity and architecture, agomelatine has also been shown to have significant phase-shifting effects that may play a role in its therapeutic effects. Older adults treated with early evening agomelatine experienced a phase-advance of approximately two hours (60). The drug has generally been well tolerated in trials with favorable side effect profiles, including minimal sexual side effects.

LY2624803 (formerly HY10275; Eli Lilly and Company) is a dual acting H_1/5-HT_{2A} antagonist originally developed by Hypnion, Inc., and sold to Eli Lilly and Company in 2007. Phase II data released in 2007 (61) on HY10275/ LY2624803 describes 52 patients with primary insomnia who were administered HY10275, 1 to 3 mg, or placebo in a randomized clinical trial. Significant reductions were observed in wake after sleep onset, which decreased in a dose-dependent manner by 62 minutes for 3 mg ($p < 0.001$) and 35 minutes for 1 mg ($p < 0.002$). Subjects with moderate to severe transient insomnia responded as well as or better than subjects with mild to moderate transient insomnia. The drug also met secondary efficacy endpoints including significant reduction in latency to persistent sleep. No adverse events were reported during the course of the trial and no evidence of next-day impairment or residual fatigue was noted. A phase II RCT of LY2624803(SLUMBER) (62), with a zolpidem comparison arm, is currently underway. Subjects include both primary and secondary insomniacs. Primary endpoint is TST.

Esmirtazapine (ORG 50081), a derivative of the widely used antidepressant, mirtazapine, is currently under development for the management of insomnia and hot flashes. Esmirtazapine is a potent 5-HT_{2A} antagonist with H_1 and α-adrenergic properties.

Initial proof-of-concept trials in primary insomnia at three dosages of the drug showed significant improvement in TST and WASO (63). A long-term safety study of two doses (1.5 and 3.0 mg) in elderly primary insomniacs is currently underway. Merck acquired Organon as part of its recent buyout of Schering-Plough and currently lists esmirtazapine in its Phase III pipeline.

ITI-007 (Intra-Cellular Therapies, Inc.) is a dual action 5-HT_{2A}/dopamine receptor phosphoprotein modulator (DPPM) agent developed for the treatment of schizophrenia. Phase 2 studies have also been conducted for sleep maintenance insomnia. ITI-007 has variable dose-dependent activity, demonstrating predominantly 5-HT_{2A} antagonism at lower dosages (1–10 mg) with increasing dopamine receptor modulation at higher dosages (up to 30 mg). Interim analysis (64) ($N = 18$), released in early 2009, of a placebo-controlled investigation of 1, 5, and 10 mg ITI-007 in sleep-maintenance insomniacs showed dose-dependent reductions of WASO and increase of slow wave sleep.

CONCLUSIONS

Current investigations of novel compounds for the treatment of insomnia hold the promise of introducing an array of new approaches to the management of this often chronic and highly prevalent condition. Many of these agents would appear to have the potential to improve sleep as defined by the conventional metrics of latency, WASO, TST, efficiency, and the like, and by virtue of their unique mechanisms, offer additional advantages not seen with BzRAs, such as enhancement of slow wave activity. Moreover, a number of these agents may offer dual action in the management of insomnia comorbid with depression, attention deficit hyperactivity disorder, hot flashes, or psychosis. However, as stated previously, the road to new drug application is fraught with many obstacles and only time will tell which of these compounds reach market.

REFERENCES

1. Roth T, Zammit GK, Scharf MB, et al. Efficacy and safety of as-needed, post bedtime dosing with indiplon in insomnia patients with chronic difficulty maintaining sleep. Sleep 2007; 30(12):1731–1738.
2. Walsh JK, Moscovitch A, Burke J, et al. Efficacy and tolerability of indiplon in older adults with primary insomnia. Sleep Med 2007; 8(7–8):753–759.
3. Rosenberg R, Roth T, Scharf MB, et al. Efficacy and tolerability of indiplon in transient insomnia. J Clin Sleep Med 2007; 3(4):374–379.
4. Scharf MB, Black J, Hull S, et al. Long-term nightly treatment with indiplon in adults with primary insomnia: Results of a double-blind, placebo-controlled, 3-month study. Sleep 2007; 30(6):743–752.
5. Lydiard RB, Lankford DA, Seiden DJ, et al. Efficacy and tolerability of modified-release indiplon in elderly patients with chronic insomnia: Results of a 2-week double-blind, placebo-controlled trial. J Clin Sleep Med 2006; 2(3):309–315.
6. Walsh JK, Thacker S, Knowles LJ, et al. The partial positive allosteric GABA(A) receptor modulator EVT 201 is efficacious and safe in the treatment of adult primary insomnia patients. Sleep Med 2009; 10(8):859–864.
7. Walsh J, Knowles LJ, Tasker T, et al. The treatment of elderly patients with primary insomnia and daytime sleepiness with EVT 201 improves sleep initiation, sleep maintenance, and daytime alertness. Sleep 2008, 31(abstract suppl):A224.
8. Zammit G, Rice K, Accomando W, et al. Effects of NG2–73 on sleep onset, quality, and next day function in a transient insomnia study. Sleep 2007; 30(abstract suppl):A239.
9. Roth T, Lankford A, Accomando WP, et al. Sleep onset and maintenance in patients with chronic insomnia treated with adipiplon in a cross-over study. Sleep 2008; 31(abstract suppl):A40–A41.
10. Neurogen announces suspension of insomnia study with adipiplon. http://www.medicalnewstoday.com/articles/114919.php. Published July 15, 2008. Accessed February 28, 2010.
11. Walsh JK, Cornette F, Staner C, et al. Pharmacodynamic profile of three novel formulations of zaleplon in normal volunteers as evaluated by the multiple sleep latency test. Sleep 2009; 32(abstract suppl):A267.
12. Gassen M, Kress A, Nedelec J, et al. Pharmacokinetic profile of single doses of zaleplon in three novel formulations in normal volunteers. Sleep 2009; 32(abstract suppl):A267.
13. http://www.novadel. com/pipeline/zolpimist.htm. Accessed October 15, 2009.
14. Staner L, Eriksson M, Cornette F, et al. Sublingual zolpidem is more effective than oral zolpidem in initiating early onset of sleep in the post-nap model of transient insomnia: A polysomnographic study. Sleep Med 2009; 10(6):616–620.
15. Roth T, Hull SG, Lankford DA, et al. Low-dose sublingual zolpidem tartrate is associated with dose-related improvement in sleep onset and duration in insomnia characterized by middle-of-the-night (MOTN) awakenings. Sleep 2008; 31(9):1277–1284.
16. Lankford DA, Corser BC, Zheng YP, et al. Effect of gaboxadol on sleep in adult and elderly patients with primary insomnia: Results from two randomized, placebo-controlled, 30-night polysomnography studies. Sleep 2008; 31(10):1359–1370.

17. Walsh JK, Mayleben D, Guico-Pabia C, et al. Efficacy of the selective extrasynaptic GABA A agonist, gaboxadol, in a model of transient insomnia: A randomized, controlled clinical trial. Sleep Med 2008; 9(4):393–402.
18. Lundahl J, Staner L, Staner C, et al. Short-term treatment with gaboxadol improves sleep maintenance and enhances slow wave sleep in adult patients with primary insomnia. Psychopharmacology (Berl) 2007; 195(1):139–146.
19. Walsh JK, Deacon S, Dijk DJ, et al. The selective extrasynaptic GABAA agonist, gaboxadol, improves traditional hypnotic efficacy measures and enhances slow wave activity in a model of transient insomnia. Sleep 2007; 30(5):593–602.
20. Deacon S, Staner L, Staner C, et al. Effect of short-term treatment with gaboxadol on sleep maintenance and initiation in patients with primary insomnia. Sleep 2007; 30(3):281–287.
21. Mathias S, Zihl J, Steiger A, et al. Effect of repeated gaboxadol administration on night sleep and next-day performance in healthy elderly subjects. Neuropsychopharmacology 2005; 30(4):833–841.
22. de Lecea L, Kilduff TS, Peyron C, et al. The hypocretins: Hypothalamus-specific peptides with neuroexcitatory activity. Proc Natl Acad Sci U S A 1998; 95(1): 322–327.
23. Sakurai T, Amemiya A, Ishii M, et al. Orexins and orexin receptors: A family of hypothalamic neuropeptides and G protein-coupled receptors that regulate feeding behavior. Cell 1998; 92(4):573–585.
24. Lin L, Faraco J, Li R, et al. The sleep disorder canine narcolepsy is caused by a mutation in the hypocretin (orexin) receptor 2 gene. Cell 1999; 98(3):365–376.
25. Chemelli RM, Willie JT, Sinton CM, et al. Narcolepsy in orexin knockout mice: Molecular genetics of sleep regulation. Cell 1999; 98(4):437–451.
26. Saper CB, Chou TC, Scammell TE. The sleep switch: Hypothalamic control of sleep and wakefulness. Trends Neurosci 2001; 24(12):726–731.
27. Marcus JN, Aschkenasi CJ, Lee CE, et al. Differential expression of orexin receptors 1 and 2 in the rat brain. J Comp Neurol 2001; 435(1):6–25.
28. Brisbare-Roch C, Dingemanse J, Koberstein R, et al. Promotion of sleep by targeting the orexin system in rats, dogs and humans. Nat Med 2007; 13(2):150–155.
29. Dingemanse J et al. Proof-of-Concept Study in Primary Insomnia Patients with Almorexant (ACT-078573): A Dual Orexin Receptor Antagonist. In: Fifth World Congress of the World Federation of Sleep Research and Sleep Medicine Societies; 2007; Cairns, Australia.
30. Almorexant. http://www1.actelion.com/en/scientists/development-pipeline/phase-3/almorexant.page. Accessed October 17, 2009.
31. Bettica P, Lichtenfeld U, Squassante L, et al. The orexin antagonist SB-649868 promotes and maintains sleep in healthy volunteers and in patients with primary insomnia. Sleep 2009; 32(abstract suppl):A252–A253.
32. Dugovic C, Shelton JE, Aluisio LE, et al. Blockade of orexin-1 receptors attenuates orexin-2 receptor antagonism-induced sleep promotion in the rat. J Pharmacol Exp Ther 2009; 330(1):142–151.
33. http://www.merck.com/research/pipeline/home.html?WT.svl=mainnav. Accessed October 20, 2009.
34. Adrien J. The serotoninergic system and sleepwakefulness regulations. In: Kales A, ed. Pharmacology of Sleep, Handbook of Experimental Pharmacology. Berlin, Germany: Springer-Verlag, 1995: 91–116.
35. Landolt HP, Meier V, Burgess HJ, et al. Serotonin-2 receptors and human sleep: Effect of a selective antagonist on EEG power spectra. Neuropsychopharmacology 1999; 21(3):455–466.
36. Viola AU, Brandenberger G, Toussaint M, et al. Ritanserin, a serotonin-2 receptor antagonist, improves ultradian sleep rhythmicity in young poor sleepers. Clin Neurophysiol 2002; 113(3):429–434.
37. Sharpley AL, Solomon RA, Fernando AI, et al. Dose-related effects of selective 5-HT2 receptor antagonists on slow wave sleep in humans. Psychopharmacology (Berl) 1990; 101(4):568–569.
38. Adam K, Oswald I. Effects of repeated ritanserin on middle-aged poor sleepers. Psychopharmacology (Berl) 1989; 99(2):219–221.
39. Paiva T, Arriaga F, Wauquier A, et al. Effects of ritanserin on sleep disturbances of dysthymic patients. Psychopharmacology (Berl) 1988; 96(3):395–399.
40. Akhondzadeh S, Malek-Hosseini M, Ghoreishi A, et al. Effect of ritanserin, a 5HT2A/2C antagonist, on negative symptoms of schizophrenia: A double-blind randomized placebo-controlled study. Prog Neuropsychopharmacol Biol Psychiatry 2008; 32(8):1879–1883.
41. Jancin B. Eplivanserin soothes insomnia without next-morning effects. Clin Psychiat News 2008; 36(11):41.
42. Erman M, Kryger M, Soubrane C, et al. A randomized double-blind placebo-controlled 12-week trial of eplivanserin in insomniac patients with sleep maintenance difficulties. Sleep 2009; 32(abstract suppl):A41.

43. Estivill E, Leger D, Soubrane C. A randomized double-blind placebo-controlled 12-week trial of eplivanserin with long-term open extension in insomniac patients with sleep maintenance difficulties: Results from the double-blind treatment period. Sleep 2009; 32(abstract suppl):A41.
44. Hindmarch I, Cattelin F. Effect of two dose regimens of eplivanserin, a new sleep agent, on sleep and psychomotor performance of healthy subjects. Sleep 2008; 2008(31):A33.
45. Hall J, Schweitzer PK, Forst EH, et al. Spectral profile of eplivanserin differs from other SWS-enhancing and hypnotic drugs. Sleep 2009; 32(abstract suppl):A37.
46. http://www.lilly.com/research/pipeline/. Accessed October 17 2009.
47. Abbas A, Roth BL. Pimavanserin tartrate: A 5-HT2A inverse agonist with potential for treating various neuropsychiatric disorders. Expert Opin Pharmacother 2008; 9(18):3251–3259.
48. Buscemi N, Vandermeer B, Hooton N, et al. The efficacy and safety of exogenous melatonin for primary sleep disorders. A meta-analysis. J Gen Intern Med 2005; 20(12):1151–1158.
49. Brzezinski A, Vangel MG, Wurtman RJ, et al. Effects of exogenous melatonin on sleep: A meta-analysis. Sleep Med Rev 2005; 9(1):41–50.
50. Rajaratnam SM, Polymeropoulos MH, Fisher DM, et al. Melatonin agonist tasimelteon (VEC-162) for transient insomnia after sleep-time shift: Two randomised controlled multicentre trials. Lancet 2009; 373(9662):482–491.
51. Feeney J, Birznieks G, Scott C, et al. Melatonin agonist tasimelteon improves sleep in primary insomnia characterized by difficulty falling asleep. Sleep 2009; 32(abstract suppl):A43.
52. Business wire: Clinical trial of treatment for sleep disorders ends in success; phase 2 discovery announces positive results for PD-6735 in primary insomnia. http://findarticles.com/p/articles/mi_m0EIN/is_2004_May_20/ai_n6036252/. Published May 20, 2004. Accessed February 24, 2010.
53. Hajak G, Rodenbeck A, Voderholzer U, et al. Doxepin in the treatment of primary insomnia: A placebo-controlled, double-blind, polysomnographic study. J Clin Psychiatry 2001; 62(6):453–463.
54. Roth T, Rogowski R, Hull S, et al. Efficacy and safety of doxepin 1 mg, 3 mg, and 6 mg in adults with primary insomnia. Sleep 2007; 30(11):1555–1561.
55. Scharf M, Rogowski R, Hull S, et al. Efficacy and safety of doxepin 1 mg, 3 mg, and 6 mg in elderly patients with primary insomnia: A randomized, double-blind, placebo-controlled crossover study. J Clin Psychiatry 2008; 69(10):1557–1564.
56. Lemoine P, Guilleminault C, Alvarez E. Improvement in subjective sleep in major depressive disorder with a novel antidepressant, agomelatine: Randomized, double-blind comparison with venlafaxine. J Clin Psychiatry 2007; 68(11):1723–1732.
57. Quera Salva MA, Vanier B, Laredo J, et al. Major depressive disorder, sleep EEG and agomelatine: An open-label study. Int J Neuropsychopharmacol 2007; 10(5):691–696.
58. Lopes MC, Quera-Salva MA, Guilleminault C. Non-REM sleep instability in patients with major depressive disorder: Subjective improvement and improvement of non-REM sleep instability with treatment (agomelatine). Sleep Med 2007; 9(1):33–41.
59. Stein DJ, Ahokas AA, de Bodinat C. Efficacy of agomelatine in generalized anxiety disorder: A randomized, double-blind, placebo-controlled study. J Clin Psychopharmacol 2008; 28(5):561–566.
60. Leproult R, Van Onderbergen A, L'Hermite-Baleriaux M, et al. Phase-shifts of 24-h rhythms of hormonal release and body temperature following early evening administration of the melatonin agonist agomelatine in healthy older men. Clin Endocrinol (Oxf) 2005; 63(3):298–304.
61. New insomnia drug well-tolerated in trials: Sleep review. http://www.sleepreviewmag.com/news/2007–01-22_01.asp. Published January 27, 2007. Accessed October 17, 2009.
62. http://clinicaltrials.gov/ct2/show/NCT00784875.
63. http://clinicaltrials.gov/ct2/show/NCT00561574.
64. Intra-cellular therapies reports positive final results of a phase II clinical trial with ITI-007 in patients with sleep maintenance insomnia. http://www.intracellulartherapies.com/investor/2009_3_10.htm. Published March 10, 2009. Accessed February 24, 2010.

38 Clinical Trials and the Development of New Therapeutics for Insomnia

Gary K. Zammit

Clinilabs, Inc., Sleep Disorders Institute, Columbia University College of Physicians and Surgeons, New York, New York, U.S.A.

The development of new therapeutics for the treatment of insomnia involves the design and execution of clinical trials. Clinical trials are research studies involving human subjects that serve to characterize drugs under development; examine their safety, tolerability, and adverse effects in healthy subjects; and document their efficacy and safety in patient populations. Clinical trials are the most important and costly phase of the drug development process. According to industry reports, the pharmaceutical industry spent $44.5 billion on research and development (R&D) in 2007 (1) with clinical development costs representing approximately 60% of these expenditures (2). The data derived from the conduct of clinical trials are critical to the delivery of new therapeutics to the market. These data ultimately drive the drug development lifecycle and provide the basis of all new drug applications (NDAs) in the United States and other regulatory environments.

A BRIEF HISTORY OF CLINICAL TRIALS

The regulations governing the conduct of clinical trials in the United States have their origins in the early 20th century. During this time, substantive legislative action was introduced to bring drug products under governmental oversight. Among the first bills to receive approval was the Federal Food and Drugs Act of 1906 (known as the Wiley Act). This Act primarily was designed to control the manufacture, sale, or transportation of adulterated, misbranded, poisonous, or deleterious foods, drugs, medicines, and liquors (3). Responsibility for the enforcement of the provisions of the Wiley Act fell under the purview of the United States Bureau of Chemistry—an early precursor of the modern-day U.S. Food and Drug Administration (FDA) (4). The Act offered important safeguards to the public and was modified several times through 1934. However, it did not require drug makers to conduct clinical trials to confirm the efficacy of drugs marketed to treat medical conditions, and it imposed no restrictions on the claims that could be made by drug sellers regarding their products. Consequently, a plethora of substances were sold to treat medical conditions without any standardized assessment of their benefits or risks. Not surprising were the many adverse events that resulted from the use of these treatments by consumers. Serious injuries, disability, and death occurred due to the use of harmful or toxic substances found in legally marketed "medications" of the day.

As the public continued to be exposed to risk related to the use of drug products, a terrible and catastrophic incident occurred that ultimately strengthened the FDA's ability to regulate drug products (5). In 1937, the Massengill Company began marketing a raspberry-flavored elixir of the antibacterial sulfa drug *sulfanilamide,* offering a new liquid formulation of a drug that previously was sold in powder form. While the introduction of this formulation initially was thought to be safe, hundreds of men, women, and children became seriously ill after using this preparation. One hundred and seven people died as a result of ingesting this product. Only later was it learned that the untested formulation was sulfanilamide diethylene glycol, a chemical solvent known to be lethal when ingested by humans. Among the charges levied against the Massengill Company under the Wiley Act was sale of a misbranded toxic substance that was an acute poison. In response to public outrage over this event, President Franklin D. Roosevelt signed the Food, Drug, and Cosmetic Act on June 25, 1938. This Act gave broad and unquestionable authority to the FDA to require manufacturers to prove that their drugs were safe before granting approval for marketing. It also gave the FDA the authority to require drug labeling that provided directions for the safe use of these products (6).

While the Food, Drug, and Cosmetic Act compelled manufacturers to document the safety of their drug products, it is remarkable that there still was no requirement that they document efficacy. Claims could be made regarding a drug's ability to treat or cure any kind of disease, even when there was no evidentiary basis for such claims. To close this loophole, policy makers eventually introduced new legislation that expanded governmental control and regulatory oversight of drug products, including requirements that certain products could be used only under the supervision of a medical professional. In particular, the 1951 Durham–Humphrey Amendment to the Food, Drug, and Cosmetic Act made certain medications available by prescription only (6). This act limited access to drug products more than ever before, but the control of drug products remained insufficient. Gaps in regulatory oversight continued to persist due to controversy over how much power the FDA should wield over private industry and health care practices. Therefore, the next truly significant milestone did not occur until 1958, after yet another catastrophe brought inadequate regulatory policies into the spotlight once again. At that time, the W.S. Merrill Company began marketing *thalidomide* in Germany as a treatment for morning sickness. Shortly thereafter, an application was filed for the approval of this drug in the United States. Some concerns regarding the safety of this drug led an astute medical officer at the FDA, Frances Kelsey, to delay thalidomide's marketing approval. Kelsey's actions are likely to have spared thousands of unborn children, as it was later learned that thalidomide had serious teratogenic adverse effects. The West German pediatrician Widukind Linz reported an association between thalidomide and the birth of nearly 4000 children exhibiting abnormal limb growth. Relatively few cases of these birth defects were reported in the United States because of Kelsey's actions, and the drug was completely removed from the market in 1961 (7). Interestingly, thalidomide later returned to the market under the brand name Thalomid, and currently is indicated for the treatment of multiple myeloma and cutaneous manifestations of moderate to severe erythema nodosum leprosum (ENL) provided that safety precautions are taken (8).

It was in a climate of concern for consumer safety that Senator Estes Kefauver held congressional hearings to address pharmaceutical industry practices regarding the development of new drug products. These hearings led to the 1962 Kefauver–Harris Amendment to the Food, Drug, and Cosmetic Act. This landmark legislation required drug manufacturers to demonstrate "substantial evidence" of a drug's efficacy for its marketed indication, in addition to requiring demonstration of its safety. Further, the Kefauver–Harris Amendment expanded the FDA's authority to regulate advertising, inspect drug manufacturing facilities, and withdraw untested drugs from the market (9,10).

Since the 1960s, many new forms of legislation and regulatory oversight have been introduced to govern the drug development and approval process. One guidance document particularly important to the field of sleep medicine was produced by the FDA in 1977, specifically relating to the development of hypnotics (11). This document provided guidelines regarding acceptable approaches to the study of investigational hypnotics in human subjects. It also offered specific recommendations regarding the types of clinical trials that should be conducted as part of a hypnotic development program, as well as the endpoints that should be considered. The durability of this document is remarkable, given that its content regarding hypnotic development remains applicable to this day. In addition to guidance on the conduct of clinical trials, the FDA recently has issued requirements for the labeling of hypnotics. In December 2006, the FDA sent letters to manufacturers of products approved for the treatment of sleep disorders indicating that they would be required to revise product labeling to include warnings about certain potential adverse events (12). Although the likelihood of the occurrence of these events was not stated in the FDA's notice, these AEs were considered significant enough to warrant a revision of the product labeling. The adverse events (AEs) of concern were

- anaphylaxis (severe allergic reaction);
- angioedema (abrupt, severe swelling, especially facial), which can occur as early as the first time the product is taken;
- complex sleep-related behaviors, which may include sleep-driving, making phone calls, and preparing and eating food (while asleep).

In conjunction with the labeling revisions required, the FDA required that each product manufacturer send letters to health care providers highlighting these changes. Manufacturers of sedative–hypnotic products also were requested to develop Patient Medication Guides for sedative–hypnotic products to inform consumers of the potential risks associated with these newly labeled adverse events.

As the FDA pursues its public health mission, it is clear that the regulatory oversight of drug development continues to be based on requirements imposed by legislation. For example, in 1981, the FDA and the Department of Health and Human Services (DHHS) revised regulations for human subject protection based on the recommendations of the 1979 Belmont Report (13). The most important revision undertaken at this time was the specification of the elements of informed consent (14). Later, in 2002, the Best Pharmaceuticals for Children Act improved the safety and efficacy of patented and off-patent medicines for children (14). These and other current requirements for the development and testing of new drug products are now specified in detail under several parts of the Code of Federal Regulations (CFR) title 21 (15). These documents have relevance for the development of sleep therapeutics, and when combined with specific guidance related to the development of hypnotics, provide science and industry with sound foundations upon which to base the development of hypnotics.

PRECLINICAL STUDIES

An important step in the development of any new therapeutic is the submission of an investigational new drug (IND) application to the FDA. This application contains information gained from preclinical studies that are required prior to the initiation of testing in human subjects. Preclinical studies fall into two categories—in vitro and in vivo. In vitro studies evaluate the effects of a drug on human or animal tissue. In vivo studies are performed in live animals, usually rats, dogs, and primates. Combined, these preclinical studies yield the pharmacology and toxicology data that form the basic safety profile of a drug (16). These data are extremely important in that they are used to select a safe starting dose for human studies, establish estimates of the toxic dose in humans, and gain a fundamental understanding of the pharmacokinetic (PK) and pharmacodynamic (PD) properties of a drug. The type of information that regulatory reviewers examine in investigational new drugs includes data from carcinogenicity studies, genotoxicity studies, toxicokinetics and pharmacokinetics, toxicity testing, reproductive toxicology, and pharmacology studies (16,17). It is interesting to note that preclinical testing represents approximately 27% of pharmaceutical R&D costs (2), and fewer than 10% of all new molecular entities (NMEs) will find their way forward from preclinical evaluation to the submission of a NDA. This is because drug manufacturers must study large numbers of drugs and apply rigid screening criteria to determine which ones they will take further into development.

Specific to the development of hypnotics, the types of preclinical studies used to examine products under consideration include tests of locomotion or myorelaxation, as these variables provide information regarding a compound's sedative properties. Examples include the rotarod test (18,19), the loaded grid test (18,20), and tests of abuse liability (21). In the rotarod test, rats are placed on a rotating surface (a rod) and faced with the challenge of remaining on the surface as it rotates. Drug-free baseline performance is assessed to determine minimum performance thresholds. Animals are then given active drug or placebo and tested to determine the amount of time they are able to remain on the rotarod. Animals that remain on the rotarod for shorter periods following drug administration may be showing evidence of myorelaxation. In the loaded grid test, animals hold on to a weighted grid with their front paws and are tested to determine the load required before they release. Again, this test is conducted so as to yield results for the baseline, placebo and drug conditions. Preclinical tests also include electroencephalographic (EEG) measures of sleep that provide indications of hypnotic activity (19,22–29). Hypnotics such as zolpidem, zaleplon, and zopiclone all have been characterized by these types of preclinical tests.

CLINICAL DEVELOPMENT PHASES

Clinical trials are conducted in three different phases prior to a drug's approval (phases I–III, Fig. 1). One additional phase (phase IV) includes studies conducted after marketing approval. Trials performed during the first of these phases of clinical development provide important

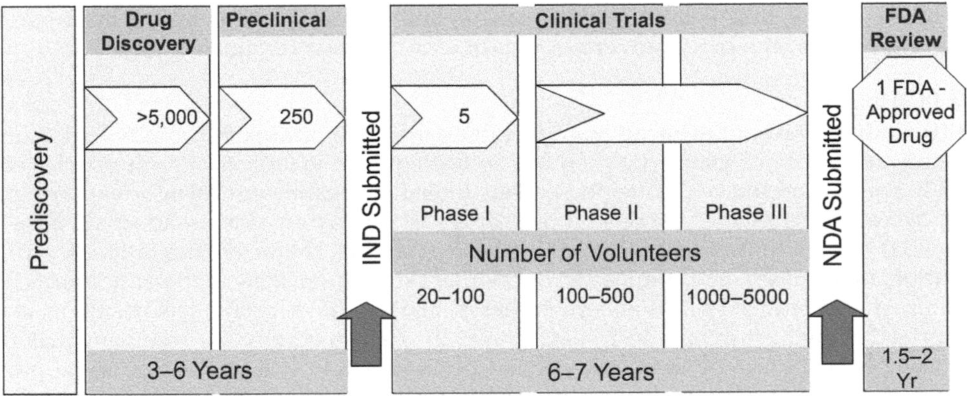

Figure 1 The R&D process—long, complex, and costly.

information that constitutes the manufacturer's evidence for carrying a drug forward, and forms the basis of the NDA that is submitted to the FDA. Although these phases are represented in consecutive order, these phases may overlap or even run concurrently. For example, a phase II study of hypnotic efficacy may be in progress when an important phase I drug–drug interaction study is initiated.

Clinical drug development is costly. An analysis conducted in 2007 estimated that the total combined cost of the preclinical and clinical trials required to bring a drug to the point of submission of an NDA is more than $1.2 billion (30). This expense includes the costs of drugs that fail to progress through the clinical development pipeline (31). For every 250 drugs that complete preclinical testing, 5 will successfully complete phase I, and only one will ultimately achieve regulatory approval (1). The four phases of clinical development are described in more detail in the following section.

Phase I Trials

In these studies, researchers test an investigational drug or device in a small group of people (20–100), usually normal health, volunteers (32). These studies are designed to determine the metabolic and pharmacologic actions of a drug in humans, the side effects associated with the drug at various doses, and if possible, to gain early evidence regarding drug effects using biomarkers or tests in small cohorts of clinical populations. Common studies conducted in this phase of drug development are first-in-human (FIH), single ascending dose (SAD), multiple ascending dose (MAD), and drug–drug interaction (DDI) studies. During phase I, sufficient information about the drug's pharmacokinetics and PD effects should be obtained to permit the design of well-controlled, scientifically valid, phase II studies. Phase I studies also evaluate drug metabolism, structure–activity relationships, and the mechanism of action in humans (33). There is a growing trend to include cohorts of patients in phase I studies, as researchers attempt to learn more about drug effects early in development.

Phase II Trials

During phase II, an investigational drug or device is given to a larger group of people (100–500) (32) to evaluate the efficacy and safety of a drug for a particular indication or indications in patients with the disease or condition under study (34). Phase II studies also aim to determine the common short-term side effects and risks associated with the drug or device under evaluation. In clinical trials of hypnotics, it is common for phase II studies to employ experimental models in healthy human subjects in order to assess efficacy, identify primary outcomes that will be used in pivotal phase III studies, and determine the types of AEs that people report. However, in this phase of drug development it is much more common to study small groups of patients, especially when no experimental models exist. Phase II offers drug manufacturers an opportunity to determine the doses that will be carried forward into phase III by weighing the trade-offs between efficacy and the risk of adverse events at each dose level evaluated.

Phase III Trials

Phase III studies represent the drug manufacturer's most important opportunity to document the efficacy and safety of their drug products by testing them in large groups of people (1000–5000) (32). Studies conducted during phase III are intended to gather critical information regarding the overall benefit–risk relationship of a drug, as well as provide an adequate basis for labeling (34). By the time a drug enters this phase of testing, characteristics of its absorption, distribution, metabolism, and elimination (ADME)are known, its likely therapeutic effects have been defined and reduced to testable hypotheses, and its safety profile has been reasonably characterized. Manufacturers who initiate phase III trials generally are confident that their product will be shown to be safe and effective, and ultimately will win regulatory approval. Even though the odds of success are much higher for a drug product at this point than when entering preclinical evaluations, only one out of every five drugs that enters phase II testing will successfully complete phase III (32).

Phase IV Trials

After a drug's NDA has been approved by the FDA, phase IV trials may be conducted to further clarify its efficacy and safety. Pharmacovigilence, pharmacoeconomic, and comparative efficacy studies are most likely to be performed during this phase of the drug development lifecycle. New and specific patient populations are likely to be studied. Elderly, pediatric, or other patient groups could become a focus of research, depending on the potential use in those patient groups. As an example, studies of therapeutics for insomnia have been conducted in special populations of patients with comorbid depression and anxiety disorders, providing invaluable information to the prescribing community. There are occasions when phase IV trials provide information that is used to revise the labeling of a drug product (e.g., the inclusion of additional adverse event information), and some phase IV trials may support a manufacturer's decision to pursue a secondary NDA (sNDA) that seeks approval for a new therapeutic indication for a drug.

STUDY DESIGNS COMMONLY USED IN THE DEVELOPMENT OF HYPNOTICS

Phase I Studies: Pharmacokinetics, Pharmacodynamics, and Interaction Studies

PK studies form the fundamental basis of most phase I testing programs. These studies examine the kinetics of drug absorption, distribution, metabolism, and excretion (ADME). Perhaps the most critical information obtained in PK studies is related to the rate of drug absorption and delivery into systemic circulation, and the rate of elimination by metabolic or excretory processes in human subjects (35). The information obtained is based on plasma concentrations at multiple time points following dosing and is reflected in outcome variables that include the maximum plasma concentration (C_{max}), time to maximum concentration (T_{max}), half-life, and area-under-the-curve (AUC)—a representation of overall drug exposure. These variables provide information that reflects the relationships between dose, time, and plasma drug levels. When appropriate, phase I studies may reveal the influences of demographic characteristics (e.g., age, gender, race, ethnicity), certain disease states, external factors, and drug binding to biological constituents (35). If hepatic metabolism and/or excretion accounts for a substantial portion (>20% of the absorbed drug) of the elimination of a parent drug or active metabolite, it is recommended that PK studies be performed in subjects with impaired hepatic functioning (36). Similarly, whenever a drug is likely to be used in patients with renal impairment, and this impairment is likely to significantly alter the PK of a drug and/or its active/toxic metabolites, or require dosage adjustment for safe and effective use, testing in patients with renal impairment is recommended (37). Finally, there may be circumstances under which it is important to perform PK studies in special populations, for example, pregnant women (38) or children (39).

PK assessments of sedative hypnotics have become increasingly important to understanding drug effects, especially since the introduction of new and novel formulations that may have specific effects on latency to sleep onset, sleep maintenance, or both. For example, the PK profiles of the original formulation of zolpidem and zolpidem ER (a reformulation of zolpidem that provides the immediate release of drug from an outer layer and a delayed release of drug from an inner core) are different from one another (40,41). These products, in turn, can be expected to be different from sublingual or other formulations of zolpidem that do not require absorption in the intestinal tract (42,43).

PK studies often are combined with PD assessments, resulting in PK/PD modeling that guides the early-phase development of a drug. In the study of sedative hypnotics, the most elegant of these is the PK/PD model developed by Greenblatt and associates. In this model, the drug being studied typically is administered to healthy adult subjects in the morning, following a full night of sleep in a controlled setting. Blood samples for PK assessments are taken predose and at several time points following dosing (e.g., before medication and at 0.5, 1, 1.5, 2, 2.5, 3, 4, 5, 6, 8, and 24 hours postdosing) (44). These PK samples may be coupled with other evaluations of sedation [e.g., electroencephalographic assessments of beta (β) activity and the Digit Symbol Substitution Test (DSST)] and various word recall instruments. The use of word recall tests is important because of the known effects of many hypnotics on memory. The timing and frequency of PK and PD sampling is determined by the experimental hypothesis appropriate to the drug or formulation. For example, when testing a hypnotic with an extended-release formulation, it may be important to assess the duration of sedative effects. The information gleaned from this evaluation may guide dose selection or formulation, or provide information regarding the residual effects investigators may observe in later-phase studies (45).

Drug–drug and food interaction studies are additional important studies conducted in phase I. Phase I drug–drug interaction trials may include evaluations of a hypnotic's interaction with cytochrome P450 (CYP) inducers (e.g., rifampin), CYP inhibitors (e.g., azoles, ritonavir, and erythromycin), histamine H_2 receptor antagonists (e.g., cimetidine and ranitidine), antidepressants, antipsychotics, antagonists of benzodiazepines, and other drugs known to cause sedation (46).Food interactions also may be studied to examine the effect of certain foods or fasting on drug absorption or metabolism (47–49). For example, grapefruit juice is a well-known inhibitor of CYP3A4 and may be expected to increase exposure to hypnotics that are metabolized through this pathway (50).

Phase II Studies: Experimental Models of Insomnia and Patient Studies

Phase II studies often are used to determine the dose of medication that will be carried forward into phase III pivotal trials, or to identify the ideal outcome measures that ultimately will be used to determine the efficacy and safety of a therapeutic. Several experimental models of transient insomnia have been well validated for use in phase II studies. These include models based on the first-night laboratory adaptation effects, phase-advanced sleep, and exposure to noise.

An experimental model based on first-night adaptation effects in a sleep laboratory environment has commonly been used to assess hypnotic efficacy. This model takes advantage of the long latency to sleep onset and sleep disruption experienced by healthy subjects during their first night in a sleep laboratory environment. One of the first studies to use this model examined temazepam's hypnotic and sleep stage effects in a parallel group study of 201 healthy, normal subjects with no sleep complaints. Each subject was randomly assigned to receive either placebo, or 7.5 to 30 mg of temazepam 30 minutes before bedtime on their first night in the sleep laboratory. Subjects were given an eight-hour sleep opportunity while polysomnographic (PSG) recordings were obtained. The PSG data revealed that total sleep time and sleep efficiency increased in a linear fashion with increasing doses of temazepam relative to placebo, providing support for the use of the "first-night" effect as a model of transient insomnia (51). This model appears particularly useful in assessing drug effects on sleep latency. One of the key trials in zolpidem's clinical development program examined the effects of zolpidem in a double-blind, parallel-group study of 462 normal volunteers. Zolpidem was tested at doses ranging from 5 to 20 mg. Statistical analysis of the 7.5-mg and 10-mg doses showed that zolpidem decreased sleep latency, increased sleep duration, and reduced the number of awakenings relative to placebo, without significant effect on next-day psychomotor performance (52). Since the original temazepam study was conducted, the model has been employed to assess the hypnotic efficacy of benzodiazepines, nonbenzodiazepines, and other drugs with novel mechanisms of action like ramelteon (53–57).

Phase-advance models have been used with success in assessing the efficacy of hypnotics in treating transient insomnia. One of the advantages of these models is that they can be used in either crossover or parallel group designs, whereas first-night models, by definition, are limited to parallel group designs only. One of the earliest studies of the phase advance model used a 180-degree shift of the sleep–wake cycle in 12 healthy subjects to determine the effects of triazolam, flurazepam, and placebo in a parallel-group design. Subjects who received placebo demonstrated significant sleep loss following the manipulation of their sleep, while the effect was attenuated for those in the active medication groups (58). One of the interesting aspects of the phase-advance model is that it may be used to assess sleep maintenance by demonstrating separation between active drug and placebo in the later portions of the sleep period (59). While the magnitude of the phase-shift has been thought to be of importance, several studies have used short phase advances in order to detect meaningful effects. For example, one study has shown that temazepam 7.5 mg and 15 mg administered to subjects in a 2-hour phase-advance paradigm had similar effects on sleep architecture 60. Statistically significant effects on LPS, TST, and other sleep variables relative to placebo have been found with other drugs, such as indiplon and gaboxadol using this model (55,61,62), occasionally coupled with the first-night model of transient insomnia (55).

There are a variety of noise models that have been used in phase II studies of insomnia. While the specific implementations may differ, these models offer a method of assessing drug effects in the presence of experimental stimuli that perturb sleep, thereby demonstrating sleep maintenance effects. One noise model involves the exposure of normal, healthy subjects to continuous white noise during the sleep period at levels sufficient to disrupt sleep [e.g., 45–75 decibels (db)] (63,64). This design may be able to detect differences between drug conditions when cyclic alternating patterns (CAP) are used (65). Another common noise model involves the use of traffic noise played during sleep, and has been shown to separate immediate-release from modified-release formulations of hypnotics (66). Problematically however, the use of the traffic noise model has not shown consistent results when separating active drug from placebo (67).

Some phase II studies require the use of patient populations rather than healthy volunteers. These studies might be used when it is desirable to test drug effects on a specific sleep outcome variable that may not be reliably produced using an experimental model, when certain crossover comparisons are of interest, or when repeated (e.g., nightly) dosing may be desired. Such studies are also useful when the identification of well-defined patient groups may provide more informative data than experimental models (68). Several double-blind, randomized, placebo-controlled clinical trials of hypnotics have employed small samples of insomnia patients to assess the efficacy and safety of hypnotics in PSG sleep laboratory studies (68–78).

Phase III Studies: PSG and Outpatient Studies

Phase III study designs are "pivotal trials" that determine the efficacy and safety of new therapeutics. Phase III studies of hypnotics commonly include large samples of people with insomnia tested in parallel-group designs, and may or may not include the use of polysomnography. (79–83). At present, PSG results appear to be required for approval of a new hypnotic by the FDA.

In the past, volunteers were enlisted to participate in trials for a short period of time. A 1997 meta-analysis of 22 double-blind, placebo-controlled studies of hypnotics showed that the longest period of treatment assessed was 35 nights, with an average period of treatment lasting 12 nights, and a median period of 7 nights (84). However, recent trends in clinical care and regulatory guidance have prompted a shift towards longer-term trials. A few phase III studies of newer hypnotics have examined their use over longer periods of time. Multiple studies have lasted up to six months, some incorporating an additional six month open-label treatment period that provides data for up to a year of usage (85–88). PSG continues to be used in some of these more lengthy evaluations to provide periodic assessments of objectively defined outcomes (89). As an example, PSG could be employed at baseline, midway through treatment, at the end of treatment, and following acute discontinuation in order to evaluate sustained efficacy, as well as tolerance or withdrawal effects that might be associated with a hypnotic (90). In contrast, other studies have relied exclusively on patient reported outcomes (PRO) (85,88,91–94). These data are important because they provide impressions regarding efficacy and safety from the patient's perspective and offer information regarding the patient's experience at home in their natural sleep setting as opposed to the artificial sleep environment of a sleep laboratory where most PSG recordings are performed.

One of the more interesting recent developments in hypnotic trials has been the use of novel study designs that have employed the "as needed," non-nightly, or non-bedtime use of hypnotics. (95–99). One study assessed the effects of non-nightly use of zolpidem 10 mg or placebo in 199 patients with primary insomnia. Patients were randomized in a parallel group design, and were instructed to take no fewer than three pills and no more than five pills per week for a period of 12 weeks. The data revealed that patients receiving zolpidem exhibited (vs. baseline) a 42% decrease in sleep latency, a 52% reduction in number of awakenings, a 55% decrease in wake time after sleep onset, and a 27% increase in total sleep time, without increases in the amount of medication used during the study interval (100).

Some studies have involved non-bedtime dosing of hypnotics. This type of evaluation is especially relevant for medications that may not have immediate sedative effects (enabling administration earlier in the day), or for medications that have rapid onset of action, metabolism, and elimination (enabling administration during nighttime awakenings). Studies employing experimentally induced awakenings in subjects with primary insomnia have examined the effects of treatment with short-acting hypnotics like zaleplon (101–104). One crossover design PSG study examined the administration of zaleplon 10 mg, zolpidem 10 mg, and placebo in 37 subjects with primary insomnia characterized by sleep maintenance difficulty. During each treatment period, subjects were seen for an eight-hour PSG recording, during which they were awakened and later given study drug or placebo. The study revealed that both zaleplon and zolpidem reduced sleep latency in the middle of the night and increased total sleep time following dosing, suggesting that after-bedtime treatment may be efficacious in treating sleep maintenance insomnia (104). This approach is not risk free however. It is notable that zolpidem was associated with poorer next-day performance and greater sleepiness on the multiple sleep latency test (MSLT) than placebo; an indicator that PK/PD relationships are important when selecting hypnotics for after-bedtime dosing. Additional studies have examined the use of middle-of-the-night dosing with other drugs using PROs, including studies of indiplon and sublingual zolpidem administered in lower doses than the oral formulation (42,105,106).

STUDY DESIGN CONSIDERATIONS

Subject Selection

The matter of subject selection is critically important to the success of clinical trials of hypnotics. When healthy subjects are being considered for inclusion in phase II studies of hypnotics, it is important that they are of the appropriate age (adult or elderly) and that they have no confounding concurrent illness, concomitant medication use, abnormal findings on physical examination, or abnormal clinical laboratory findings. Since recent FDA guidance now requires manufacturers to assess the cardiac safety of all new drugs that have systemic exposure (107), electrocardiographic (ECG) assessments are important in selecting subjects appropriate for study.

Among the unique aspects of subject selection for hypnotic studies are those related to subjects' sleep habits. When selecting healthy subjects for clinical trials, one must consider subjects' usual bedtimes, rise times, napping, recent travel across multiple time zones, use of stimulants such as caffeine or nicotine, and the use of alcohol or other substances that might affect sleep. Some studies that have used experimental models of insomnia have been careful to exclude otherwise healthy subjects who may be sleep deprived. Assessments used to identify sleep deprivation include the Epworth Sleepiness Scale (108,109), Stanford Sleepiness Scale, and the MSLT (110,111).

When identifying patients with primary insomnia to participate in phase II or III trials, the selection criteria are of utmost importance. First and foremost, it is important that the characteristics of the patient population be clearly specified. Most trials of hypnotics performed for registration purposes have studied patients with primary insomnia, most often defined by *Diagnostic and Statistical Manual of Mental Disorders*, version IV (*DSM-IV*) criteria. There are relatively minor, but important, differences between *DSM-IV* criteria for primary insomnia and other diagnostic nomenclatures also used to identify insomnia complaints. The *International Statistical Classification of Diseases and Related Health Problems, 10th Revision* (*ICD-10*) specifies criteria for "nonorganic insomnia" that stipulate that symptoms must be present at least three times per week for at least one month, while the *DSM-IV* criteria specify a duration of one month or longer but do not require a minimum number of times per week. In contrast to both the *DSM-IV* and *ICD-10*, the Research Diagnostic Criteria (RDC) for insomnia disorder do not specify a duration criterion. Therefore, the fundamental diagnostic definition of insomnia used in a trial must be thoughtfully considered. The use of centralized interviews may be one way to minimize variability in diagnostic ratings of insomnia made by clinicians, similar to those used in clinical trials in other therapeutic indications (112).

Once the insomnia diagnosis is specified, it is important to consider the types of symptoms that patients must have in order to participate in the trial. For example, if a clinical trial is intended to assess the effects of a drug on sleep latency, the study protocol should require subjects to report difficulty falling asleep. Similarly, if the clinical trial is intended to assess the effects of a drug on sleep maintenance, the study protocol is likely to require subjects to report wakefulness during the sleep period. The frequency and severity of the sleep problems required for inclusion depends on the specific objectives of the protocol. Some recent studies assessing drug effect in patients with sleep maintenance insomnia have required both a sleep latency and wakefulness after sleep onset (WASO) of ≥20 minutes as measured by polysomnography during the screening process (68,113).

The clinical trial protocol typically provides an exhaustive list of specific inclusion and exclusion criteria for study subjects. All of these criteria must be met in order to enroll subjects into a study. The determination that these criteria are met usually is based on an office visit ("screening visit") during which a clinician obtains all pertinent history and a physical examination, clinical laboratory tests, ECG, and other assessments are performed. The first office visit is when written informed consent is obtained from the subject, prior to performing any study-related activity. Failure to meet all inclusion and exclusion criteria may result in a protocol violation, which may result in the exclusion of a subject from analysis.

It has become a common practice to include PSG screening nights in PSG trials of hypnotics. These screening nights serve to confirm that subjects meet certain PSG inclusion/exclusion criteria prior to randomization to active drug or placebo, and improve the likelihood that trial participants mirror the insomnia diagnosis that investigators wish to evaluate. Studies designed to assess the effect of a hypnotic on reducing sleep latency commonly require a minimum LPS criterion on PSG screening nights. For example, a mean LPS of ≥20 minutes on two or three PSG screening nights, with no night less than 15 minutes might be employed. Studies designed to assess the effect of a hypnotic on sleep maintenance often employ a minimum criterion for WASO. For example, a mean WASO of ≥60 minutes on two or three PSG screening nights, with no night less than 45 minutes might be required for trial participation. Note that these criteria are dependent on the scientific hypothesis being tested and are not hard-and-fast standards imposed by industry. In addition to such PSG inclusion criteria, there are PSG exclusion criteria. The most common PSG exclusion criteria involve the exclusion of subjects who have an apnea/hypopnea index (AHI) >10 or a periodic limb movement with arousal index (PLMAI) >10. Some upward adjustments to these thresholds may be warranted when working with elderly samples.

Multicenter Trials

Phase I studies often are conducted at single sites. However, as drugs enter phase II development, clinical trials usually are assigned to a small number of specialized investigator sites. Hypnotic studies typically might include six to eight investigator sites, all likely to have experienced, trained staff and PSG recording capability. The use of multiple sites for phase II studies provides geographic reach, enhances the accrual of study subjects from diverse populations, and enables the study to progress more rapidly than those conducted at a single center. Further along this continuum, phase III studies often involve such large samples that it is necessary to enlist the assistance of a much larger number of investigator sites. At this point in the development process, dozens of sites representing a multinational assembly of investigators may be employed to execute pivotal phase III studies of hypnotics.

One of the most important considerations when conducting multicenter trials relates to the standardization of clinical trial methodology. It is desirable for all investigators in a multicenter trial to collect data in a uniform manner. Standardization of data collection processes contributes to data quality, minimizes confounds, and reduces variance. The ultimate goal is to have all investigator sites operating as a unified group so that results from a patient enrolled at one site are comparable to the results expected if the same patient was enrolled at any other study site. The foundation of such synchrony lies in the study protocol that specifies study procedures. In hypnotic drug trials, study protocols often include specific instructions for the collection of PSG or other outcome data. Highly specialized PSG recording manuals commonly accompany clinical study protocols for hypnotics. Training of investigators and site staff on these procedures significantly contributes to the ability of investigators to standardize data collection at their sites.

In recent years, multicenter trials have increasingly relied on centralized services in order to standardize data collection and processing methodologies. Such centralized services may include centralized subject assessment and diagnosis (which may now be performed using Web-based or live interview services), centralized randomization and drug allocation, centralized subject assessments, and centralized clinical laboratory and electrocardiographic (ECG) services. The use of such services has not only enforced standardization but has also proved helpful in reducing errors, minimizing variance in datasets, and establishing a single location for data management and auditing. One centralized service specific to studies of hypnotics relates to the use of centralized PSG scoring services. Such centralized services often are used to confirm that subjects meet PSG inclusion/exclusion criteria and ensure that PSG scoring is performed in accordance with a uniform standard.

Outcome Variables

The goals of traditional hypnotic therapy primarily relate to reducing latency to sleep onset or reducing wakefulness during the sleep period. The most commonly used primary outcome variables in traditional PSG hypnotic studies have been latency to persistent sleep (LPS), total sleep time (TST), sleep efficiency, and number of awakenings. These outcome variables have been used in trials of benzodiazepines, nonbenzodiazepines (zolpidem, zaleplon, zopiclone), and novel therapeutics such as ramelteon and doxepin. More recent focus on the prevalence and impact of sleep-maintenance insomnia has led to the development of hypnotics that address this type of sleep complaint. In PSG studies of drug effects on sleep maintenance, the most commonly used outcome variable is WASO. WASO has been used as a primary outcome variable in pivotal trials of both zolpidem ER and eszopiclone. Self-reported measures of sleep latency, total sleep time, and sleep maintenance complement objective PSG outcome variables. These self-reported measures may be used either in the context of PSG trials or, separately, in outpatient studies with no PSG component. Traditionally, these variables have been collected using sleep diaries. More recently it has become common to obtain patient-reported data using electronic or integrated voice response system (IVRS) technology. Table 1 provides a summary of common primary and secondary outcome variables used in PSG and outpatient studies of hypnotics.

Within recent years there has been increasing recognition that insomnia complaints regarding sleep "quantity" (e.g., LPS, WASO) may include disruptions of sleep not detected by traditional sleep stage scoring alone. These disruptions may be concurrent with, or independent of, complaints of poor quality or nonrestorative sleep. Preliminary evidence of these disruptions has sparked an interest in examining sleep microarchitecture. Such trials might involve careful assessment of slow wave sleep activity measured during stages 3 and 4 sleep or throughout the entire sleep period, or may focus on other measurable aspects of sleep through the use of power spectral analysis (114) or scoring of cyclic alternating patterns (CAPs) (64,115–117). At present, these newer outcome variables are not commonly used clinical trial endpoints, but further exploration may lead to their consideration as outcomes for insomnia treatment studies.

Other potential treatment outcomes for insomnia may include measures of daytime functioning or health. Functional outcomes might assess next-day well-being, sleepiness, fatigue, or performance on various psychomotor or memory assessments—all of which may be important to understand the clinical utility and proper labeling of hypnotics. For example, recent clinical studies of hypnotics have begun to demonstrate that improvements following hypnotic treatment may be associated with less napping and significantly higher ratings of daytime alertness, sense of physical well-being, and quality-of-life (118). Finally, health outcomes might represent an important new focus of hypnotic treatment. Recent data suggesting that sleep deprivation is related to impairments in glucose metabolism (119–121), obesity and diabetes risk (122,123), hypertension (124,125), cardiac arrythmias (126,127), and mortality (128) may increase the frequency with which health outcomes are included in hypnotic trials.

While one primary objective of clinical trials is to assess efficacy, the other is to assess safety. Safety outcomes in trials of hypnotics frequently include assessments of adverse events and serious adverse events, and involve specific measures of sedation, cognitive functioning, psychomotor functioning, and withdrawal. Adverse events are any untoward experience in a clinical trial participant, whether or not the experience is believed to be related to the investigational drug (129). Serious adverse events (SAEs) are adverse events that result in death or are life-threatening, result in hospitalization or prolongation of an existing hospitalization, result in significant disability or incapacity, or result in congenital abnormalities or birth defects (129). These AEs and SAEs are reported by investigators and are carefully considered by regulatory authorities when reviewing NDAs. In hypnotic trials, assessments of self-reported sedation might be captured as AEs, especially if it occurs during the day. Objective measures of sedation might further include the Digit Symbol Substitution Test (DSST), Symbol Copying Test (SCT), or word recall tests. These tests often are performed at baseline, immediately after drug administration, and in the morning following awakening in order to assess next-day, residual impairment (8.5 hours or more after dosing). Some studies have used the multiple sleep latency test to assess residual sleepiness. Safety assessments also might be performed during the typical nighttime sleep period in order to determine a drug's effect on cognitive or psychomotor performance during awakenings. As an example, some recent studies have used computerized dynamic posturography to assess balance and postural control following middle-of-the-night awakenings of healthy elderly and those with insomnia following bedtime dosing with hypnotic agents.

Specialty Populations

There are a number of health conditions that commonly are comorbid with insomnia. They include obstructive sleep apnea (OSA) (130), chronic obstructive pulmonary disease (COPD) (131), pain, menopause (132,133), and psychiatric illness such as depression (134) or anxiety (135). Therefore, the assessment of hypnotic efficacy and safety in insomnia comorbid with these other conditions is an important aspect of hypnotic life cycle management. Depression is among the most commonly associated conditions comorbid with insomnia, giving rise to studies of the combination use of antidepressants and hypnotics. The use of zolpidem was examined in SSRI-treated patients with persistent comorbid insomnia (134). Patients who participated in this study were diagnosed with depression, treated stably with the SSRIs fluoxetine, sertraline, or paroxetine, and complained of sleep-onset difficulty or inadequate sleep time at least three nights a week with daytime impairment. Over a four-week period, treatment with zolpidem 10 mg lengthened sleep time, improved sleep quality, reduced the number of awakenings, and improved multiple measures of daytime functioning as compared to placebo.

A recent study evaluated the coadministration of eszopiclone 3 mg with the SSRI fluoxetine in major depressive disorder (MDD) patients over an 8-week period (136). Compared to fluoxetine alone, the fluoxetine–eszopiclone group demonstrated statistically significant improvements in all sleep parameters evaluated at all time points. Measures included sleep latency, wake time after sleep onset, total sleep time, sleep quality, and depth of sleep. Importantly, eszopiclone also resulted in a greater treatment response to fluoxetine as measured by improvements on the Hamilton Depression Rating Scale (HAM-D-17) and two clinical global impression scales (CGI-I and CGI-S). Furthermore, a significantly greater percentage of individuals in the cotherapy group were classified as responders (59% vs. 48%) and remitters (42% vs. 33%) at the end of the study.

There are a limited number of clinical trials of subjects with insomnia and comorbid anxiety. One double-blind, randomized, placebo-controlled, parallel-group study examined the efficacy of eszopiclone combined with escitalopram in adult patients with insomnia and generalized anxiety disorder (GAD) (135). Patients received 10 mg of escitalopram oxolate for 10 weeks and were randomized to also receive either 3 mg of eszopiclone ($n = 294$) or placebo ($n = 301$) nightly for the first 8 weeks. For the last two weeks, eszopiclone was replaced with a single-blind placebo. Sleep, daytime functioning, psychiatric measures, and adverse events were assessed throughout the 10-week period. The results showed that, compared with treatment with placebo and escitalopram, coadministration of eszopiclone and escitalopram resulted in significantly improved sleep and daytime functioning ($P < 0.05$), greater improvements in total Hamilton Anxiety Scale (HAM-A) scores at each week ($P < 0.05$) and at weeks 4 through 10, and greater improvements on the Clinical Global Impressions (CGI) of Improvement ($P < 0.02$). Overall, the data obtained for the treatment of insomnia and comorbid psychiatrics conditions suggest that study designs like these will become increasingly valuable during phases IIIb and IV development, and may be used to document the efficacy and safety of hypnotics in insomnia comorbid with other conditions. Such documentation adds to the clinical understanding of the potential uses of hypnotics and also helps to differentiate hypnotics from each other.

In addition to the comorbidities presented here, the clinical trials of insomnia in special populations may represent an important area of focus for future clinical trials. In the future, subjects with histories of alcohol or drug problems, or those with Alzheimer's disease or other forms of dementia, may become routinely included in clinical trials. In addition, children with insomnia might be considered a population of interest for clinical trials, given that no hypnotics have been specifically indicated for the treatment of pediatric insomnia.

CONCLUSION

Clinical trials for hypnotics occur in a well-controlled regulatory environment. These trials represent the method by which the efficacy and safety of new drug treatments for insomnia are determined. The development of new hypnotics includes both preclinical (animal) and clinical (human) studies, the latter being grouped into three phases that occur prior to the submission of an NDA, and a fourth phase that occurs following the approval of a drug product. The successful completion of a hypnotic development program involves the careful consideration of subject and patient populations, study designs, methodology, and study endpoints. While regulatory guidance and precedents exist, our expanding knowledge of insomnia, its morbidities, and its pathophysiology will undoubtedly lead to new clinical development strategies for hypnotics and the development of new therapeutics that treat insomnia and its morbidities.

REFERENCES

1. Pharmaceutical Research and Manufacturers of America (PhRMA). Washington, DC: PhRMA Annual Survey, 2008.
2. Pharmaceutical Research and Manufacturers of America (PhRMA). Washington, DC: PhRMA Report, 2006.
3. U.S. Food and Drug Administration (FDA). Federal Food and Drugs Act of 1906 (The "Wiley Act"), Public Law Number 59–384, 34 Stat. 768 (1906), 1906.
4. U.S. Food and Drug Administration (FDA). History of the FDA. 2008. http://www.fda.gov/oc/history/historyoffda/default.htm.
5. Ballentine C. Taste of Raspberries, Taste of Death: The 1937 Elixir Sulfanilamide Incident. 1981.
6. U.S. Food and Drug Administration (FDA). History of the FDA: The 1938 Food, Drug, and Cosmetic Act. 2008.
7. Daemmrich A. A tale of two experts: Thalidomide and political engagement in the United States and West Germany. Soc Hist Med 2002; 15(1):137–158.
8. Celgene Corporation. Thalomid (thalidomide) Capsules. 2009.
9. Krantz JC Jr. New drugs and the Kefauver-Harris amendment. J New Drugs 1966; 6(2):77–79.
10. Krantz JC Jr. The Kefauver-Harris amendment after sixteen years. Mil Med 1978; 143(12):883.
11. Center for Drug Evaluation and Research (CDER). Guidelines for the clinical evaluation of hypnotic drugs. In: U.S. Department of Health, Education, and Welfare, ed. 1977.
12. U.S. Food and Drug Administration (FDA). FDA Requests Label Change for All Sleep Disorder Drug Products. FDA News 2007.
13. National Institutes of Health. Research TNCftPoHSoBaB. The Belmont Report: Ethical Principles and Guidelines for the Protection of Human Subjects of Research, the National Research Act (Pub. L. 93–348), 1979.

14. U.S. Food and Drug Administration (FDA). Milestones in U.S. Food and Drug Law History. 2005.
15. U.S. Department of Health and Human Services (DHHS). Code of Federal Regulations (CFR), Title 21.
16. U.S. Department of Health and Human Services. Guidance for Industry, Investigators, and Reviewers; Exploratory IND Studies. U.S. Department of Health and Human Services, 2006. Accessed 23 May, 2008.
17. Ng R. Drugs, From Discovery to Approval. Hoboken, NJ: John Wiley & Sons, 2004.
18. Sanger DJ, Morel E, Perrault G. Comparison of the pharmacological profiles of the hypnotic drugs, zaleplon and zolpidem. Eur J Pharmacol 1996; 313(1–2):35–42.
19. Ebert B, Anderson NJ, Cremers TI, et al. Gaboxadol—a different hypnotic profile with no tolerance to sleep EEG and sedative effects after repeated daily dosing. Pharmacol Biochem Behav 2008; 90(1):113–122.
20. Griebel G, Perrault G, Tan S, et al. Comparison of the pharmacological properties of classical and novel BZ-omega receptor ligands. Behav Pharmacol 1999; 10(5):483–495.
21. Dhawan K, Dhawan S, Chhabra S. Attenuation of benzodiazepine dependence in mice by a tri-substituted benzoflavone moiety of *Passiflora incarnata* Linneaus: A non-habit forming anxiolytic. J Pharm Pharm Sci 2003; 6(2):215–222.
22. Alexandre C, Dordal A, Aixendri R, et al. Sleep-stabilizing effects of E-6199, compared to zopiclone, zolpidem and THIP in mice. Sleep 2008; 31(2):259–270.
23. Saitou K, Kaneko Y, Sugimoto Y, et al. Slow wave sleep-inducing effects of first generation H1-antagonists. Biol Pharm Bull 1999; 22(10):1079–1082.
24. Shinomiya K, Shigemoto Y, Okuma C, et al. Effects of short-acting hypnotics on sleep latency in rats placed on grid suspended over water. Eur J Pharmacol 2003; 460(2–3):139–144.
25. Shinomiya K, Shigemoto Y, Omichi J, et al. Effects of three hypnotics on the sleep-wakefulness cycle in sleep-disturbed rats. Psychopharmacology (Berl) 2004; 173(1–2):203–209.
26. Visser SA, Wolters FL, van der Graaf PH, et al. Dose-dependent EEG effects of zolpidem provide evidence for GABA(A) receptor subtype selectivity in vivo. J Pharmacol Exp Ther 2003; 304(3):1251–1257.
27. Winsky-Sommerer R, Vyazovskiy VV, Homanics GE, et al. The EEG effects of THIP (gaboxadol) on sleep and waking are mediated by the GABA(A)delta-subunit-containing receptors. Eur J Neurosci 2007; 25(6):1893–1899.
28. Michaud JC, Muyard JP, Capdevielle G, et al. Mild insomnia induced by environmental perturbations in the rat: A study of this new model and of its possible applications in pharmacological research. Arch Int Pharmacodyn Ther 1982; 259(1):93–105.
29. Noguchi H, Kitazumi K, Mori M, et al. Electroencephalographic properties of zaleplon, a non-benzodiazepine sedative/hypnotic, in rats. J Pharmacol Sci 2004; 94(3):246–251.
30. Di Masi JA, Grabowski HG. The cost of biopharmaceutical R&D: is biotech different? Managerial and Dec Econ 2007; 28(4–5):469–479.
31. Sachs G. United States: Healthcare Services: CROs, 2007.
32. Pharma. Pharma Annual Report. Washington, DC: 2008.
33. Center for Drug Evaluation and Research (CDER).
34. National Institutes of Health (NIH). Glossary of Clinical Trial Terms. 2008.
35. Center for Drug Evaluation and Research (CDER). Guideline for the Format and Content of Human Pharmacokinetics and Bioavailability Section of an Application. 1987.
36. Center for Drug Evaluation and Research (CDER). Guidance for Industry. Pharmacokinetics in Patients with Impaired Hepatic Function: Study Design, Data Analysis, and Impact on Dosing and Labeling. 2003.
37. Center for Drug Evaluation and Research (CDER). Guidance for Industry: Pharmacokinetics in Patients with Impaired Renal Function: Study Design, Data Analysis, and Impact on Dosing and Labeling. 1998.
38. Center for Drug Evaluation and Research (CDER). Guidance for Industry: Pharmacokinetics in Pregnancy: Study Design, Data Analysis, and Impact on Dosing and Labeling. 2004.
39. Center for Drug Evaluation and Research (CDER). Draft Guidance for Industry General Considerations for Pediatric Pharmacokinetic Studies for Drugs and Biological Products. 2003.
40. Zammit G. Zolpidem extended-release: Therapy for sleep induction and sleep maintenance difficulties. Expert Opin Drug Metab Toxicol 2008; 4(3):325–331.
41. Greenblatt DJ, Legangneux E, Harmatz JS, et al. Dynamics and kinetics of a modified-release formulation of zolpidem: Comparison with immediate-release standard zolpidem and placebo. J Clin Pharmacol 2006; 46(12):1469–1480.
42. Roth T, Hull SG, Lankford DA, et al. Low-dose sublingual zolpidem tartrate is associated with dose-related improvement in sleep onset and duration in insomnia characterized by middle-of-the-night (MOTN) awakenings. Sleep 2008; 31(9):1277–1284.

43. Staner L, Eriksson M, Cornette F, et al. Sublingual zolpidem is more effective than oral zolpidem in initiating early onset of sleep in the post-nap model of transient insomnia: A polysomnographic study. Sleep Med 2008.
44. Greenblatt DJ, Harmatz JS, von Moltke LL, et al. Comparative kinetics and dynamics of zaleplon, zolpidem, and placebo. Clin Pharmacol Ther 1998; 64(5):553–561.
45. Hindmarch I, Legangneux E, Stanley N, et al. A double-blind, placebo-controlled investigation of the residual psychomotor and cognitive effects of zolpidem-MR in healthy elderly volunteers. Br J Clin Pharmacol 2006; 62(5):538–545.
46. Hesse LM, von Moltke LL, Greenblatt DJ. Clinically important drug interactions with zopiclone, zolpidem and zaleplon. CNS Drugs 2003; 17(7):513–532.
47. Greenblatt DJ, Patki KC, von Moltke LL, et al. Drug interactions with grapefruit juice: An update. J Clin Psychopharmacol 2001; 21(4):357–359.
48. Shader RI, Greenblatt DJ. Fruit juices and pharmacology. J Clin Psychopharmacol 1997; 17(4):245–246.
49. Yamazaki A, Kumagai Y, Fujita T, et al. Different effects of light food on pharmacokinetics and pharmacodynamics of three benzodiazepines, quazepam, nitrazepam and diazepam. J Clin Pharm Ther 2007; 32(1):31–39.
50. Sugimoto K, Araki N, Ohmori M, et al. Interaction between grapefruit juice and hypnotic drugs: Comparison of triazolam and quazepam. Eur J Clin Pharmacol 2006; 62(3):209–215.
51. Roehrs T, Vogel G, Sterling W, et al. Dose effects of temazepam in transient insomnia. Arzneimittelforschung 1990; 40(8):859–862.
52. Roth T, Roehrs T, Vogel G. Zolpidem in the treatment of transient insomnia: A double-blind, randomized comparison with placebo. Sleep 1995; 18(4):246–251.
53. Erman MK, Erwin CW, Gengo FM, et al. Comparative efficacy of zolpidem and temazepam in transient insomnia. Hum Psychopharmacol 2001; 16(2):169–176.
54. Rosenberg R, Caron J, Roth T, et al. An assessment of the efficacy and safety of eszopiclone in the treatment of transient insomnia in healthy adults. Sleep Med 2005; 6(1):15–22.
55. Rosenberg R, Roth T, Scharf MB, et al. Efficacy and tolerability of indiplon in transient insomnia. J Clin Sleep Med 2007; 3(4):374–379.
56. Tietz EI, Roth T, Zorick FJ, et al. The acute effect of quazepam on the sleep of chronic insomniacs. A dose-response study. Arzneimittelforschung 1981; 31(11):1963–1966.
57. Zammit G, Schwartz H, Roth T, et al. The effects of ramelteon in a first-night model of transient insomnia. Sleep Med 2008.
58. Seidel WF, Roth T, Roehrs T, et al. Treatment of a 12-hour shift of sleep schedule with benzodiazepines. Science 1984; 224(4654):1262–1264.
59. Seidel WF, Cohen SA, Bliwise NG, et al. Dose-related effects of triazolam and flurazepam on a circadian rhythm insomnia. Clin Pharmacol Ther 1986; 40(3):314–320.
60. Erman MK, Loewy DB, Scharf MB. Effects of temazepam 7.5 mg and temazepam 15 mg on sleep maintenance and sleep architecture in a model of transient insomnia. Curr Med Res Opin 2005; 21(2):223–230.
61. Walsh JK, Mayleben D, Guico-Pabia C, et al. Efficacy of the selective extrasynaptic GABA A agonist, gaboxadol, in a model of transient insomnia: A randomized, controlled clinical trial. Sleep Med 2008; 9(4):393–402.
62. Walsh JK, Schweitzer PK, Sugerman JL, et al. Transient insomnia associated with a 3-hour phase advance of sleep time and treatment with zolpidem. J Clin Psychopharmacol 1990; 10(3):184–189.
63. Terzano MG, Parrino L, Fioriti G, et al. Modifications of sleep structure induced by increasing levels of acoustic perturbation in normal subjects. Electroencephalogr Clin Neurophysiol 1990; 76(1):29–38.
64. Terzano MG, Parrino L, Boselli M, et al. Changes of cyclic alternating pattern (CAP) parameters in situational insomnia under brotizolam and triazolam. Psychopharmacology (Berl) 1995; 120(3): 237–243.
65. Parrino L, Boselli M, Spaggiari MC, et al. Multidrug comparison (lorazepam, triazolam, zolpidem, and zopiclone) in situational insomnia: Polysomnographic analysis by means of the cyclic alternating pattern. Clin Neuropharmacol 1997; 20(3):253–263.
66. Hindmarch I, Legangneux, E, Stanley N. A randomized, double-blind, placebo-controlled, 10-way crossover study shows that a new zolpidem modified-release formulation improves sleep maintenance compared to standard zolpidem. Sleep 2004; 27:A55.
67. Cluydts R, De Roeck J, Cosyns P, et al. Antagonizing the effects of experimentally induced sleep disturbance in healthy volunteers by lormetazepam and zolpidem. J Clin Psychopharmacol 1995; 15(2):132–137.
68. Erman MK, Zammit G, Rubens R, et al. A polysomnographic placebo-controlled evaluation of the efficacy and safety of eszopiclone relative to placebo and zolpidem in the treatment of primary insomnia. J Clin Sleep Med 2008; 4(3):229–234.

69. Monti JM, Attali P, Monti D, et al. Zolpidem and rebound insomnia—a double-blind, controlled polysomnographic study in chronic insomniac patients. Pharmacopsychiatry 1994; 27(4):166–175.
70. Herrmann WM, Kubicki ST, Boden S, et al. Pilot controlled double-blind study of the hypnotic effects of zolpidem in patients with chronic "learned" insomnia: Psychometric and polysomnographic evaluation. J Int Med Res 1993; 21(6):306–322.
71. Declerck AC, Ruwe F, O'Hanlon JF, et al. Effects of zolpidem and flunitrazepam on nocturnal sleep of women subjectively complaining of insomnia. Psychopharmacology (Berl) 1992; 106(4):497–501.
72. Cohn JB, Wilcox CS, Bremner J, et al. Hypnotic efficacy of estazolam compared with flurazepam in outpatients with insomnia. J Clin Pharmacol 1991; 31(8):747–750.
73. Elie R, Lavoie G, Bourgouin J, et al. Zopiclone versus flurazepam in insomnia: Prolonged administration and withdrawal. Int Clin Psychopharmacol 1990; 5(4):279–286.
74. Nair NP, Schwartz G, Dimitri R, et al. A dose-range finding study of zopiclone in insomniac patients. Int Clin Psychopharmacol 1990; 5(suppl 2):1–10.
75. Ponciano E, Freitas F, Camara J, et al. A comparison of the efficacy, tolerance and residual effects of zopiclone, flurazepam and placebo in insomniac outpatients. Int Clin Psychopharmacol 1990; 5(suppl 2):69–77.
76. Cohn JB. Double-blind crossover comparison of triazolam and lorazepam in the posthypnotic state. J Clin Psychiatry 1984; 45(3):104–107.
77. Roth T, Rogowski R, Hull S, et al. Efficacy and safety of doxepin 1 mg, 3 g, and 6 mg in adults with primary insomnia. Sleep 2007; 30(11):1555–1561.
78. Roth T, Seiden D, Wang-Weigand S, et al. A 2-night, 3-period, crossover study of ramelteon's efficacy and safety in older adults with chronic insomnia. Curr Med Res Opin 2007; 23(5):1005–1014.
79. Scharf MB, Roth T, Vogel GW, et al. A multicenter, placebo-controlled study evaluating zolpidem in the treatment of chronic insomnia. J Clin Psychiatry 1994; 55(5):192–199.
80. Fabre LF Jr, Brachfeld J, Meyer LR, Slowe IA, et al. Multi-clinic double-blind comparison of triazolam (Halcion) and placebo administered for 14 consecutive nights in outpatients with insomnia. J Clin Psychiatry 1978; 39:679–682.
81. Walsh JK, Targum SD, Pegram V, et al. A multi-center clinical investigation of estazolam: Short-term efficacy. Curr Ther Res 1984; 36:866–874.
82. Walsh JK, Soubrane C, Roth T. Efficacy and safety of zolpidem extended release in elderly primary insomnia patients. Am J Geriatr Psychiatry 2008; 16(1):44–57.
83. Zammit G, Erman M, Wang-Weigand S, et al. Evaluation of the efficacy and safety of ramelteon in subjects with chronic insomnia. J Clin Sleep Med 2007; 3(5):495–504.
84. Nowell PD, Mazumdar S, Buysse DJ, et al. Benzodiazepines and zolpidem for chronic insomnia: A meta-analysis of treatment efficacy. JAMA 1997; 278(24):2170–2177.
85. Krystal AD, Erman M, Zammit GK, et al. Long-term efficacy and safety of zolpidem extended-release 12.5 mg, administered 3 to 7 nights per week for 24 weeks, in patients with chronic primary insomnia: A 6-month, randomized, double-blind, placebo-controlled, parallel-group, multicenter study. Sleep 2008; 31(1):79–90.
86. Walsh JK, Krystal AD, Amato DA, et al. Nightly treatment of primary insomnia with eszopiclone for six months: Effect on sleep, quality of life, and work limitations. Sleep 2007; 30(8):959–968.
87. Scharf MB, Black J, Hull S, et al. Long-term nightly treatment with indiplon in adults with primary insomnia: Results of a double-blind, placebo-controlled, 3-month study. Sleep 2007; 30(6):743–752.
88. Krystal AD, Walsh JK, Laska E, et al. Sustained efficacy of eszopiclone over 6 months of nightly treatment: Results of a randomized, double-blind, placebo-controlled study in adults with chronic insomnia. Sleep 2003; 26(7):793–799.
89. Zammit GK, McNabb LJ, Caron J, et al. Efficacy and safety of eszopiclone across 6-weeks of treatment for primary insomnia. Curr Med Res Opin 2004; 20(12):1979–1991.
90. Roth T, Soubrane C, Titeux L, et al. Efficacy and safety of zolpidem-MR: A double-blind, placebo-controlled study in adults with primary insomnia. Sleep Med 2006; 7(5):397–406.
91. Hajak G, Clarenbach P, Fischer W, et al. Zopiclone improves sleep quality and daytime well-being in insomniac patients: Comparison with triazolam, flunitrazepam and placebo. Int Clin Psychopharmacol 1994; 9(4):251–261.
92. Dominguez RA, Goldstein BJ, Jacobson AF, et al. Comparative efficacy of estazolam, flurazepam, and placebo in outpatients with insomnia. J Clin Psychiatry 1986; 47(7):362–365.
93. Scharf MB, Roth PB, Dominguez RA, et al. Estazolam and flurazepam: A multicenter, placebo-controlled comparative study in outpatients with insomnia. J Clin Pharmacol 1990; 30(5):461–467.
94. Ancoli-Israel S, Walsh JK, Mangano RM, et al. Zaleplon: A novel nonbenzodiazepine hypnotic, effectively treats insomnia in elderly patients without causing rebound effects. Prim Care Companion J Clin Psychiatry 1999; 1(4):114–120.

95. Cluydts R. Zolpidem 'as needed': Methodological issues and clinical findings. CNS Drugs 2004; 18(suppl 1):25–33; discussion 43–45.
96. Hajak G, Geisler P. Experience with zolpidem 'as needed' in primary care settings. CNS Drugs 2004; 18(suppl 1):35–40; discussion 1, 3–5.
97. Walsh JK, Roth T, Randazzo A, et al. Eight weeks of non-nightly use of zolpidem for primary insomnia. Sleep 2000; 23(8):1087–1096.
98. Hajak G, Cluydts R, Declerck A, et al. Continuous versus non-nightly use of zolpidem in chronic insomnia: Results of a large-scale, double-blind, randomized, outpatient study. Int Clin Psychopharmacol 2002; 17(1):9–17.
99. Roth T, Hauri P, Zorick F, et al. The effects of midazolam and temazepam on sleep and performance when administered in the middle of the night. J Clin Psychopharmacol 1985; 5(2):66–69.
100. Perlis ML, McCall WV, Krystal AD, et al. Long-term, non-nightly administration of zolpidem in the treatment of patients with primary insomnia. J Clin Psychiatry 2004; 65(8):1128–1137.
101. Danjou P, Paty I, Fruncillo R, et al. A comparison of the residual effects of zaleplon and zolpidem following administration 5 to 2 h before awakening. Br J Clin Pharmacol 1999; 48(3):367–374.
102. Walsh JK, Pollak CP, Scharf MB, et al. Lack of residual sedation following middle-of-the-night zaleplon administration in sleep maintenance insomnia. Clin Neuropharmacol 2000; 23(1):17–21.
103. Hindmarch I, Patat A, Stanley N, et al. Residual effects of zaleplon and zolpidem following middle of the night administration five hours to one hour before awakening. Hum Psychopharmacol 2001; 16(2):159–167.
104. Zammit GK, Corser B, Doghramji K, et al. Sleep and residual sedation after administration of zaleplon, zolpidem, and placebo during experimental middle-of-the-night awakening. J Clin Sleep Med 2006; 2(4):417–423.
105. Farber RH, Burke PJ. Post-bedtime dosing with indiplon in adults and the elderly: Results from two placebo-controlled, active comparator crossover studies in healthy volunteers. Curr Med Res Opin 2008; 24(3):837–846.
106. Roth T, Zammit GK, Scharf MB, et al. Efficacy and safety of as-needed, post bedtime dosing with indiplon in insomnia patients with chronic difficulty maintaining sleep. Sleep 2007; 30(12): 1731–1738.
107. Center for Drug Evaluation and Research (CDER). Guidance for Industry: E14 Clinical Evaluation of QT/Qtc Interval Prolongation and Proarrhythmic Potential for Non-Antiarrhythmic Drugs. In: U.S. Department of Health and Human Services, FADA, ed.; 2005.
108. Johns MW. A new method for measuring daytime sleepiness: The Epworth Sleepiness Scale. Sleep 1991; 14(6):540–545.
109. Johns MW. Reliability and factor analysis of the Epworth Sleepiness Scale. Sleep 1992; 15(4):376–381.
110. Carskadon MA, Dement WC, Mitler MM, et al. Guidelines for the multiple sleep latency test (MSLT): A standard measure of sleepiness. Sleep 1986; 9(4):519–524.
111. Thorpy MJ. The clinical use of the Multiple Sleep Latency Test. The Standards of Practice Committee of the American Sleep Disorders Association. Sleep 1992; 15(3):268–276.
112. Kobak KA, DeBrota D, Engelhardt N, et al. Site vs. centralized raters in a clinical depression trial. In: 46th Annual Meeting of the National Institutes of Health, New Clinical Drug Evaluation Unit,; 2006; Boca Raton, FL.
113. McCall WV, Erman M, Krystal AD, et al. A polysomnography study of eszopiclone in elderly patients with insomnia. Curr Med Res Opin 2006; 22(9):1633–1642.
114. Monti JM, Alvarino F, Monti D. Conventional and power spectrum analysis of the effects of zolpidem on sleep EEG in patients with chronic primary insomnia. Sleep 2000; 23(8):1075–1084.
115. Ozone M, Yagi T, Itoh H, et al. Effects of zolpidem on cyclic alternating pattern, an objective marker of sleep instability, in Japanese patients with psychophysiological insomnia: A randomized crossover comparative study with placebo. Pharmacopsychiatry 2008; 41(3):106–114.
116. Terzano MG, Parrino L. Clinical applications of cyclic alternating pattern. Physiol Behav 1993; 54(4):807–813.
117. Terzano MG, Parrino L, Spaggiari MC, et al. CAP variables and arousals as sleep electroencephalogram markers for primary insomnia. Clin Neurophysiol 2003; 114(9):1715–1723.
118. Scharf M, Erman M, Rosenberg R, et al. A 2-week efficacy and safety study of eszopiclone in elderly patients with primary insomnia. Sleep 2005; 28(6):720–727.
119. Knutson KL, Spiegel K, Penev P, et al. The metabolic consequences of sleep deprivation. Sleep Med Rev 2007; 11(3):163–178.
120. Knutson KL, Van Cauter E. Associations between sleep loss and increased risk of obesity and diabetes. Ann N Y Acad Sci 2008; 1129:287–304.
121. Van Cauter E, Holmback U, Knutson K, et al. Impact of sleep and sleep loss on neuroendocrine and metabolic function. Horm Res 2007; 67(suppl 1):2–9.

122. Gangwisch JE, Heymsfield SB, Boden-Albala B, et al. Sleep duration as a risk factor for diabetes incidence in a large U.S. sample. Sleep 2007; 30(12):1667–1673.
123. Gangwisch JE, Malaspina D, Boden-Albala B, et al. Inadequate sleep as a risk factor for obesity: Analyses of the NHANES I. Sleep 2005; 28(10):1289–1296.
124. Gangwisch JE, Heymsfield SB, Boden-Albala B, et al. Short sleep duration as a risk factor for hypertension: Analyses of the first National Health and Nutrition Examination Survey. Hypertension 2006; 47(5):833–839.
125. Gottlieb DJ, Redline S, Nieto FJ, et al. Association of usual sleep duration with hypertension: The Sleep Heart Health Study. Sleep 2006; 29(8):1009–1014.
126. Ozer O, Ozbala B, Sari I, et al. Acute sleep deprivation is associated with increased QT dispersion in healthy young adults. Pacing Clin Electrophysiol 2008; 31(8):979–984.
127. Sari I, Davutoglu V, Ozbala B, et al. Acute sleep deprivation is associated with increased electrocardiographic P-wave dispersion in healthy young men and women. Pacing Clin Electrophysiol 2008; 31(4):438–442.
128. Gangwisch JE, Heymsfield SB, Boden-Albala B, et al. Sleep duration associated with mortality in elderly, but not middle-aged, adults in a large US sample. Sleep 2008; 31(8):1087–1096.
129. Center for Drug Evaluation and Research (CDER). Guidance for Industry: E6 Good Clinical Practice: Consolidated Guidance. In: U.S. Department of Health and Human Services, FADA, ed., 1996.
130. Kryger M, Wang-Weigand S, Roth T. Safety of ramelteon in individuals with mild to moderate obstructive sleep apnea. Sleep Breath 2007; 11(3):159–164.
131. Cohn MA, Morris DD, Juan D. Effects of estazolam and flurazepam on cardiopulmonary function in patients with chronic obstructive pulmonary disease. Drug Saf 1992; 7(2):152–158.
132. Dorsey CM, Lee KA, Scharf MB. Effect of zolpidem on sleep in women with perimenopausal and postmenopausal insomnia: A 4-week, randomized, multicenter, double-blind, placebo-controlled study. Clin Ther 2004; 26(10):1578–1586.
133. Soares CN, Joffe H, Rubens R, et al. Eszopiclone in patients with insomnia during perimenopause and early postmenopause: A randomized controlled trial. Obstet Gynecol 2006; 108(6):1402–1410.
134. Asnis GM, Chakraburtty A, DuBoff EA, et al. Zolpidem for persistent insomnia in SSRI-treated depressed patients. J Clin Psychiatry 1999; 60(10):668–676.
135. Pollack M, Kinrys G, Krystal A, et al. Eszopiclone coadministered with escitalopram in patients with insomnia and comorbid generalized anxiety disorder. Arch Gen Psychiatry 2008; 65(5):551–562.
136. Fava M, McCall WV, Krystal A, et al. Eszopiclone co-administered with fluoxetine in patients with insomnia coexisting with major depressive disorder. Biol Psychiatry 2006; 59(11):1052–1060.

39 Practice Models

Michael J. Sateia
Department of Psychiatry, Dartmouth Medical School, Lebanon, New Hampshire, U.S.A.

INTRODUCTION

Acute and chronic insomnia are prevalent in a multitude of medical settings. The degree of relevance of this disorder to the particular medical care being delivered will vary substantially from one setting to another. Nevertheless, it is incumbent on health care providers of all types to recognize the potential importance of this problem and the influence it may have on care delivery and outcome, and to be familiar with at least the basics of assessment and management. Chronic insomnia is associated with increased health care utilization, chronic illness, and high rates of disability and functional impairment (1,2) (see also chapter 3). As outlined in previous chapters, the condition may also predispose to psychiatric disorders (3,4), alter pain thresholds (5), and perhaps, adversely affect cardiovascular function (6), to name but a few of the possible consequences.

Recognizing the presence of an insomnia problem is a relatively straightforward process, in that it requires only a complaint of sleep disturbance, despite adequate opportunity to sleep, that is associated with daytime consequences (7). Despite the relative simplicity of the general diagnosis, we know that most individuals with the problem are not identified. Health care providers are constantly assailed with the need to do more and more in a health care environment that allows them less and less time per patient. In this climate of competition for the attention of providers (and patients), it is necessary to make the case for why this particular problem warrants precious time. Ultimately, this requires demonstration that intervention enhances outcome in one or more spheres. At present, the field of sleep medicine is still some distance from making that case in a convincing manner. The same, of course, may be said for a host of other common health care practices. Nevertheless, data on outcomes in current therapeutic research, though spotty, suggest that identification and treatment improves health and function (8–10).

The extent to which insomnia is identified and addressed can be expected to vary widely from one medical discipline to another. Although the greatest management expertise presumably resides within sleep medicine, there can be little doubt that the great majority of insomnia is encountered in primary care and mental health practices. Therefore, it is necessary to consider what levels of intervention can reasonably be expected in these varied settings. A simple goal would be mere identification of a chronic sleep problem, but the extant data suggest that current practice is far from achieving this goal. Neither physicians nor patients seem particularly inclined to bring this issue to medical attention, despite the fact that some patients, when asked, report insomnia as a very significant symptom (11).

What, then, are realistic expectations at a primary care level? Routine health screening should include, at a minimum, an inquiry regarding the patient's sleep. This brief query, coupled with determination of daytime consequences and adequacy of opportunity to sleep (i.e., time in bed under conducive circumstances), is sufficient to establish the presence of an insomnia problem. Primary care providers can also be expected to ascertain the duration of the problem. Management of an acute problem is likely to be quite different from that of one that has been present for years or decades.

ACUTE INSOMNIA IN THE PRIMARY CARE SETTING

The vast majority of acute or transient insomnia does not come to medical attention. However, when short-term sleep disturbance is a source of significant distress or daytime dysfunction, physicians may be called on to respond. Current practice typically consists of reassurance and, in some cases, pharmacological recommendations. Most recent data indicate that these recommendations are quite often for over-the-counter (OTC) products (antihistamine or melatonin) or off-label use of sedating antidepressants (12). Patients may have initiated self-medication with alcohol or OTC products, including herbal supplements.

Optimal management of short-term insomnia is reasonably straightforward. It is necessary to consider what current stresses or conditions may have precipitated the sleep problem. The presence of other common and readily treatable illness such as major depression must be considered. If the insomnia is, indeed, an adjustment disturbance, several straightforward approaches are indicated. First, consideration of whether the patient requires further assistance in coping effectively with the current stress. Brief stress management counseling in the office or referral for more specialized mental health counseling are options. On occasion, daytime pharmacotherapy (antianxiety medication) may be indicated. Second, sleep education is likely to reduce the likelihood of an acute disorder evolving into chronic insomnia. These principles are discussed in detail in chapter 23. Preventing the development of factors that are likely to perpetuate the insomnia by encouraging maintenance of a regular schedule and stimulus control measures is particularly important. Finally, consideration must be given to pharmacological aid. As noted, patients may already be self-medicating. Although specific practice parameters regarding pharmacological management of adjustment insomnia do not exist, most sources suggest that self-medicating is generally not advisable. Alcohol, the most common form of self-medication for insomnia, clearly is contraindicated (chapters 16 and 36) and efficacy of OTC products is not well established (chapter 36). When patient and physician agree that the degree of distress or dysfunction warrants use of a sleep aid, a benzodiazepine receptor agonist (BzRA) or melatonin agonist hypnotic is indicated (13). The efficacy of these drugs is well established and, when used and monitored properly, they carry limited clinical risk. The most critical aspect of choosing a specific hypnotic medication is matching the duration of the clinical action of the drug to the sleep complaint. This issue is discussed at greater length in preceding chapters. Perhaps most importantly, follow-up in the primary care setting is critical. This should include (1) review of the current status of the insomnia; (2) inquiry regarding precipitating conditions; (3) continued sleep hygiene and stimulus control education; (4) determination of effectiveness and side effects of medication; (5) tapering and discontinuation of hypnotic medication as exacerbating events and sleep disturbance resolve, with education regarding possible transient rebound insomnia.

CHRONIC INSOMNIA IN PRIMARY CARE

Most insomnia complaints that come to medical attention are chronic in nature (14). While the greatest expertise in assessment and treatment of chronic insomnia lies with sleep medicine physicians and behavioral sleep medicine specialists, sheer numbers dictate that initial evaluation and treatment for the great majority will occur in primary care offices. Identification of a chronic insomnia problem in this setting should be followed by consideration of potential etiologies. The general etiologic categories to be considered for chronic insomnia are (1) primary insomnia; (2) insomnia comorbid with medical, neurological, psychiatric, or substance use/abuse conditions; (3) sleep–wake schedule disorders; (4) insomnia comorbid with other sleep disorders (e.g., breathing, movement, environmental). Primary care providers can be expected to identify comorbid factors such as chronic pain, major psychiatric disorders, substances, or other medical and neurological problems, which may contribute to the insomnia. These factors are discussed extensively in preceding chapters. Screening for primary sleep disorders, especially breathing and movement disorders, is required. In most cases, positive screens should prompt referral to a sleep specialist.

Therapy for chronic insomnia can be complex. It could be argued that the optimal treatment for these patients would be in a comprehensive sleep center with available expertise in cognitive behavioral treatment of insomnia. As is the case with many common conditions though, a majority of these patients are and will continue to be managed by their primary provider. Therefore, a realistic set of guidelines is necessary. These, in effect, can be distilled into three major areas: (1) managing comorbid conditions; (2) pharmacotherapies; and (3) psychological and behavioral therapies.

Comorbidities

Certainly, primary care physicians should address those common comorbidities that are within the realm of their expertise—conditions such as major depression, substance abuse, pain, gastro-esophageal reflux disorder (GERD), nocturia, nocturnal respiratory distress (e.g., asthma), or endocrine disease. A review of medications with consideration of possible offending substances is likewise appropriate. When comorbidities such as this are identified and a suspicion of causal linkage to the insomnia exists, primary care providers have traditionally been inclined to focus primarily on treating the comorbidity, with the expectation that the sleep problem, as a "secondary" symptom, would resolve. More recent evidence indicates the need for a paradigm shift in this respect (15). Studies in several key areas, particularly depression and pain, suggest that optimal outcome may be achieved by concurrent treatment of not only the comorbid condition, but the insomnia as well (16,17). Treatment for the insomnia may be psychological/behavioral, pharmacological, or both.

Cognitive Behavioral Therapy

Guidelines for the treatment of chronic insomnia indicate that all patients, whenever possible, receive cognitive behavioral treatment for insomnia (CBT-I). (13) An abundant research demonstrates the early and long-term effectiveness of these modalities (18,19). Unfortunately, a substantial gap exists between the academic and the real world application of CBT-I. Identification of a skilled CBT-I therapist has been difficult to impossible for most clinicians in general practice. There are, perhaps, more viable options available, although none have seen widespread implementation. Some well-meaning clinicians will attempt to address certain cognitive or behavioral aspects of chronic insomnia with brief discussion and education concerning sleep hygiene. While such education may be quite helpful in preventing an acute insomnia problem from becoming chronic, there is inadequate evidence to support education as an effective strategy for chronic insomnia, alone or combined with medication (18). A number of specific CBT approaches have proven efficacy and an attempt needs to be made to deliver this to as many patients as possible.

One option for the primary health care provider is to attempt to deliver some form of these therapies from their office practice. It seems quite unlikely that many physicians are going to have the time or inclination to learn and deliver this care themselves. However, there is some evidence, as discussed in previous chapters, that providers other than doctoral level individuals can be educated to offer these treatments in an effective manner (8,20). Educational programs for would-be therapists are available on a regular basis and manualized treatment approaches can make delivery somewhat more straightforward (8,21). Brief (3–5 sessions) group CBT-I, offered by a nurse or other qualified health care professional, on a quarterly basis, for example, could offer relief to significant numbers of individuals with chronic insomnia. There are also a number of self-help, internet-based CBT approaches, sometimes coupled with phone intervention (18,22–27). Assessment of these programs suggests some promising results and primary physicians and patients with limited access to alternatives may consider this approach. Having said that, it is likely that patients with the most severe chronic insomnia problems will require the skills of a highly experienced expert in this area. Many of these experts are specifically certified as behavioral sleep medicine specialists by the American Academy of Sleep Medicine (AASM), and most are attached to accredited comprehensive sleep centers. Establishment of stronger alliances between these sleep centers and the primary or specialty care practices in their communities could serve as a foundation for identifying or developing resources for provision of effective CBT-I.

Prescribing Hypnotics

The decision regarding prescription of medication for chronic insomnia patients is a complex one. Numerous factors influence this decision. These include (1) patient preference; (2) prior experience with medication and results of this; (3) willingness to engage in CBT-I; (4) availability of CBT clinicians; (5) contraindications to use of hypnotics or other sedating medications. Many physicians are reluctant to prescribe medication for chronic insomnia, based on fears of dependency and tolerance. The practice of recommending OTC medication (commonly antihistamine compounds) or sedating antidepressants, in all likelihood, reflects the belief that these agents are safer alternatives to approved BzRA medications. Unfortunately, the efficacy of these alternatives is not well established in chronic insomnia, and it is not clear that they are intrinsically "safer" than standard hypnotics (28). Therefore, current AASM guidelines recommend that when medications are prescribed for chronic insomnia, the first-line choice should be an appropriate shorter-acting BzRA (13). The more important issues, perhaps, for health care providers with respect to prescribing these medications are (1) patient education regarding goals, expectations, and side effects of medication; (2) use of minimal effective dosages of a medication with a duration of action appropriate to the insomnia complaint; (3) implementation of effective psychological and behavioral therapies; (4) tapering and discontinuation of medication in conjunction with (3); and (5) continued follow-up during and after medication trials. Alternative pharmacotherapies are addressed briefly in the following section on mental health models and more extensively elsewhere in this text.

Combined Treatment

Clinicians must recognize that when hypnotic medication is prescribed for chronic insomnia, it should, whenever possible, be accompanied by CBT-I. The primary reason for this dictum is that current data make clear that short-term trials of sleep medication, while effective during the period of active administration, do not typically produce sustained improvement of the sleep disturbance (18,29,30). Evidence is also clear that CBT-I does produce durable change. Thus, in the absence of these nonpharmacological therapies, clinicians are frequently left in the uncomfortable position of either discontinuing medication, with resulting recrudescence of the problem, or maintaining chronic hypnotic use.

For some time, there has been debate over whether combining pharmacotherapy with CBT-I is advantageous or, alternatively, counterproductive. Proponents of combined treatment argue that medication may provide faster relief and enhance patient confidence in their ability to sleep, thus reinforcing gains associated with CBT. Opponents suggest that patients may misattribute gains to medication, rather than to CBT, be less motivated to implement skills effectively, and thus, be more prone to relapse with discontinuation of the medication. The evidence on this is mixed. The most widely cited study of combined treatment (18) found that combined therapy was associated with a trend toward greater improvement immediately posttreatment than either treatment alone, but the longer-term outcome with combined treatment was more variable than with CBT alone. Another study found no advantage of combined treatment over CBT alone (29).

Chronic Hypnotic Usage

Even under the best of circumstances, some patients who have received adequate assessment and treatment, including skilled CBT-I, will continue to suffer from insomnia without the assistance of medication. Some of these patients will be well controlled on medication without significant side effects or complications. Recent randomized, placebo-controlled studies have confirmed long-term efficacy of newer generation BzRAs without significant dosage escalation, side effect, withdrawal, or rebound insomnia complications (31,32). Therefore, it seems reasonable to consider long-term use of hypnotics in CBT treatment-refractory patients. When sleep medications are to be used chronically, the clinician must follow several practices, all involving ongoing follow-up, to ensure optimal outcome. These include (1) verifying that the medication is still effective; (2) making certain that no significant side effects or complications have developed (this would include indication of dosage escalation); (3) reassessing for the emergence of new comorbidities that may complicate the management; (4) encouraging the continued employment of cognitive behavioral strategies; (5) periodically readdressing the possibility that medications may be tapered or discontinued.

Chronic Hypnotic Discontinuation

Providers are frequently confronted with established chronic hypnotic usage in insomnia patients who have never received treatment other than pharmacotherapy and who are often not experiencing adequate relief of the sleep problem even with regular use of medication. The general mind-set among many clinicians is that this chronic reliance on sleeping pills is an undesirable practice; however, the provider is frequently trapped between a desire to minimize long-term complications or dependency risks (i.e., discontinue the medication) and a patient who is desperate for relief from insomnia. To further complicate this scenario, patients often report that the current medication, and many prior ones, are ineffective, but will resist efforts to discontinue them. In turn, this may prompt further and increasingly desperate efforts on the part of the prescriber to find an effective medication or combination of medications. While pharmacotherapy has a legitimate place in the treatment of chronic insomnia, as discussed, it is seldom the case that rapid turnover polypharmacy, in its own right, is the solution for chronic insomnia. Efforts to simplify and discontinue medications in this population may be the more advantageous therapeutic strategy in many cases. Given the fact that the improvements seen with short-term medication trials alone are not generally sustained in chronic insomnia patients, it is hardly surprising that primary care providers would often meet resistance and be frustrated in efforts to achieve medication tapering or discontinuation without providing the patient with effective alternative therapies. A growing body of evidence clearly defines the effectiveness of CBT-I in promoting successful tapering and discontinuation of chronic hypnotic medication (18).

One study (33) demonstrated a twofold higher rate of complete hypnotic discontinuation in older chronic hypnotic users when CBT-I (small group format × 8 weeks) was utilized in combination with medication tapering (77% discontinuation) versus tapering alone (38%). This differential was even greater at 12-month follow-up (70% vs. 24%). These observations have been extended in a separate study to assess the combination of self-help CBT with tapering (34). These two conditions produced comparable rates of reduction in hypnotic usage, although sleep efficiency increased and wake time decreased in the CBT group. However, the sleep-related improvements in the CBT group may reflect primarily the effects of restricted time in bed. In a similar investigation (35) of BZD discontinuation in patients with anxiety disorder or insomnia, treatment as usual (tapering and physician counseling) was compared to tapering coupled with either group support or group CBT). Both group support and CBT produced significantly higher rates of discontinuation (85% and 83%, respectively) than treatment as usual (39%). Of note, however, is the fact that rates for group support (in which any specific recommendations were specifically prohibited) were equivalent to those for CBT. A more recent placebo-controlled investigation (36) suggests that administration of melatonin in conjunction with tapering may promote higher rates of hypnotic discontinuation in an elderly population than tapering alone.

In summary, while some patients may benefit from chronic use of sleep medications, many others have not received adequate evaluation or nonpharmacological therapies. Ultimately, a number of chronic insomnia sufferers will not respond adequately to the level of treatment offered by primary care providers. In such cases, consideration should be given to referral to a specialist in sleep medicine. This is discussed further in later sections.

CHRONIC INSOMNIA IN THE MENTAL HEALTH SETTING

Insomnia is considered an intrinsic component of many major psychiatric conditions. As discussed earlier, this gives rise to the view, still widely held by mental health professionals, that the sleep-related symptoms will resolve with treatment of the primary mental illness alone. While this is indeed true in many cases, especially acute, short-lived disorders such as a single major depressive episode, many psychiatric conditions are recurrent or chronic in nature and provide ample opportunity for development of factors that perpetuate chronic insomnia. As discussed previously, recent evidence supports the notion that pharmacological or behavioral treatment of insomnia, concurrent with treatment of the psychiatric disorder, may produce improved outcome for both sleep and psychiatric parameters (16,17). Further fueling the need for such concurrent intervention is the observation that residual sleep disturbance conveys an increased risk for persistence or recurrence of mental illness (37–39). Finally, adequate sleep is likely to bolster coping mechanisms, enhance compliance with mental health treatment, and generally improve quality of life in patients with serious mental illness.

The principles of treatment for chronic insomnia comorbid with psychiatric disorders are much the same as those outlined above in the primary care section. However, several additional considerations are worthy of note. For many years, the efficacy of CBT-I was demonstrated in sample populations of patients with primary insomnia alone. Significant doubt existed as to whether or not these therapies would be successful in patient with the added complexities of mental disorders. On the basis of a number of trials (27,40–42) (see also chapter 30), it now seems quite clear that insomnia comorbid with psychiatric conditions has outcomes that are quite comparable to those observed in primary insomnia. Widespread application of group CBT-I by psychologists or psychiatric nurses in community mental health settings, inpatient or partial hospitalizations, or rehabilitation programs might provide significant benefit, but initiation of such endeavors is in its infancy, at best.

Patients with chronic psychiatric disorders often exhibit many complicating factors that must be addressed if sleep disturbance is to improve. Substance abuse may be foremost among these. The characteristics and management of insomnia comorbid with alcohol and drug abuse is discussed in detail in chapter 16. As a result of isolation and lack of social zeitgebers, patients with chronic psychiatric illness are prone to circadian disorders such as delayed or irregular sleep–wake rhythms. Special consideration must be given to the impact of psychotropic medications on sleep–wake function. The contribution of certain symptoms associated with specific psychiatric disorders to insomnia may also need to be addressed. One of the most common examples of this is recurrent nightmares in patients with posttraumatic stress disorder. In recent years, two therapies have shown particular promise in managing nightmares. The α_1-adrenergic antagonist, prazosin, has been shown to not only reduce nightmare frequency, but also to improve sleep in post-traumatic stress disorder (PTSD) patients (43,44). Likewise, the cognitive-behavioral therapy of imagery rehearsal and desensitization shows similar outcomes (45,46). Other symptoms such as nocturnal panic attacks or hallucinations may also require specific treatment focus.

Pharmacotherapy for insomnia in the setting of mental illness requires special considerations. In many cases, the primary psychopharmacological treatment may be a sedating compound, which can be administered at bedtime and may significantly aid sleep. Examples of this would include sedating antidepressant medications such as mirtazapine, or antipsychotic medications including many first-generation neuroleptics as well as second-generation drugs such as quetiapine, olanzapine, or risperidone. Mood-stabilizing agents may also provide substantial sedative effect, which may be used to good advantage at bedtime. Certainly, combined use of these medications for psychiatric indications and sleep disturbance may be quite appropriate and may simplify the medication regimen.

Beyond this combined indication, however, there are many patients who require the addition of a sedating medication primarily for the indication of insomnia. Psychiatrists, like many primary care physicians, often prescribe off-label use of sedating antidepressants such as trazodone (47–50), or sedating antipsychotics, especially quetiapine (51–53). These agents and others are discussed in detail in chapter 34. While these agents may have certain advantages in this population, it is important for practitioners to recognize that there has been very limited assessment of these drugs, often in uncontrolled studies, with regard to their efficacy in chronic insomnia. For this reason, guidelines suggest that BzRAs or ramelteon are the treatments of choice for chronic insomnia, including those cases comorbid with mental disorders. Having said that, it must also be recognized that in patients with high potential for abuse, such drugs may be contraindicated.

THE ROLE OF SLEEP MEDICINE

When patients with chronic insomnia cannot be effectively evaluated and/or treated in other settings, they should be referred to a comprehensive sleep center for specialized care. The role of the sleep specialist is threefold: (1) more detailed assessment of the problem; (2) employment of polysomnography, when indicated; and (3) more specialized, expert therapy, which includes follow-up to the point of problem resolution or maximum therapeutic benefit.

While it is within the expected purview of primary care or mental health providers to identify the most common and straightforward comorbidities of chronic insomnia and to obtain a basic characterization of the complaint, sleep specialists are trained to identify and integrate the numerous and often complex medical, psychiatric, and behavioral components of chronic insomnia. The intricacies of this are described elsewhere in the "Evaluation" section (chapter 9) of this volume. It is also the primary responsibility of the sleep specialist to effectively screen for other primary sleep disorders, most notably breathing and movement abnormalities that may contribute to insomnia. Suspicion of these disorders is the major indication for polysomnography in patients with chronic insomnia (54). Interpretation of the significance of the results of sleep studies and development of multicomponent, phased treatment approaches is a key aspect of sleep medicine's role in the overall management of chronic insomnia.

Most patients referred to sleep centers for chronic insomnia have received some form of pharmacotherapy before they arrive. It is the responsibility of the sleep specialist to review these therapies, to determine what has and has not been effective, to implement new pharmacological approaches, and to discontinue those medications that are ineffective or contraindicated. Beyond this, comprehensive sleep medicine programs must be able to provide the highest level of cognitive behavioral therapy, integrated with other components of treatment. Ideally, centers could provide individual treatment by a behavioral sleep medicine specialist for all referred patients. Given the scarcity of this resource, though, even these programs must think in terms of brief, group therapy as an entry-level treatment for at least some chronic insomnia patients. Ongoing monitoring and follow-up, medication tapering accomplished in concert with CBT-I, and management of other comorbid sleep disorders are also essential. Finally, if effective diagnosis and management of chronic insomnia is to occur, specialized centers need to provide outreach to primary care, psychiatric and other practices in their regions. These outreach efforts should include raising awareness of the frequency and significance of this condition, providing simplified evaluation and diagnostic approaches, and clarifying the role of pharmacological and psychological/behavioral therapies in the management of chronic insomnia. In light of the paucity of available CBT-I, sleep centers should also be prepared to work with nurses and other health care workers to provide training in entry-level CBT-I and consultation when greater expertise is required.

CONCLUSIONS

Modern medicine, despite its many advances, is not providing reliable detection or effective treatment for the vast majority of people with chronic sleep disturbance. This probably reflects some degree of indifference to the problem, stemming from lack of education and awareness, as well as uncertainty regarding the appropriate assessment and management. The net result of this is unnecessary suffering, increased health care utilization, and in all likelihood, increased risk for significant medical and psychiatric disorders. Chronic insomnia is probably preventable for many, although we lack the large-scale public health interventions necessary to test this assertion. Likewise, the great majority of established chronic sleep disturbance does not come to medical attention. The economic cost of this enormous gap in loss of productivity, accidents, OTC and self-help therapies, and increased health care utilization numbers in the billions. Yet, capturing the attention of those affected and their care providers remains a daunting task.

Unfortunately, while medicine struggles to manage numerous problems that have no effective treatments, this readily treatable disorder is largely ignored. However, sleep medicine must come to terms with the fact that, while we have made great strides in developing and testing efficacious therapies that can produce long-term improvement, we lag far behind in identifying or developing the resources necessary to effectively deliver these therapies to even a small percentage of the affected population. It seems likely that health care providers would be far more prepared to address the issue of chronic insomnia if a clear treatment pathway and necessary resources were available to them. Absent this, we should expect little change in the current dynamic.

REFERENCES

1. Simon GE, VonKorff M. Prevalence, burden, and treatment of insomnia in primary care. Am J Psychiatry 1997; 154(10):1417–1423.
2. Terzano MG, Parrino L, Cirignotta F, et al. Studio Morfeo: insomnia in primary care, a survey conducted on the Italian population. Sleep Med 2004; 5(1):67–75.
3. Breslau N, Roth T, Rosenthal L, et al. Sleep disturbance and psychiatric disorders: A longitudinal epidemiological study of young adults. Biol Psychiatry 1996; 39(6):411–418.
4. Weissman MM, Greenwald S, Nino-Murcia G, et al. The morbidity of insomnia uncomplicated by psychiatric disorders. Gen Hosp Psychiatry 1997; 19(4):245–250.
5. Roehrs T, Hyde M, Blaisdell B, et al. Sleep loss and REM sleep loss are hyperalgesic. Sleep 2006; 29(2):145–151.

6. Phillips B, Mannino DM. Do insomnia complaints cause hypertension or cardiovascular disease? J Clin Sleep Med 2007; 3(5):489–494.
7. American Academy of Sleep Medicine. International Classification of Sleep Disorders. Diagnostic and Coding Manual, 2nd ed. Westchester, IL: American Academy of Sleep Medicine, 2005.
8. Espie CA, Fleming L, Cassidy J, et al. Randomized controlled clinical effectiveness trial of cognitive behavior therapy compared with treatment as usual for persistent insomnia in patients with cancer. J Clin Oncol 2008; 26(28):4651–4658.
9. Botteman MF, Ozminkowski RJ, Wang S, et al. Cost effectiveness of long-term treatment with eszopiclone for primary insomnia in adults: A decision analytical model. CNS Drugs 2007; 21(4):319–334.
10. Foley DJ, Vitiello MV, Bliwise DL, et al. Frequent napping is associated with excessive daytime sleepiness, depression, pain, and nocturia in older adults: Findings from the National Sleep Foundation '2003 Sleep in America' Poll. Am J Geriatr Psychiatry 2007; 15(4):344–350.
11. Ancoli-Israel S, Roth T. Characteristics of insomnia in the United States: Results of the 1991 National Sleep Foundation Survey. I. Sleep 1999; 22(suppl 2):S347–S353.
12. Morlock RJ, Tan M, Mitchell DY. Patient characteristics and patterns of drug use for sleep complaints in the United States: Analysis of National Ambulatory Medical Survey data, 1997–2002. Clin Ther 2006; 28(7):1044–1053.
13. Schutte-Rodin S, Broch L, Buysse D, et al. Clinical guideline for the evaluation and management of chronic insomnia in adults. J Clin Sleep Med 2008; 4(5):487–504.
14. Morgan K, Clarke D. Longitudinal trends in late-life insomnia: Implications for prescribing. Age Ageing 1997; 26(3):179–184.
15. National Institutes of Health. National Institutes of Health State of the Science Conference statement on Manifestations and Management of Chronic Insomnia in Adults, June 13–15, 2005. Sleep 2005; 28(9):1049–1057.
16. Fava M, McCall WV, Krystal A, et al. Eszopiclone co-administered with fluoxetine in patients with insomnia coexisting with major depressive disorder. Biol Psychiatry 2006; 59(11):1052–1060.
17. Manber R, Edinger JD, Gress JL, et al. Cognitive behavioral therapy for insomnia enhances depression outcome in patients with comorbid major depressive disorder and insomnia. Sleep 2008; 31(4): 489–495.
18. LeBlanc M, Beaulieu-Bonneau S, Merette C, et al. Psychological and health-related quality of life factors associated with insomnia in a population-based sample. J Psychosom Res 2007; 63(2): 157–166.
19. Murtagh DR, Greenwood KM. Identifying effective psychological treatments for insomnia: A meta-analysis. J Consult Clin Psychol 1995; 63(1):79–89.
20. Espie CA, Inglis SJ, Tessier S, et al. The clinical effectiveness of cognitive behaviour therapy for chronic insomnia: Implementation and evaluation of a sleep clinic in general medical practice. Behav Res Ther 2001; 39(1):45–60.
21. Edinger JD, Sampson WS. A primary care "friendly" cognitive behavioral insomnia therapy. Sleep 2003; 26(2):177–182.
22. Kaneita Y, Ohida T, Uchiyama M, et al. The relationship between depression and sleep disturbances: A Japanese nationwide general population survey. J Clin Psychiatry 2006; 67(2):196–203.
23. Krahn LE, Miller BW, Bergstrom LR. Rapid resolution of intense suicidal ideation after treatment of severe obstructive sleep apnea. J Clin Sleep Med 2008; 4(1):64–65.
24. van Straten A, Cuijpers P, Smit F, et al. Self-help treatment for insomnia through television and book: A randomized trial. Patient Educ Couns 2009; 74(1):29–34.
25. Morin CM, Mimeault V, Gagne A. Nonpharmacological treatment of late-life insomnia. J Psychosom Res 1999; 46(2):103–116.
26. van Straten A, Cuijpers P. Self-help therapy for insomnia: A meta-analysis. Sleep Med Rev 2009; 13(1):61–71.
27. Rybarczyk B, Stepanski E, Fogg L, et al. A placebo-controlled test of cognitive-behavioral therapy for comorbid insomnia in older adults. J Consult Clin Psychol 2005; 73(6):1164–1174.
28. Meolie AL, Rosen C, Kristo D, et al. Oral nonprescription treatment for insomnia: An evaluation of products with limited evidence. J Clin Sleep Med 2005; 1(2):173–187.
29. Jacobs GD, Pace-Schott EF, Stickgold R, et al. Cognitive behavior therapy and pharmacotherapy for insomnia: A randomized controlled trial and direct comparison. Arch Intern Med 2004; 164(17):1888–1896.
30. Sivertsen B, Overland S, Neckelmann D, et al. The long-term effect of insomnia on work disability: The HUNT-2 historical cohort study. Am J Epidemiol 2006; 163(11):1018–1024.
31. Krystal AD, Thakur M, Roth T. Sleep disturbance in psychiatric disorders: Effects on function and quality of life in mood disorders, alcoholism, and schizophrenia. Ann Clin Psychiatry 2008; 20(1): 39–46.

32. Krystal AD, Walsh JK, Laska E, et al. Sustained efficacy of eszopiclone over 6 months of nightly treatment: Results of a randomized, double-blind, placebo-controlled study in adults with chronic insomnia.Sleep 2003; 26(7):793–799.
33. Baillargeon L, Landreville P, Verreault R, et al. Discontinuation of benzodiazepines among older insomniac adults treated with cognitive-behavioural therapy combined with gradual tapering: A randomized trial. CMAJ 2003; 169(10):1015–1020.
34. Belleville G, Guay C, Guay B, et al. Hypnotic taper with or without self-help treatment of insomnia: A randomized clinical trial. J Consult Clin Psychol 2007; 75(2):325–335.
35. O'Connor K, Marchand A, Brousseau L, et al. Cognitive-behavioural, pharmacological and psychosocial predictors of outcome during tapered discontinuation of benzodiazepine. Clin Psychol Psychother 2008; 15(1):1–14.
36. Garzon C, Guerrero JM, Aramburu O, et al. Effect of melatonin administration on sleep, behavioral disorders and hypnotic drug discontinuation in the elderly: A randomized, double-blind, placebo-controlled study. Aging Clin Exp Res 2009; 21(1):38–42.
37. Dombrovski AY, Mulsant BH, Houck PR, et al. Residual symptoms and recurrence during maintenance treatment of late-life depression. J Affect Disord 2007; 103(1–3):77–82.
38. Dombrovski AY, Cyranowski JM, Mulsant BH, et al. Which symptoms predict recurrence of depression in women treated with maintenance interpersonal psychotherapy? Depress Anxiety 2008; 25(12):1060–1066.
39. Pigeon WR, Hegel M, Unützer J, et al. Is insomnia a perpetuating factor for late-life depression in the IMPACT cohort? Sleep 2008; 31(4):482–488.
40. Edinger JD, Olsen MK, Stechuchak KM, et al. Cognitive behavioral therapy for patients with primary insomnia or insomnia associated predominantly with mixed psychiatric disorders: A randomized clinical trial. Sleep 2009; 32(4):499–510.
41. Espie CA, MacMahon KM, Kelly HL, et al. Randomized clinical effectiveness trial of nurse-administered small-group cognitive behavior therapy for persistent insomnia in general practice. Sleep 2007; 30(5):574–584.
42. Rybarczyk B, Lopez M, Benson R, et al. Efficacy of two behavioral treatment programs for comorbid geriatric insomnia. Psychol Aging 2002; 17(2):288–298.
43. Taylor FB, Martin P, Thompson C, et al. Prazosin effects on objective sleep measures and clinical symptoms in civilian trauma posttraumatic stress disorder: A placebo-controlled study. Biol Psychiatry 2008; 63(6):629–632.
44. Raskind MA, Peskind ER, Hoff DJ, et al. A parallel group placebo controlled study of prazosin for trauma nightmares and sleep disturbance in combat veterans with post-traumatic stress disorder. Biol Psychiatry 2007; 61(8):928–934.
45. Moore BA, Krakow B. Imagery rehearsal therapy for acute posttraumatic nightmares among combat soldiers in Iraq. Am J Psychiatry 2007; 164(4):683–684.
46. Krakow B, Zadra A. Clinical management of chronic nightmares: Imagery rehearsal therapy. Behav Sleep Med 2006; 4(1):45–70.
47. Schwartz T, Nihalani N, Virk S, et al. A comparison of the effectiveness of two hypnotic agents for the treatment of insomnia. Int J Psychiatr Nurs Res 2004; 10(1):1146–1150.
48. Kaynak H, Kaynak D, Gozukirmizi E, et al. The effects of trazodone on sleep in patients treated with stimulant antidepressants. Sleep Med 2004; 5(1):15–20.
49. Saletu-Zyhlarz GM, Anderer P, Arnold O, et al. Confirmation of the neurophysiologically predicted therapeutic effects of trazodone on its target symptoms depression, anxiety and insomnia by post-marketing clinical studies with a controlled-release formulation in depressed outpatients. Neuropsychobiology 2003; 48(4):194–208.
50. Nierenberg AA, Adler LA, Peselow E, et al. Trazodone for antidepressant-associated insomnia. Am J Psychiatry 1994; 151(7):1069–1072.
51. Philip NS, Mello K, Carpenter LL, et al. Patterns of quetiapine use in psychiatric inpatients: An examination of off-label use. Ann Clin Psychiatry 2008; 20(1):15–20.
52. Wiegand MH, Landry F, Bruckner T, et al. Quetiapine in primary insomnia: A pilot study. Psychopharmacology (Berl) 2008; 196(2):337–338.
53. Endicott J, Rajagopalan K, Minkwitz M, et al. A randomized, double-blind, placebo-controlled study of quetiapine in the treatment of bipolar I and II depression: Improvements in quality of life. Int Clin Psychopharmacol 2007; 22(1):29–37.
54. Chesson AL Jr,Ferber RA, Fry JM, et al. The indications for polysomnography and related procedures. Sleep 1997; 20(6):423–487.

Appendix: Resources

WEBSITES

http://www.sleepeducation.com – the public education site of the American Academy of Sleep Medicine (AASM) includes detailed information on the causes and treatments of insomnia and other sleep disorders.

http://www.aasmnet.org – the American Academy of Sleep Medicine professional site includes detailed information on accreditation of sleep centers, professional education programs and resources, clinical standards and useful information for the health professional within and outside the field.

http://www.sleepcenters.org – this AASM site provides a roster of accredited sleep centers across the United States.

http://www.sleepresearchsociety.org/ – the Sleep Research Society is the major professional organization of sleep researchers. The site includes educational opportunities and products and additional resources for sleep researchers.

http://www.nhlbi.nih.gov/about/ncsdr/index.htm – the National Center on Sleep Disorders Research (NCSDR) is a division within the National Heart, Lung and Blood Institute (NHLBI). This site provides public and professional education and research information.

http://www.sleepfoundation.org – the National Sleep Foundation engages in public education and information gathering through its annual national sleep survey.

http://www.americaninsomniaassociation.org – the American Insomnia Association is a patient-based organization which is dedicated to advancing identification and treatment of insomnia through public and professional education and research.

http://www.absm.org/BSM Specialists.htm – the American Board of Sleep Medicine (ABSM) maintains a list of certified behavioral sleep medicine specialists nationwide.

http://www.absm.org/Diplomates/listing.htm – the ABSM also maintains a list of health professionals certified by this board.*

*Since 2007, the board certification examination in sleep medicine is offered by the American Board of Internal Medicine, in conjunction with other primary specialty boards. Rosters of physicians certified since 2007 by these respective boards can be found on the web sites of those organizations.

SELF-HELP BOOKS AND MANUALIZED TREATMENT APPROACHES FOR CHRONIC INSOMNIA

No More Sleepless Nights by Peter Hauri and Shirley Linde

Sleep Manual: Training Your Mind and Body to Achieve the Perfect Night's Sleep by Wilfred R. Pigeon

Say Good Night to Insomnia by Gregg D. Jacobs

The Insomnia Answer: A Personalized Program for Identifying and Overcoming the Three Types of Insomnia by Paul Glovinsky and Art Spielman

Cognitive Behavioral Treatment of Insomnia: A Session-by-Session Guide by Michael L. Perlis, Carla Jungquist, Michael T. Smith, and Donn Posner

Overcoming Insomnia: A Cognitive-Behavioral Therapy Approach Workbook (Treatments That Work) by Jack D. Edinger and Colleen E. Carney

The Insomnia Workbook: A Comprehensive Guide to Getting the Sleep You Need by Stephanie Silberman and Charles Morin

The Harvard Medical School Guide to a Good Night's Sleep (Harvard Medical School Guides) by Lawrence Epstein and Steven Mardon

Index

Note: Page numbers followed by f, n, and t indicate figures, notes, and tables, respectively.

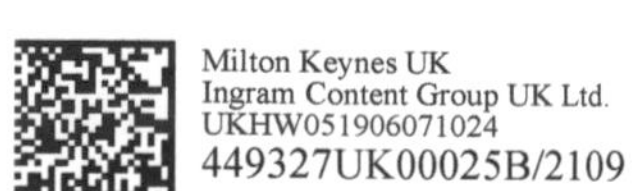
Milton Keynes UK
Ingram Content Group UK Ltd.
UKHW051906071024
449327UK00025B/2109

9 780367 384166